W9-APR-865

About the cover: The Star of Life logo is internationally identified for emergency medical services (EMS) and is synonymous with emergency medicine. The veterinary medicine caduceus and the equine schema represent equine veterinary medicine—connected, they signify equine emergencies.

Atropine

bronchodilation   0.6 m/ 1000 # IV, im

Manual of
Equine
Emergencies
Treatment and Procedures

Manual of
Equine
Emergencies
Treatment and Procedures

Second Edition

James A. Orsini, DVM, Dipl ACVS
Associate Professor of Surgery
New Bolton Center
School of Veterinary Medicine
University of Pennsylvania
Kennett Square, Pennsylvania

Thomas J. Divers, DVM, Dipl ACVIM, ACVECC
Professor, Large Animal Medicine
New York State College of Veterinary Medicine
Department of Clinical Studies
Cornell University
Ithaca, New York

With 245 illustrations

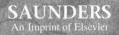

SAUNDERS
An Imprint of Elsevier

SAUNDERS
An Imprint of Elsevier

The Curtis Center
Independence Square West
Philadelphia, Pennsylvania 19106

MANUAL OF EQUINE EMERGENCIES Second Edition

Copyright © 2003 by Elsevier All rights reserved.
Original figures and tables in Chapter 57 copyright Jonathan M. Naylor.

No part of this publication may be reproduced or transmitted in any form or by any means, electronic or mechanical, including photocopying, recording, or any information storage and retrieval system, without permission in writing from the publisher.

Permissions may be sought directly from Elsevier's Health Sciences Rights Department in Philadelphia, PA, USA: phone: (+1) 215 239 3804, fax: (+1) 215 239 3805, email: health-permissions@elsevier.com. You may also complete your request on-line via the Elsevier homepage (http://www.elsevier.com), by selecting 'Customer Support' and then 'Obtaining Permissions'.

NOTICE

Pharmacology is an ever-changing field. Standard safety precautions must be followed, but as new research and clinical experience broaden our knowledge, changes in treatment and drug therapy may become necessary or appropriate. Readers are advised to check the most current product information provided by the manufacturer of each drug to be administered to verify the recommended dose, the method and duration of administration, and contraindications. It is the responsibility of the treating veterinarian, relying on experience and knowledge of the patient, to determine dosages and the best treatment for each individual patient. Neither the publisher nor the editor assumes any liability for any injury and/or damage to persons or property arising from this publication.

THE PUBLISHER

Previous edition copyrighted 1998

Library of Congress Cataloging-in-Publication Data

Orsini, James A.
    Manual of equine emergencies: treatment and procedures / James A. Orsini, Thomas J. Divers.—2nd ed.
        p. cm.
    Includes bibliographical references.
    ISBN-13: 978-0-7216-9298-2   ISBN-10: 0-7216-9298-2
    1. Horses—Diseases. 2. Veterinary emergencies. I. Divers, Thomas J. II. Title.

SF951 .077 2002
636.1'089—dc21   2002030931

Senior Editor: Elizabeth M. Fathman
Managing Editor: Teri Merchant
Publishing Services Manager: Pat Joiner
Project Manager: Keri O'Brien
Designer: Mark A. Oberkrom
Cover Art: Molly Higgins

EH/RDC

Printed in the United States of America

Last digit is the print number.   9   8   7   6   5   4   3

In loving memory of **Anne** *and* **Robert** *– who are greatly missed*
and
Spot *– for his love of children and John and Marianne*

Contributors

Fairfield T. Bain, DVM, Dipl ACVIM, ACVP, ACVECC
Staff Internist/Director of Clinical Laboratory
Hagyard-Davidson-McGee Associates
Lexington, Kentucky;
Adjunct Professor of Pathology
Department of Pathobiology
University of Tennessee
Knoxville, Tennessee
Interpretation of Acid-Base Values, CBC & Chemistry

T. Douglas Byars, DVM, Dipl ACVIM, ACVECC
Director, Equine Internal Medicine
Hagyard-Davidson-McGee Associates
Lexington, Kentucky
Foal Diarrhea, Coagulopathies

Alexander deLahunta, DVM, ACVIM, PhD
James Law Professor of Veterinary Anatomy
Department of Biomedical Science
Cornell University College of Veterinary Medicine
Ithaca, New York
Evaluation of Horses with Suspected Neurologic Dysfunction

Thomas J. Divers, DVM, Dipl ACVIM, ACVECC
Professor, Large Animal Medicine
New York State College of Veterinary Medicine
Department of Clinical Studies
Cornell University, Ithaca, New York
Respiratory Diseases, Diarrhea, Neurology, Hepatic Failure, Anemia, Pharmacology, Urinary Diseases, Toxicology, Euthanasia, Shock and Systemic Inflammatory Response Syndrome, Temperature-Related Problems, Emergency Drug Dosages

David L. Foster, DVM
Morganville, New Jersey
Dental Emergencies and Procedures, Aging/Teeth

Rebecca M. Gimenez, PhD
Editor, *Equine and Bovine Magazine*
Editor, *American Academy of Veterinary Disaster Medicine*
Instructor, Large Animal Emergency Rescue
NDMS/Veterinary Medical Assistance Team-3
Adjunct Faculty, Anderson College
Pendleton, South Carolina
Disaster Medicine

Tomas Gimenez, Dr. Med. Vet.
Professor, Animal and Veterinary Sciences Department
Clemson University;
Large Animal Emergency Rescue Instructor
NDMS/Veterinary Medical Assistance Team-3
Clemson, South Carolina
Disaster Medicine

Robin D. Gleed, BVSc, MRCVS, DVA, Dipl ACVA, ECVA, MRCA
Associate Professor of Clinical Sciences
Department of Clinical Sciences
Cornell University College of Veterinary Medicine
Ithaca, New York
Anesthesia for Field Emergencies

Robert B. Hillman, DVM, MS, Dipl ACT
Senior Clinician Emeritus
Cornell University College of Veterinary Medicine
Ithaca, New York
Reproductive System

David M. Hood, DVM, PhD
Hoof Diagnostic and Rehabilitation
   Clinic
College Station, Texas
Laminitis

Kent A. Humber, DVM, MS, Dipl ACVIM
Rancho Sante Fe, California
Cytology

Nita L. Irby, DVM, Dipl ACVO
Cornell University College of Veterinary
   Medicine
Ithaca, New York
Procedures Section/Ophthalmology

J. Edward Kirker, DVM
Pharmacy Director
Cornell University College of Veterinary
   Medicine
Ithaca, New York
*Pharmacology and Adverse Drug
   Reactions*

Christine Kreuder, VMD
School of Veterinary Medicine
University of California at Davis
Davis, California
*Emergency Medical and Surgical
   Principles and Procedures*

**Tim Mair, BVSc, PhD, Dipl ECEIM,
   MRCVS**
Bell Equine Veterinary Clinic
Mereworth, Kent, United Kingdom
Emergency Diseases Seen in Europe

Richard A. Mansmann, VMD, PhD
Chapel Hill, North Carolina
Disaster Medicine

**C. Wayne McIlwraith, BVSc, MS, PhD,
   DSc, FRCVS, Dipl ACVS**
Professor of Surgery
Director of Orthopaedic Research
Department of Clinical Sciences
College of Veterinary Medicine
Colorado State University
Fort Collins, Colorado
Musculoskeletal Emergencies

James N. Moore, DVM, PhD, ACVS
Professor of Large Animal Surgery
University of Georgia
Department of Clinical Studies
College of Veterinary Medicine
Athens, Georgia
*Gastrointestinal Emergencies & Other
   Causes of Colic*

P.O. Eric Mueller, DVM, PhD, Dipl ACVS
Associate Professor of Large Animal
   Surgery
University of Georgia
Department of Large Animal Medicine
College of Veterinary Medicine
Athens, Georgia
*Gastrointestinal Emergencies & Other
   Causes of Colic*

**Jonathan M. Naylor, BSc, DVM, PhD,
   Dipl ACVIM, ACVN**
Professor, Department of Large Animal
   Clinical Sciences
Western College of Veterinary
   Medicine
University of Saskatchewan,
   Saskatoon, Saskatchewan, Canada
*Nutritional Guidelines for the
   Sick/Injured Horse*

James A. Orsini, DVM, Dipl ACVS
Associate Professor of Surgery
New Bolton Center
School of Veterinary Medicine
University of Pennsylvania
Kennett Square, Pennsylvania
*Procedures Section, Musculoskeletal
   Emergencies, Reproductive System,
   Appendices, Emergency Drug
   Dosages*

Jonathan E. Palmer, VMD, Dipl ACVIM
Associate Professor of Medicine
Director of Neonatology/Perinatology
   Programs
Connelly Intensive Care Unit
New Bolton Center
School of Veterinary Medicine
University of Pennsylvania
Kennett Square, Pennsylvania
*Perinatology and Foal Cardiopulmonary
   Resuscitation*

Robert H. Poppenga, DVM, PhD
Associate Professor
Chief, Toxicology Laboratory
New Bolton Center
School of Veterinary Medicine
University of Pennsylvania
Kennett Square, Pennsylvania
Toxicology

Virginia B. Reef, DVM, Dipl ACVIM
Mark Whittier & Lila Griswald Allam
    Professor
Director of Large Animal Cardiology and
    Ultrasonography
Chief, Section of Sports Medicine &
    Imaging
New Bolton Center
University of Pennsylvania
Kennett Square, Pennsylvania
Cardiology and Ultrasonography

Thomas L. Seahorn, DVM
Hagyard-Davidson-McGee Associates
Lexington, Kentucky
Equine Respiratory Emergencies

Donald H. Schlafer, DVM, PhD, ALVP
Professor of Comparative Reproductive
    Biology
Cornell University
College of Veterinary Medicine
Ithaca, New York
Reproductive System

Ted S. Stashak, DVM, MS, Dipl ACVS
Professor of Surgery, Veterinary
    Teaching Hospital
Department of Clinical Sciences
College of Veterinary Medicine and
    Biomedical Sciences
Colorado State University
Fort Collins, Colorado
Integumentary System

Ann Townsend, LVT, AAS
Veterinary Technician
Supervisor, Equine/Farm Animal
    Anesthesia
Cornell University College of Veterinary
    Medicine
Ithaca, New York
*Anesthesia for Field Emergencies and
    Euthanasia*

Michael Tomasic, VMD, Dipl ACVA
Veterinary Pain Management
Santa Fe, New Mexico
*Pain Management/Procedures
    Epidural Catheter Placement*

**Pamela A. Wilkins, DVM, PhD,
    Dipl ACVIM, ACVECC**
Assistant Professor, Large Animal
    Medicine
New Bolton Center
School of Veterinary Medicine
University of Pennsylvania
Kennett Square, Pennsylvania
Neonatology

Preface

The first edition of the *Manual of Equine Emergencies* was well received, with more than 5000 copies distributed, as well as Spanish and French translations. We believe this indicates the value of the subject matter for our colleagues and friends. As with any first edition, we found room for improvement; we labored tirelessly to revise and update the content and fine-tune the format in the second edition.

NEW AND UPDATED TOPICS

- All chapters have been updated, and new information has been added on emergency ultrasonography, perinatology, bleeding disorders, interpretation of laboratory results, diseases specific to Europe, new procedures, pain management, fluid therapy, and additional color plates.
- The toxicology chapter has been expanded to include many more poisonous plants, with the addition of distribution maps to help identify those problematic plants in your area.
- The number of outstanding contributing authors was increased, with many from private practice. Again, we thank our colleagues and authors for their excellent contributions!
- All the current products cited in the book have been updated for accurate listings, company names, addresses, phone numbers, and fax and e-mail details where available. We recognize there are other products used in clinical practice and request that if you have something that works better for you that is not included in the book, please share this information with us so that we can incorporate it in a future edition.
- The Equine Emergency Drugs: Approximate Dosages table has been extensively revised and updated, including 18 additional drugs. Our goal was to make this one of the most valuable additions to the book. We recommend that you check all the product information currently provided by the manufacturer regarding each drug.

IMPROVED FORMAT

Key information is easier to find. Our goal is that you will quickly find all the information needed to manage any equine emergency in a precise, state-of-the-art format.

- The gray banner down the pages of the Equine Emergency Drugs table makes this table easy to locate and practical for everyday use.
- The logo ▶ along the left-hand column of the page throughout the book is a new addition to call attention to "must know" information—especially valuable in any emergency setting.
- Also see the handy tabs in the right-hand page column to rapidly identify the topic covered in that particular chapter of the book. Our goal is to help you find the information you need as fast as possible.
- The inside front cover now lists the table of contents to enable quick look-up of all topics. The hotline numbers have been moved to the inside back cover.

We strived for ease of use and comprehensive coverage for our readers. We trust that *Manual of Equine Emergencies* will be your "*vade mecum*"—book carried constantly for use. We wish you trouble-free emergencies.

James A. Orsini
Thomas J. Divers

Acknowledgments

The second edition of our book required the combined efforts of many of our colleagues, veterinary students, support staff, and friends. The high quality of our book is a result of the outstanding chapters from the many contributing authors who are experts in their field. Everyone was loyal and encouraging in the completion of this edition, and for this we are genuinely thankful and deeply indebted.

Dr. Orsini would also like to acknowledge the outstanding support and cherished friendship of John and Marianne Castle, Mary Alice Malone, Margaret Duprey, Allaire duPont, Ellen and Herb Moelis, Vonnie and Larry Steinbaum, Marian and Gib McIlvain, The Noble Family, Dr. Roy Pollock, a visionary; Dr. John Lee, who read every page of the first edition and made practical criticisms that were incorporated into the second edition; Drs. Tracy Norman and Julie Engiles; and veterinary students Marie (Mimi) Haddock and Lynne (Lexie) Stine, who double-checked every detail for accuracy.

We would also like to acknowledge all our previous house officers, fellow equine clinicians, and many teachers who have given so generously in our educational and professional development, specifically Drs. Willard H. Daniels, William J. Donawick, Charles F. Ramberg, and Wayne S. Schwark for Dr. Orsini; Drs. Dilmus Blackmon, Brad Smith, Gary Carlson, Lisle George, Robert Whitlock, Bud Tennant, and Doug Byars for Dr. Divers.

The expert staff at Elsevier Health Sciences is first rate and guided us throughout the process. Without their untiring efforts and expertise this edition would have never made the established goals and timetable; thanks to Linda Duncan, Publishing Director; Liz Fathman, Senior Editor; Teri Merchant, Managing Editor; and Keri O'Brien, Project Manager. This wonderful staff at Elsevier Science (W.B. Saunders Company), notably Teri Merchant and Keri O'Brien, once again permitted editorial freedom to make last-minute additions to ensure the timeliness of the book in all aspects.

Thanks also to Amy Lanfair, Joyce Reyner, and Ann Littlejohn for helping meet the deadlines to the publisher; Jean Young, AVT, and Robin McGrath, AVT, for validating the manufacturers' listings and; of course, our right-hand assistants, Debbie Lent and Margie Schwartz, who once again provided excellent editorial, organizational, and motivational skills to assist us with this project.

Most important, we appreciate our families: Nita, Shannon, Bobby, Toni, and Colin, who arranged their lives to suit us, and parents Hattie and Sal, who continually provide love, encouragement, and advice about life.

James A. Orsini
Thomas J. Divers

Contents

Plate 1. Stylohyoid osteoarthropathy. Endoscopic examination of the right guttural pouch of a 22-year-old Warmblood with acute facial paralysis and vestibular dysfunction. There is obvious proliferation of the most proximal part of the stylohyoid bone. Attempts at manual manipulation of the hyoid bone during endoscopy did not reveal movement of the stylohyoid bone at the temporohyoid junction, suggesting bony fusion.

Plate 2. This a funduscopic photograph of a horse with equine motor neuron disease. The brown "streaking" in both the tapetal and nontapetal area is lipofuscin deposition in the retinal pigment epithelium, resulting from prolonged and severe vitamin E deficiency and oxidative damage. This finding can be seen with the ophthalmoscope in approximately 50% of cases of equine motor neuron disease.

Plate 3. A, Four weeks before this photo was taken, a 3-year-old Warmblood stallion sustained iatrogenic blunt trauma to the eye. Consolidating subretinal hemorrhage is evident at the left, with resolving peripapillary retinal and choroidal edema. **B,** One year after injury, a classic "butterfly" lesion is evident (peripapillary choroidal atrophy and scarring).

Plate 4. Eye of a 2-year-old Thoroughbred colt with severe subconjunctival emphysema secondary to dorsal orbital rim fracture involving the frontal sinus.

Plate 5. Severe corneal stromal ulceration, with severe keratomalacia, hypopyon, and early corneal neovascularization. The cornea did not retain fluorescein stain before referral. A ç-shaped tear in the loose corneal epithelium, evident dorsally, occurred during the examination.

Plate 6. Eye of a 4-month-old Thoroughbred filly with a 5-mm diameter superficial corneal ulcer of 3 days' duration. The lesion developed an acute increase in edema, a change in contour, and a mucoid appearance, indicating active keratomalacia. *Staphylococcus aureus* was cultured.

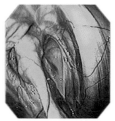

Plate 1

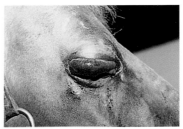

Plate 4

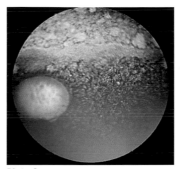

Plate 2

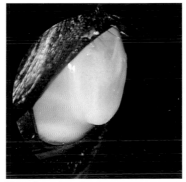

Plate 5

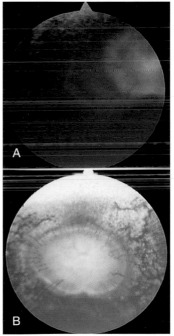

A

B

Plate 3

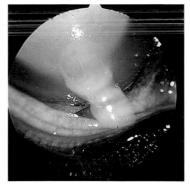

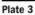

Plate 6

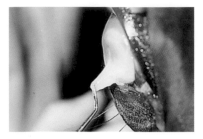

Plate 7. Eye of a 12-year-old Thoroughbred gelding with a severe corneal ulcer of 8 days' duration. A toothed forceps is being used to elevate the malacic cornea for debridement with ophthalmic scissors.

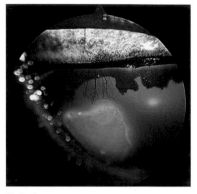

Plate 9. Eye of a 9-month-old Thoroughbred filly with a 10-day history of corneal disease that began as a superficial erosion in the dorsotemporal perilimbal cornea. Photo illustrates the caseous, white surface exudate and severe corneal neovascularization.

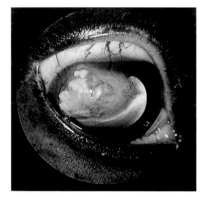

Plate 8. Eye of a 12-year-old Thoroughbred mare with an 8-week history of a superficial corneal ulcer that began in the ventrotemporal perilimbal cornea and gradually progressed centrally.

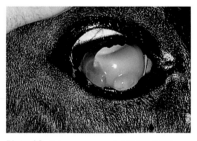

Plate 10. Severe corneal edema with bullae formation in the right eye of a weanling Thoroughbred filly. She was one of 18 Thoroughbred weanlings from a group outbreak of acute unilateral or bilateral corneal edema (mild-to-extremely severe), some cases of which involved concurrent retinal detachments. An etiology was not conclusively determined.

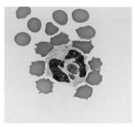

Plate 11. Wright-Giemsa stain of a blood smear of an adult horse from northern Virginia with fever and leg edema. The light blue bodies in the neutrophil are *anaplasma Phagocytophilia* morulae.

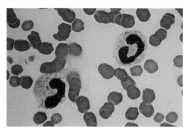

Plate 12. Wright Giemsa stain of a blood smear of a horse with colitis. The lower neutrophil is curved and nonsegmented (a band neutrophil) and the cytoplasm of both neutrophils have foamy vacuolation and purplish staining granules (toxic granulation), suggesting severe toxemia.

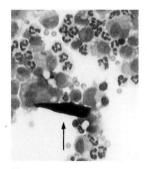

Plate 13. Peritoneal fluid (400 ×). A mixture of nondegenerate neutrophils and macrophages. One eosinophil is present. The arrow points to a keratin flake (rolled-up squamous epithelial cell). A small number of erythrocytes are present in the background.

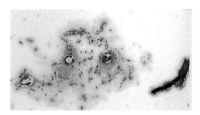

Plate 14. Peritoneal fluid (400 ×). Ruptured intestine.

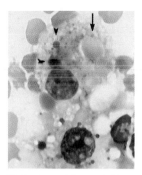

Plate 15. Peritoneal fluid (1000 ×). Macrophages containing erythrocytes *(arrow)* and hemosiderin pigment *(arrowheads)*. The cells demonstrate erythrocytophagia and provide evidence of hemorrhage into the sample site.

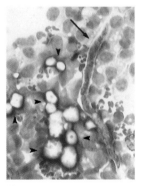

Plate 16. Peritoneal fluid (400×). Mixture of macrophages and nondegenerate neutrophils. A *Setaria* sp. microfilaria is present *(arrow)*. Several talc crystals *(arrowheads)* are demonstrated. Note that the talc crystals are out of focus, whereas the cellular structures are in focus. Compare with Plate 17.

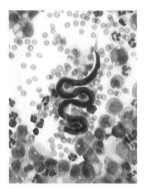

Plate 18. Peritoneal fluid (400×). *Setaria* sp. microfilaria. A mixture predominantly of macrophages, along with nondegenerate neutrophils and erythrocytes, is present.

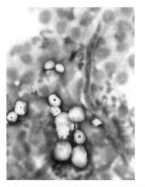

Plate 17. Peritoneal fluid (400×). Same microscopic field as Plate 16; however, the focus has been changed to show the three-dimensional depth and central nidus of the talc crystals.

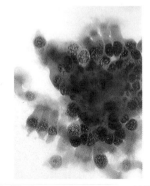

Plate 19. Transtracheal aspirate (400×). A sheet of normal ciliated columnar epithelial cells.

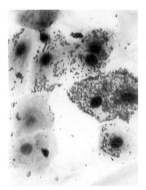

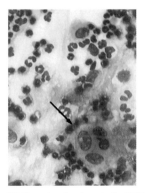

Plate 20. Transtracheal aspirate (400×). Keratinized squamous epithelial cells with large numbers of a mixed population of adherent extracellular bacteria. The pink material in the background is mucus. This is compatible with oropharyngeal contamination of the sample.

Plate 22. Transtracheal aspirate (1000×). Increased numbers of neutrophils, abundant mucus, and pulmonary macrophages are present. One multinucleate giant cell *(arrow)* is demonstrated. No microorganisms are present. The diagnosis is suppurative inflammation. The presence of multinucleate giant cells indicates chronicity. The sample is compatible with chronic obstructive pulmonary disease (COPD).

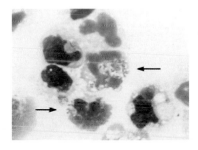

Plate 21. Transtracheal aspirate (1000×). Degenerated neutrophils containing intracellular bacteria (cocci in pairs and rods). Note the swollen appearance of the nuclear chromatin (karyolysis) and the more eosinophilic staining character compared with nondegenerate neutrophils. Cytoplasmic vacuolization is a common feature. The diagnosis is septic suppurative inflammation.

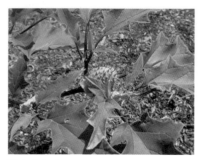

Plate 23. *Datura stramonium* seed capsule

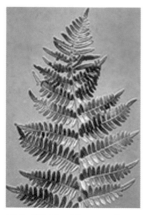

Plate 26. *Pteridium aquilinum*

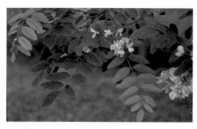

Plate 24. *Robinia pseudoacacia*

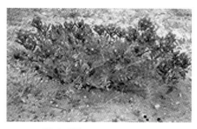

Plate 27. *Astragalus* spp

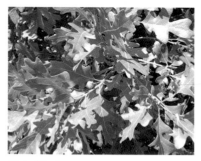

Plate 25. *Quercus gambelli* or scrub oak

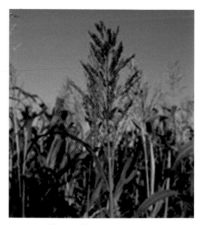

Plate 28. *Sorghum* spp

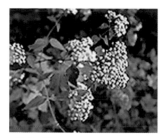

Plate 29. *Eupatorium rugosum*

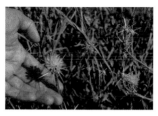

Plate 30 *Centaurea solstitialis*

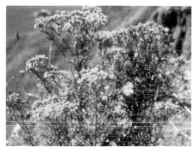

Plate 31. *Senecio jacobea*

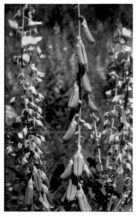

Plate 32. *Crotalaria spectabilis*

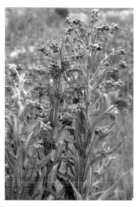

Plate 33. *Cynoglossum officinale*

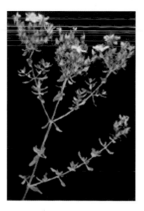

Plate 34.
*Hypericum
perforatum*

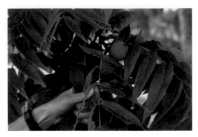

Plate 35. *Juglans nigra*

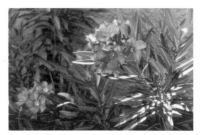

Plate 38. *Nerium oleander*

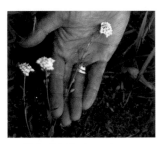

Plate 36. *Berteroa incana*

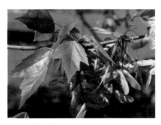

Plate 39. *Acer rubrum*

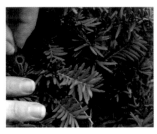

Plate 37. *Taxus cuspidata*

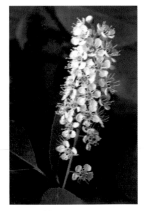

Plate 40. *Prunus serotina*

Emergency Medical and Surgical Principles and Procedures

General Diagnostic and Therapeutic Procedures

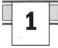 **1** Blood Collection

James A. Orsini and Christine Kreuder

VENIPUNCTURE

Blood collection from a vein is a routine procedure commonly performed during patient examination. Many diagnostic tests require either whole blood or serum and specific additives to prevent coagulation (Table 1–1).

External Jugular Vein

The external jugular vein is most accessible and is easily found within the jugular groove along the ventral aspect of the neck. The vein is safely punctured in the cranial half of the neck where muscle (omohyoideus muscle) interposes between the vein and the underlying carotid sheath containing the carotid artery. The vein distends rapidly with firm pressure applied near the thoracic inlet. Stroking the vein distally causes motion waves higher up, which is helpful if the distended vein is not easily seen.

TABLE 1–1. Blood Tubes for Diagnostic Procedures

Color of Top of Vacutainer Tube	Additive	Analysis Possible
Red or red/black	None	Chemistry studies; viral antibody studies; cross match[*]
Purple	Na EDTA	Hematology studies—CBC and platelet counts Immunohematology; Coombs' test; fluid cytology; cross match[*]
Green	Na heparin	Chemistry studies; blood gases
Yellow	Acid citrate dextrose	Cross match[*]; blood typing
Blue	Na citrate	Coagulation studies—fibrinogen, PT, PTT, AT III
Gray	Na fluoride/ K oxylate	Glucose measurement

Na, Sodium; *EDTA*, ethylenediaminetetraacetic acid; *CBC*, complete blood cell count; *PT*, prothrombin time; *PTT*, partial thromboplastin time; *AT III*, antithrombin III; *K*, potassium.
[*]Both red or red/black and purple required.

Equipment
- 20- to 25-gauge, 1- to 1.5-inch (2.54- to 3.75-cm) Vacutainer* needle (or a 10-ml syringe and 20-gauge needle for fractious patients)
- Vacutainer cuff
- Appropriate Vacutainer tube or tubes

Procedure
- Screw the protected, short end of the needle into the Vacutainer cuff.
- Distend the vein and swab the venipuncture site with alcohol.
- The needle is aligned parallel with the vein opposite the direction of the blood flow.
- Insert the needle through the skin at a 45-degree angle and then redirect it in a parallel direction once the vein lumen has been entered.
- Attach the Vacutainer tube by pushing the cover of the tube onto the short, protected needle in the Vacutainer cuff. The vacuum draws blood into the tube to the appropriate level. If additional tubes are needed, switch tubes while leaving the needle and cuff in place.

Transverse Facial Vein

The transverse facial vein in the head is commonly used in adults or nonfractious patients or both to sample very small volumes of blood for a packed cell volume (PCV) or total solids (TS) determination. The vein runs ventral to the facial crest and parallel to the transverse facial artery.

Equipment
- 22- to 25-gauge, 1- to 1.5-inch (2.5- to 3.75-cm) needle
- 3-ml syringe
- Appropriate Vacutainer or hematocrit tube or tubes

Procedure
- Swab the area beneath the facial crest with alcohol.
- Align the needle perpendicular to the skin beneath the facial crest, and push the needle through the skin until bone is encountered.
- Attach the syringe and withdraw the needle while aspirating until the needle is in the vein lumen.
- A Vacutainer needle and tube may be used to collect blood.

Other Sites for Venipuncture (Fig. 1-1)
- The **superficial thoracic vein** in the cranial and ventral third of the thorax caudal to the point of the elbow
- The **cephalic vein** on the medial aspect of the forelimb
- The **medial saphenous vein** on the medial aspect of the hindlimb

If the sample is collected in a syringe, immediately transfer it to a Vacutainer tube, because the sample begins to clot as soon as it is drawn. Push the needle through

---

*Vacutainer needles, cuffs, and blood tubes. Becton-Dickinson Vacutainer Systems, Rutherford, NJ 07070.

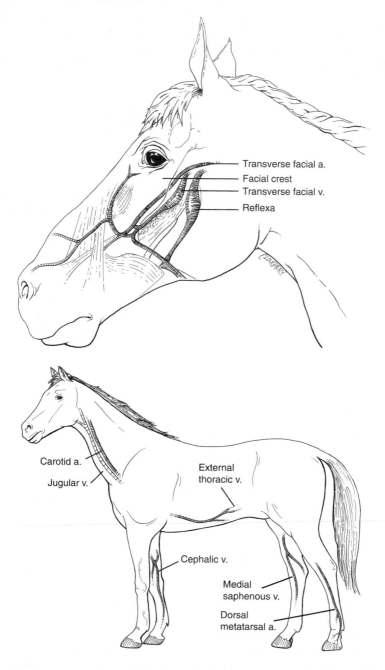

FIGURE 1-1. Veins and arteries used for blood collection.

the cover of the Vacutainer tube and let the vacuum draw the blood from the syringe. Actively pushing blood into the tube damages the blood cells. Mix the anticoagulant into the sample by gently rotating the tube upside down several times. The sample should last for several hours if properly mixed and kept cool. Serum should be separated from whole blood by means of centrifugation if the sample is to sit for longer than several hours, to prevent hemolysis. Hemolysis has a significant effect on many values, such as calcium (increased), chloride (decreased), creatinine (increased), alkaline phosphate (increased), potassium (increased), and lactate dehydrogenase (increased). Slides for a differential are best made soon after the sample is obtained.

Complications

A **hematoma** often forms if a large-gauge needle is used or if the vein is excessively traumatized and blood continues to escape from the venipuncture site. *Keeping the head elevated and applying direct pressure to the puncture site minimizes this complication.*

Thrombosis of the vein is an uncommon complication that can occur if the vascular endothelium is damaged from repeated venipuncture. **Septic thrombophlebitis** occurs if the site becomes infected.

ARTERIAL PUNCTURE

Arterial puncture is most commonly performed for blood gas analysis, which is an excellent indicator of respiratory and metabolic conditions. Several arteries are suitable for sampling (see Fig. 1–1). The **carotid artery** is accessible in the caudal third of the neck.

Equipment

- 20- or 25-gauge, 1- to 1.5-inch (2.54- to 3.75-cm) needle
- Heparinized plastic syringe
- Gauze sponges soaked in alcohol
- Green top (heparin) Vacutainer tube

Procedure

- The carotid pulse is palpable within the jugular groove. The carotid artery lies slightly dorsal and immediately deep to the jugular vein.
- Clean the area thoroughly with alcohol gauze sponges. While palpating the pulse, puncture the artery with the needle. If the artery has been punctured, bright red blood flows rapidly from the needle.
- Attach a syringe and aspirate a sample. Remove air from the syringe immediately. If blood gas analysis is planned, it should be performed within minutes, or the sample should be placed in a heparin Vacutainer tube and cooled.
- As soon as the needle is withdrawn, apply digital pressure over the puncture site with a gauze sponge for several minutes.

Other Sites for Arterial Puncture

- The **facial artery,** as it courses from under the mandible to the facial crest, is punctured easily in a heavily sedated or anesthetized patient.
- The **dorsal metatarsal artery,** which courses laterally and distally from the cranial aspect of the proximal metatarsus, is the preferred site in recumbent foals.

- The **transverse facial artery** is caudal to the lateral canthus (see Fig. 1–1).
- The **brachial artery** serves as an alternate site in foals and can be located on the medial surface in the middle of the humerus.

Complications

- As with venipuncture, the most common complication is **hematoma** formation. Use the smallest-gauge needle possible to minimize vessel trauma, applying pressure to the artery until bleeding stops.
- Local skin infiltration of 2% local anesthetic directly over the site for needle puncture improves patient compliance and thus decreases injury to the vessel wall.

---

2 Medication Administration

James A. Orsini and Christine Kreuder

Multiple routes of administration exist for equine pharmaceuticals. Each route affects the pharmacokinetics of a drug. The pharmaceutical package insert describes the routes available and is a valuable source of information.

ORAL DRUG ADMINISTRATION

The oral route is the most convenient route of administration and causes the fewest complications. This route is ideal for client/owner drug administration. Drugs with an oral preparation come in tablets, granules, powders, suspensions, and pastes.

Many horses eat powders, granules, and crushed tablets mixed with a palatable food (sweet feed, pellets, chopped apples, and applesauce).

For difficult or anorectic patients, an alternative is to mix the powder or dissolve the tablets in water and administer using a dose syringe.* Adding molasses, syrup, or baby carrot food increases palatability and therefore encourages acceptance by the patient. Medications in paste or suspension form should be administered as follows:

- Properly restrain the head.
- Make sure the mouth is cleared of food.
- Carefully place the dose syringe between the buccal mucosa and the molars, and angle it over the tongue. Gently grasp the tongue and pull it forward and out of the way before placing the syringe in the mouth to ensure that the medicine remains in the mouth.
- Spread the medicine evenly over the back of the tongue and dispense slowly to encourage swallowing.

---

*Dose syringe with catheter tip (60 or 35 ml), Monoject. Sherwood Medical, St. Louis, MO 63103.

Administration through a **nasogastric tube** is useful for individuals who refuse dosage in the preceding manner or who need delivery of a large volume of medication. Nasogastric tubing also ensures that the entire dose is delivered.

- See Nasogastric Tube Placement (Chapter 18, p. 81)
- Medication is delivered easily with a large, 400-ml dose syringe* that fits on the end of most nasogastric tubes.
- After administering the medication, deliver a dose syringeful of water, then air, to ensure that all drug has cleared the tubing.
- Leave the syringe attached or kink the tube when removing it to reduce the risk of aspiration.

Complications

The complete dose often is not delivered unless administered through a nasogastric tube.

Some drugs are inactivated in the stomach of herbivores, so check to be sure that the drug is for oral use in horses.

Use of the oral route results in high drug levels in the gastrointestinal tract, which can alter the normal bacterial flora and cause diarrhea or colic.

INTRAMUSCULAR ADMINISTRATION

Intramuscular administration typically causes slower absorption than does use of the intravenous route, results in lower peak blood levels, and allows less frequent administration. As with oral administration, many owners are comfortable administering drugs intramuscularly. Several large muscle masses are suitable for drug administration (Fig. 2–1).

- Small volumes (10 ml or less) may be administered in the neck in the indented triangular space that lies above the cervical vertebrae, below the nuchal ligament, and a handbreadth in front of the cranial border of the scapula.
- The lower halves of the semitendinosus and semimembranosus muscles are suitable for large volumes. Proper restraint of the horse is needed, and the person dispensing the drug should stand as close to the horse's side as possible to avoid personal injury.
- Large volumes may be administered in the pectoral muscles (pectoralis descendens) between the front limbs.

Procedure

- Clean the site with an alcohol- or chlorhexidine-soaked swab until the gross dirt is removed.
- Use a 1.5-inch, 22-, 20-, 19-, or 18-gauge needle, depending on the viscosity of the medicine to be delivered.
- Quickly stick the needle through the skin up to the hub.

---

*400-ml nylon dose syringe. J.A. Webster, Inc., 86 Leominster Road, Sterling, MA 01564-2198; (800) 225-7911.

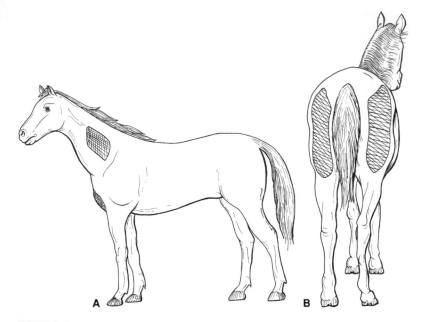

FIGURE 2-1. Sites for intramuscular drug delivery. **A,** Lateral view. **B,** Posterior view.

- Attach the drug-filled syringe to the needle and aspirate to ensure that the needle is not in a vessel.
- Ideally, administer no more than 5-10 ml in any one site. For large volumes, the needle may be redirected without leaving the skin after each 5- to 10-ml aliquot.
- When dosing must be repeated, rotate between muscle groups to avoid repeated injury to any one muscle.

Complications

Abscess formation is an occasional complication. Clean the skin thoroughly before injecting, and choose a site that is easily drained if this complication occurs.

Muscle **soreness,** specifically neck soreness, is fairly common and is related to drug irritation and associated inflammation, the volume administered, and the site of administration. Injection sites in high-motion areas should be avoided. Avoid repeated **intramuscular** injection in foals.

Severe **drug reactions** can occur if certain drugs (e.g., procaine penicillin G) are accidentally injected in a vessel.

INTRAVENOUS ADMINISTRATION

Use of the intravenous route provides immediate blood levels of the drug but typically requires more frequent administration. Medication must be administered slowly (at a rate of approximately 1 ml per 5 seconds) or diluted in sterile water or saline solution, especially if the particular drug is known to cause any type of adverse reaction.

The external jugular vein is most commonly used for medication delivery. Venipuncture should only be in the cranial third of the neck. See Fig. 1–1 for the location of venipuncture sites.

Equipment

- Alcohol-soaked gauze
- 18-, 19-, or 20-gauge 1.5-inch (3.75-cm) needle
- Syringe with medication

Procedure

- Clean site with an alcohol wipe until gross dirt is removed.
- Ideally, detach the syringe from the needle. While holding off the vein below the venipuncture site, align the needle directly over the vein, opposite the blood flow. Experienced clinicians prefer to leave the syringe attached to the needle.
- Push the needle through the skin and enter the vein; blood fills the hub of the needle if the needle is in the vein. If blood is pulsing from the hub of the needle, an artery may have been accidentally entered, and the needle must be redirected. Venipuncture is commonly performed with the syringe and needle attached; however experience is needed to ensure that medication is not accidentally administered into an artery.
- Once the needle has been properly placed, attach the syringe to the needle without changing the needle position. Always check correct placement of the needle by drawing back on the syringe and confirming a flashback of blood in the syringe before injecting the solution. Recheck the position of the needle between injections of each 5 ml.
- Frequent and long-term administration of intravenous drugs requires an indwelling catheter to reduce injury to the vein and improve patient cooperation. See intravenous catheter placement (Chapter 3, p. 11).

Complications

CAUTION: Accidental **intraarterial** injection is **life-threatening** with most substances. Using a large-bore needle and entering the vein with the needle detached increases the likelihood of detecting arterial puncture (see Chapter 52, p. 450).

Accidental delivery of a caustic substance (e.g., phenylbutazone, thiopental) outside the vein can result in **necrosis** and **sloughing** of the surrounding skin.

Thrombosis and **infection** of the vein are uncommon. The risk increases with frequent venipuncture, especially if the medication is known to be irritating to the vessel lumen.

TOPICAL ADMINISTRATION

Medication may be administered topically using the skin, eyes, and mucous membranes and within body cavities (intravaginal, intrauterine, intracystic, intramammary, and intrarectal) for a direct local effect. Drugs approved for topical use are special preparations in ointments, creams, pastes, sprays, and powders. Possible general effects should be considered because many drugs are absorbed systemically. Certain oral medications (e.g., metronidazole/aspirin) may be made into solution and delivered per rectum in patients who are receiving nothing by mouth.

RECTAL ADMINISTRATION

Rectal administration of drugs is used to produce local or systemic effects. Absorption is inconsistent but can be useful in patients unable to take medications by mouth (e.g., postoperatively).

Drugs can be suspended in 1-2 oz (30-60 ml) of water and introduced rectally through a soft feeding tube and 60-ml syringe.

TRANSDERMAL/CUTANEOUS ADMINISTRATION

Use of the transdermal or cutaneous dosage form, in which the drug is incorporated in a stick-on patch and applied to an area of thin skin, is increasingly more common in clinical practice. Drugs administered by this route include fentanyl, scopolamine, nitroglycerin, and estrogen.

INTRASYNOVIAL ADMINISTRATION

The decision to administer drugs intraarticularly should be made after considering the potential complications of altering the intraarticular environment. Direct intrasynovial administration naturally produces much higher drug levels in a joint than does use of the systemic route and is commonly used in the treatment of degenerative joint disease and infectious arthritis. Medications to be injected intraarticularly should be considered carefully for their potential to cause irritation or inflammation. It is safest to use only drugs specifically labeled for intraarticular use. Certain acids or bases may be modified by the addition of a buffering solution before intrasynovial injection. Sites for intraarticular injection and the relevant anatomic features are described in Chapter 23 (p. 93).

INTRATHECAL ADMINISTRATION

The intrathecal route of drug administration is used only to achieve direct spinal analgesia, perform myelography, or treat meningoencephalitis. Medication is administered directly into the subarachnoid space. See Chapter 32 for equipment needs, procedure, and potential complications (p. 120).

EPIDURAL ADMINISTRATION

Epidural drug administration is used for anesthesia for urogenital surgery and pain management. Medications injected into the epidural space include local anesthetics (lidocaine, mepivacaine, and bupivacaine) and α_2-adrenergic agents (xylazine) and narcotics (morphine). The sacrococcygeal interspace or the first and second coccygeal interspaces (more common) are sites for epidural injection.

Equipment
- Stocks for restraint
- Twitch, sedation, or both (detomidine/xylazine and butorphanol tartrate)
- Clippers
- Material for sterile scrub
- Sterile gloves
- 2% local anesthetic, 5-ml syringe, and 22-gauge, 1-inch needle

- 18-gauge, 10.2-cm, thick-walled Tuohy needle; 18-gauge Teflon epidural catheter with stylet or 18-gauge, 1.5-inch (3.75-cm) needle
- 12-ml syringe (sterile)

Procedure

- Restrain the patient in stocks. Sedate using xylazine, 0.2-1.1 mg/kg IV, and butorphanol, 0.01-0.1 mg/kg IV to effect.
- Clip and aseptically prepare an area over the first coccygeal interspace. The first coccygeal interspace (Co_1-Co_2) is the first palpable depression on the midline caudal to the sacrum.
- 1-2 ml of 2% bupivacaine (Carbocaine) is injected subcutaneously to desensitize the skin.
- A stab incision is made through the skin to facilitate passage of the epidural needle. An 18-gauge (Periflex*) Tuohy needle is inserted on the midline into the interspace and directed cranially and ventrally at a 45-degree angle to the rump. Entrance into the epidural space is confirmed by a loss of resistance to passage of the needle; correct placement of the needle is confirmed by the ability to inject 5-10 ml of air without resistance.
- Thread an 18-gauge, polyethylene epidural catheter (Accu-Bloc Periflex*) through the Tuohy needle into the epidural space and secure it to the skin for repeated drug administration.
- If an 18-gauge 1.5-inch (3.75-cm) hypodermic needle is used for the procedure, a stab incision is not required.

Complications

Incomplete block can be caused by the presence of congenital membranes, adhesions from previous epidural procedures, location of the epidural catheter or needle in the ventral epidural space, or escape of the epidural catheter tip through the intervertebral foramen.

---

3 Intravenous Catheter Placement

James A. Orsini and Christine Kreuder

Intravenous catheters are used for the administration of large volumes of fluids or frequent dosing of intravenous medications. The size and catheter type needed depends on the intended use. Large-gauge, 5-inch (12.5-cm) catheters (14-, 12-, or 10-gauge) are used to administer intravenous fluids rapidly to adults. Bilateral jugular venous catheters may be used for rapid, large-volume fluid replacement in the treatment of severely dehydrated patients. Large-bore catheters are more likely to cause thrombophlebitis, cellulitis, or both. A 16-gauge, 5-inch catheter is used if

---

*Burrow Accu-Bloc Periflex, 18-gauge polyethylene epidural catheter. Burrow Medical, Inc., 824 Twelfth Avenue, Bethlehem, PA 18018; (800) 359-2439.

intravenous access is required specifically for frequent dosing of medications. A 16-gauge, 5-inch catheter is also appropriate for foals. Catheters are available for short-term* and long-term[†] use. Short-term catheters are left in for a maximum of 3 days, whereas long-term catheters are maintained for several weeks. The jugular vein is most accessible for catheter placement. If the jugular vein cannot be used, the cephalic and lateral thoracic veins are suitable alternatives for catheters.

> **NOTE:** The following technique applies to simple over-the-needle catheter placement. Guidewire catheters[‡] are available in longer lengths and for long-term use. Instructions for placement accompany each catheter.

Equipment
- Material for a sterile scrub
- Clippers
- Sterile gloves
- Appropriate over-the-needle catheter
- Heparin saline flush (2000 units of heparin in 500 ml of saline solution)
- 2-0 nonabsorbable suture
- Rapid-acting glue (cyanoacrylate)
- 20- or 35-ml syringe and 18-gauge needle with heparin saline flush
- Extension set[§] filled with heparin saline solution
- Intermittent injection cap[#]
- Elasticon roll**

Procedure
- Choose an area in the cranial third of the jugular groove for catheter placement.
- Clip or shave the area to be aseptically prepared.
- Perform a sterile scrub in the area for the catheter and an area 10-15 cm distal, where the jugular vein is to be temporarily occluded.
- Fill extension set tubing with heparin saline solution.
- Sterile gloves should be worn to minimize contamination of the catheter shaft.
- Remove the protective sleeve on the catheter and loosen the cap on the stylet. The catheter should be handled **ONLY** at the **hub.**
- Distend the jugular vein by placing three fingers in the jugular groove distal to the catheter site.
- The catheter should be angled so that it is parallel to the jugular groove and following the flow of blood in the vein.

---

*Abbocath-T radiopaque FEP Teflon IV catheter. Abbott Hospitals, Inc., North Chicago, IL 60064.

[†]Milacath polyurethane catheter-over-needle. Mila International, Inc., 7604 Dixie Highway, Florence, KY 41042; (859) 371-1722, (888) 645-2468.

[‡]Guidewire catheters (14- or 16-gauge, 8-inch). Mila International, Inc., 7604 Dixie Highway, Florence, KY 41042; (859) 371-1722, (888) 645-2468. Single- and double-lumen styles available.

Central venous catheter (16-gauge, 8-inch). Arrow International, Inc., 3000 Bernville Road, Reading, PA 19605; (610) 378-0131.

[§]Extension set (7-inch or 30-inch). Abbott Laboratories, North Chicago, IL 60064.

Large animal extension set (large-bore, 7-inch). International Win, Ltd., 340 North Mill Road, Suite 6, Kennett Square, PA 19348; (800) 359-4946.

[#]Injection (along with Luer-Lok). Baxter Healthcare Corp., Deerfield, IL 60015.

**Elasticon. Johnson and Johnson Medical, Inc., Arlington, TX 76004-3130.

- Enter percutaneously at a 45-degree angle, and advance the catheter and stylet until blood appears at the catheter hub. When the catheter is within the vein lumen, angle the catheter parallel to the jugular groove and advance the catheter and stylet 2-5 cm; separate the catheter and stylet and slide the catheter down the vein lumen, holding the stylet in place. The catheter should advance without resistance. Remove the stylet.
- Attach the extension set tubing and injection cap.
- Use the syringe with the heparin flush to aspirate blood into the extension set to ensure the catheter is in the vein. Blood should flash back easily. Flush the catheter with heparin saline solution.
- Use cyanoacrylate adhesive to anchor the catheter hub to the skin (optional).
- Secure the catheter hub to the skin using suture, taking care not to kink the catheter or puncture the jugular vein. Additionally secure the extension set to the skin in several places.
- The extension set is usually left exposed for ease of inspection for catheter-associated problems or covered by a sterile dressing and an Elasticon bandage placed around the neck. To deliver fluids, remove the injection cap and attach the extension set to an intravenous administration set.*

CATHETER USE AND MAINTENANCE

Injection caps should be replaced daily or as needed.

The injection port should be wiped with an alcohol swab before each needle insertion.

All catheters need to be flushed with 5-7 ml of heparin saline solution every 4-6 hours to maintain patency.

Patency should be checked each time the catheter is flushed and before administration of any medications. Check patency by attaching a syringe filled with heparin saline solution and aspirate to achieve a flashback of blood; slowly inject in 5-7 ml of heparin saline solution. Failure to achieve a flashback may be due to

- Clotted blood in the catheter
- Kinking of the catheter or extension set
- Loose attachment of the injection cap or extension set
- Positional effect of the patient's head or neck

If no flashback is seen, gently inject 5-7 ml of heparin saline solution into the catheter and draw back. The catheter may need to be replaced if a flashback is not confirmed.

When administering medication through a catheter, choose an injection port close to the catheter, clamp off any fluids that are flowing through the catheter, and check for a flashback, followed by injecting 5 ml of heparin saline solution before the first drug, between each drug, and after the last drug is administered. Certain drugs precipitate when mixed (see Chapter 52, p. 650). Flushing between each drug minimizes this complication. Drugs should be administered slowly, at a rate of 1 ml per 5 seconds. Medications known to cause adverse systemic reactions should be administered even slower and diluted.

---

*Stat large animal IV set (large-bore, 10 feet long). International Win, Ltd., 340 North Mill Road, Suite 6, Kennett Square, PA 19348; (800) 359-4946.

When replacing a catheter, use an alternate vein to minimize phlebitis. If possible, do not catheterize the same venipuncture site until the venipuncture site is healed. Use a long-term catheter if venous access is required for more than 6 days, to avoid injury to the vein.

Complications

Thrombophlebitis, phlebitis, or **local cellulitis** is a common complication of long-term venous access (catheterization).

Examine the catheter site twice daily for swelling, heat, and pain. A small circle of reactive skin at the site of skin puncture is normal, but any thickening at this site and any associated heat or pain are abnormal and require immediate removal of the catheter. Phlebitis can be a cause of fever and an increase or decrease in nucleated cell count.

Phlebitis usually is responsive to local therapy (hot packing, topical dimethyl sulfoxide [DMSO]) but must be monitored closely because complete blockage of the vein with a septic thrombus, abscess, and secondary bacteremia or septicemia may entail more aggressive treatment. Antimicrobial treatment should be directed against *Staphylococcus* spp. pending culture and susceptibility results.

Embolization of the catheter can occur if the catheter is accidentally severed or breaks off. This is an uncommon occurrence if the catheter is examined for holes and kinks and replaced as needed. Chest radiographs can be used to locate the catheter with surgical retrieval if the catheter is in the jugular vein or heart. A catheter in the lung generally does not cause any long-term problems.

4 Intraosseous Infusion Technique

James A. Orsini and Christine Kreuder

Intraosseous infusion technique (IIT) is an alternative method for rapid delivery of fluids and medications to patients receiving neonatal intensive care when intravenous access is not possible. Access to the central circulation is through the intramedullary vessels in the bone marrow, which do not collapse because of the rigid bony shell that maintains the vascular space. The absorption rate of medications is similar to that with the intravenous route of administration. IIT is used in human medicine in the care of patients with cardiac arrest, hypovolemic shock, and circulatory collapse.

Equipment
- Material for sterile scrub
- Clippers
- Sterile gloves
- Sedative: xylazine and butorphanol
- Local anesthesia: 2% mepivacaine (Carbocaine)
- #15 scalpel blade
- #4 (28-mm) Steinmann pin and Jacobs chuck

- 12- or 14-gauge intraosseous needles/Sur-fast Cook* intraosseous needle
- 14-gauge, 0.5-inch (1.25-cm) stainless steel needle
- Heparin saline solution
- Crystalloid solution, lactated Ringer's solution
- Sterile wrap

Procedure
- Sedate foal with xylazine (0.5-1.1 mg/kg IV) and butorphanol (0.01-0.04 mg/kg IV).
- The foal is placed in right or left lateral recumbency.
- Sterile preparation of the intraosseous site on the tibia is the proximal medial one third of bone 3 cm distal to the tendinous (flat area devoid of vessels) band of the semitendinosus muscle.

CAUTION: A branch of the saphenous vein crosses the tibia 2 cm distal to the infusion site. The nutrient foramen is 2-3 cm distal to the infusion site near the popliteal line in the center of the tibial shaft.

- Infiltrate skin, subcutaneous tissues, and periosteum with 2% mepivacaine (Carbocaine) over the intraosseous site.
- With the #15 scalpel blade, incise the skin and subcutaneous tissues.
- Use a #4 Steinmann pin and Jacobs chuck to penetrate the tibial cortex by positioning the pin at a 90-degree angle to the bone, applying a downward pressing and twisting motion against the bone until a loss of resistance is felt.
- Entrance into the medullary cavity is confirmed by placing a 14-gauge, 0.5-inch (1.25-cm) stainless steel needle into the cavity and aspirating blood or marrow contents.
- Flush the needle with 5-10 ml of heparin saline solution.
- The intraosseous needle can be removed after infusion of a maximum of 1 L of crystallized solution or secured in place. It should be flushed with heparin saline every 4-6 hours to maintain patency.
- Place a sterile wrap over the intraosseous site to maintain sterility.

Complications
Subperiosteal or subcutaneous leakage of fluids or malposition of the intraosseous needle can result in partial occlusion of the needle.

Tibial fractures can be caused by poor needle placement.

Soft tissue swelling, cellulitis, and periosteal reactions are usually a temporary problem, lasting no more than 60 days.

---

*Sur-fast. Cook Critical Care, Inc., Bloomington, IN 47401.

5 | Regional Perfusion

James A. Orsini

Regional perfusion generally is used to manage specific problems such as septic arthritis/tenosynovitis, bursitis, osteomyelitis, and other soft-tissue infections. It is the delivery of antibiotics under pressure to the affected region of a limb through an artery or vein. The goal is to achieve high concentrations of an antibiotic or antibiotics in an area that is usually poorly perfused by the systemic circulation and/or to produce a concentration gradient that forces high doses of the infused drug from the vascular space into the interstitial spaces. Delivery of the drug is customarily performed using an intravenous catheter in a superficial vein or with a catheter adapter placed in a 4.5-mm hole drilled in the bone (see intraosseous infusion technique, p. 14), to access the medullary cavity. Regardless of the method used, this procedure is more commonly performed under general, regional, and/or local anesthesia. The treated limb is tightly wrapped with an Esmarch bandage proximal to the access point to the venous system and the site of infection. This is necessary to occlude the superficial venous system and open the collateral osseous venous circulation. Perfusions should be administered over 30 minutes with a maximum perfusion pressure of 450 psi.

Equipment

- General, regional and/or local anesthesia (see Chapter 56, p. 00)
- Material for a sterile scrub
- Clippers
- Sterile gloves
- Appropriate over-the-needle catheter (20-23 gauge)
- Heparin saline flush (2000 units of heparin in 500 ml of saline solution)
- 2-0 nonabsorbable suture
- Cyanoacrylate glue or similar adhesive if catheter is to remain in place for any period of time
- 20- or 35-ml syringe and 18-gauge needle with heparin saline flush
- Extension set primed with heparin saline solution
- Elasticon tape
- Esmarch bandage
- Rubber surgical tubing tourniquet
- 60 ml of balanced electrolyte solution containing the equivalent of one parenteral antimicrobial agent dose for infusion

Procedure (see Chapter 36, p. 273)

- Place the patient under general anesthesia if required.
- Aseptically prepare the skin overlying the catheter insertion site.
- Introduce the catheter into the selected vein percutaneously or by direct cutdown.
- Apply the Esmarch bandage above the site selected for perfusion—above and below the perfusion site if the site is more proximal on the limb.
- Using rubber surgical tubing as a tourniquet, wrap the leg twice and secure the tourniquet in place.

- Remove the Esmarch bandage.
- Perfuse the limb with 60 ml of a balanced electrolyte solution administering one systemic dose of the selected antimicrobial agent. The choice of antimicrobial agent(s) for treatment depends on culture and susceptibility results. Examples of antimicrobials used in perfusate include the aminoglycosides (gentamicin and amikacin), beta-lactams (penicillins, cephalosporins, carbapenems, monobactams), and vancomycin.
- Inject the perfusate over 1 minute.
- Remove the tourniquet 30 minutes after injection of the perfusate.
- Suture the skin (cutdown), and/or cover the injection site with a sterile bandage.

Complications

Improper placement of the tourniquet can result in diffusion of the drug above the tourniquet.

Leaving the tourniquet on longer than 30 minutes can result in vessel and nerve injury.

---

6 Bacterial, Fungal, and Viral Infection Diagnoses

James A. Orsini and Christine Kreuder

Laboratory confirmation of an etiologic agent often is necessary in the management of infectious diseases. Bacterial and fungal infections are difficult to differentiate, and bacterial culture and sensitivity results are essential for specific antibiotic therapy. A suspected pathogen may not be isolated owing to improper sample collection or handling procedures, weak virulence of a pathogen relative to the contaminants, and concurrent antibiotic therapy. To interpret results correctly, the clinician must have a working knowledge of the likely pathogens at a particular site, the normal flora associated with the site, common environmental contaminants, and the probability of accurate laboratory identification. Patient history and physical examination also must be applied to interpretation of laboratory results. All collected samples for submission should be clearly labeled.

Equipment

- The equipment and techniques used for collection of synovial, peritoneal, cerebrospinal, and pleural fluids, transtracheal aspiration, and bronchoalveolar lavage (BAL) samples are described as separate procedures.

BACTERIAL SAMPLES

NOTE: The collection and transport system depends on the bacteria suspected (aerobic versus anaerobic). Anaerobic infection occurs frequently in peritonitis, pleuritis, osteomyelitis, adult pneumonia, and abscesses.

- Culturette collection and transport system* for aerobic or facultative anaerobic samples
- Port-A-Cul tube† for anaerobic samples
- Blood culture bottle‡ for blood samples
- Gram stain and microscope slides

FUNGAL SAMPLES
- Sterile vial
- Gram stain and microscope slides

VIRAL SAMPLES
- Culturette collection and transport system
- Viral transport medium§
- Vacutainer tubes#; plain (red top) and EDTA (purple top) are most commonly used for blood samples. Citrate or heparin tubes may be needed for certain viral isolation tests; request information from the diagnostic laboratory
- Icepacks and Styrofoam container for transport

Procedure
BACTERIAL SAMPLES
- Collect the sample using sterile technique.
- Culture the site of interest before debridement or manipulation.
- Ideally, the patient has not received antibiotic therapy for 24 hours before culture sampling.
- Use cotton swabs to culture **abscesses, wounds, pustules,** or sites without fluid.
- Choose an abscess or pustule that is intact and uncontaminated for culture samples.
- A sterile #15 scalpel blade is best to incise the abscess.
- Select the appropriate swab depending on whether aerobic, anaerobic, or both cultures are desired.
- Moisten the swab with the transport medium before collecting the sample. Many microbes are highly susceptible to desiccation.
- Sample the wall of the abscess or pustule, because the center may be sterile. Culture the deepest, least contaminated part.
- Once the sample is collected, immediately place the swab in the transport medium and seal the container. Obligate anaerobes do not survive more than 20 minutes in room air.
- If possible, aspirate fluid from abscesses or pustules using a sterile needle and syringe and submit this to the laboratory.
- Transport fluid samples of **exudate, transtracheal wash,** and BAL samples, **synovial fluid, cerebrospinal fluid, pleural fluid,** and **peritoneal fluid** in the syringe used for collection; see individual procedure for method of collection.

---

*Culturette collection and transport system. Becton-Dickinson Microbiology Systems, Cockeysville, MD 21030.
†Port-A-Cul tube. BBL Division of Becton-Dickinson, Cockeysville, MD 21030.
‡Septi-check BB blood culture bottle. Roche Diagnostic Systems, Indianapolis, IN 46256.
§Viral transport medium is supplied by diagnostic laboratories upon request.
#Vacutainer tubes. Becton-Dickinson Vacutainer Systems, Rutherford, NJ 07070.

Remove the air from the syringe and cap the syringe with a sterile needle. If anaerobes are suspected, bend the needle back on itself or preferably place the sample into a Port-A-Cul tube. NOTE: *Do not refrigerate Port-A-Cul samples for anaerobic cultures.* Place the sample in a blood culture bottle if the samples are not to be processed for more than 12 hours. This dilutes the antibacterial factors that normally occur in these fluids.

- **Urine** samples degrade rapidly. Transport the sample in a syringe or sterile vial and refrigerate. The sample does not last more than 2 days. See urinary tract catheterization procedure (p. 90) for method of collection. **Request colony counts on isolated organisms.**

- **Blood** samples (10-20 ml) should be placed directly into special blood culture bottles. Clip the hair and perform a sterile scrub at the venipuncture site. Use a syringe to aspirate the blood, and change needles before injecting the blood into the culture bottle. Collecting several culture specimens during a 24-hour period is indicated if bacterial growth does not occur initially and bacteremia is highly suspected. Polymerase chain reaction (PCR) testing for organisms in blood (e.g., *Ehrlichia risticii*) is best performed from EDTA samples.

- **Feces** can be collected into a clean container. Because the gastrointestinal tract has normal bacterial flora, request isolation of specific species only. If attempting to isolate *Salmonella* species, submit five separate culture specimens obtained 12 hours apart or a single sample for PCR testing. If a delay in processing is expected, place the sample in an enrichment broth* for *Salmonella*. *Clostridium difficile* and *perfringens* toxins can be detected in the stool without any special storage and/or handling.

- **Uterine** cultures can be collected with a sterile guarded swab† with a protective cap. Preferably, the mare is in estrus, so the cervix is open. Wash the perineum with antiseptic solution and rinse with water. Use sterile gloves. Place a small amount of sterile lubricating jelly‡ (nonspermicidal) on one hand and insert the gloved, lubricated hand into the vagina. Gently dilate the cervix with one finger and guide the swab into the cervix with the other hand. Once the swab is in the uterus, push the swab out through the protective cap, obtain a sample, and retract the swab into the guarded sleeve before removing it from the uterus. Break off the swab, place it in a Culturette transport system, and moisten the sample.

- Transport solid tissue samples in the smallest sterile container possible. Add sterile saline solution to the sample to prevent desiccation. Keep the sample refrigerated.

- Routine samples taken at **necropsy** include lung, liver, lymph nodes, sections of gastrointestinal tract, gross lesions, and organs suspected because of clinical signs. Accurate samples cannot be obtained from individuals dead more than 4 hours.

- The sooner the samples are processed, the more accurate are the results.

- Laboratory results may require 3-6 days.

---

*Difco. BBL Division of Becton-Dickinson, Cockeysville, MD 21030.

†Double-guarded uterine swab. Hartford Veterinary Supply, 9100 Persimmon Tree Road, Potomac, MD 20854.

‡K-Y lubricating jelly. Johnson and Johnson Medical, Inc., Arlington, TX 76004-3130.

H-R lubricating jelly. Carter Products, Division of Carter-Wallace, Inc., New York, NY 10105.

- A separate swab is used to make a slide at the time of collection. Roll the swab onto the slide. Fluids should be spread in a thin layer on the slide. Tissue samples should be compressed on the slide and removed to make an impression smear. Allow the slide to air dry, stain with Gram stain. Gram-positive bacteria stain blue or purple, and Gram-negative bacteria stain pink or red. Assess bacterial morphologic features, reaction to Gram stain, relative number of each type of bacterium, inflammatory cells, and phagocytosis.

FUNGAL SAMPLES

- Collect fungal specimens in the same manner as bacterial samples. Use syringes and sterile containers for transport.
- The **skin** is sampled by plucking hairs and performing a skin scrape of the suspected lesion. Use a #10 scalpel blade to scrape the skin at the edge of the lesion. Place mineral oil on the skin to minimize loss of the sample. Submit the hair, skin scrapings, and scalpel blade in a sterile vial.
- Laboratory results may take up to 2-3 weeks.
- Use Gram stain to look for evidence of a fungal infection (spores, hyphae, filamentous rows of coccoid cells). This is particularly important for suspected fungal keratitis (see Chapter 41).

VIRAL SAMPLES

- Obtain viral samples as soon as a viral disease is suspected because the highest yield is in the early stages of infection. Horses that are in contact with those showing clinical signs should be sampled because they are likely to be in an early stage of infection.
- The testing laboratory should be called in advance for information on sample sites, collection, and handling techniques for a specific virus and to request viral transport media.
- Sample sites most often affected by the infection are mucosal vesicles, nasal secretions, transtracheal wash or BAL samples, feces, and so on. Use a moistened swab for sample collection. A fluid sample is preferred. Scraping or biopsy of the lesion also is appropriate.
- Place the sample in viral transport medium and refrigerate as soon as possible. If the sample will not be processed within 4 hours, freeze the specimen and ship in dry ice.
- **Blood** samples are useful because most infections have a viremic stage. Divide 12-20 ml of blood into plain Vacutainer tubes (for serum) and 10 ml into EDTA tubes. Do not freeze blood samples for shipment.
- Virus isolation results take 2-8 weeks. Fluorescent antibody testing, if available, may speed the diagnosis.
- Paired serum antibody titers are used to confirm a laboratory diagnosis. Antibody titers should be taken 2-4 weeks apart: acute phase and convalescent phase. A fourfold increase in antibody titer is considered diagnostic of a recent exposure.

7 Biopsy Techniques

James A. Orsini and Christine Kreuder

Tissue biopsy often is helpful in antemortem diagnosis of disease. The different procedures sometimes are invasive and therefore are used for treatment or prognosis purposes only. Biopsy techniques are discussed for the different tissues.

NOTE:

- Samples should be sent to a veterinary pathologist or specialist with the appropriate information.
- Biopsy specimens should be less than 1 cm × 1 cm for proper formalin fixation.
- The formalin to tissue volume ratio is 10:1.
- Samples should not be allowed to freeze during transport.

SKIN BIOPSY

Skin biopsy is used in cases of undiagnosed skin disease because of treatment failure or persistent clinical signs. Biopsy should be performed early, within 3 weeks, because the histopathologic findings are difficult to interpret in chronic cases. Punch biopsy or wedge biopsy (elliptical incision) usually is performed. Punch biopsy is preferred, except for sampling of vesicular, bullous, or ulcerative lesions, for which a wedge biopsy is more useful.

Equipment

- 6- or 8-mm cutaneous biopsy punch* or a #15 scalpel blade for wedge biopsy
- 2% local anesthetic, 25-gauge needle, and 3-ml syringe
- Rat-toothed forceps
- Metzenbaum scissors
- Needle holders
- Sterile gauze sponges
- 2-0 absorbable suture
- 10% buffered formalin

Procedure

- Select areas representative of disease. A biopsy should include the lesion, point of transition, and normal skin.
- Do not wash or scrub the intended sample site, to prevent disruption of the tissue architecture.
- A local anesthetic is infiltrated in the subcutaneous tissue beneath the area for the biopsy. Do not inject directly through the intended sample. Mark the area anesthetized.
- **Punch biopsy:** Select the site and rotate the biopsy punch while applying firm pressure until the instrument cuts through the dermis. Because the biopsy spec-

---

*Baker's biopsy punch. Baker Cummins Dermatologicals, Inc., Miami, FL 33178; (800) 347-4474.

imen is adherent to subcutaneous fat, grasp it with a forceps and separate it with a scissors.
- **Wedge biopsy:** Use a scalpel blade to make an elliptical skin incision and cut the subcutaneous fat with scissors to free the sample.
- **Be careful not to create a tissue artifact.**
- Place the sample on a tongue depressor, subcutaneous-fat side down, and immerse the tongue depressor in formalin. The tongue depressor preserves sample architecture during transport. Michel medium is for immunofluorescence tests and is not a good preservative for histopathologic testing.
- The wound is closed with a simple interrupted or cruciate suture pattern. Large wedge biopsy requires a two-layer closure.

Complications

Infection is rare; avoid biopsies over joint capsules or contaminated areas. If **dehiscence** occurs, clean daily. Healing is by secondary intention. *If a large wedge biopsy is in a high-motion area, restrict exercise for 1 week to decrease the risk of dehiscence.*

BIOPSY OF MASS, NODULE, AND CYST

Cutaneous masses, nodules, and cysts are sampled by means of aspiration or excisional biopsy. Fine-needle aspiration yields a cellular sample and is differentiated cytologically as infectious, allergic, parasitic, or neoplastic. Excisional biopsy requires complete removal of a mass for treatment. Histopathologic examination is used to confirm a diagnosis.

Equipment
FINE-NEEDLE ASPIRATION
- 20-gauge, 1- to 1.5-inch (2.5 to 3.75-cm) needle and 20-ml syringe
- Microscope slides

EXCISIONAL BIOPSY
- Material for sterile scrub
- 2% local anesthetic
- #10 blade and handle
- Rat-toothed forceps
- Metzenbaum scissors
- Needle holder and suture scissors
- Sterile 4 × 4 gauze sponges
- Container with 10% buffered formalin
- 1-0/2-0 absorbable suture

Procedure
FINE-NEEDLE ASPIRATION
- Insert the needle with attached syringe into the center of the mass.
- The sample material is aspirated into the needle and not into the syringe barrel.
- The needle is redirected several times without leaving the mass or contaminating the aspirate with normal tissue. If blood contaminates the sample, repeat the procedure with a new needle and syringe. Release the negative pressure before withdrawing.

- A slide for cytologic examination is made by disconnecting the needle, filling the syringe with air, reattaching the needle, and expelling the needle contents onto a slide. Smear the aspirate for blood, or compress it between two slides and pull them apart. Allow the slides to air dry.
- A fluid-filled mass or cyst is aspirated in a similar manner, sampling 1-2 ml of fluid to make a smear.
- Stain the slides with Wright or Diff-Quick stain. Send stained and unstained slides to pathologist.

EXCISIONAL BIOPSY
- Perform a sterile scrub of the mass to be excised. Do not scrub if the surface is important for histologic interpretation.
- Inject a local anesthetic into the subcutaneous tissue or create a ring block.
- Make an elliptical incision around the mass and undermine the subcutaneous tissue with scissors.
- Place the tissue in formalin. If the mass is larger than 1 cm diameter, fillet it longitudinally into 1-cm-wide sections.
- The subcutaneous and skin layers are closed; a horizontal or vertical mattress pattern in the skin relieves tension.
- Exercise is restricted to handwalking for 7-10 days.

Complications
See earlier, Skin Biopsy, Complications.

LYMPH-NODE ASPIRATION
Fine-needle aspiration of enlarged or abnormal lymph nodes is adequate for cytologic examination and can be helpful in differentiating infectious and neoplastic causes of lymphadenopathy. Complications are unusual.

Equipment
- 22-gauge, 1.5-inch (3.75-cm) needle
- 10 ml syringe
- Microscope slides

Procedure
- Stabilize the lymph node with one hand, and insert the needle with attached syringe into the center of the lymph node.
- Please read description for Fine-Needle Aspiration technique.
- Allow the slides to air dry. Stain slides with Diff-Quick. Send stained and unstained slides to a pathologist experienced in reading equine cytologic samples, because the cytologic diagnosis of lymphosarcoma is difficult in the horse.

RENAL BIOPSY
Biopsy of the kidney is unusual because renal disease is well characterized with serum chemistry and renal function tests. Indications include renal masses and undiagnosed causes of renal failure. Percutaneous renal biopsy entails some risk and is performed when the information is likely to affect the outcome. The right

kidney is easily viewed with ultrasound, and biopsy should be performed with ultrasound guidance to obtain an accurate sample and decrease the risk of complications. Biopsy of the left kidney is performed using ultrasound guidance.

Equipment

- Sedative (xylazine hydrochloride and butorphanol tartrate)
- 14-gauge, 6-inch (15-cm) biopsy needle*
- #15 scalpel blade
- Clippers
- Material for a sterile scrub
- Sterile gloves
- 2% local anesthetic, 25-gauge needle, and 3-ml syringe
- Sterile sleeve and sterile lubricant for ultrasound-guided biopsy of the right kidney
- 10% buffered formalin

Procedure

- Sedate patient to minimize motion during the procedure.

RIGHT KIDNEY ULTRASOUND-GUIDED BIOPSY

- The right kidney is located between the 15th and 17th intercostal spaces ventral to the lumbar processes.
- Clip the hair over the area and perform a sterile scrub.
- Place the ultrasound transducer in a sterile sleeve and identify a site to sample away from the renal vessels.
- A local anesthetic is injected subcutaneously at the biopsy site; repeat the sterile scrub.
- With sterile, gloved hands, make a stab incision and advance the biopsy needle through the stab incision to the kidney.
- A second person can perform ultrasound guidance during the biopsy. The needle appears as a hyperechoic line on the ultrasound screen.

NOTE: Be familiar with operation of the selected biopsy unit.
- Place the biopsy specimen in 10% formalin.

LEFT KIDNEY BIOPSY

- The left kidney is more loosely attached to the abdominal wall and may require stabilization per rectum during the biopsy procedure. Successful biopsy of the left kidney requires ultrasound guidance.
- Skin preparation and biopsy techniques are identical to those of the ultrasound-guided biopsy for the right kidney. The kidney must remain motionless during needle placement.

Complications

Infection and **peritonitis** occur if sterile technique is not maintained or if the rectum is perforated. *If rectal tissue or feed material is found, begin systemic*

---

*Tru-Cut biopsy needle. Baxter Healthcare Corp., Pharmaseal Division, Mundelein, IL 60060.

antibiotic therapy. Do not perform a biopsy on a suspected renal abscess, because of the risk of infection.

Hemorrhage is a serious complication if the needle penetrates the renal artery or vein or one of the accessory arteries entering the caudal pole of the kidney. All patients should be closely monitored for several days with serial packed cell volume (PCV) and total protein (TP) determinations. *A clotting profile should be performed before the renal biopsy.*

Hematuria is not uncommon and generally resolves spontaneously.

LIVER BIOPSY

Percutaneous biopsy of the liver is a simple procedure indicated in the treatment of patients with undiagnosed liver disease. Histopathologic findings often can define the liver disease as infectious, toxic, or obstructive/congestive. **NOTE:** A specific diagnosis is made in a few diseases. Ultrasound should be used to ensure that the biopsy specimen is obtained from an affected section of liver.

Equipment
- Sedative (xylazine hydrochloride and butorphanol tartrate)
- 14-gauge, 6-inch (15-cm) biopsy needle
- #15 scalpel blade
- Clippers
- Sterile scrub
- 2% local anesthetic, 25-gauge needle, and 3-ml syringe
- Sterile gloves
- 10% buffered formalin

Procedure
- Perform clotting times (prothrombin time [PT] and partial thromboplastin time [PTT]) and platelet count before biopsy of the liver.
- Using ultrasound, view a portion of the liver between the sixth and fifteenth intercostal spaces of the right lower to upper abdomen. Clip the hair, and select a section of liver for biopsy.
- Perform liver biopsy "blindly" (without ultrasound) from the right fourteenth intercostal space in a line drawn from the point of the shoulder to the tuber coxae. Occasionally the liver cannot be seen on the right, and it is necessary to perform a biopsy of the liver, under ultrasound guidance, on the left at the level of the elbow, just caudal to the diaphragm.
- Sedate the patient for the procedure.
- Clip the hair and perform a sterile scrub at the selected site.
- Inject a local anesthetic subcutaneously; perform a second sterile scrub.
- With sterile gloved hands, make a stab incision, insert the biopsy needle into the incision, and advance it in a cranial and ventral direction.

NOTE: Know the operation of the biopsy needle before using it.
- Place the biopsy in 10% formalin.

Complications
Hemorrhage occurs if the liver disease is affecting the clotting profile. *Assess clotting time before biopsy.* MONITOR all patients for signs of hemorrhage for

48 hours after the procedure. *If platelet count is normal, bleeding is uncommon even in the face of prolonged PT and PTT times.*

Infection (cellulitis, peritonitis) is unlikely if sterile technique is maintained. Do not perform biopsy on liver abscesses. *Accidental biopsy of the colon mandates antibiotic therapy.*

LUNG BIOPSY

Percutaneous biopsy of the lung is used in the evaluation of patients with diffuse lung disease if radiography, ultrasonography, and bronchoalveolar lavage do not provide a diagnosis.

The procedure is relatively safe and easy to perform although deaths have occurred.

Equipment

- Sedative (xylazine hydrochloride)
- Material for a sterile scrub
- Clippers
- Sterile gloves
- 2% local anesthetic, 22-gauge, 1.5-inch (3.75-cm) needle, and 3-ml syringe
- #15 scalpel blade
- 14-gauge, 15-cm Tru-Cut biopsy needle
- 2-0 nonabsorbable suture on a straight or curved needle
- 10% buffered formalin

Procedure

- Sedation is determined by the temperament of the patient.
- The most common site for biopsy, when lung disease is diffuse, is the right 7th or 8th intercostal space. Place the needle approximately 8 cm above the level of the olecranon and at the cranial aspect of the rib to avoid the intercostal vessels.
- Clip the hair and perform a gross scrub.
- A local anesthetic is infiltrated into the subcutaneous tissues and parietal pleura.
- Perform a sterile scrub at the site of needle puncture.
- With sterile gloved hands, make a stab incision through the skin and muscle.
- Advance the biopsy needle through the skin, muscle layer, and parietal pleura in a cranial and medial direction and continue during end inspiration for an additional 2 cm into lung parenchyma.

NOTE: Be familiar with operation of the biopsy unit.
- Place the tissue in formalin.
- Close the skin incision using a simple cruciate pattern.

Complications

A small volume of air may leak into the thorax before the skin is closed and should not cause a problem. Hemoptysis may occur and is rarely a problem. Fatal tension pneumothorax rarely occurs after lung biopsy (see Chapter 43, p. 501).

BONE MARROW BIOPSY

Bone marrow biopsy is a useful procedure to determine causes for changes in peripheral blood cell count or cell morphology. The finding of neoplastic or abnormal cells in the circulating blood is an indication for bone marrow biopsy. This procedure is used to differentiate primary hematopoietic disease (lymphosarcoma, multiple myeloma, myeloproliferative disease), compensatory marrow changes (iron deficiency anemia, anemia of chronic disease), and red cell hypoplasia following erythropoietin use. Bone marrow is analyzed by means of core aspiration or biopsy. A sample for complete blood cell count (CBC) drawn at the time of biopsy should be sent with the biopsy sample.

Equipment
- Sedative (xylazine hydrochloride and butorphanol tartrate)
- Material for a sterile scrub
- Clippers
- Sterile gloves
- 2% local anesthetic, 25-gauge needle, and 3-ml syringe
- #15 scalpel blade
- 15-gauge, 2-inch (5-cm) bone marrow needle* for marrow aspiration or 11-gauge, 4-inch (10-cm) bone marrow needle for marrow biopsy
- 12-ml Luer-Lok syringe with anticoagulant (10% disodium EDTA), Petri dish, and microscope slides if aspiration is performed (more commonly used of the two procedures)
- 10% buffered formalin if a biopsy specimen is submitted

Procedure
- The sternebrae is the most common site; the marrow cavity lies just below the periosteum. The tuber coxae is also used for biopsy in individuals less than 4 years.
- Sedation is recommended.
- A local anesthetic is infiltrated into the subcutaneous tissues and periosteum.
- Clip the hair and perform a sterile scrub.
- With sterile, gloved hands, make a small stab incision.

FOR BONE MARROW ASPIRATION
- Insert the needle and stylet through the skin and advance to the periosteum. A rotational motion is needed to advance the needle through the cortex and into the marrow cavity.
- Remove the stylet and attach the syringe. Aspirate the bone marrow with negative pressure on the plunger; aspirations should be short and gentle. Excessive negative pressure results in blood contamination of the sample.
- Place the sample in a Petri dish. Remove the marrow spicules and place them on a microscope slide. Prepare a squash smear by positioning one slide on top of the

---

*Jamshidi disposable bone marrow biopsy/aspiration needle. Baxter Healthcare Corporation, Deerfield, IL 60015.

other and gently pulling them apart. Send both stained (Diff-Quick) and unstained slides to the laboratory.

FOR BONE MARROW BIOPSY
- Insert the biopsy needle through the skin and advance to the cortex with a forceful rotational movement.
- Remove the stylet, and advance the needle 2 cm.
- A rotational thrust of the needle should detach the specimen; withdraw the needle.
- The stylet is used to push the biopsy specimen out of the needle and into a formalin container.

Complications
Hemorrhage can occur and rarely is clinically significant unless the patient has thrombocytopenia or another clotting deficiency.

　　Osteomyelitis is rare.

MUSCLE BIOPSY

Histopathologic examination of muscle samples is useful whenever disease of muscle fibers, neuromuscular junctions, or peripheral nerves is suspected. This is a minor surgical procedure performed on a standing horse. Samples of diseased and normal muscle should be collected. If polysaccharide storage myopathy is suspected, biopsy of the semimembranosus muscle is required. For motor neuron disease, the biopsy is performed on the muscle at the tail head (sacrocaudalis dorsalis medialis).

> **NOTE:** Formalin may not be the preservative of choice, depending on the specific analysis. Contact the pathology laboratory before performing a muscle biopsy for preservative recommendations.

Equipment
- Material for sterile scrub
- Clippers
- Sterile gloves
- 2% local anesthetic, 25-gauge needle, and 5-ml syringe
- #10 scalpel blade and handle
- Metzenbaum scissors
- Tongue depressor
- 0 or 2-0 absorbable and nonabsorbable suture
- Appropriate fixative

Procedure
- Sedation as determined by the temperament and state of debilitation of the patient.
- The sample should be approximately 5 mm wide, 20 mm long, and 5 mm thick and should be parallel to the direction of the diseased muscle fibers.
- Clip hair and perform a gross scrub at the biopsy site.
- Infiltrate a local anesthetic into the subcutaneous tissues. *Do not* inject anesthetic into the muscle; this affects the histopathologic findings.
- Perform a sterile scrub.
- With sterile, gloved hands, incise the skin over the muscle belly. Use blunt dissection to separate the skin from the muscle belly. Remove a muscle sample using sharp dissection.

- Secure the sample to a tongue depressor or Rayport muscle biopsy clamp* with stay sutures to prevent sample shrinkage.
- Suture the incision in two layers to minimize dead space.

Complications
Infection is very uncommon but dehiscence of semimembranosus muscle can occur.

ENDOMETRIAL BIOPSY

Endometrial biopsy is a useful tool to evaluate infertility. **NOTE:** Rule out pregnancy before biopsy to avoid accidental abortion. The procedure is best performed during estrus.

Equipment
- Sedative (xylazine hydrochloride and butorphanol tartrate)
- Scrub material
- Sterile sleeve (shoulder length)
- Sterile lubricant[†]
- 70-cm alligator punch[‡] (sterile)
- Bouin fixative

Procedure
- Sedation is recommended, with the mare restrained in stocks with a twitch.
- The mare's tail is tied to the side.
- Scrub the perineum with a dilute antiseptic solution (povidone-iodine or chlorhexidine) and rinse with water.
- With a sterile, gloved arm, digitally dilate the cervix and gently guide the biopsy instrument through the cervix.
- Advance the biopsy instrument into the uterus and with the gloved arm in the rectum, confirm instrument placement.
- Via rectal palpation, depress a portion of the uterine mucosa between the jaws of the biopsy instrument to obtain the sample.
- Place the sample in the appropriate fixative and process within 24 hours.

Complications
Abortion can occur if the mare is pregnant at the time of biopsy. *Perform a complete reproductive examination before biopsy.* The cervix should be closed if the mare is pregnant.

Endometritis can occur if bacterial pathogens are introduced into the uterus.

---

*Rayport muscle biopsy clamp; Order No. SU130-1111 (10mm), SU130-1112 (12mm), SU130-1113 (16mm); Allegiance Health Care, 100 Raritan Center Parkway, Edison, NJ 08837; (800) 964-5227.

[†]K-Y lubricating jelly. Johnson and Johnson Medical, Inc., Arlington, TX 76004-3130.
H-R Lubricating Jelly. Carter Products, Division of Carter-Wallace Inc., New York, NY 10105.

[‡]Jackson uterine biopsy forceps. Jorgensen Laboratories, Inc., 1450 North Van Buren Avenue, Loveland, CO 80538; (970) 669-2500.

8 Endoscopy Techniques

James A. Orsini and Christine Kreuder

Endoscopy is now performed routinely in equine practice and is an extremely valuable tool. Endoscopy allows direct examination of the upper and lower airway, esophagus, stomach, duodenum, urethra, and bladder. This procedure can be used to explain changes found on radiographic and ultrasound examination and to identify lesions that are not detectable using other methods. Samples (biopsy specimens and aspirates) can be obtained transendoscopically for culture and cytologic and histopathologic examination. Regardless of the system examined, endoscopic examination should be performed systematically. A thorough knowledge of applied anatomy is necessary to "drive" the endoscope and to differentiate normal from abnormal.

Many of the flexible endoscopes used in equine practice have been designed for use in humans. Flexible endoscopes are either fiberoptic endoscopes or videoendoscopes. Both are easily adapted for procedures on horses. A fiberoptic endoscope is portable and considerably less expensive than a videoendoscope but produces inferior image quality. The image is viewed through an eyepiece on the endoscope, so only one person can view the examination unless the endoscope is adapted for a teaching head. A videoendoscope has excellent image quality that is projected onto a monitor. The examination can be seen by all and can be recorded. The unit is generally not easily suited for field use because it is not portable. Endoscopes should have a biopsy channel and a system for air and water delivery. The size of the endoscope required depends on the anatomic site examined and the size of the patient. This is addressed with the description of the endoscopic examination for each system.

Equipment

- Appropriately sized flexible endoscope, flexible fiberoptic endoscope,* or videoendoscope†
- Saline bowl with warm water
- Biopsy forceps, grasping forceps, polypectomy snares, and polyethylene tubing, which are accessories available with each unit
- 30-ml syringe for transendoscopic aspirates

General Procedure

- Two or three persons are needed to perform endoscopic examinations.
- Sedation, a twitch, or both may be needed depending on the patient and the system examined. The patient is best restrained in stocks or in a stall.

---

*Flexible fiberoptic endoscopes: 11-mm outer diameter, 100-cm long; 12-mm outer diameter, 160-cm long; and 8-mm outer diameter, 150-cm long. Karl Storz Veterinary Endoscopy-America, Inc., 175 Cremona Drive, Goleta, CA 93117; (800) 955-7832.

†Flexible videoendoscopes: GIF Type Q140 Gastrointestinal Videoscope (9.8-mm outer diameter, 200-250 cm long), SIF 100 (11.2-mm outer diameter, 300-cm long), and CF 100 TL (12.9-mm outer diameter, 200- or 300-cm long). Available by special order from Olympus America, Inc., 2 Corporate Center Drive, Melville, NY 11747; (516) 844-5000.

- The endoscope should be arranged to minimize danger to the operators, patient, and equipment.
- Familiarity with the mechanics of the endoscope is necessary, as is manipulation of the endoscope tip in all directions. The air and water controls are operated from the handpiece; typically, the red button delivers air and the blue button delivers water.
- Lubricate the endoscope with warm water or a small amount of sterile lubricating jelly* (avoid the tip of the endoscope).
- Passage of the endoscope is described separately for each system.
- Water delivered to the tip of the endoscope cleans the lens; air is delivered to dilate the cavity and improve the examination.
- Biopsy is performed by means of advancing the biopsy instrument through the biopsy channel until it protrudes 2-3 cm beyond the tip of the endoscope. Manipulate the instrument to obtain a sample and withdraw. Place the specimen in appropriate fixative.
- Transendoscopic **aspiration** is performed by means of passing sterile polyethylene tubing through the biopsy channel until it protrudes 2-3 cm beyond the tip of the endoscope. Aspirate a sample using a 30-ml syringe. Administering sterile saline solution frequently facilitates the aspiration. Place the sample directly onto slides or into an EDTA Vacutainer tube.
- The endoscope should be cleaned with antiseptic solution and rinsed after each use.

ENDOSCOPIC EXAMINATION OF THE AIRWAY

Endoscopy of the airway is indicated in the evaluation of patients with nasal discharge, epistaxis, coughing, dyspnea, dysphagia, facial asymmetry, respiratory noise, or exercise intolerance. This is the method of choice for diagnosing ethmoid hematoma, laryngeal hemiplegia, epiglottic entrapment, dorsal displacement of the soft palate (DDSP), guttural pouch empyema and mycosis, exercise-induced pulmonary hemorrhage (EIPH), and tracheal trauma or stricture. This procedure also assists in the diagnosis of paranasal sinusitis and pulmonary infection or abscess.

- The endoscope should be 150-200 cm long and 9 mm in outside diameter for examination of the lower airway; a 9-mm-diameter endoscope is the largest that can be safely passed in a foal.
- Do not sedate the patient, if possible, because sedation can affect the function of the pharynx and the larynx. Sedation is recommended for examination of the lower airway to reduce coughing.
- Pass the endoscope into a nostril and systematically evaluate the upper airway structures, taking care not to injure the ethmoid turbinates. Maintain a clear line of vision during the entire examination. The trachea is entered by means of passing the scope between the arytenoid cartilages. Tracheal rings are seen if the scope has been properly introduced. Note any abnormal discharge, mucosal inflammation, cysts, or masses.

---

*K-Y lubricating jelly. Johnson and Johnson Medical, Inc., Arlington, TX 76004-3130.
H-R lubricating jelly. Carter Products, Division of Carter-Wallace, Inc., New York, NY 10105.

CAUTION: The scope can retroflex in the pharynx and enter the oral cavity, causing damage to the instrument. Ensure an unobstructed view to prevent this problem.

- Pass the endoscope into the pharynx using either nostril.
- The nasomaxillary opening is located in the caudal middle meatus and can be reached with a 9-mm-diameter scope. Drainage from the paranasal sinuses into the middle meatus may be seen in cases of sinusitis.
- Entering the guttural pouch is aided with a biopsy instrument or brush as a guide, or it can be performed by means of passing a Chambers catheter up the opposite nostril and "flipping" open the opposite pouch opening.
- Spray the trachea with 4-6 ml of sterile 2% lidocaine through the biopsy channel to decrease coughing if the lower respiratory tract is examined.

ENDOSCOPIC EXAMINATION OF THE GASTROINTESTINAL TRACT

Endoscopy allows examination of the esophagus, stomach, duodenum, rectum, and distal small colon. It is the method of choice for confirming the presence of gastric and duodenal ulceration and can aid in the diagnosis of rectal tears.

- The endoscope must be 225-300 cm long for complete examination of the stomach and duodenum in adults. A 200-cm endoscope is the minimal length for cursory examination of the stomach in an adult.
- Adults should be fasted for 8-12 hours before gastroscopy and weanling foals fasted for 6-8 hours. If the duodenum is being examined, longer fasting periods may be required (24 hours for adults). Do not fast nursing foals.
- Sedation is generally required.
- See Nasogastric Tube Placement (p. 81) for passage of the endoscope into the esophagus. Confirm entrance into the esophagus to prevent damage to the endoscope.

CAUTION: Retroflexion of the long endoscopes in the pharynx and entering the oral cavity can be avoided if the view is clear and unobstructed at all times.

- To prevent damage to the endoscope, a short nasogastric tube may be passed into the proximal esophagus and used as a cannula.
- Insufflation assists passage and examination of the esophagus, cardiac sphincter, and stomach.

ENDOSCOPIC EXAMINATION OF THE URINARY TRACT

- The endoscope should be at least 100 cm long and 9 mm or less in diameter for examination of the urethra and bladder.
- Perform the procedure using aseptic technique.
- Cold-sterilize the endoscope in Cidex disinfectant for 30 minutes. Flush the biopsy channel.
- Sedation is recommended for stallions and geldings. Administer 0.4-0.6 mg/kg xylazine, 0.01 mg/kg butorphanol, and 0.02 mg/kg acepromazine (geldings only) IV for restraint and relaxation.
- Perform a sterile scrub of the distal penis and external urethral process, catheterize the bladder, and evacuate the urine. See Urinary Tract Catheterization (p. 90).

- Using sterile gloves, lubricate the length of the endoscope, avoiding the tip.
- Advance the endoscope using the same technique as described for catheterization of the bladder.
- Systematically evaluate the urethra and the bladder, using insufflation to improve the examination. Insufflation normally causes the urethral vessels to appear engorged.

Complications
With prolonged air insufflation of the urethra, arterial air embolism and death can occur.

---

9   Use of Ultrasonography
Virginia B. Reef

ULTRASOUND EXAMINATION

The ultrasound examination is a noninvasive method of obtaining rapid diagnostic information in the emergency setting. Ultrasonography is particularly useful in the rapid assessment of the horse presenting with:

- Trauma
- An acute abdomen
- Respiratory distress
- Evaluating fetal well-being in high-risk pregnant mares
  Echocardiography is useful for assessing the horse with cardiovascular emergencies and is discussed beginning on p. 133.

Patient Preparation

The best images are obtained by clipping the hair from the skin over the area to be examined using a #40 surgical clipper blade.

- Shaving the skin is usually not necessary.
- If clipping is not an option, wetting the hair and skin thoroughly with warm water along the lay of the hair or spraying the area with alcohol may be sufficient for a diagnostic quality image.
- The skin should be scrubbed clean with surgical soap and water.
- Ultrasound coupling gel should be applied to the skin.
- If there is an acute laceration or puncture wound, the exam should be performed *aseptically*, using sterile ultrasound gel or sterile K-Y jelly and a sterile ultrasound "condom" or surgical glove to cover the transducer.

EMERGENCY MUSCULOSKELETAL EXAMINATIONS

Ultrasonographic assessment of horses with a recent history of trauma, severe lameness, or a penetrating wound or laceration helps the clinician differentiate areas of muscle injury from injury to bone, tendons, ligaments, joints, tendon sheaths, or the surrounding soft tissue structures. Fractures can be diagnosed in

PROCEDURES

horses in which routine radiographs are not diagnostic or in patients with fractures in areas that are not amenable to routine radiography. In a horse with a laceration or a penetrating wound, the extent of damage to the synovial and tendinous or ligamentous structures in the area can be evaluated and the presence and location of foreign material can be determined.

Normal Ultrasonographic Findings in the Equine Musculoskeletal System

Each tendon and ligament should be evaluated in two mutually perpendicular planes. The normal size, shape, and sonographic characteristics should be similar between the same anatomic tissues in opposing limbs. The unaffected limb can be used as a control, if necessary.

- Most tendons and ligaments have a homogeneous echoic appearance with a parallel fiber pattern.
  - The proximal suspensory ligament has a more heteroechoic appearance caused by varying amounts of muscle fibers, connective tissue, and fat at the origin and in the proximal suspensory body.
  - The biceps tendon also contains connective tissue and fat and therefore has a slightly more heterogeneous ultrasonographic appearance.
- The tendon sheath appears as a thin echoic structure with a thinner hypoechoic lining. There is normally minimal anechoic intrathecal fluid.
  - A small collection of anechoic fluid is normally imaged in the carpal sheath between the deep digital flexor tendon and inferior check ligament.
- A bursa is a potential space that normally contains little or no discernible fluid.

The normal ultrasonographic appearance of muscle and bone is unique to each and should be compared with that in the contralateral limb, if abnormalities are suspected.

- Normal muscle has a unique speckle pattern when imaged in its short axis and a unique striated pattern when imaged in its long axis.
- The normal bony surface echo is a thin echoic line of uniform thickness, which is smooth, except in the region of normal bony protuberances.
  - Articular cartilage is anechoic and varies in thickness, depending upon its location.
  - A soft tissue layer immediately adjacent to the bone is present in all nonarticular areas.

Each joint has a characteristic ultrasonographic appearance with varying thickness of the joint capsule and synovium but should be similar in both limbs.

- The joint capsule is a slightly thicker, echoic, usually curvilinear structure with a thin layer of hypoechoic synovium within.
- The joint fluid is anechoic.

Abnormal Ultrasonographic Findings in the Musculoskeletal System

Indications for an emergency musculoskeletal ultrasonographic examination include marked swelling with associated heat and sensitivity, severe lameness, a laceration, a penetrating wound, or a suspected fracture that is not seen radiographically or is in an area in which radiographic images cannot be obtained.

Severe Tendinitis or Desmitis

Marked enlargement of a tendon or ligament with complete disruption of its fiber pattern is consistent with rupture of the tendon or ligament. The injured tendon may appear *anechoic, hypoechoic,* or *echoic* depending on how much time has elapsed since the injury and if an organized clot is contained within the lesion. Significant peritendinous or periligamentous soft tissue swelling is usually present.

- Fetlock drop is found with severe suspensory desmitis and superficial digital flexor tendinitis.
- The toe flipping up with weight bearing is consistent with rupture of the deep digital flexor tendon.
- Subluxation of the proximal interphalangeal joint occurs with severe oblique distal sesamoidean desmitis and rupture of the superficial digital flexor tendon in the pastern.
- Flexion of the stifle with extension of the hock is consistent with a ruptured peroneus tertius tendon.

Severe Tenosynovitis or Bursitis

Marked distention of the tendon sheath or bursa with fluid and fibrin is consistent with a septic tenosynovitis or bursitis and can occur in horses with recent intrathecal or intrabursal hemorrhage or active, nonseptic inflammation within the tendon sheath or bursa.

- Fibrin appears as filmy, hypoechoic strands or clumps within the synovial fluid.
- Fluid in an infected tendon sheath or bursa can appear anechoic, hypoechoic, or echoic depending on the protein content and cellularity of the synovial fluid.
- Acute bleeding into a synovial structure usually has a swirling echoic appearance. Anechoic fluid with hypoechoic loculations and echoic masses is consistent with recent hemorrhage.
- Disruptions of the tendon sheath or bursa resulting in the formation of a synovial fistula are identified by the discontinuity in the tendon sheath or bursa and the adjacent, usually anechoic, periarticular fluid accumulation.

Myositis and Muscle Rupture

Enlargement of the affected muscle belly occurs with myositis. The ultrasound changes in muscle echogenicity, and the presence or absence of muscle striations, are indicative of the type of muscle pathology present.

- Muscle edema results in the muscle appearing less echoic than normal, but retaining its normal striations.
- Increased muscle echogenicity with loss of the normal striations is consistent with a postanesthetic myopathy.
- A more heterogeneous sonographic appearance with loss of the normal muscle fiber pattern is consistent with a necrotizing myositis.
  - The detection of pinpoint hyperechoic echoes consistent with free gas in the muscle or muscle fascia, and in the absence of a tract lined with gas associated with a penetrating wound, is consistent with a *Clostridial myositis* (Fig. 9–1).
- Cavitation of the most severely affected muscle often is seen associated with liquefaction necrosis.

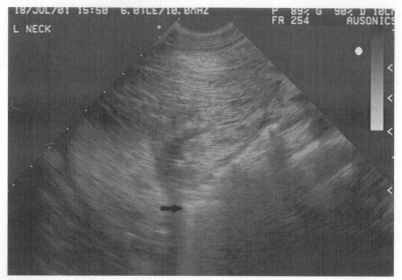

FIGURE 9-1. Sonogram of the left side of the neck obtained from a horse with acute *Clostridial myositis*. Note the hyperechoic free gas echoes *(arrow)* in the muscle casting gray acoustic shadows and obliterating the deeper musculature. The adjacent muscles are more echoic than normal and hypoechoic fluid is evident in the fascial planes.

Areas of muscle fiber disruption are the most common muscle injuries detected ultrasonographically. Muscle tears in horses are most frequently seen in the hind limb and shoulder muscles. The affected muscles can be diagnosed by carefully tracing the involved muscles from their origin to insertion.

- Anechoic fluid-filled areas with hypoechoic loculations are imaged within the muscle belly.
- Large anechoic loculated fluid-filled areas are usually imaged between the adjacent muscle fascia and in the adjacent subcutaneous tissues.
- The free edge of a completely disrupted muscle may be imaged floating in the anechoic loculated fluid.
- Echoic masses consistent with clot are often imaged within the intramuscular, interfascial, or subcutaneous hematoma.
  - Acoustic shadows may be cast from the far side of these clots as they become more organized.

Muscle neoplasms, particularly hemangiosarcomas, should *always* be considered in the differential diagnosis of horses with acute severe muscle disruption, especially when multiple sites are involved.

- Individuals with skeletal muscle hemangiosarcoma often have discrete echoic masses in the muscle; however, anechoic loculated heterogeneous masses may be imaged in areas of tumor necrosis (Fig. 9–2).

Fractures

The ultrasonographic diagnosis of a fracture depends on imaging the fracture line or fracture fragment in two mutually perpendicular ultrasound planes.

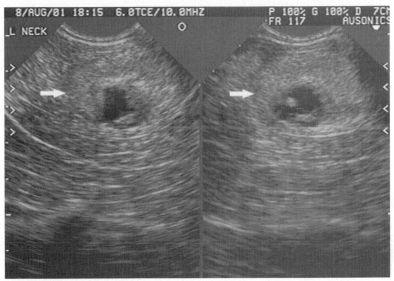

FIGURE 9-2. Sonograms of the left side of the neck obtained from a horse with disseminated skeletal muscle hemangiosarcoma. Note the echoic round to oval mass in the superficial musculature (*arrows*) with the anechoic area of cavitation (necrosis and hemorrhage).

- A nondisplaced fracture is diagnosed when there is a break in the normal hyperechoic bony surface echo in an area where there is not a normal vascular channel.
- A hyperechoic bony structure casting an acoustic shadow that is distracted from the underlying parent portion of the bone in two mutually perpendicular ultrasound planes is consistent with a displaced fracture fragment (Fig. 9-3).
- Anechoic loculated fluid is usually present in the adjacent soft tissues.
  - Echoic masses are frequently detected within the anechoic loculated fluid that is consistent with a clot.
- Disruption of the surrounding musculature is commonly imaged with comminution or displacement of the fracture fragment.

Severe Synovitis

Marked distention of the joint with fluid and fibrin is indicative of a severe synovitis.

- Flocculent, hypoechoic to echoic synovial fluid may be imaged in septic arthritis.
- A hemarthrosis is suggested by the presence of large quantities of uniformly echoic synovial fluid, particularly in individuals with periarticular hematomas.
- Thickening of the synovium is also frequently imaged in patients with severe synovitis, regardless of its etiology.
- Marked periarticular hypoechoic soft tissue swelling is usually present surrounding the joint capsule in individuals with severe synovitis.
  - Anechoic loculated fluid surrounding the joint is most consistent with a traumatic synovitis.

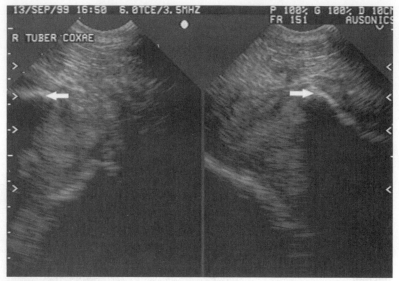

FIGURE 9-3. Sonograms of the right tuber coxae fracture with marked ventral displacement of the fracture fragment. The fractured tuber coxae is easily seen in both views (*arrows*), and disruption of the adjacent musculature is visible.

- Disruptions of the joint capsule resulting in the formation of a synovial fistula are identified by the discontinuity in the joint capsule and the adjacent periarticular fluid accumulation.

    Joint instability or radiographic findings of avulsion fractures associated with the origin or insertions of the collateral ligaments should prompt sonographic evaluations of the collateral ligaments associated with that joint, looking for disruption of the fibers of the collateral ligament.
    - Enlargement of the collateral ligament, with disruption of its fiber pattern and a decrease in its echogenicity, is consistent with collateral desmitis. The ligament may be difficult or impossible to identify in areas of complete rupture. Comparison to the contralateral limb is helpful in deciding on the degree of injury sustained.

Lacerations and Puncture Wounds

Ultrasonographic examination of puncture wounds and lacerations should be done after aseptic preparation of the area. *Puncture wounds should be examined ultrasonographically before a contrast study is performed because the air injected with the contrast media impairs visualization of the underlying structures, limiting the usefulness of the ultrasonographic examination.* The sonographic examination should begin superficially and gradually progress deeper until the full extent of the tract is found.

- The tracts usually appear as hypoechoic linear or tubular paths containing various amounts of anechoic fluid and hyperechoic gas.

- Hyperechoic free gas echoes are usually seen at the skin surface of the puncture wound or laceration and decrease in number as the tract or laceration extends deeper. These gas echoes are usually pinpoint and cast small gray acoustic shadows.
- A foreign body appears as an echoic to hyperechoic structure within the tract of the puncture wound or laceration.
  - Wood, the most common foreign body detected in horses, is hyperechoic and casts a strong black acoustic shadow from its near surface.
  - A needle, nail, wire, and BB gun pellets produce the typical metallic reverberation artifact.
  - Tubular hyperechoic structures that cast weak acoustic shadows may represent a piece of hoof.
- Always look for more than one foreign body.
- The type of foreign body and the position of the ultrasound beam relative to the foreign body determine the type of acoustic shadow cast by the foreign body.

EMERGENCY ABDOMINAL EXAMINATIONS

- Diagnostic ultrasound is helpful in the assessment of the foal or adult with an acute abdomen.
- The findings on ultrasonographic examination help differentiate surgical from medical causes of colic.
- Diagnostic ultrasonography provides a window for noninvasive evaluation of the gastrointestinal viscera and abdominal organs.
- Transrectal ultrasonographic examination of abnormalities detected on rectal palpation can also be performed to further clarify the rectal findings.

Normal Ultrasonographic Findings in the Equine Gastrointestinal Tract

Both large and small intestinal echoes are imaged from the ventral abdomen in the foal, whereas in the adult, only large intestinal echoes are usually imaged from this window. A few loops of jejunum may be imaged in the midventral abdomen in some adults. Only large intestinal echoes are usually imaged in the intercostal spaces (ICSs) and the flank.

- Large intestinal echoes are recognized by their large semicircular, sacculated appearance.
- The large intestinal wall is hypoechoic to echoic with a hyperechoic gas echo from the mucosal surface that normally measures 3 mm or less in thickness.
- Peristaltic activity is normal.
- The right dorsal colon is imaged ventral to the liver in the tenth-to-fourteenth ICSs.
- The cecum is imaged in the right paralumbar fossa.

The gastric fundic echo is imaged as a large semicircular structure medial to the spleen at the level of the splenic vein in the left ninth-to-twelfth ICS ventral to the diaphragm and ventral lung.

- The wall of the stomach is hypoechoic to echoic with a hyperechoic gas echo from the mucosal surface and can measure up to 7.5 mm in thickness.

The duodenum is imaged medial to the right lobe of the liver, adjacent to the right dorsal colon, beginning at approximately the tenth ICS and can be followed caudally around the caudal pole of the right kidney.

- It appears as a small oval or circular structure (when sliced in its short axis) with a hypoechoic to echoic wall ≤3 mm thick.
- The duodenum usually appears partially collapsed with regular waves of fluidy ingesta imaged during real-time scanning.

The jejunum is rarely visualized in the adult except adjacent to the stomach and occasionally in the midventral to caudal left side of the abdomen, whereas in the foal the jejunum is readily seen along the floor of the ventral abdomen.

- The small intestinal echoes are recognized by their small tubular and circular appearance.
- The wall of the jejunum is hypoechoic to echoic with a hyperechoic echo from the mucosal surface and is usually ≤3 mm thick.
- Some anechoic fluidy ingesta and hyperechoic "gassy" ingesta is often imaged in the lumen of the jejunum.
- Peristaltic waves are normally seen.

The ileum is rarely imaged transcutaneously but may be imaged transrectally in the adult as a slightly thicker (4-5 mm), more muscular segment of small intestine in the dorsal caudal abdomen with visible peristaltic activity.

Only a small amount of anechoic fluid is usually imaged within the peritoneal cavity cranioventrally.

Abnormal Ultrasonographic Findings in the Equine Gastrointestinal Tract

Marked increases in the thickness of the intestinal wall, coupled with marked distention of the lumen and a lack of visible peristaltic activity, are ultrasonographic indications of significant intestinal compromise. Marked fluid distention of the stomach should prompt nasogastric decompression.

Herniation

Surgical colic is caused by herniation of the abdominal viscera into thoracic cavity, scrotum, umbilicus, or through the body wall.

UMBILICAL

- Gastrointestinal viscera, peritoneal fluid, or omentum imaged in the external umbilicus.
- Measure the size of the hernia.
- Determine the viability of entrapped or incarcerated intestine.
  - Measure wall thickness and intestinal distention, and evaluate peristalsis.
- If hernia is complicated, look for internal umbilical remnant infection, subcutaneous abscess, and/or enterocutaneous fistula.

INGUINAL

- Gastrointestinal viscera or omentum imaged in the enlarged scrotal sac.
- Determine viability of the entrapped or incarcerated intestine.
  - Measure wall thickness and intestinal distention and evaluate peristalsis.

- Perform a rectal examination in the stallion and evaluate the small intestine to determine the degree of distention proximal to the obstruction.

DIAPHRAGMATIC
- Gastrointestinal viscera, omentum, or abdominal organs imaged in the thoracic cavity.
- A rent in the diaphragm is usually a result of a herniated viscera displacing the lung dorsally.
- The approximate size of the hernia can be estimated by the number of ICSs affected and whether it is imaged on one or both sides of the thorax.
- Determine the viability of entrapped or incarcerated intestine (Fig. 9-4).
  □ Measure wall thickness and intestinal distention and evaluate peristalsis.
- A diaphragmatic hernia could be missed ultrasonographically if located in the center of the diaphragm and the herniated viscera were not in contact with the thoracic wall.

Abdominal Wall Hernias and Rupture of the Prepubic Tendon
- Determine the viability of entrapped or incarcerated intestine.
  □ Measure wall thickness and intestinal distention and evaluate peristalsis.
- Identify the intestine involved and the presence and locations of adhesions.
- Evaluate the muscles and/or tendon of the abdominal wall.
  □ Measure the size of the defect and evaluate the edges of the hernial ring.

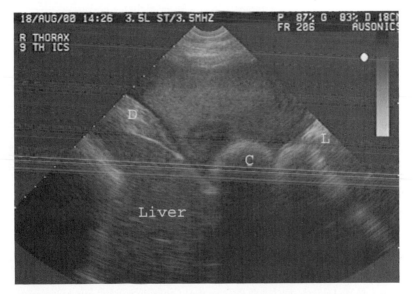

FIGURE 9-4. Sonogram of the right side of the thorax obtained in the ninth intercostal space from a horse with a diaphragmatic hernia. The right side of the image is dorsal and the left side is ventral. Notice the echoic swirling fluid consistent with a hemothorax *(top)*, the white hyperechoic circular sacculated colon *(C)* in the thoracic cavity adjacent to the lung *(L)*, and the muscular part of the diaphragm *(D)* dorsal to the liver.

Nephrosplenic Ligament Entrapment

Ultrasonographic findings consistent with a nephrosplenic ligament entrapment include:

- An inability to see the tail of the spleen or left kidney transcutaneously.
- The identification of ingesta and/or gas-filled large bowel in the left caudodorsal abdomen.
- The dorsal splenic border appears horizontal and is ventrally displaced to the middle of the abdomen.

The sonogram can be used to determine if treatment with phenylephrine, followed by lunging or rolling the horse, has successfully corrected the nephrosplenic ligament entrapment.

Sand Colic

- Small, pinpoint granular hyperechoic echoes, casting multiple acoustic shadows, imaged in the ventral most portion of the affected intestine.
- Loss of normal sacculations in the affected portion of large intestine as it is flattened by the weight of the intraluminal sand.
- Markedly decreased or absent peristaltic movements of the sand containing ventral portion of the colon.

Enterolithiasis

- Rarely shows up in images as the affected colon is not usually seen from a transcutaneous or rectal "window."
- A large, hyperechoic mass, casting a strong acoustic shadow imaged within the lumen of the intestine, if the affected portion of intestine is adjacent to the ventral body wall.
- Wall thickness may be increased.
- Decreased to absent peristalsis in the affected segment of intestine.

Intussusception

- Characteristic ultrasonographic findings associated with the invagination of one loop of intestine (intussusceptum) into another loop of intestine (intussuscipiens).
  - Target or "bull's eye" sign in the affected portion of intestine (Fig. 9–5).
  - The strangulated intestine usually has thickened, edematous, hypoechoic walls
  - Little or no peristaltic activity imaged in the affected portion of intestine.
  - Often fibrin is imaged between the intussusceptum and intussuscipiens.
  - Distended, fluid-filled intestine is imaged proximal to a strangulated portion of intestine.
- *Jejunal intussusception* is usually imaged from the ventral-most portion of the abdomen, and is most common in foals.
- *Ileal intussusception* is usually imaged rectally or transcutaneously in the caudodorsal abdomen and is most common in yearlings and young horses.
- *Large bowel intussusception* usually involves the ileum and large bowel and is most frequently imaged from the right side of the abdomen because the cecum or right ventral colon is involved. It is most common in adult horses.

Strangulating Small Intestinal Disorders and Small Intestinal Volvulus

- Characteristic ultrasonographic findings:
  - The strangulated small intestine usually has thickened, edematous, hypoechoic walls with little or no peristaltic activity.

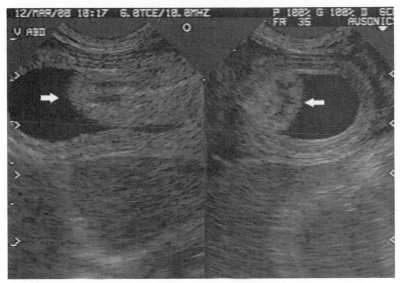

FIGURE 9-5. Sonograms of a jejunal-jejunal intussusception obtained from a foal. Notice the target or "bull's eye" appearance of the short axis section *(right image)* of the jejunum at one end of the intussusception. The arrow points to the intussusceptum.

- □ Small intestinal loops are turgid and fluid filled.
- □ Luminal contents are anechoic or layered with echoic ventral particulate ingesta.
- □ Distended, fluid-filled small intestine is imaged proximal to the strangulated small intestine.
- ▪ Distended, thick-walled small intestine most frequently detected in the ventral portion of the abdomen due to their increased weight.
- ▪ Sonographic evaluation of the equine abdomen is an excellent diagnostic tool for the detection of small intestinal distention and wall thickening and determining the need for surgical intervention.
- ▪ Diagnosis of the specific cause of strangulation is often not possible.

Intestinal Masses
- ▪ Ultrasonographic findings with intraluminal, intramural, or mesenteric masses obstructing the passage of ingesta:
  - □ Focal, mural anechoic to echoic masses within the intestinal wall that often compromise the lumen of the affected portion of intestine.
  - □ Echoic areas of narrowed irregular bowel wall have been imaged in horses with mural stricture.
  - □ Thickening of the wall of the ileum is indicative of ileal hypertrophy, detectable transrectally and transcutaneously.
  - □ Intraluminal hemorrhage appears as echogenic clots or echoic swirling fluid.
- ▪ Mural masses in the adult may be:
  - □ Abscesses
  - □ Intestinal carcinoids

- ▫ Leiomyomas
- ▫ Granulomas
- ▫ Hematomas
- ▫ Fibrosis
- Mural masses in foals or young horses may be abscesses.
- Diffuse thickening of the bowel has been seen with hypoxic injury to the bowel or enterocolitis.

Impaction

Characteristic ultrasonographic findings of impaction include:

- A round or oval echoic distended viscus, lacking sacculations, often measuring 20-30 cm or more in the adult.
- Meconium appears as hypoechoic, echoic, or hyperechoic masses in the lumen of the large colon, small colon, or rectum.
  - ▫ The bladder can be used as an "acoustic window" to evaluate the rectum and small colon immediately dorsal to it.
- Ascarids appear as hyperechoic to echoic tubular structures that are often knotted into a mass in the lumen of the intestine.
  - ▫ Isolated ascarid worms are often imaged in fluid-distended colon.
- Intestinal wall thickness may be normal or increased.
- A large acoustic shadow cast from the impacted ingesta adjacent to the colonic mucosa.
- Distention of the colon proximal to the impaction is usually present, making ultrasonographic evaluation of the impaction easier.
- Little or no peristaltic activity of the affected intestine.
- Impactions can only be imaged transcutaneously when the impacted large colon or cecum is adjacent to the body wall or fluid is interposed between the affected portion of the intestine and the body wall.
- Usually can be imaged from the flank or side of the abdomen in horses with cecal or right dorsal colon impactions.
- Small colon impactions have been imaged from the flank in miniature horses.
- In adults, small or large colon impactions can be imaged transrectally if palpable.

Medical Colic

ENTEROCOLITIS

Characteristic ultrasonographic findings of enterocolitis include:

- Increased peristalsis
- Fluid distension of the intestinal tract
- The intestinal wall may be thickened and more hypoechoic than normal, particularly with severe inflammatory bowel disease
- "Shreds" of intestinal mucosa may be imaged in the intestinal lumen.
- Marked fluid distension of the stomach should prompt nasogastric decompression.

DUODENITIS

Characteristic ultrasonographic findings of duodenitis include:

- Fluid distension of the duodenum
- Usually decreased or absent duodenal motility consistent with an ileus
- ± Thickening of the duodenal wall

- ± Duodenal stricture

± CHOLANGIOHEPATITIS AND ELEVATED BILIARY ENZYMES
Characteristic ultrasonographic findings include:

- Hepatomegaly
- Increased echogenicity of the hepatic parenchyma
- Biliary distension and echoic bile within biliary tree
- ± Thickening of the bile ducts
- ⊥ Hepatoliths

Gastric Distention and Delayed Gastric Emptying
Ultrasonographic findings include:

- Circular to oval gastric echo distended with anechoic to hypoechoic fluid or echoic to hyperechoic ingesta, seen on the left side of the abdomen.
  - Echoic fluid or hypoechoic fluid containing echoic lumps in foals is milk.
  - Layering of the dorsal gas, ventral fluid, and, if present, even more ventral ingesta is often imaged.
- Imaging the gastric echo over five or more ICSs on the left side of the abdomen is consistent with marked gastric distention.
- Imaging the gastric echo on the right side of the abdomen is rare and is consistent with severe gastric distention.
- A markedly enlarged gastric echo filled with hyperechoic material casting an acoustic shadow extending over five or more ICSs on the left side of the abdomen is detected with gastric impaction.
- A mass with a complex pattern of echogenicity in the wall of the stomach, often with invasion into the adjacent spleen or liver parenchyma, is consistent with a gastric squamous cell carcinoma. It is most common in older horses.
- Gastric emptying problems identified when large amounts of ingesta persist unchanged in the stomach in a fasted, anorexic or "refluxing" individual on repeat examinations.

Right Dorsal Colitis
Ultrasonographic findings include:

- Thickening of the wall of the right dorsal colon with mucosal irregularities.
- Evaluate the right dorsal colon in the right twelfth or thirteenth ICSs directly ventral to the liver and the duodenum.

Verminous Arteritis
Ultrasonographic findings include:

- Thick-walled artery
- Large plaquelike or mass lesions along the intimal surface of the vessel, invading the arterial lumen
- Verminous arteritis can be imaged ultrasonographically if the affected vessel is depicted transrectally

Abdominal Abscess
Characteristic ultrasonographic findings include:

- Abdominal abscesses are anechoic, hypoechoic, or filled with echoic material and are often multiloculated, especially in the foal with *Rhodococcus equi* infections.

- Hyperechoic echoes representing free gas may be detected suggesting concurrent anaerobic infection.
- Large or small intestine may be adhered to the wall of the abscess and its movement restricted.
- Abdominal abscesses in foals are detected in the ventral abdomen associated with *Rhodococcus equi* abscesses involving the mesenteric lymph nodes.
- In the adult, abdominal abscesses may be detected in the ventral abdomen, but are also frequently found dorsally associated with the root of the mesentery, cecum and large colon.
- Abdominal abscesses are frequently reported in the adult and associated with the liver.

Peritonitis

Characteristic ultrasonographic appearance:

- Anechoic, hypoechoic, or echoic fluid.
- ± Flocculent, composite fluid.
- ± Fibrin and/or adhesions between the serosal surfaces of the intestine and the abdominal wall.
- Free gas echoes and particulate echogenic debris are consistent with a ruptured viscus (Fig. 9–6).
- The abdomen, gastrointestinal, and abdominal viscera should be thoroughly examined for the source of the peritonitis such as an abdominal abscess or devitalized area of bowel.

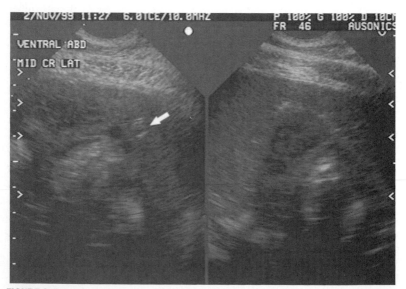

FIGURE 9-6. Sonograms of a devitalized loop of small intestine with a leak causing peritonitis. The devitalized loop of jejunum is markedly thickened with a hypoechoic to echoic wall. The arrow points to the hyperechoic free gas echoes trapped on the serosal surface of the jejunum in the fibrin layer surrounding the intestine. The peritoneal fluid is more echoic than normal, consistent with peritonitis.

Hemoperitoneum

- Homogeneous, hypoechoic to echoic swirling cellular fluid is consistent with hemoperitoneum.
- The spleen, liver, and kidneys should be carefully examined to be sure that a rupture of one of these organs is not the cause of the hemoperitoneum.
  □ Anechoic, loculated fluid within the spleen, liver, or kidney or in the subcapsular space is indicative of organ trauma.
- A very small spleen supports splenic contraction associated with significant blood loss.
- Rupture of the middle uterine artery often results in a large volume of blood in the broad ligament with a smaller quantity of blood free in the peritoneal cavity.

EMERGENCY URINARY SYSTEM EXAMINATIONS
Normal Sonographic Findings in the Equine Bladder

The equine urinary bladder is a round to oval fluid-filled structure with a hypoechoic to echoic bladder wall. The urine contained within the foal's urinary bladder should be anechoic, whereas the urine contained in the adult urinary bladder has a composite echoic appearance caused by the mucus and crystalluria.

Uroperitoneum

Uroperitoneum is a large accumulation of the urine within the peritoneal cavity associated with a defect in the urinary tract, which allows urine to flow into the peritoneal cavity.

- Uroperitoneum occurs most frequently in the equine neonate in the immediate postpartum period.
- In the adult, uroperitoneum is most common in the postpartum mare.
- The location of the urinary tract defect can be determined by the sonographic appearance of the urinary bladder, ureters, urachus, and retroperitoneal space.
- A large quantity of fluid in the peritoneal cavity is consistent with uroperitoneum.
- The fluid is usually anechoic but becomes more echoic as the uroperitoneum becomes more long-standing and a chemical peritonitis develops.
- The gastrointestinal viscera normally float in the peritoneal fluid and urine contained within the peritoneal cavity.
- A folded, collapsed urinary bladder is consistent with a rupture of the urinary bladder (Fig. 9-7).
- Fluid around the urachus and in the retroperitoneal space along the ventral abdomen with an intact urinary bladder is indicative of a defect in the urachus.
- Retroperitoneal fluid around the kidney with an intact urinary bladder is consistent with a ureteral defect.

ULTRASONOGRAPHY IN HIGH-RISK PREGNANCIES
Fetal Well-Being in High-Risk Pregnancies

Ultrasonographic evaluation of the fetus and its intrauterine environment from a transcutaneous and transrectal approach provide the clinician with important information when evaluating the high-risk pregnant mare. Severe illness of the mare, premature udder development, premature lactation, or an abnormal vaginal discharge should prompt a complete transcutaneous and transrectal ultrasonographic evaluation of the fetus to determine its well-being. Prompt intervention may improve the

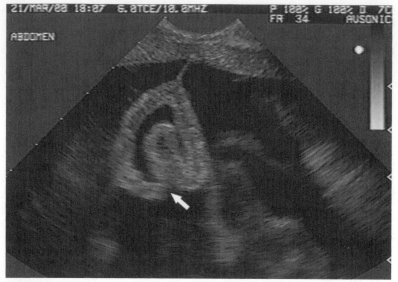

FIGURE 9-7. Transverse sonogram of the urinary bladder obtained from a foal with uroperitoneum and a ruptured bladder. Notice the collapsed and folded appearance of the bladder. Although it appears as if the rupture may be located on the dorsal surface of the bladder *(arrow)*, the defect is not readily visible. Surrounding the bladder is a large volume of anechoic fluid within the peritoneal cavity; the gastrointestinal viscera are floating in this fluid.

outcome for foals born to high-risk mares. The normal late gestation mare has a single fetus in anterior presentation, dorsopubic position. The nonfetal horn is usually evident from the ventral abdominal window in late gestation.

Biophysical Profile

The equine biophysical profile consists of seven parameters which, if normal, support the delivery of a normal fetus (Table 9–1). Each of these parameters is assigned a score of 2 if it is normal and 0 if it is abnormal for a "perfect" biophysical profile of 14. The equine biophysical profile consists of:

- **Breathing movements:** Regular breathing movements should be present in the late gestation fetus.
- **Cardiac rate and rhythm:** The mean resting fetal heart rate in the late gestation equine fetus is 75 beats/minute with a heart rate range detected ultrasonographically of ± 15 beats/minute and a regular rhythm. If the gestation is prolonged, the fetal heart rate continues to slow to as low as 57 beats/minute if the gestation length is <320 days. The heart rate can slow to 50 beats/minute if the gestation length is 320-360 days; and as low as 41 beats/minute if the gestation length is >360 days.
- **Fetal aortic diameter:** The fetus in late gestation should have an aortic diameter that is approximately 23 mm.
- **Fetal movement and tone:** The normal fetus is active during the examination with periods of activity imaged for more than 50% of the scanning time. The normal fetus has muscular tone and should not appear flaccid.

TABLE 9–1. Equine Biophysical Profile

Calculation of Biophysical Profile. Assign 2 Points to Each Category if All Evaluations Normal; Assign 0 Points to Each Category if One of Evaluations is Abnormal.

Fetal or Maternal Measurement	Patient	Abnormal
FETAL HEART RATE (HR) AND RHYTHM	—	0
Rhythm		Irregular or absent
Low HR <320 days gestation (bpm)	—	<57
Low HR 320–360 days gestation (bpm)	—	<50
Low HR >360 days gestation	—	<41
High (postactivity) HR (bpm)	—	>126
HR range (bpm)	—	>50 or <5
Fetal Breathing		0
Rhythm	—	Irregular or absent
FETAL AORTIC DIAMETER	—	0
Y = 0.00912 * X + 12.46	Y ± 4 * S.E.(5.038)	> or <Y ± * S.E.(5.038)
FETAL ACTIVITY AND TONE	—	0
Fetal activity		Absent
Fetal tone		Absent
FETAL FLUID DEPTHS	—	0
Maximal allantoic fluid depth (cm)	—	<4.7 or >22.1
Maximal amniotic fluid depth (cm)	—	<0.8 or >18.5
UTEROPLACENTAL THICKNESS	—	0
Uterus and chorioallantois (mm)	—	<3.9 or >21
UTEROPLACENTAL CONTACT	—	0
Areas of discontinuity	—	Large
Biophysical profile score	—	≤10 = negative outcome; 12 = high risk for negative outcome

BPM, Beats per minute; *Y*, predicted aortic diameter; *X*, pregnant mare's weight in lbs; *, multiplied by; *SE*, standard error.

- **Fetal fluids:** There should be ample quantition of amniotic and allantoic fluid that surround the normal late term fetus. There should be between 0.8-14.9 cm of amniotic fluid and 4.7-22.1 cm of allantoic fluid surrounding the normal fetus.
- **Uteroplacental thickness:** The normal mean thickness of the uterus and the chorioallantois combined should be 11.5 mm.
- **Uteroplacental separation:** The uterus and chorioallantois should be closely associated with one another with no imaged areas of separation or only small focal areas imaged.

Abnormal Fetal and Maternal Findings in the High-Risk Pregnant Mare

- The inability to image the nonfetal horn in late gestation is a good ultrasonographic indication of a twin pregnancy.

- The detection of two contiguous chorioallantoic membranes, usually perpendicular to the uterus, also signals the presence of a twin pregnancy.
- The imaging of two separate thoraxes confirms the presence of twin fetuses; two different fetal heart rates are usually detected if the fetuses are both alive.
- The fetal aortic diameters and thoracic diameters generally differ in size, with one of the twins smaller than the other.
- The twin fetuses may have different presentations, with the posterior presentation abnormal.
- If the head of the fetus is imaged in late gestation from the ventral abdominal window, the mare is likely to need assistance at the time of delivery.
- Torsion of the umbilical cord with marked distention of the urinary bladder has been identified in fetuses in utero and has resulted in the abortion or death of the fetus.
- Other fetal abnormalities may also be identified that may affect fetal health.
- Thickening of the amnion is also abnormal and may be detected in mares with a severe placentitis.
- Increased echogenicity of the fetal fluids may be seen in mares with placentitis or meconium stained fetus.
- Increased echogenicity of the fetal fluids has not been correlated with an adverse outcome in the late gestation fetus, only when these findings are detected earlier in gestation.

Abnormal Biophysical Profile

If only two or more of the seven parameters are abnormal (a score of 10), the foal delivered is likely to be compromised.

- **Breathing movements:** Irregular or absent fetal breathing movements is abnormal in the late gestation fetus. This abnormality may be associated with acute intrauterine hypoxia.
- **Cardiac rate and rhythm:** A heart rate of <57 beats/minute is abnormal for calculation of the biophysical profile if the gestation length is <320 days; a heart rate of <50 beats/minute is abnormal if the gestation length is 320-360 days; and a heart rate of <41 beats/minute is abnormal if the gestation length is >360 days. An irregular heart rhythm, a heart rate in excess of 126 beats/minute or a heart rate range in excess of 50 beats/minute or less than 5 beats/minute is also abnormal in the late gestation fetus. These abnormalities may be associated with acute intrauterine hypoxia.
- **Fetal aortic diameter:** An aortic diameter of <18 mm or greater than 27 mm is abnormal in the late gestation fetus. A smaller than normal aortic diameter is indicative of intrauterine growth retardation or the presence of twins.
- **Fetal movement and tone:** Absent fetal activity or a flaccid appearance to the fetus is abnormal. These abnormalities may be associated with acute intrauterine hypoxia.
- **Fetal fluids:** Hydrops should be considered when there are >14.9 cm of amniotic fluid (hydrops amnii) or >22.1 cm of allantoic fluid (hydrops allantois) that surround the fetus. A fetus that is not surrounded by adequate amounts of fetal fluids (<0.8 cm amniotic or <4.7 cm allantoic) is distressed.
  - Intrauterine hypoxia and premature rupture of the fetal membranes may be responsible for the decreased quantities of fetal fluid.
- **Uteroplacental thickness** A combined uteroplacental thickness of <3.9 mm or >21 mm is abnormal for the calculation of the biophysical profile. *Treatment of*

the mare for suspected placentitis is often initiated when the combined uteroplacental thickness is 15 mm or greater.

- **Uteroplacental separation:** Premature placental separation is supported when there is a large and/or progressive area of separation between the uterus and chorioallantois.

EMERGENCY THORACIC EXAMINATIONS

Thoracic ultrasonography is very helpful in assessing the foal or adult with severe lower respiratory tract problems. Almost the entire thorax can be evaluated ultrasonographically, including the cranial mediastinal region. The affected side or sides of the thorax, and also "pinpointing" the location of lesions, can be determined in most individuals because the involved lung segment is usually pleural based. The character of pleural fluid can be determined ultrasonographically; the type, severity of underlying pulmonary parenchymal disease can be diagnosed and differentiated:

- Consolidation
- Pleuropneumonia
- Abscesses
- Granulomas
- Tumors in the lung or pleural cavity
- Penetrating thoracic wounds
- Diaphragmatic hernias

The thoracic ultrasound examination findings can be used to formulate a more accurate prognosis for survival and to select appropriate treatment, as well as monitoring response to therapy. Survival of horses with pleuropneumonia is more likely if pleural fluid, fibrin, loculations, free gas echoes, or parenchymal necrosis are not detected on the initial ultrasonographic examination.

Normal Ultrasonographic Appearance of the Lung and Pleural Cavity

The lung is seen on both sides of the thorax from the sixteenth to seventeenth ICS cranially to the fourth ICS. The cranial mediastinum is pictured only from the right third ICS in normal horses. The lung covers the cranial and caudal mediastinum in most individuals, although a hypoechoic soft tissue mass (thymus) may be imaged in youngsters ventral and medial to the right apical lung lobe and cranial to the heart. Fatty tissue may also be seen in this area and around the heart, most commonly detected in ponies and fat horses. Fat is usually slightly more heterogeneous and echogenic than thymus and continues caudally around the heart into the caudal mediastinum.

- The normal visceral pleural edge of the lung is a straight hyperechoic line with characteristic equidistant reverberation air artifacts indicating normal aeration of the pulmonary periphery.
- In real-time, the visceral pleural edge of the lung glides ventrally across the diaphragm with inhalation and dorsally with exhalation, *"the gliding sign."*
- No pleural fluid or a small accumulation (up to 3.5 cm) of anechoic pleural fluid in the most ventral portions of the thorax may be detected.
- The curvilinear diaphragm is thick and muscular ventrally and thin and tendinous caudodorsally.

Pleural Disease
PLEURAL EFFUSION
Characteristic ultrasonographic findings include:

- Anechoic, hypoechoic, or echoic space between the lung (visceral pleura), thoracic wall (parietal pleura), diaphragm, heart, and on either side of the mediastinal septum.
- Composite fluids are complex and more echogenic than normal, containing fibrin, cellular debris, a higher cell count and total protein concentration, and/or gas.
- Sonographic patterns of pleural fluid include anechoic, complex nonseptated, and complex septated fluid.
  - Anechoic fluid represents a transudate or modified transudate.
  - Increased echogenicity of the fluid indicates an increased cell count or total protein concentration.
  - Blood within the pleural cavity (hemothorax) has a hypoechoic to echogenic swirling pattern and may be septated.

NOTE: Hemangiosarcoma should always be considered in the differential diagnosis of hemothorax.

  - Clotting in pleural fluid appears as soft, echoic masses.
- The cells and cellular debris in pyothorax are more echogenic, heavier, and in the most ventral location, whereas the less cellular fluid or gas cap is detected dorsally.
- Fibrin appears hypoechoic with a filmy to filamentous or frondlike appearance.
- Fibrous adhesions are rigid and echoic, often distorting the structures to which they are attached during one phase of respiration and restricting pulmonary mechanics.
- Free gas within the fluid (polymicrobullous fluid) is imaged as small, very bright, pinpoint, hyperechoic echoes within pleural fluid.
  - More free gas echoes are imaged dorsally in the pleural fluid.
  - The microbubble echoes move in various directions depending on respiratory motion, cardiac motion, and the patient's movements.
  - The free gas echoes adhere to the fibrinous pleural surfaces and initially may only be detected adjacent to fibrin.
  - Free gas echoes may be compartmentalized in only one portion of the thorax.
  - Free gas echoes are usually caused by an anaerobic infection within the pleural cavity (Fig. 9–8).
- The largest accumulation is ventral.
- Compression of normal lung (compression atelectasis), retraction of the lung toward the pulmonary hilus, and a ventral lung tip that floats in the surrounding fluid, if there is no ventral consolidation of the lung.
- The pericardial-diaphragmatic ligament, a normal pleural reflection of the parietal pleura over the diaphragm and heart, is pictured as a thick membrane floating in pleural fluid.
- The thoracocentesis should be performed several centimeters above the normal ventral margin of the thorax caudal to the heart where nonloculated pleural fluid or the largest pocket of loculated fluid is imaged (usually the seventh ICS).
- Care should be used so that the thoracocentesis does not occur immediately adjacent to the heart or too ventrally in the thorax in a patient with a large pleural effusion (below the ventral attachment of the diaphragm to the chest wall).

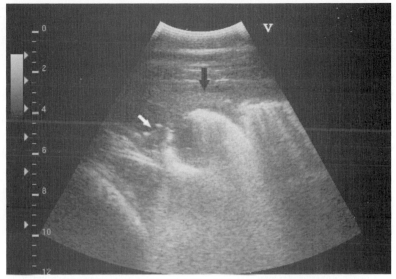

FIGURE 9-8. Sonogram of the right side of the thorax obtained from a horse with anaerobic pleuropneumonia. Note the hypoechoic consolidated lung *(black arrow)* and the sonographic air bronchogram visible as a tubular hyperechoic structure within the consolidated lung. The hyperechoic free air in the pleural space *(white arrow)* is associated with the fibrin strands present on the axial surface of the lung. These sonographic findings are consistent with an anaerobic fibrinous pleuropneumonia.

- Loculations between the parietal and visceral pleural surfaces of the lung, diaphragm, pericardium, and inner thoracic wall limit pleural fluid drainage.
- The fluid level and the extent of pulmonary parenchymal consolidation or abscessation present, generally corresponds to the volume of pleural fluid recovered by thoracentesis.
  - Less than 1 liter of fluid with pleural fluid only around the cranioventral lung tip.
  - A pleural fluid line level with the point of the shoulder corresponds to the recovery of 1-5 liters of pleural fluid/side.
  - A pleural fluid line to midthorax corresponds to 5-10 liters of pleural fluid/side.
  - A pleural fluid line to the top of the thorax corresponds to 20-30 liters of pleural fluid/side.
- The detection of fibrinous pleuropneumonia, with or without loculations, warrants a guarded prognosis initially and the initiation of broad-spectrum antimicrobial therapy, after obtaining a transtracheal fluid aspirate and pleural fluid aspirate for culture and susceptibility testing.
- If free gas echoes are detected in pleural fluid, a guarded to grave prognosis should be given and broad spectrum antimicrobial therapy, including appropriate coverage for anaerobic microorganisms (e.g., metronidazole), initiated immediately before results of culture and susceptibility testing are available.
- The cost effectiveness of treatment must be considered because horses with anaerobic pleuropneumonia are likely to require a longer period of

antimicrobial treatment and are unlikely to return to their prior performance level, if they survive.

Pneumothorax

Characteristic ultrasonographic findings with free air dorsally in the thoracic cavity include:

- A soft tissue density echo detected between the dorsal free gas echo and the ventral aerated lung echo in the area of pulmonary atelectasis.
- A gas-fluid interface with hydropneumothorax (pleural effusion and pneumothorax).
- The gas-fluid interface moves simultaneously in a dorsal to ventral direction with respiration, the *"curtain sign,"* reproducing the movements of the diaphragm.
  - Best seen with pleural effusion, parenchymal consolidation, or atelectasis.
- A bronchial-pleural fistula is the most common cause for hydropneumothorax.
- A pneumothorax without pleural effusion is more difficult to detect ultrasonographically because gas free in the pleural cavity and air within the lung both have the characteristic hyperechoic reflection and reverberation artifacts with periodicity.
  - Small hypoechoic irregularities with *comet tail* artifacts are absent dorsally in the area of the pneumothorax.
- To detect pneumothorax in patients without pleural effusion, the scan should begin at the most dorsal aspect of the thorax and continue ventrally, looking for a break in the characteristic reverberation air artifact.

Noneffusive Pleuritis

- Fibrin without fluid between the pleural surfaces is more difficult to detect because there is no fluid separating parietal and visceral pleural surfaces.
- Examine the parietal and visceral pleural interface carefully during inspiration and expiration, evaluating lung movement relative to the parietal pleura.
- Characteristic ultrasonographic findings include:
  - Rough or erratic movement of the visceral pleural lung surface across the parietal pleura.
  - Absence of any movement between these surfaces during respiration is consistent with dry pleuritis or adhesions.
  - Ensure that the patient is taking deep breaths because shallow respiration may mimic a dry pleuritis.

Pulmonary Disease

Compression Atelectasis

Compression atelectasis occurs whenever the lung parenchyma is collapsed by fluid, air, or viscera (in individuals with diaphragmatic hernia) occupying space in the thorax normally containing the lung.

Characteristic ultrasonographic findings include:

- The lung is collapsed and without air, leaving this portion of lung hypoechoic (echogenicity of soft tissue).
- The atelectic lung is retracted toward the hilus.
- Linear air echoes may be imaged in larger airways and squeeze together as they converge toward the root of the lung.
- The atelectic lung floats on top of and within the pleural fluid.

Consolidation Atelectasis

Characteristic ultrasonographic findings:

- An irregular visceral pleura with radiating comet tail artifacts is a nonspecific finding seen in individuals with acute or mild pneumonia.
- Irregular anechoic to hypoechoic areas surrounded by normally aerated lung.
- ± Sonographic air bronchograms, pictured as distinctive hyperechoic linear air echoes in anechoic or hypoechoic lung.
- ± Sonographic fluid bronchograms, pictured as nonpulsatile, anechoic tubular structures in anechoic or hypoechoic lung.
- ± Fluid bronchiectasis, represented as an enlarging diameter of the fluid bronchogram toward the periphery.
- Both air and fluid bronchograms become larger as they converge toward the root of the lung.
- The consolidation is usually cranioventral with the right lung more commonly and more severely affected.
- Often, if the ultrasound examination is performed very early in the course of the disease and the pneumonia is severe, it appears less extensive and later tends to coalesce into larger areas of consolidation.
- The small hypoechoic areas of early consolidation may be seen only during exhalation.
- A large area of consolidated lung is usually wedge-shaped, poorly defined, and hypoechoic.
- Hepatization of lung parenchyma occurs with severe consolidation, resulting in an ultrasonographic appearance similar to that of the liver.
- Multiple small hyperechoic gas echoes in a severely consolidated or hepatized lung are suggestive of an anaerobic pneumonia.
- A rounded or bulging anechoic area suggests severe consolidation, often progressing to pulmonary necrosis or abscess formation.
- A gelatinous-appearing lung occurs with parenchymal necrosis. These necrotic areas either cavitate and form an abscess, or rupture into the pleural space creating a bronchial-pleural fistula.
- The detection of parenchymal necrosis also warrants a grave-to-guarded prognosis initially. Individuals with parenchymal necrosis should also be treated aggressively with broad-spectrum antimicrobials targeted for anaerobes.
- The cost effectiveness of treatment should be considered because horses with parenchymal necrosis are likely to require a long period of antimicrobial treatment and are unlikely to return to their prior performance level, if they survive.
- The number of treatment days is also likely to be longer for horses with pleuropneumonia when fibrin, loculations, pulmonary parenchymal necrosis, or abscesses are detected ultrasonographically.

Bronchial-Pleural Fistula or Abscess

A bronchial-pleural fistula is a communication between a bronchus and the pleural cavity that results in a pneumothorax. It is usually the result of a necrotizing pneumonia that becomes a walled off bronchial-pleural abscess.

Characteristic ultrasonographic findings include:

- A cavitation involving the visceral edge of the lung with hyperechoic air echoes and sonolucent fluid echoes imaged in real time and moving from the gelatinous area of pulmonary necrosis into the pleural space
- ± Pleural effusion

Pulmonary Abscess

A pulmonary abscess is a cavitary area in the lung parenchyma lacking bronchi or vessels and filled with purulent fluid.

Characteristic ultrasonographic findings include:

- An anechoic or hypoechoic area lacking air or fluid bronchograms with acoustic enhancement of lung deep to the sonolucent area
- The material contained may vary from anechoic to hyperechoic, depending on the type of exudate present.
- ± Loculations or compartmentalization of the abscess
- ± Encapsulation (uncommon)
- ± Hyperechoic free gas echoes mixed with the exudate, suggesting anaerobic infection
- ± A dorsal gas cap, indicative of a bronchial communication and probable anaerobic infection
- In foals with multiple *Rhodococcus equi* abscesses, many involve the pulmonary periphery and therefore are detectable ultrasonographically.

Pulmonary Fibrosis or Diffuse Granulomatous Disease, Metastatic Neoplasia

Characteristic ultrasonographic findings include:

- Small hypoechoic to echoic soft tissue masses scattered throughout the lung periphery.
- Usually homogeneous, rarely heterogeneous.
- Lack bronchial and normal vascular structures within the masses.

Cranial Mediastinal Abscess

Characteristic ultrasonographic findings include:

- Walled off, usually encapsulated mass of hypoechoic to echoic fluid and fibrin cranial to the heart.
- Caudal displacement of the heart occurs and signs of cranial vena cava obstruction develop in patients with large cranial mediastinal abscesses.

Cranial Mediastinal Neoplasia

Neoplastic infiltration of the lymphoid tissue in the cranial mediastinal, caudal cervical, or bronchial lymph nodes results in a large space-occupying mass in the cranial mediastinum.

Characteristic ultrasonographic appearance includes:

- Homogeneous or heterogeneous hypoechoic to echoic soft tissue mass displacing the lung dorsally and the heart caudally.
- The mass usually occupies the entire cranial mediastinum, obliterating the normal mediastinal septum.
- Usually associated with a large anechoic pleural effusion.
- Caudal displacement of the heart occurs.
- The mass is usually lymphosarcoma, although may be seen in individuals with mesothelioma or hemangiosarcoma.
- The mass can usually be imaged from either third ICS and may extend dorsally and cranially toward the thoracic inlet and up the ventral neck with cervical lymph node involvement.

SUMMARY

Ultrasonography is valuable in the emergency setting because it is a noninvasive imaging modality that can be used in a wide variety of areas, helping the clinician determine the etiology of the crisis and providing useful diagnostic information that can help formulate a prognosis and treatment plan.

SUGGESTED REFERENCES:

Reef VB: Musculoskeletal ultrasonography. In Reef VB, editor: *Equine diagnostic ultrasound,* Philadelphia, 1998, WB Saunders, pp 39-186.

Reef VB: Thoracic ultrasonography. In Reef VB, editor: *Equine diagnostic ultrasound,* Philadelphia, 1998, WB Saunders, pp 187-214.

Reef VB: Abdominal ultrasonography. In Reef VB, editor: *Equine diagnostic ultrasound,* Philadelphia, 1998, WB Saunders, pp 273-363.

Reef VB: Pediatric abdominal ultrasonography. In Reef VB, editor: *Equine diagnostic ultrasound,* Philadelphia, 1998, WB Saunders, pp 364-403.

Reef VB: Fetal ultrasonography. In Reef VB, editor: *Equine diagnostic ultrasound,* Philadelphia, 1998, WB Saunders, pp 425-445.

Reef VB: Ultrasonography of small parts. In Reef VB, editor: *Equine diagnostic ultrasound,* Philadelphia, 1998, WB Saunders, pp 480-547.

PROCEDURES

Respiratory System

10 Nasotracheal and Orotracheal Tube Placement

James A. Orsini and Christine Kreuder

Establishing an airway is the first step for a patient exhibiting respiratory distress (cyanotic mucous membranes, respiratory stridor, apnea). Intubation is the most rapid and least invasive method and is performed through the nose or mouth. Tracheotomy is used in patients with obstruction of the upper airway. Nasotracheal intubation is preferred to orotracheal intubation because it can be performed on a conscious horse, and the tube can be left in place indefinitely. General anesthesia is required for orotracheal intubation. For an anesthetized patient, orotracheal intubation is preferred because a larger endotracheal tube can be used for oxygen supplementation (p. 64) or assisted ventilation (p. 65).

NASOTRACHEAL INTUBATION
Equipment
- Sedatives (xylazine hydrochloride and butorphanol tartrate)
- Appropriately sized nasotracheal tube
  □ Adults, 11- to 14-mm internal diameter*
  □ Foals, 7- to 12-mm internal diameter†
- Lubricating jelly‡ or warm water
- White tape
- 20-ml syringe

Procedure
- Sedation may be required for an adult. Sedation is generally unnecessary for foals. Suggested adult (physiologically stable) dose: 0.3-0.5 mg/kg xylazine and 0.01-0.02 mg/kg butorphanol IV.

---

*Cuffed endotracheal tubes. Cook Veterinary Products, PO Box 489, Bloomington, IN 47402; (800) 457-4500.

†Cuffed nasotracheal tubes for foals. Cook Veterinary Products, PO Box 489, Bloomington, IN 47402; (800) 457-4500.

‡K-Y lubricating jelly. Johnson and Johnson Medical, Inc., Arlington, TX 76004-3130.

CAUTION: Sedation or tranquilization of a dyspneic patient may lead to cardiopulmonary depression, increased upper airway resistance, and apnea.

- Lubricate the tube sparingly or place in warm water.
- Reflect the alar fold of the nostril and insert the tube medially along the ventral nasal meatus.
- Extend and elevate the head to allow easier access to the trachea and to prevent the tube from being swallowed.
- Advance the tube into the pharynx. *Do not use force.* If resistance is encountered, rotate and advance. If still meeting resistance, use a smaller-diameter tube.
- Confirm that air is flowing through the tube, which indicates correct placement.
- Use an air-filled syringe to inflate the cuff to the point at which air cannot escape around the tube.

CAUTION: Do not inflate the cuff past the point where resistance is first encountered.

- Secure the tube by placing tape around the tube end and tying it to the horse's halter.

OROTRACHEAL INTUBATION
Equipment
- Drugs for general anesthesia (xylazine hydrochloride and ketamine for adults, diazepam and ketamine for physiologically stable foals)
- Appropriately sized orotracheal tube with inflatable cuff[*]
  - □ Adults, 18- to 28-mm internal diameter
  - □ Foals, 8- to 11-mm internal diameter
- Oral speculum PVC pipe, 5-cm diameter, 4-5 cm long, wrapped with white tape
- Lubricating jelly[†]
- 20- or 30-ml syringe, not Luer-Lok

Procedure
- General anesthesia should be used if the patient is fully conscious. Recommended dose for adults: 1 mg/kg xylazine IV for sedation followed by 2 mg/kg ketamine IV. Recommended dose for foals: 0.1 mg/kg diazepam IV **slowly** for sedation, followed by 1 mg/kg ketamine IV **slowly**.

CAUTION: Intubate **as soon as** the patient is anesthetized. Equipment for cardiopulmonary resuscitation should be available.

- Dorsiflex the head and pull the tongue out through the interdental space.
- Place the speculum between the lower and upper incisors.

---

[*]Cuffed endotracheal tubes. Cook Veterinary Products, PO Box 489, Bloomington, IN 47402; (800) 457-4500.

[†]K-Y lubricating jelly. Johnson and Johnson Medical, Inc., Arlington, TX 76004-3130.

H-R Lubricating jelly. Carter Products Division of Carter-Wallace, Inc., New York, NY 10105.

- Sparingly lubricate the endotracheal tube.
- Advance the tube through the center of the speculum. If resistance is encountered, rotate and advance the tube gently. If the patient repeatedly swallows, administer 0.1-mg/kg doses of ketamine IV until swallowing stops; allow 2-3 minutes for effect.
- The endotracheal tube placement is confirmed by demonstrating air moving through the tube. The tube should *not* be palpable in the proximal cervical area.
- Use a 20-ml syringe to inflate the cuff until resistance is encountered.
- Maintain general anesthesia while the orotracheal tube is in place.

Complications

Overinflation of the endotracheal tube cuff can cause pressure necrosis of the tracheal mucosa and sloughing. In the most severe cases, tracheal stenosis may result. *Do not inflate the cuff beyond the point where resistance is first met.*

An excessively long tube may terminate in a main stem bronchus with ventilation of only a portion of the pulmonary tree.

Hemorrhage from trauma to nasal mucosa occurs commonly during nasotracheal intubation. Generally, this is not clinically significant.

---

11 Transtracheal Aspiration and Bronchoalveolar Lavage

James A. Orsini and Christine Kreuder

TRANSTRACHEAL ASPIRATION

Transtracheal aspiration is a simple, commonly used technique for assessing disease in the lower respiratory tract. The fluid obtained from aspiration is a mixture of secretions and cellular material that has collected in the distal trachea. Results of cytologic examination of the aspirate determine the type and severity of inflammation and the level of the respiratory tract involved. The upper respiratory tract is host to a large bacterial population, and culture results of specimens from the nares or guttural pouch are difficult to interpret. Transtracheal aspiration bypasses the upper respiratory tract and is the best method for obtaining a representative sample for culture. Tracheal aspirates also can be retrieved through a flexible, fiberoptic endoscope biopsy channel; a sterile endoscopic catheter is available for sampling via the endoscope.* Results of cultures are not as reliable when sampling via the biopsy channel. Using an endoscope allows the clinician to see the area being sampled and avoids complications from tracheal puncture.

---

*Endoscopic Microbiology Aspiration Catheter (Reorder No.: EMCA800), Mila International, Inc., 7604 Dixie Highway, Florence, KY 41042; (859) 371-1722, (888) 645-2468.

Equipment

- Twitch (sedation usually is unnecessary unless the patient is very young, difficult to restrain, or coughs excessively during the procedure; xylazine hydrochloride [0.3-0.5 mg/kg] with butorphanol tartrate [0.01-0.02 mg/kg] IV is recommended for restraint and as a cough suppressant)
- Clippers
- Material for sterile scrub
- Sterile gloves
- 16-gauge through-the-needle catheter* with or without a 7-inch (17.5-cm) extension set[†]
- 60-ml syringe (sterile)
- An alternative is a 12-gauge nondisposable needle and 5F polyethylene tubing
- 100-ml sterile 0.9% saline solution without bacteriostatic agent
- Plain and EDTA Vacutainer tubes[‡]
- Port-a-Cul culture system[§]

Procedure

- Clip and sterilely prepare a 10-cm area on the ventral midline of the middle third of the trachea.
- Palpate the trachea with sterile gloves and stabilize it with one hand.
- Face the cannula bevel downward and place the catheter through the skin and **between tracheal rings** into the tracheal lumen (Fig. 11–1).
- Feed the catheter down the trachea to the thoracic inlet and remove the stylet. Coughing may cause the catheter to retroflex into the pharynx and become contaminated.
- Attach the syringe and rapidly inject 20-30 ml of sterile saline solution.
- Aspirate the fluid injected into the sampling syringe; only a portion of the fluid instilled is retrievable.
- Inject another aliquot of fluid through the catheter if the sample collected is inadequate. Do not inject more than 100 ml total volume. Reposition or slowly withdraw the catheter to assist aspiration of the sample.
- Carefully withdraw the catheter after obtaining the sample.
- If the sample contains any purulent debris, an antibiotic should be infiltrated subcutaneously at the puncture site. Apply a sterile dressing for 24 hours.

Complications

Catheter laceration and loss into the airway can occur. The catheter almost always is coughed out within 30 minutes.

Subcutaneous **abscess** or **cellulitis** can occur at the site of needle puncture. In severe cases, infection may extend to the mediastinum. *Administer systemic antimicrobial therapy. Apply a hot pack, and paint DMSO over the infected site.* If needed, incise for drainage.

---

*Intracath intravenous catheter placement unit. Deseret Medical, Inc., Becton-Dickinson and Company, Sandy, UT 84070.

[†]7-inch (17.5 cm) or 30-inch (75 cm) extension set. Abbott Laboratories, North Chicago, IL 60064.

[‡]Vacutainer. Becton-Dickinson Vacutainer Systems, Rutherford, NJ 07070.

[§]Port-a-Cul. Becton-Dickinson Microbiology Systems, Cockeysville, MD 21030.

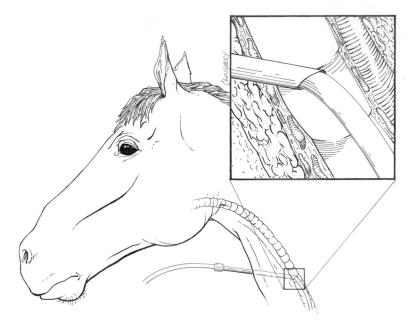

FIGURE 11–1. Technique for transtracheal aspiration and washing. Through-the-needle catheter is placed between tracheal rings.

Subcutaneous **emphysema** around the trachea is common and can result in **pneumomediastinum.** It is rarely a problem unless the patient is in respiratory distress.

Damage to the tracheal rings can result in **chondritis** or **chondroma** formation. **Stenosis** of the tracheal lumen would be the most severe sequela.

BRONCHOALVEOLAR LAVAGE

Bronchoalveolar lavage (BAL) is used to sample the terminal airway and associated alveoli. It is an excellent method for evaluating pathologic changes in the most distal portion of the respiratory tract. Because only a limited section of the lung can be evaluated and the sample is generally not as suitable for culture as is aspirate, BAL should be performed as an adjunct to transtracheal aspiration. BAL may be performed blindly or with endoscopic guidance.

Equipment
- Sedatives (xylazine hydrochloride and butorphanol tartrate)
- 3-m BAL catheter* **or** 2- to 3-m, 9-mm-diameter flexible fiberoptic endoscope†
- 2% mepivacaine (Carbocaine) hydrochloride or 2% lidocaine (Xylocaine)

---

*240- to 300-cm (2.4- to 3-m) BAL Catheter. Cook Veterinary Products, Inc., 1100 W. Morgan St., Spencer, IN 47460; (800) 826-2380, order VPBAL-300.

†GIF 130 gastroscope (2 or 3 m long, 9.8 mm outer diameter). Olympus America, Inc., 2 Corporate Center Drive, Melville, NY 11747; (516) 844-5000.

- Sterile 60-ml syringe
- 300-ml sterile 0.9% saline solution without bacteriostatic agent, warmed to body temperature
- Plain and EDTA Vacutainer tubes

Procedure

- Sedation usually is required. Recommended doses: 0.4-0.6 mg/kg xylazine with 0.01-0.02 mg/kg butorphanol IV.
- If using a BAL catheter, extend the horse's head and gently pass the catheter through the nose and into a terminal airway. Wedge the catheter into the bronchus of a lower lung lobe. The main disadvantage to this procedure is that the location of the catheter is not specifically known.
- If using an endoscope, clean the biopsy channel of the endoscope with antiseptic solution and rinse with sterile water. Pass the endoscope (see Chapter 8, p. 30), and gently wedge it into the smallest-diameter bronchus. At this point, 20-30 ml of lidocaine can be injected through the biopsy channel to minimize excessive coughing.
- Infuse 50-ml aliquots of sterile saline solution until a representative sample is collected. Do not infuse more than 300 ml.
- If undue coughing occurs consider increasing the sedation and/or infuse 5 ml of dilute mepivacaine.
- Place sample in an EDTA Vacutainer tube (purple top) for cytologic analysis.

RESPIRATORY FLUID ANALYSIS

A direct smear of the fluid can be made if the sample appears cellular; otherwise the sample is centrifuged, and the centrifugate is placed on a glass slide. The slide prep may be air dried and stained with Wright stain. Cytologic examination should include a differential cell count, degenerative status of the cells, and an assessment of the bacterial component. Total cell counts are not meaningful because the density of the cell population varies with the amount of saline solution retrieved. The differential cell count should be determined, although the aspiration reflects only a small segment of the pulmonary tree in both transtracheal aspiration and BAL. Normal results of BAL, in particular, do not rule out lung disease, because a normal section of lung can accidentally be lavaged.

Normal aspirate contains strands of mucus. Columnar epithelial cells and pulmonary alveolar macrophages are the predominant cell types. Lymphocytes may account for 40% of the population in a BAL sample. Neutrophils and eosinophils are normally less than 5% of the differential. The presence of a few degenerate neutrophils is normal. Increased numbers of nondegenerate neutrophils are common in chronic obstructive pulmonary disease (COPD), whereas a large population of degenerate, toxic neutrophils is present with septic bronchitis or pneumonia. An infectious process is supported by the presence of intracellular bacteria. The presence of squamous epithelial cells, usually in rafts or rolled into a cigar shape, indicates either pharyngeal contamination or metaplasia in the lower respiratory tract from chronic irritation or inflammation. Curschmann spirals are coiled mucus plugs from terminal airways and sometimes are signs indicating chronic inflammation. Pulmonary hemorrhage is detected by means of finding hemosiderin-laden alveolar macrophages. Free bacteria and fungal elements are common in normal samples. For a morphologic description of cell types and their role in disease processes, see Beech (1991).

The transtracheal aspirate should be submitted for aerobic and anaerobic culture. Gram stain is useful in determining initial antibiotic therapy while awaiting culture results. The significance of the results should be interpreted in conjunction with cytologic findings, because contamination is always a possibility, and the normal trachea can contain bacteria.

REFERENCES

Beech J: *Equine respiratory disorders,* Philadelphia, 1991, Lea & Febiger.
Darien BJ, Brown CM, Walker RD, Williams MA, Derkson FJ: A tracheoscopic technique for obtaining uncontaminated lower airway secretions for bacterial culture in the horse, *Equine Vet J* 22:170-173, 1990.
Hoffman AM, Viel L: Techniques for sampling the respiratory tract of horses, *Vet Clin North Am Equine Pract* 13:463-475, 1997.
Sweeney CR, Sweeney RW, Benson CE: Comparison of bacteria isolated from specimens obtained by use of endoscopic guarded tracheal swabbing and percutaneous tracheal aspiration in the horse, *J Am Vet Med Assoc* 195:1225-1229, 1989.

12 Nasal Oxygen Insufflation

James A. Orsini and Christine Kreuder

Oxygen administration is more frequently used to treat neonatal foals than it is to treat adults but is therapeutic for both. Supplementation of oxygen should be based on clinical signs and results of blood gas analysis. Hypoxia is suspected in patients with pneumonia, pulmonary edema, hemolytic anemia, marked blood loss, obstructive pulmonary disease, hypoventilation, and recumbency-associated or neonatal ventilation/perfusion mismatch. Nasal oxygen insufflation is beneficial to all patients undergoing general anesthesia. Increasing the concentration of oxygen in the inspired air increases blood PaO_2 levels. Patients with severe parenchymal disease may not respond to nasal oxygen administration.

Equipment
- Oxygen source (high-pressure oxygen cylinder*)
- Oxygen flowmeter/humidifier (humidifier should be filled with sterile water)
- Oxygen tubing (2-4 m) to extend from the flowmeter to the patient
- Nasal catheter[†]
- 1-inch (2.5 cm) white tape
- Examination gloves
- 2-0 nonabsorbable suture on a straight needle

---

*High-pressure oxygen cylinder (size E is small and portable). Oxygen supply service is available through local health care companies. Reusable oxygen cylinders are provided.
†Nasal catheter "Levin tubes" 235200-160. Rusch, Inc., Duluth, GA 30136; (800) 553-5324.

Procedure

- Attach the humidifier to the flowmeter on the oxygen source.
- Connect the nasal catheter to the oxygen tubing, then connect the oxygen tubing to the humidifier.
- Using the nasal catheter, measure the distance between the nostril and the medial canthus. This is the approximate distance to the nasopharynx.
- Reflect one nostril and place the catheter along the ventral meatus (the most ventral and medial portion of the nasal passage) and into the nasopharynx.
- Place a butterfly square of tape around the tubing (approximately 6 cm from the nostril), then reflect the tubing around and suture the tape to the nostril. Gloves are optional but recommended for handling suture material. Tubing may have to be sutured in several places.
- Set the flow of oxygen between 5 and 15 L/min, depending on the size and needs of the patient.
- Check the setup frequently (every 2 hours) to ensure tube patency. Replace the nasal catheter daily.

NOTE: This may increase FiO_2 to only ±30%. Use of two catheters and two lines may result in an additional increase to ±40%.

 # 13 Assisted Ventilation

James A. Orsini and Christine Kreuder

Assisted ventilation is used in the care of patients with apnea, hypoventilation, persistent fetal circulation, or respiratory distress not corrected by placement of an endotracheal tube and oxygen supplementation. Clinical disorders inducing hypoventilation include foal maladjustment syndromes, respiratory disease resulting in decompensation, thoracic injury or disease, diaphragmatic herniation, and botulism. Persistent cyanotic mucous membranes and dyspnea or an arterial PCO_2 greater than 60 mm Hg are strong clinical indicators of hypoventilation and tissue hypoxia. Short-term ventilation is relatively easy, whereas long-term ventilation is expensive and labor intensive, requiring 24-hour nursing care and sophisticated equipment.

NOTE: Unless the patient is semiconscious or unconscious, a **neuromuscular blocking agent** is needed before assisted ventilation. Assisted ventilation can be performed for a standing patient but is not well tolerated. **Endotracheal intubation** (or tracheotomy) must be performed before an attempt is made to ventilate. Placement of a cuffed, wide-diameter orotracheal tube is preferred (p. 59).

Equipment

- Oxygen cylinder* with a regulator† that has a flowmeter and a DISS fitting for a demand valve (small "E" cylinder is portable)

---

*Oxygen supply service is available through local health care companies. Reusable oxygen cylinders are provided.

†LSPO2 Regulator 270-020. Allied Health, St. Louis, MO; (800) 444-3960.

- Regulator for E cylinder with **both** a flowmeter giving 1, 2, 4, 6, 10, 15, and 25 LPM and a DISS connection for a demand valve
- One of the following methods for delivering positive-pressure ventilation:
  - □ Oxygen demand valve*
  - □ Ambu bag with an adapter for oxygen insufflation (for foals only)
  - □ Appropriately sized nasogastric tube if the Ambu bag, or an endotracheal tube, is not available

Procedure

- Intubate the patient and inflate the cuff of the endotracheal tube (p. 59).

VENTILATION WITH A DEMAND VALVE

- Attach the demand valve to the oxygen cylinder.
- Open the tank by turning the valve on the tank regulator counterclockwise.
- Attach the demand valve directly to the endotracheal or tracheotomy tube.
- Ventilation is achieved by pressing the button on the demand valve. The demand valve delivers oxygen at 160 L/min. Monitor the chest expansion, then release; exhalation occurs passively.
- Generally, allow **2-3 seconds** to deliver one breath to an adult; to a foal, allow **significantly** less time. It is safest to watch the chest rise and end inspiration as soon as the chest nears full expansion.

CAUTION: Do not overinflate the lungs; overinflation causes barotrauma. This can readily occur in foals when a demand valve is used. Therefore, an Ambu bag is preferred for foal resuscitation.

- If the chest does not rise, check for leaks and tube placement. Confirm that the esophagus has not been accidentally intubated. This can be established by seeing and/or palpating the tube or by use of a capnograph to monitor exhaled carbon dioxide.
- For an adult, deliver **10-12 breaths per minute;** for a foal, deliver **15-20 breaths per minute.**
- The demand valve can be used to assist ventilation if the patient breathes independently. The demand valve triggers automatically when inspiration begins and shuts off when exhalation begins. This method increases airway resistance and the work of breathing and should be discontinued as soon as the patient is able to breathe room air.
- A full E oxygen cylinder contains ~600 L of O_2 and lasts **only** 15-20 minutes in resuscitation of an adult.

VENTILATION WITH AN AMBU BAG IN FOALS

- Attach the Ambu bag to the endotracheal or tracheotomy tube.
- Place the oxygen insufflation tube (see Chapter 47) into the reservoir of the Ambu bag to increase inspired O_2 concentration.
- Open the oxygen tank and turn the flowmeter to 15 L/min.
- Compress the Ambu bag until full expansion of the lungs is achieved.
- Exhalation is passive through a valve on the Ambu bag.
- Administer approximately **20 breaths per minute.**

---

*LSP Demand Valve (with 6-ft [1.8-m] hose and female DISS fitting) 063-03. Must specify 160 LPM when ordering. Allied Health, St. Louis, MO; (800) 444-3960.

VENTILATION WITH A NASOGASTRIC TUBE AND DEMAND VALVE

- Intubate the patient with a clean, lubricated nasogastric tube (see intubation procedure, p. 81). Do not advance beyond the midcervical area of the trachea.
- Attach the free end of the tube to the oxygen cylinder regulator.
- Open the regulator on the tank to a maximal flow rate.
- Occlude both nares and watch the chest rise to full inflation, which can take as long as 8 seconds in an adult, depending on lung compliance. **Do not overinflate the lungs.**
- Once the lungs are inflated, open the nostrils to allow passive exhalation.
- Deliver **10-12 breaths per minute** to an adult and **15-20 breaths per minute** to a foal.
- The E oxygen cylinder lasts **only** 10-15 minutes at maximal flow.

Complications

Overinflation of the lungs results in barotrauma and injury to the alveoli and, possibly, pulmonary emphysema.

---

14 ⊟ Tracheotomy

James A. Orsini and Christine Kreuder

Tracheotomy is performed on an emergency basis when acute respiratory obstruction occurs. This procedure establishes an airway that bypasses the larynx and nasal passages and can be lifesaving if there is an obstruction of the upper respiratory tract. Tracheotomy provides a direct route for manual ventilation regardless of the cause of respiratory distress. Tracheotomy occasionally is indicated before recovery from operations on the larynx or nasal passage when respiratory obstruction is anticipated.

Equipment

- Clippers
- Material for sterile scrub
- 2% local anesthetic, 5- to 10-ml syringe, and 22-gauge, 0.5-inch (1.25-cm) needle
- Sterile gloves
- #10 scalpel blade and handle
- Appropriately sized tracheotomy tube*
- Size 0 nonabsorbable suture on a straight needle

Procedure

- Sedate patient if circumstances allow.

---

*Tracheotomy tube (18-mm or 28-mm internal diameter). Jorgensen Laboratories, Inc., 1450 North Van Buren Avenue, Loveland, CO 80538; (970) 669-2500.

LANDMARKS: The trachea is easily palpated directly on the ventral midline of the neck. Isolate a section of the trachea between the upper and middle third of the neck in a horse and middle of the neck in a pony.

- Clip the surgical area and prepare with a sterile scrub.
- Inject 5-10 ml of local anesthetic into the subcutaneous tissue over the trachea. The bleb should be 5-7 cm long on the midline.
- With sterile gloved hands, grasp the trachea and make a 5-cm incision through the skin and subcutaneous tissue with a scalpel blade.
- Bluntly dissect the underlying muscle bellies; retract each muscle belly laterally until the trachea is located on the midline (Fig. 14–1).
- Incise the tracheal annular ligament **between** two cartilage rings. The incision should be parallel to the cartilage rings and thus perpendicular to the skin incision. The incision should be only long enough to allow passage of the tracheal tube and should not exceed more than a third of the circumference of the trachea (see Fig. 14–1).

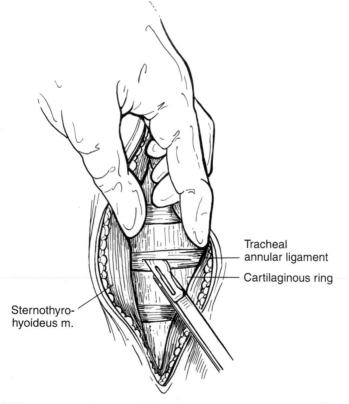

Tracheal annular ligament

Cartilaginous ring

Sternothyro-hyoideus m.

FIGURE 14-1. Surgical technique for tracheotomy. Make a vertical incision in the skin, divide the sternothyrohyoideus muscle, and horizontally incise an annular ligament to allow passage of the tracheotomy tube.

- Insert the tracheal tube through the incision and suture in place.
- Suction and clean or replace the tracheotomy tube daily, because it can become obstructed easily.
- The tracheotomy tube should be large enough to fill the tracheotomy site and must not extend beyond the bifurcation of the trachea to ensure that all lung fields are ventilated.

> In a **life-threatening** emergency, sterile technique is abandoned, any sharp object is used to incise in the described procedure, and any tube available (stomach tube, garden hose, and so on) may be used to establish an airway initially.

Complications

Wound infection can occur, particularly if sterile technique is not used. The airway is a contaminated environment, and the tracheotomy site should be cleaned several times daily until the wound has healed.

Subcutaneous **emphysema** is likely if air can move around the outside of the tube. The air is a problem only if it carries infection with it or if it dissects along tissue planes, leading to pneumomediastinum, pneumothorax, or both.

Tracheal **stricture** is possible as the tracheal mucosa contracts during healing. Granulation tissue is produced intraluminally and can contribute to luminal narrowing if excessive.

15 Paranasal Sinus Trephination

James A. Orsini and Christine Kreuder

Trephination, or creating a hole in the bone overlying the paranasal sinuses for access to the sinus cavity, is a procedure used for diagnosis and treatment of paranasal sinus disease. Clinical signs suggestive of sinus disease (nasal discharge, facial asymmetry) are frequently supported by abnormal findings on radiographs that help localize the disease to a particular sinus. If findings on radiographs are normal or inconclusive, exploratory sinoscopy of the frontal and caudal maxillary sinuses can be performed through a small trephination site. If a bacterial infection is suspected, sinocentesis provides a laboratory sample suitable for cytologic examination and culture and sensitivity determinations. Trephination with sinus lavage is the treatment of choice for patients with chronic sinusitis and associated empyema that are refractory to systemic antibiotic therapy.

The **frontal sinus** is dorsal and medial to the orbit. The left and right frontal sinuses are separated by a median septum. The frontal sinus communicates with the caudal maxillary sinus through the frontal maxillary opening. Sinoscopy of both the frontal and caudal maxillary sinuses is most easily performed by means of trephination of the frontal sinus (Ruggles, 1994).

The **maxillary sinus** is paired and is rostral and ventral to the orbit. It is divided into rostral and caudal compartments by an incomplete oblique septum. Both compartments communicate with the ventral nasal meatus through the nasomaxillary opening. Because of its more ventral location, the maxillary sinus is usually the site of greatest fluid accumulation in sinusitis. Ideally, both compartments should be cultured and lavaged, but lavage of the rostral compartment only can provide satisfactory results.

Equipment

- Sedative (xylazine hydrochloride or detomidine)
- Clippers
- 2% local anesthetic, 25-gauge, ⅝-inch (1.6-cm) needle, 3-ml syringe
- Material for a sterile scrub
- Sterile gloves
- #15 scalpel blade with handle
- The **trephine** used depends on availability and the size of the hole required
  - For sinus lavage: 2.5-, 3.2-, or 4.5-mm (³⁄₁₆-¼ inch) drill bit and drill or 2.0- to 4.5-mm (⁵⁄₃₂, ³⁄₁₆, or ¼ inch) Steinmann pin* with Jacobs chuck†
  - For passage of a 4-mm endoscope: 6.34-mm Steinmann pin with Jacobs chuck.

FOR SINOCENTESIS AND SINUS LAVAGE

- Intravenous catheter‡ (14-gauge, 2-inch [5 cm] long); remove stylet and cut end so that the catheter is only ¾ inch (1.9 cm) long
- 2-0 nonabsorbable suture
- 5-ml syringe
- EDTA (purple top) Vacutainer tube§ for cytologic examination
- Culturette# or Port-a-Cul** culture system or both
- 1 L of saline solution with 0.5-1% povidone-iodine (Betadine) and a 30-inch (75 cm) extension set†† for sinus lavage

Procedure

- May be done on a standing sedated patient or with general anesthesia. For sedation, administer 0.01-0.02 mg/kg detomidine IV **or** 0.4-0.7 mg/kg xylazine IV.
- See Fig. 15–1 for trephination sites for each paranasal sinus.
- Choose a trephination site and infiltrate 2 ml of 2% local anesthetic subcutaneously into the periosteum.
- Clip a 5-cm area and perform a sterile scrub.
- Maintaining aseptic technique, make a 0.5- to 1.5-cm stab incision (depending on the portal size required).
- Using a Steinmann pin ⅛-¼ inch (0.3-0.6 cm) or a 3.2-mm drill bit, drill a hole in the bone overlying the sinus perpendicular to the bone surface.

---

*Steinmann pin (size 2.5, 3.2, 4.5, or 6.34 mm). Synthes (USA), P.O. Box 1766, 1690 Russell Road, Paoli, PA 19301-0800; (800) 523-0322.

†Jacobs chuck. A. J. Buck and Son, Inc., 11407 Cronhill Drive, Owings Mills, MD 21117; (800) 638-8672; (Fax) (410) 581-1809.

‡Abbocath-T radiopaque FEP Teflon IV catheter (14-gauge, 2-inch long). Abbott Hospitals, Inc., North Chicago, IL 60064.

§Vacutainer tubes. Becton-Dickinson Vacutainer Systems, Rutherford, NJ 07070.

#Culturette collection and transport system. Becton-Dickinson Microbiology Systems, Cockeysville, MD 21030.

**Port-a-Cul tube. BBL Division of Becton-Dickinson and Co., Cockeysville, MD 21030.

††30-inch extension set. Abbott Laboratories, North Chicago, IL 60064.

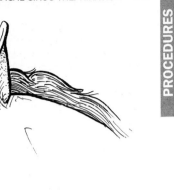
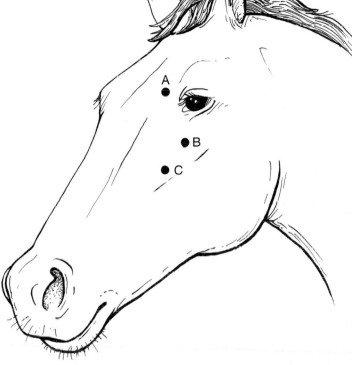

FIGURE 15-1. Sites for paranasal sinus trephination in an adult. *A*, **Frontal sinus.** Draw a horizontal line from midline to the medial canthus and trephine at a location 1 cm caudal to the midpoint of this line. *B*, **Caudal maxillary sinus.** Trephine at a location 3 cm rostral from the medial canthus and 3 cm dorsal from the facial crest. *C*, **Rostral maxillary sinus.** Trephine at a location half the distance along a line drawn from the medial canthus to the rostral end of the facial crest.

CAUTION: Be careful not to overdrill the bone and traumatize the sinus cavity. The bone is only a few millimeters thick, and drilling should stop as soon as there is loss of resistance. When a drill bit is used, there is a greater chance of breaking the drill bit if the patient moves.

FOR SINOCENTESIS AND SINUS LAVAGE
- Insert the catheter and attempt to seat the injection portal into the bone.
- Attach a 5-ml syringe to the catheter and aspirate any fluid within the sinus. If no fluid is obtained, infiltrate 30 ml of warm sterile saline solution before reaspirating. A sample for cytologic examination should be collected at this time.

- Once a sample is obtained, attach the extension set to the catheter, and flush the dilute povidone-iodine solution into the sinus. The saline solution, and any purulent exudate is lavaged from the sinus through the nasal passages if the nasomaxillary opening is patent (Merriam, 1993).
- If repeated lavage is needed, suture the catheter to the skin. If not, remove the catheter and place several interrupted sutures in the skin. If purulent material has exited from the trephination site, clean the area, and place topical antibiotics in the wound before suture placement.

Complications

Wound infection or **abscess** formation can occur at the trephination site. *Lance the abscess or remove the sutures and allow the area to drain and heal by secondary intention.* Clean aseptically and apply topical antibiotics until the area is healed.

Epistaxis occurs if the sinus mucosa is excessively traumatized during trephination or catheter placement.

REFERENCES

Merriam JG: Field sinusotomy in the management of chronic sinusitis and alveolitis. In *39th annual convention proceedings of the American Association of Equine Practitioners,* San Antonio, Texas, 1993.

Ruggles AJ: Endoscopic examination of the paranasal sinuses in the horse. In *22nd annual surgical forum of the American College of Veterinary Surgeons,* Washington, DC, 1994.

16 Thoracocentesis and Chest Tube Placement

James A. Orsini and Christine Kreuder

Thoracocentesis is the aspiration of fluid from the thoracic cavity. It serves both diagnostic and therapeutic functions. The procedure is easily performed on a standing horse and is indicated whenever pleural effusion is suspected on the basis of findings at auscultation of the chest, on radiographs, or at ultrasound examination. Pleural effusion most often accompanies pleuropneumonia, formation of a pleural abscess, and neoplasia. Analysis of pleural fluid differentiates these problems and can be lifesaving if the effusion compromises respiratory function.

Equipment

- Clippers
- Material for sterile scrub
- Local anesthetic
- 5-ml syringe and 25-gauge, ⅝- inch (1.6-cm) needle
- Sterile scalpel blade (#12) and handle (#3)

- Sterile metal teat cannula (2½-4 inches [6.2-10 cm] long)* or metal bitch urinary catheter (10.5 inches [26.2 cm] long).† Blunt-tipped cannulas are less likely to lacerate the lung.
- Three-way stopcock‡ or extension set tubing§
- 60-ml syringe
- Nonabsorbable size 0 suture
- Chest tube# with or without Heimlich one-way valve** for repeated drainage
- Plain and EDTA Vacutainer tubes††
- Port-a-Cul (aerobic/anaerobic) culture system‡‡

Procedure

- Sedation is usually not necessary unless the patient is intractable. Recommended dosage: 0.3-0.5 mg/kg xylazine with 0.01-0.025 mg/kg butorphanol IV.
- Choose a site for thoracocentesis on the basis of results of auscultation of dull lung fields and radiographic or ultrasound examination. Fluid usually collects ventrally. A common site for thoracocentesis is the lower third of the thorax between the 7th and 8th intercostal spaces. Both sides of the chest should be aspirated if bilateral effusion is suspected, because in general a healthy horse has an intact mediastinum.

CAUTION: Avoid the heart when placing the needle ventrally. Ultrasound guidance is recommended for precise needle placement.

- Clip and prepare the site aseptically.
- Inject 5-10 ml of local anesthetic subcutaneously and into the intercostal muscle. Perform final skin preparation.
- Make a stab incision through the skin and fascia at the cranial aspect of the rib to avoid the intercostal vessels and nerves, which are located on the caudal border.
- Maintaining aseptic technique, hold the cannula and attach a three-way stopcock or tubing with the end clamped to prevent pneumothorax if negative pressure exists in the thoracic cavity.
- Insert the cannula into the skin incision and push through the intercostal muscle. A sudden decrease in tension is felt as the pleural space is entered.
- Attach a 60-ml syringe to the stopcock or tubing. Aspiration should yield fluid if an effusion is present. Rotation or redirection of the cannula often is needed. If fluid is freely flowing, it can be siphoned off into a bucket.

---

*Ideal udder infusion cannula. Butler Company, 5000 Bradenton Avenue, P.O. Box 7153, Dublin, OH 43017-0753.

†Metal bitch urinary catheter. Jorgensen Laboratories, Inc., 1450 North Van Buren Avenue, Loveland, CO 80538; (970) 669-2500.

‡Pharmaseal K75 3-way stopcock. Baxter Healthcare Corp., Pharmaseal Co., Mundelein, IL 60060.

§Extension set, 7 or 30 inch. Abbott Laboratories, North Chicago, IL 60064.

#Thal-Quick chest drainage catheter set (24-36 French, 41-cm long). Cook Veterinary Products, PO Box 489, Bloomington, IN 47402; (800) 457-4500.

**Heimlich chest drainage valve. Cook Veterinary Products, PO Box 489, Bloomington, IN 47402; (800) 457-4500.

††Vacutainer. Becton-Dickinson Vacutainer Systems, Rutherford, NJ 07070.

‡‡Port-a-Cul. Becton-Dickinson Microbiology Systems, Cockeysville, MD 21030.

- Keep the tubing or stopcock closed when not removing fluid to prevent aspiration of air and iatrogenic pneumothorax.
- Once fluid is no longer retrievable, place a pursestring suture around the cannula and tighten as the cannula is removed. If septic fluid is removed, infiltrate antibiotics in and around the incision, apply an antiseptic or antibiotic ointment, and bandage the wound.

CHEST TUBE PLACEMENT

Repeated drainage often is necessary, particularly when large volumes of fluid are present or infection is suspected. For these patients, an indwelling human chest tube is required.

- Choose the smallest-size tube that allows fibrinous material to pass through.
- Follow the instructions for chest tube placement that accompany the product. A one-way valve can be used to maintain negative pressure.
- Use a pursestring suture to attach the tube to the skin; tie the free suture ends around the tube several times in a locking pattern, or use rapid-acting glue.
- Clamp and seal the tube when it is not being used.
- The chest tube may be left in place for up to 1 month. It generally is changed every 2-3 days because fibrinous debris occludes the lumen. Sinus tracts that form around the tube often heal spontaneously after tube removal.

PLEURAL FLUID ANALYSIS

Only 1-2 ml of straw-colored fluid is retrieved from a normal pleural cavity. Color, opacity, volume, and odor are useful parameters. Yellow, opaque fluid with fibrinous clots suggests a septic exudate. The presence of foul-smelling effusion correlates well with the presence of anaerobic bacterial colonization. A relatively clear to serosanguineous exudate occasionally is seen in neoplastic processes. Often neoplastic cells are shed into the pleural fluid and can be identified at cytologic examination. Cytologic examination (with a total cell count and differential) and measurement of total protein should be performed to classify the effusion definitively. The normal total protein level is less than 2.5 gm/dl, and the total nucleated cell count is typically less than 8000 cells per microliter. Neoplastic disease often has a significant inflammatory component and can mimic an infectious process. Specimens for anaerobic and aerobic cultures should be submitted to the laboratory if infection is suspected.

Complications

Pneumothorax can occur when air enters the pleural cavity if the cannula is placed too dorsally during thoracocentesis. The thorax normally has negative pressure, and when fluid has been removed, the thorax should return to negative pressure. *To correct pneumothorax, aspirate air dorsally in the same manner that fluid is aspirated.*

Hemothorax can occur if a large vein or artery is punctured during insertion of a cannula. *Avoid the lateral thoracic vein (in the ventral third of the thorax) and always enter along the cranial margin of a rib.*

If the heart is accidentally punctured during cannula placement, **fatal cardiac arrhythmia** can result. *Avoid the cranial/ventral aspect of the thorax and use ultrasound guidance.*

Hypovolemia occasionally results when large volumes (10-20 L) are removed by means of thoracocentesis. In rare instances, horses collapse if fluid is removed too rapidly, because fluid shifts from the circulating volume into the thorax. *Fluid therapy should be instituted to replace the volume lost.*

Gastrointestinal System

17 Aging Guidelines and Dentistry

David L. Foster

- Aging of horses by the teeth becomes less exact as the individual advances in years.
- Bracketing into 0-2 years, 3-10 years, 10-20 years, and >20 years is generally a useful starting point.
- Specific aging of the horse is accomplished by:
  - Noting the eruption of the deciduous incisors
  - Shedding of the juvenile incisors
  - Eruption and wear of the permanent incisors

Once the deciduous incisors are shed and the permanent incisors are erupted, aging is less clear with advancing age. The degree of wear, general shape, length, and other features all contribute to suggest an approximate age. As the horse ages, small variations of the teeth, oral configuration, and diet contribute to the appearance, angulation, and wear of the teeth.

General guidelines are described as follows:

- **FOALS** use the "rule of 8"
  - First incisors erupt at 8 days
  - Second incisors erupt at 8 weeks
  - Third incisors erupt at 8 months
- Two-year-olds shed the central incisors
- Three-year-olds shed the second incisors
- Four-year-olds shed the third incisors
- Five-year-olds have erupted all permanent incisors
- Seven-year-olds have all the incisors erupted, and the corner mandibular incisors (303/403) have their table surface in wear and a large central "cup"
- Ten-year-olds: Galvayne's groove appears on 103/203 (maxillary I3); 301/401 and 302/402 have developed a "round" table surface. All cups are lost from the mandibular incisors.
- Greater than 10 years of age it becomes increasingly more difficult to accurately determine age by dental examination.
- The length, angulation, degree of wear, and shape of incisors are "markers" of an individual's age, but become increasingly unreliable with advancing age.

USING TATTOOS AND BRANDS TO AGE HORSES

Several horse breed registries mark the year of birth in the tattoo or freeze brand applied to their horses.

Thoroughbreds

- All racing Thoroughbreds in the United States receive a lip tattoo.
- A letter followed by four or five numbers (representing the registration number) completes the tattoo.
- The letter denotes the year of birth: A-1971 through Z 1996; all letters of the alphabet are used.
- The alphabet is repeated every 26 years; all Thoroughbreds born in 1997 are tattooed beginning with the letter A; 1998-B; 1999-C; and so on (Box 17–1).
- An exception is made for foreign-bred horses who, once properly identified, receive a lip tattoo beginning with an asterisk followed by a number and no letter; this serves as the full registration number.

Standardbreds

- The Standardbred tattoo system can be used to determine the year of birth. However, it is an idiosyncratic system and is difficult to apply in the field without a tattoo list.
- In the United States, a system is used that records the full registration number, a letter to denote the year of birth, and four more characters, one of which may be another letter (Table 17–1).
- Standardbreds rotate the year of birth letter from the first position to the last in the tattoo character series once all letters are used. Not all letters of the alphabet are used in any given series.
- Any Standardbred born after 1995 may have its identification markings as either a lip tattoo or a freeze brand applied to the upper right side of the neck.
- For example, 4321A could be a lip tattoo assigned to a horse born in 1961.
- A Standardbred born in 1995 could have either a lip tattoo or a freeze brand of P4321.

BOX 17–1. Thoroughbred Tattoos

A=1971, 1997	N=1984
B=1972, 1998	O=1985
C=1973, 1999	P=1986
D=1974, 2000	Q=1987
E=1975, 2001	R=1988
F=1976, 2002	S=1989
G=1977, 2003	T=1990
H=1978	U=1991
I=1979	V=1992
J=1980	W=1993
K=1981	X=1994
L=1982	Y=1995
M=1983	Z=1996

Arabian Horse Registry of America/United States Bureau of Land Management Registry

- Employs a freeze-brand encryption to identify both full- and partial-bred Arabian horses and mustangs (Fig. 17–1).
- The first figure represents the breed.
- If the figure is rotated to the right (clockwise), it represents a half-breed.
- The next stacked figures represent the year of birth and are followed by the animal's registration number.

Racing Quarter Horses

- Racing Quarter Horses are identified by lip tattoos, but they do not indicate the year of birth, as in Thoroughbreds and Standardbreds.

EQUINE DENTAL NOMENCLATURE

There are two nomenclature systems used for horses:

- Anatomical descriptive system (Fig. 17–2)
- Triadan (numeric) nomenclature system (Fig. 17–3)

Communication between professionals, accurate record keeping, and organized oral examinations all benefit from the use of a concise nomenclature system.

TABLE 17–1. Standardbred Tattoos

Born in 1981 or earlier:	Born in 1982 or later:
First three digits are numbers. The fourth can be a letter or a number. The fifth is a letter indicating year of foaling. *The letters M,N,O,Q, and U are not used.*	The first character is a letter, indicating year of foaling. The second can be a letter or a number. The last three digits are numbers. *The letters I,O,Q, and U are not used.*
A=1961	A=1982
B=1962	B=1983
C=1963	C=1984
D=1964	D=1985
E=1965	E=1986
F=1966	F=1987
G=1967	G=1988
H=1968	H=1989
I=1969	J=1990
J=1970	K=1991
K=1971	L=1992
L=1972	M=1993
P=1973	N=1994
R=1974	P=1995
S=1975	R=1996
T=1976	S=1997
V=1977	T=1998
W=1978	V=1999
X=1979	W=2000
Y=1980	X=2001
Z=1981	Z=2002

In 2003, the year of birth letter will revert to the fifth or last character.

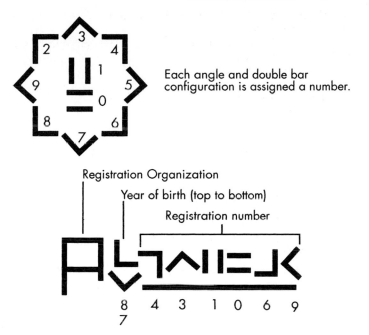

Each angle and double bar configuration is assigned a number.

Registration Organization

Year of birth (top to bottom)

Registration number

8 4 3 1 0 6 9
7

FIGURE 17–1. Freeze branding system for breed registration can be useful in individual age identification. A number is assigned to each angle or double bar configuration *(top)*. Sample registration is depicted below the freeze branding system. (Courtesy Michael Q. Lowder, DVM, MS.)

In the **anatomical** system (Fig. 17–2), a letter defines the type of tooth being described. All lowercase letters used denote deciduous teeth, capital letters permanent teeth: I, incisors; C, canines; P, premolars; and M, molars. A number is then assigned to the letter that denotes the location of the tooth in the oral cavity (e.g., first molar, second incisor). The oral cavity is divided into four quadrants. The horse's right maxillary arcade is the first arcade. The other three quadrants are assigned sequentially in a clockwise manner from the examiner's position. The anatomical letter then has the positional number placed around the letter to represent the location of the tooth. For example,

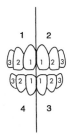

a right mandibular second incisor would be defined as $_2$I; a left maxillary second incisor would be defined as I^2.

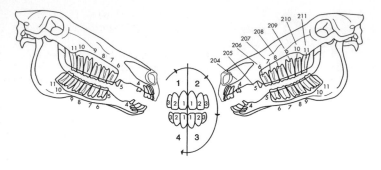

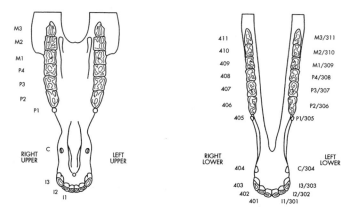

FIGURE 17–2. Numbering and anatomical descriptive systems used to identify equine teeth.

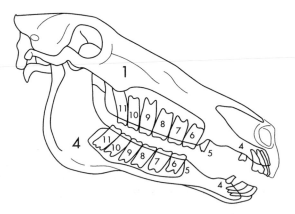

FIGURE 17–3. In the Triadan system, juvenile or deciduous teeth are identified by replacing the first digit with 5, 6, 7, or 8. For example, 203 for the permanent tooth would be identified by the number 603 for the deciduous tooth.

PROCEDURES

The right mandibular arcade of an adult male would be noted in the anatomical system as follows: $_1$I, $_2$I, $_3$I, $_1$C, $_2$P, $_3$P, $_4$P, $_1$M, $_2$M, $_3$M (assuming that the first premolar is not present).

The **Triadan digital nomenclature system** assigns a three-digit number to each tooth (Fig. 17–3). The first number defines the quadrant in which the tooth resides. The quadrants are numbered one through four starting with the horse's right maxillary arcade and progressing clockwise relative to the examiner, as is the case for the anatomical nomenclature system. The following two numbers in this system define the position of the tooth relative to the centerline of the oral cavity. The first or central incisor is assigned "01," the next (middle) incisor "02," and so on. The right mandibular arcade of an adult male would be described in the Triadan system as follows: 401, 402, 403, 404, 406, 407, 408, 409, 410, 411. This supposes that 405 (the lower first premolar or wolf tooth) is not present.

18 Nasogastric Tube Placement

James A. Orsini and Christine Kreuder

Placement of a nasogastric tube often is used for the administration of large volumes of oral medication(s), fluids, and electrolytes. This is also an important diagnostic and therapeutic procedure in the care of a horse with signs of colic. A tube is passed to determine whether fluid has accumulated in the anterior gastrointestinal tract. The fluid is removed to relieve the pressure on the stomach and the associated pain due to dilatation of the stomach. Nasogastric intubation also is necessary in suspected cases of choke to relieve the obstruction in the esophagus. Every clinician develops his/her own technique for passing a nasogastric tube. The following description may be useful for the less experienced.

Equipment

- Nasogastric tube (sized appropriately)
- Bucket half-filled with warm water
- 400-ml nylon dose syringe*

Procedure

- Immerse the nasogastric tube in warm water until it is clean and flexible.
- Adequately restrain the horse. This may require a chain shank over the nose or under the lip, a twitch, or both.
- Stand on the horse's left, place the right hand over the nose, and use the thumb to reflect the alar fold of the left nostril dorsally. Do not obstruct airflow in the right nostril.
- Using the left hand, guide the tube ventrally and medially along the ventral nasal meatus. The middle nasal meatus is immediately dorsal and must be avoided.
- Advance the tube slowly, and refrain from forcing the tube if excessive resistance is encountered. If the patient is tossing its head, hold the tube in the nostril using the thumb of the right hand.

---

*400-ml nylon dose syringe. J.A. Webster, Inc., 86 Leominster Road, Sterling, MA 01564-2198; (800) 225-7911.

- The tube encounters some resistance as it passes over the epiglottis. Most horses swallow the tube immediately. Try to pass the tube on the patient's first swallow, because subsequent attempts to stimulate swallowing become progressively more difficult. Keep the end of the tube in front of the epiglottis while waiting for the horse to swallow. Gently bumping the epiglottis with the end of the tube or blowing into the tube to trickle water down the pharynx may encourage some patients to swallow. If no swallow reflex is elicited, attempt to pass the tube using the other nostril.
- Be absolutely certain the tube is in the esophagus and not in the trachea. There are several ways to ensure correct placement. All the following must be confirmed before the tube is advanced farther and before any medication is delivered:
  □ Some resistance is encountered when the tube moves down the esophagus. The tube passes down the trachea relatively easily, and the tracheal rings are palpable.
  □ Negative pressure is obtained with suction if the tube is in the esophagus because the lumen collapses. Suction on the end of a tube in the trachea does not cause negative pressure.
  □ The end of the tube is seen advancing down the neck to the left of midline. The tube is not seen if it is in the trachea. If the tube is not apparent, it must be palpated as it passes through the thoracic inlet or, more likely, as it rests beside the rostral trachea (usually to the left). Exact tube placement is confirmed by gently pushing the trachea dorsally with one hand, while using the fingertips to feel the tube in the esophagus. This is the most reliable assessment of correct tube placement. A small percentage of horses have a right-sided esophagus.
- Blow into the tube to facilitate advancement through the cardia into the stomach. Once the tube is in the stomach, gas that smells like ingesta is emitted, and blowing on the end of the tube produces an audible bubbling noise. This is final test to insure that the tube is indeed in the stomach.
- Attempt to obtain reflux before administering large volumes of fluid. To obtain reflux, create a siphon by establishing a column of water between the stomach and the outside. Administer a dose syringeful of warm water to fill the tube, aspirate a small amount of fluid, detach the syringe, and lower the tube end. Several tries usually are needed before gastric fluid is siphoned off the stomach.
- If no net reflux is obtained, administer medication warmed to body temperature into the tube. Lift the tube end above the patient's head to complete delivery of the medication. Before removing the tube, lower the tube end to ensure that there is not excessive pressure on the stomach.
- Crimp the tube or leave the dose syringe attached during removal so that fluid does not drain into the pharynx or nasal passages.

A normal horse usually refluxes less than 2 L of fluid. Measure the amount of fluid pumped into the stomach to calculate the volume of fluid retrieved as reflux. Medication should not be delivered to patients with large volumes of reflux because it is not absorbed and increases the pressure on the stomach wall. Excessive reflux indicates ileus, an abnormal secretory process in the anterior gastrointestinal tract (anterior enteritis), or an obstructive process (usually in the small intestine). The volume, appearance, and odor of the fluid are important parameters to assess when treating a horse with colic. Patients with a large quantity of reflux should have a nasogastric tube left in place and secured to the halter to prevent gastric rupture. Retrieval of reflux should be repeated every few hours in these cases.

Complications

Accidentally administering a large volume of fluid into the lungs of a patient can be fatal. For this reason, one must literally "see, feel, smell, and hear" the tube in the correct position.

Hemorrhage from the nose is an occasional complication. The conchal mucosa is extremely vascular and is easily injured. Almost all nosebleeds eventually stop.

If a nosebleed occurs, rinse the tube and attempt to pass it gently through the other nostril.

A smaller-diameter tube is less likely to damage the mucosa. Also, make sure that the tube has no nicks or sharp edges that could cause mucosal injury.

If bleeding continues for more than 10-15 minutes or is believed excessive, an intranasal spray of 10 mg phenylephrine hydrochloride diluted in 10 ml of sterile saline solution can be infused through a nasal catheter.

---

19 Abdominocentesis and Peritoneal Fluid Analysis

James A. Orsini and Christine Kreuder

Peritoneal fluid analysis is an excellent measure of gastrointestinal disease. This procedure is indicated whenever a patient has acute or intermittent abdominal pain, diarrhea, or chronic weight loss.

Equipment

- Twitch (sedation is generally not necessary)
- Clippers
- Material for sterile scrub
- Sterile gloves
- Sterile 18-22-gauge, 1.5-inch (3.8-cm) needles *or* metal teat cannula (3.75-inches [9.4 cm] long)* for foals or metal bitch urinary catheter (10.5 inch [26.3 cm] long)† for larger or obese horses
- 2% local anesthetic (with 25-gauge needle and 3-ml syringe)
- #15 blade if using a cannula or urinary catheter
- Sterile gauze sponge
- EDTA and plain Vacutainer tubes‡ for analysis
- Sterile vial, Port-a-Cul culture and transport system§ or blood culture bottle# for culture and sensitivity

---

*Ideal udder infusion cannula. Butler Company, 5000 Bradenton Avenue, P.O. Box 7153, Dublin, OH 43017-0753.

†Metal bitch urinary catheter. Jorgensen Laboratories, Inc., 1450 North Van Buren Avenue, Loveland, CO 80538; (970) 669-2500.

‡Vacutainer. Becton-Dickinson Vacutainer Systems, Rutherford, NJ 07070.

§Port-a-Cul. Becton-Dickinson Microbiology Systems, Cockeysville, MD 21030.

#Septi-check, BB blood culture bottle. Roche Diagnostic Systems, Indianapolis, IN 46256.

PROCEDURES

Procedure

- Choose an area in the most dependent portion of the abdomen (usually directly on the midline 5 cm caudal to the xiphoid). A right paramedian approach may be used to avoid the spleen.
- Clip or shave the area chosen for abdominocentesis.
- Perform a sterile scrub.
- Place twitch.
- Glove and maintain sterility throughout the procedure.
- While standing next to the patient, insert the needle with a quick thrust through the skin and linea alba. If drops of abdominal fluid are not seen at the needle hub, reposition and rotate the needle or attach a syringe and aspirate. If necessary, place a second needle a few inches from the first to release the negative pressure in the abdomen.
- Consider ultrasound examination to locate fluid pockets; however, peritoneal fluid can still be obtained even if not seen after ultrasound evaluation.
- If abdominal fluid is not obtained, use a teat cannula or a stainless steel bitch urinary catheter to reach the peritoneal cavity. *A small-diameter teat cannula is recommended for foals because their intestinal wall is thin and easily lacerated.*
  - ▫ Place a subcutaneous bleb of local anesthesia.
  - ▫ Make a small stab incision with a #15 blade through the skin and subcutaneous tissue.
  - ▫ To reduce blood contamination from the incision, push the tip of the cannula through a sterile sponge.
  - ▫ Gently insert the cannula or urinary catheter into the incision. Some force is required to push the blunt-tipped instrument through the linea alba. A marked loss of resistance is felt once the abdomen is entered.
  - ▫ Allow the abdominal fluid to drip directly into EDTA Vacutainer tubes with or without culture material.

PERITONEAL FLUID ANALYSIS

Changes in peritoneal fluid are recognized fairly quickly after the onset of gastrointestinal disease (Table 19–1). In cases of acute obstruction or strangulating obstruction, changes in peritoneal fluid are seen several hours after the onset of clinical signs. More insidious lesions, such as nonstrangulating obstruction, enteritis, and peritonitis, are likely to produce changes in the peritoneal fluid before or concurrent with clinical signs. Inguinal herniation, intussusception, and entrapment of diseased bowel in the omental bursa or epiploic foramen may initially result in local peritonitis with normal peritoneal fluid.

Normal peritoneal fluid is clear and light yellow. Color and specific gravity are easily assessed and are the most predictive of the severity of the lesion. Normal specific gravity is 1.005 mg/dl. Increased turbidity results from increased protein or cellular content, which may be caused by septic peritonitis or inflammation of a segment of intestine. The color of the fluid reflects the type of cells present. Cloudy white-to-yellow fluid or exudate represents large numbers of white blood cells, as in septic peritonitis. In an abdominal crisis, segments of bowel become compromised once there is diminished venous and lymphatic drainage from the bowel segment. Initially transudate, red blood cells, and protein leak out of vessels. An elevated total protein level and red blood cell count in serosanguineous fluid often are the first changes seen. Peritoneal fluid becomes white or yellow as bowel becomes

TABLE 19–1. Correlation of Peritoneal Fluid Parameters and Intraperitoneal Disorders

Condition	Appearance*	Total Protein* (g/dl)	Total Nucleated Cells/L*	Cytologic Findings*
Normal[†]	Yellow, clear	<2.0	<7.5 x 10⁹	40%-80% neutrophils 20%-80% mononuclear
Nonstrangulating obstruction	Yellow, clear to slightly turbid	<3.0	<3.0-15.0 x 10⁹	Predominantly neutrophils (well preserved)
Strangulating obstruction	Red-brown, turbid	2.5-6.0	5.0-50.0 x 10⁹	Predominantly neutrophils (degenerate)
Proximal duodenitis-jejunitis	Yellow-red, turbid	3.0-4.5	<10.0 x 10⁹	Predominantly neutrophils (well preserved)
Bowel rupture	Red-brown, green, turbid with or without particulate matter	5.0-6.5	>20.0 x 10⁹ (20-150 x 10⁹)	>95% neutrophils (severely degenerate); intracellular and extracellular bacteria, with or without plant matter
Septic peritonitis	Yellow-white, turbid	>3.0	>20.0 x 10⁹ (20-100 x 10⁹)	Predominantly neutrophils (degenerate)
Postceliotomy	Yellow-red, turbid	Variable	Variable	Predominantly neutrophils (slight to moderate degenerate); no intracellular bacteria
Enterocentesis	Brown-green, with or without particulate matter	Variable	<1.0 x 10⁹	Free bacteria, few cells, plant matter
Intraabdominal hemorrhage	Dark red	Initially similar to peripheral blood, WBC count increases with time		PCV less than PCV of peripheral blood, erythrocytophagia, few to no platelets

PCV, Packed cell volume.
NOTE: Absence of gross or cytologic abnormalities in the peritoneal fluid does not rule out compromised intestine.
*Most common findings; exceptions can occur.
[†]Including peripartum mares.

ischemic and necrotic and white blood cells begin to leave the vessels. Necrotic bowel also leaks bacteria and endotoxin, accelerates chemotaxis of white blood cells and increases the turbidity and white blood cell count. Red-brown or green-colored fluid may indicate rupture of the stomach or intestine and may contain plant material. Dark red fluid may be obtained when a vessel or the spleen is entered. In rare instances, hemoperitoneum results from rupture of a vessel; the sample contains no platelets and may have evidence of erythrophagocytosis. The packed cell volume (PCV) may be compared with that of a systemic sample to differentiate samples from the spleen (PCV is higher) and from a vessel (PCV is the same).

A direct smear is made with Wright or Gram stain or both. Cytologic examination should include a white blood cell count and differential and evaluation of cellular degeneration and the presence of bacteria and food particles. White blood cell counts are normally lower in foals. A moderate amount of blood contamination in the sample (not more than 17%) should not affect any parameters except the number of red blood cells. White blood cell count and total protein levels are elevated in a patient that has undergone abdominal surgery even with manipulation of the intestines only. A sample with increased white blood cell numbers in which most neutrophils appear toxic and degenerate is evidence of septic peritonitis, even if the sample is obtained after celiotomy.

Complications

Cellulitis or **abscess** formation can occur after a break in sterile technique or removal of septic or purulent peritoneal fluid.

Accidental **enterocentesis** (aspiration of bowel contents) is not uncommon but rarely causes a problem other than sample contamination. *A blunt-tipped cannula decreases the likelihood of bowel puncture. Ultrasound-guided abdominocentesis is useful in foals to prevent intestinal laceration.*

Accidental **splenic aspiration** causes sample contamination.

Omental herniation may occur in foals after abdominocentesis in the rostral to middle abdomen performed with a teat cannula. Transect the omentum at or near the body wall, apply an antiseptic cream or ointment, and cover with an abdominal bandage.

REFERENCES

Freden GO, Provost PJ, Rand WM: Re-evaluating the clinical application of abdominal fluid analysis in the equine colic patient. Presented at the 5th Equine Colic Research Symposium, Athens, Georgia, 1994.

Malark JA, Peyton LC, Galvin MJ: Effects of blood contamination on equine peritoneal fluid analysis, *J Am Vet Med Assoc* 201:1545-1548, 1992.

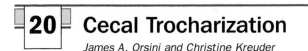

20   Cecal Trocharization

James A. Orsini and Christine Kreuder

Cecal trocharization is performed to decompress the cecum in patients with cecal tympany. Cecal gas distention is suspected in colicky patients when a ping is heard on simultaneous percussion and auscultation in the right paralumbar fossa and confirmed with rectal palpation. Cecal tympany can be a primary or secondary disorder. Decompression stimulates cecal motility and relieves the pain caused by cecal distention. The procedure helps normalize intraabdominal pressure and improves venous return and ease of breathing. This procedure is frequently performed on surgical patients before general anesthesia. If the patient is not a surgical candidate, trocharization can resolve colic in simple cases of tympany or certain colonic displacements.

Equipment
- Twitch
- Clippers
- Material for sterile scrub
- 2% local anesthetic, 5-ml syringe, and 22-gauge, 1.5-inch (3.8-cm) needle
- Sterile gloves
- 16-gauge, 5-inch (12.5-cm) pliable intravenous catheter*
- 7-inch (17.5-cm) extension set†
- Small cup of tap water

Procedure
- Consider use of a twitch if the patient is not sedated. Sedation is generally not necessary.
- Clip an area in the right paralumbar fossa where the "ping" is best heard.
- Infiltrate 3-5 ml of local anesthetic subcutaneously and in the underlying muscle at the trocharization site.
- Perform a sterile scrub.
- Wearing sterile gloves, insert the catheter and stylet through the skin, subcutaneous tissue, and abdominal muscle. The catheter should remain perpendicular to the skin. Remove the plastic cap on the catheter; if the catheter is in the cecum, gas escapes. When the catheter is in the cecum, remove the stylet entirely or withdraw the stylet approximately 0.5 inch to prevent collapse of the catheter by the abdominal wall.
- Attach the extension set and place the free end in the cup of water. Bubbles are produced as long as gas is being removed from the cecum; suction may be used if available.
- If gas is no longer retrievable, withdraw the catheter; do not attempt to redirect the catheter.

---

*Abbocath-T radiopaque FEP Teflon IV catheter. Abbott Hospitals, Inc., North Chicago, IL 60064.

†Extension set, 7-inch. Abbott Laboratories, North Chicago, IL 60064.

Complications

Low-grade, localized **peritonitis,** which can affect peritoneal fluid parameters, is expected to occur after this procedure. Clinical evidence or subsequent complications are rare. Signs of infection should raise suspicion, however, and be managed promptly with the appropriate therapy. *Injecting antibiotics (ampicillin, neomycin, or gentamicin) through the catheter during removal may minimize this complication.* Repeating trocharization is **not recommended,** because clinical peritonitis can develop.

Local **cellulitis** or **abscess** can occur at the trocharization site. The inflammation is usually self-limiting but should be monitored and managed appropriately.

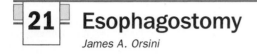

21 Esophagostomy

James A. Orsini

Esophagostomy is indicated for the placement of an indwelling feeding tube and is performed with local or general anesthesia depending on the temperament of the patient, the type of obstruction, cost, and the surgeon's preference. Because of the potential need for ventral drainage and the increased risk of cellulitis associated with a lateral approach to the cranial esophagus, an 8-10 cm longitudinal skin incision is made along the ventral midline. This site is used to aid in ventral drainage if the incision is left to heal by secondary intention or if dehiscence of the primary incision occurs. Placement of a nasogastric tube before surgery is recommended to identify the esophagus and minimize the dissection of surrounding tissues.

Procedure

- Make the surgical approach from either side of the neck (Fig. 21–1).
- *Cranial third of the esophagus:* Reflect the cutaneous colli muscle dorsally, the sternocephalicus muscle and jugular vein ventrally, and the brachiocephalacus and omohyoideus muscles dorsally.
- *Middle third of the cervical portion of the esophagus:* Separate the paired sternothyrohyoideus muscles and retract the trachea to the right of midline.
- *Caudal third of the cervical esophagus:* Use a ventrolateral approach with the incision ventral to the left jugular vein to access the esophageal portion lying dorsal to the trachea.

CAUTION: The vagosympathetic trunk and recurrent laryngeal nerve must be identified and avoided during the surgical procedure.

- *Thoracic esophagus:* Use a left rib resection for access to this portion of the esophagus.
- Perform careful dissection of the adventitia to expose the esophagus. Identify and gently retract the carotid sheath, which contains the vagosympathetic trunk and recurrent laryngeal nerve and artery.
- To incise the muscular layer of the esophagus, grasp the mucosa with an Allis tissue forceps and enlarge the incision so that the esophagus is separated into two distinct layers consisting of the muscle and the mucosa and submucosa.
- Pass a stomach tube in a normograde direction, and suture the tube to the skin.

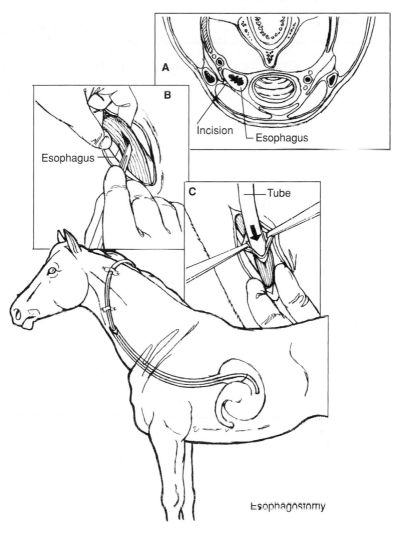

A

B

Esophagus

Incision └ Esophagus

C ── Tube

Esophagostomy

FIGURE 21-1. Technique of esophagostomy for placement of an indwelling feeding tube.

Complications

Even with delicate tissue handling, laryngeal hemiplasia from damage to the recurrent laryngeal nerve can be a sequela to the surgery.

REFERENCES

Freeman DE: Standing surgery of the neck and thorax, *Vet Clin North Am* 7:603-626, 1991.
Fubini SL, Starrak GS, Freeman DE: Esophagus. In Auer JA, Stick JA: *Equine Surgery,* ed 2, Philadelphia, 1999,WB Saunders.

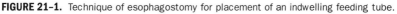

Genitourinary System

22 Urinary Tract Catheterization

James A. Orsini and Christine Kreuder

Urinary tract catheterization assures an accurate, uncontaminated urine sample in a convenient manner. A midstream, free-catch urine sample is adequate for urinalysis but is less suitable for culture. The same technique is used for passage of the fiberoptic or videoendoscope in performing cystoscopy or urethroscopy.

Equipment
- Sedative or tranquilizer (xylazine hydrochloride, butorphanol tartrate, and acepromazine)
- Tail tie for mares
- Sterile gloves
- Lubricating jelly*
- Appropriate urinary catheter (sterile)
  □ Stallions and geldings: 9-mm outer diameter urinary catheter[†]
  □ Mares: 11-mm outer diameter urinary catheter[‡]
- 60-ml catheter-tip syringe[§] (sterile)
- 3 sterile vials for urinalysis, cytologic examination, and culture specimens

Procedure
MALE CATHETERIZATION
- Stallions and geldings usually need sedation and tranquilization for restraint and extrusion of the penis. (Recommended dosage: 0.3-0.5 mg/kg xylazine, 0.01-0.02 mg/kg butorphanol, combined with 0.02 mg/kg acepromazine IV)
- Scrub the penis with a dilute antiseptic solution (povidone-iodine or chlorhexidine) and rinse with water.
- Wear sterile gloves while minimally lubricating the catheter.
- Stabilize the penis with one hand and gently advance the catheter through the urethral opening.

---

*K-Y lubricating jelly. Johnson and Johnson Medical, Inc., Arlington, TX 76004-3130. H-R lubricating jelly. Carter Products, Division of Carter-Wallace, Inc., New York, NY 10105.

[†]Stallion Foley catheter (28F Foley). Cook Veterinary Products, PO Box 489, Bloomington, IN 47402; (800) 457-4500.

[‡]Mare urinary catheter. Jorgensen Laboratories, Inc., 1450 North Van Buren Avenue, Loveland, CO 80538; (970) 669-2500. Uterine flushing tube (33F, 80 cm long). Cook Veterinary Products, PO Box 489, Bloomington, IN 47402; (800) 457-4500.

[§]Monoject 60-ml syringe with catheter tip. Sherwood Medical, St. Louis, MO 63103.

- Advance the catheter approximately 50-70 cm. The catheter should glide through the urethra easily until the urethral sphincter is contacted. Injection of 60 ml of air and/or 10 ml of lidocaine into the urethra may aid passage through the sphincter.
- If urine does not flow freely when the catheter has reached the bladder, gently aspirate with a 60-ml syringe.
- Place samples directly into the sterile vials for urinalysis, cytologic examination, culture and colony count.

FEMALE CATHETERIZATION
- Sedation is generally not needed, although use of a twitch is recommended.
- Wrap the tail and pull it to the side.
- Scrub the perineum with a dilute antiseptic solution (povidone-iodine or chlorhexidine) and rinse with water.
- Wearing sterile gloves, minimally lubricate the catheter.
- Place a hand within the vagina and locate the urethral opening on the floor of the vagina. Insert one finger into the urethra and gently guide the catheter with the other hand.
- Advance the catheter approximately 5-10 cm. If urine does not flow freely, aspirate with a 60-ml syringe.
- Place samples in appropriate containers.

URINALYSIS

Urinalysis is useful in the diagnosis of both lower and upper urinary tract disorders. Each sample should be submitted for a complete urinalysis, cytologic examination, and bacterial culture with **colony count**. A urine sample should be examined within 20 minutes of collection or be refrigerated immediately. Gross evaluation of equine urine is difficult because of the high mucus content. Pigmenturia is easily seen but must be differentiated from hematuria, hemoglobinuria, and myoglobinuria by means of microscopic examination.

A urine dipstick is routinely used to determine pH, protein content, glucose, bilirubin, and the presence of pigments. A refractometer is used to determine specific gravity. The specific gravity of the urine of adults is normally between 1.008 and 1.045; that of the urine of foals is between 1.001 and 1.025. Highly concentrated urine is often caused by decreased water intake. If urinary specific gravity remains isosthenuric (equal to blood specific gravity of 1.010) despite changes in water intake or a water deprivation test, significant renal disease should be suspected.

Normal urine should not contain protein, glucose, or bilirubin. If a dipstick is used, protein may be falsely elevated if the urine is highly concentrated or very alkaline. Protein is detected if there is pigmenturia or inflammation or infection in the urinary tract. Absolute (true) proteinuria should be quantitated with mechanical methods and is seen with glomerulonephritis and amyloidosis. Glucosuria occurs in hyperglycemia with normal renal function. If the blood glucose level is normal, glucosuria is highly suggestive of renal tubular disease. Pigmenturia occurs with myolysis (muscle damage), hemolysis (bilirubinuria and hematuria), cystitis (secondary to urinary calculi), pyelonephritis, and rarely, neoplasia. Normal equine urine is alkaline; adult urinary pH is 7.5-8.5, foal urinary pH is 5.5-8.0. Increased acidity occurs with strenuous exercise, metabolic acidosis, and starvation.

Cytologic examination of the urine is important in differentiating urinary tract inflammation and infection. Slides should be made from the sample centrifugate, air dried, and stained with Wright or Diff-Quik stain. Five red blood cells and five white blood cells per high-power field ($\times 1000$) are normal. More than 10 red blood cells per field suggests hemorrhage, and more than 10 white blood cells per field suggests inflammation. If inflammation is present, a Gram stain should be performed to look for bacteria. Bacteria should not be detected in normal urine if the sample is collected using aseptic technique. Assessment of bacterial morphology helps in instituting antibiotic therapy before culture results are obtained. Casts (cellular debris shed from the renal tubules) indicate renal tubular damage. Calcium carbonate crystals are common and considered within normal limits unless clinical signs suggest the presence of urinary calculi.

Complications

Infection of the lower urinary tract can occur if sterile technique is not maintained, particularly if the bladder is atonic.

Musculoskeletal System

23 Local Anesthesia for the Diagnosis of Lameness

James A. Orsini and Christine Kreuder

Local anesthesia is a diagnostic tool used to help localize lameness or confirm examination findings. Perineural anesthesia infiltrates the sensory fibers of a nerve and desensitizes specific anatomic regions in a systematic manner. A thorough knowledge of applied neuroanatomy is required for performance and accurate interpretation of nerve blocks. Intrasynovial anesthesia is more specific and is used to localize lameness within joints, tendon sheaths, and bursae. Anesthesia may be placed directly into a joint, bursa, or tendon sheath and often alleviates intrasynovial pain more completely than nerve blocks do.

CAUTION: Trotting a horse after placement of local anesthesia is contraindicated if a fracture is suspected. Radiography and/or nuclear scintigraphy are recommended before regional anesthesia in these cases to rule out an incomplete fracture and prevent catastrophic bone failure after desensitization. Local anesthesia may be used if the horse is severely lame (grades 4-5 out of 5) to localize the lameness by determining whether weight bearing or soundness at a slow walk is achievable. Stall confinement with or without mild tranquilization is necessary until the effects of the block wear off.

Equipment

- Twitch (optional)
- Material for sterile scrub
- 2% mepivacaine* local anesthetic. Most commonly used because it causes less tissue reaction and has a rapid onset of action, which lasts 60-90 minutes. Lidocaine[†] also is a well-suited local anesthetic. Bupivacaine[‡] lasts 4-6 hours and should be used when longer-lasting anesthesia is desired.
- Sterile disposable 18- to 25-gauge needles and an assortment of 3- to 60-ml syringes (not Luer-Lok); see the illustrations for exact needle and syringe size required for each block.

---

*Carbocaine-V (2% mepivacaine hydrochloride). The Upjohn Company, Kalamazoo, MI 49001.

[†]Anthocaine (2% lidocaine hydrochloride). Anpro Pharmaceutical, Arcadia, CA 91006.

[‡]Marcaine (0.5% bupivacaine hydrochloride). Abbott Laboratories. North Chicago, IL 60064.

- Clippers and sterile gloves for intrasynovial procedures.

Procedure

- See Figs. 23–1 through 23–3 for sites and landmarks for perineural anesthesia, size of needle recommended, and amount of local anesthesia required. Begin with the most distal block, regardless of the clinical impressions, and move proximally until the lameness is eliminated. Perineural anesthesia is less specific in the proximal limb.
- Scrub the injection sites to remove gross contamination, and wash hands.
- Place twitch. Sedation or tranquilization is not recommended because both affect interpretation of the block.
- Once the nerve is palpated, place the needle with a quick stick through the skin, attach the syringe with anesthetic, aspirate to rule out intravascular placement, and inject anesthetic around the nerve. If resistance is encountered, the needle may be in a ligament, tendon, or intradermal tissue and should be repositioned. The volume of local anesthetic agent ranges from 2 ml to 5 ml per site.
- Allow 5-10 minutes before testing skin sensation for anesthesia effect. Check for deep pain with hoof testers, flexion, and deep palpation.
- Repeat the lameness examination and assess improvement (0%-100%).

INTRASYNOVIAL ANESTHESIA

- See Figs. 23–4 through 23–10 for sites and landmarks for intrasynovial (intra-articular) anesthesia, size of the needle recommended, and amount of local anesthetic needed for each joint.
- Joint blocks may be used in conjunction with perineural anesthesia if only partial relief of the lameness is achieved and a joint is believed to be contributing to the lameness. The technique is similar to that for perineural anesthesia, except aseptic technique and patient restraint are essential.
- Clip and shave the site for needle placement.
- Perform a sterile scrub at the site of injection and the landmarks to be palpated before injection.
- Wear sterile gloves to handle the syringe and needle and to palpate the landmarks.
- Use an unopened bottle of local anesthetic. One needle should be used to fill the syringe and another for joint injection. Needles and syringes should remain sterile.
- Place a twitch for restraint.
- Detach the needle from the syringe and place the needle with a quick stick through the skin. If the needle has been placed successfully, synovial fluid appears at the hub of the needle in most cases. Digital pressure on the joint capsule encourages synovial fluid to flow from the needle. Care should be used in needle placement to prevent damage to the articular cartilage and surrounding soft tissue.
- Collect and analyze synovial fluid. (See arthrocentesis procedure, p. 105.)
- Once the needle is in place, attach the syringe and rapidly inject the anesthetic. There should be minimal resistance to injection. If resistance is encountered, detach the syringe and redirect the needle without exiting the skin. Holding on to the hub of the needle with one hand and injecting with the other facilitates rapid detachment of the syringe should the patient move.
- The volume of the anesthetic injected intrasynovially varies from joint to joint.

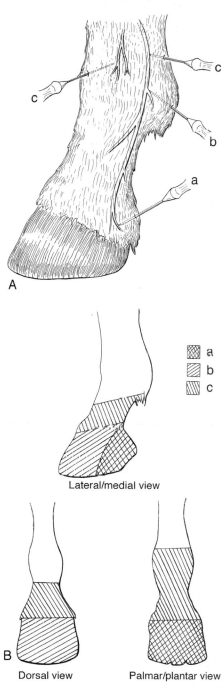

A

Lateral/medial view

B

Dorsal view   Palmar/plantar view

FIGURE 23-1. A, Sequential sites for perineural anesthesia of the distal limb.

a. **Palmar digital nerve block** (25-gauge, ⅝-inch [1.6-cm] needle). The posterior digital nerve runs along the medial and lateral borders of the deep digital flexor tendon. The nerves are easily palpable within a neurovascular bundle. The nerve is palmar to the digital vein and artery (VAN relationship). Elevate the foot and block the nerve with 2-3 ml of local anesthetic just above the collateral cartilages.

b. **Abaxial sesamoid nerve block** (25-gauge, ⅝-inch [1.6-cm] needle). The palmar digital nerves are easily palpable on the abaxial surfaces of the sesamoid bones. Hold the limb in a flexed position and deposit 3-4 ml of local anesthetic over each nerve.

c. **Low palmar and palmar metacarpal nerve blocks** (25-gauge, ⅝-inch [1.6-cm] needle). The palmar nerve runs in the medial and lateral groove between the suspensory ligament and the deep digital flexor tendon. Block the palmar nerve with 3-4 ml of local anesthetic above the level of the bell of the splint bone (to avoid the digital tendon sheath). Block the palmar metacarpal nerve as it emerges distally from the bell of the splint bone with 2-3 ml of local anesthetic. This block may be performed with the limb in a flexed or standing position. Note: The plantar and plantar metatarsal nerves of the hindlimb are blocked in a similar manner. For complete anesthesia of the distal hindlimb, the medial and lateral dorsal metatarsal nerves must be blocked with 2 ml of local anesthetic on either side of the long digital extensor tendon just above the fetlock.

B, Hash marks represent the affected area of limb.

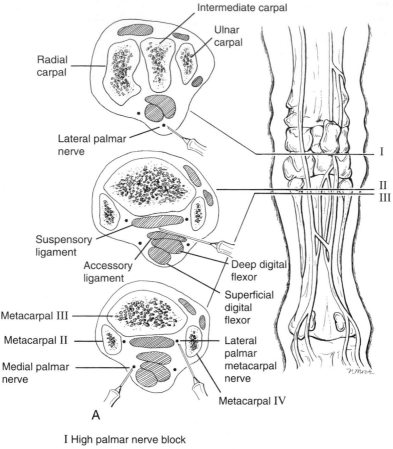

I High palmar nerve block
II High suspensory block
III High palmar and palmar metacarpal nerve block

FIGURE 23-2. Sequential sites for perineural anesthesia of the proximal forelimb.
A, High palmar and palmar metacarpal nerve blocks (22-gauge, 1.5-inch [3.6-cm] needle). The palmar nerves lie beneath a dense fascial sheath between the deep digital flexor tendon and the suspensory ligament. Use 3-5 ml of local anesthetic to block the lateral nerve at the level of the distal accessory carpal bone and the medial nerve at the level of the medial splint bone head. A subcutaneous bleb should *not* appear if the fascial sheath has been successfully penetrated. The palmar metacarpal nerves course axially to the splint bones and should be blocked with 3-5 ml of local anesthetic below the head of each splint bone.

CAUTION: Inadvertent anesthesia of the carpal sheath, carpometacarpal joint, or middle carpal joint can occur when one deposits local anesthetic in the palmar carpometacarpal region. As a precaution, a sterile skin preparation and sterile technique should be used when these blocks are performed. If lameness is successfully blocked with anesthesia of this region, anesthesia of the middle carpal joint is indicated to confirm placement of anesthetic.

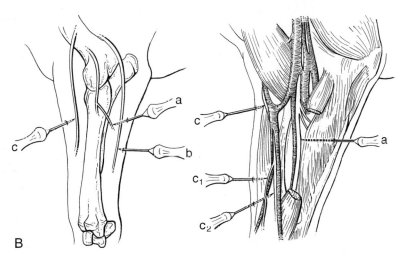

B

FIGURE 23-2. *(Cont'd)* **B, Median, ulnar, and medial cutaneous antebrachial nerve blocks** (20- or 22-gauge, 1.5-inch [3.6-cm] needle). Block the median nerve with 10 ml of local anesthetic in the posterior medial aspect of the radius approximately 10 cm proximal to the chestnut (*a*). Block the ulnar nerve with 8 ml of local anesthetic in the groove between the flexor carpi ulnaris and the ulnarls lateralis muscles, approximately 10 cm proximal to the accessory carpal bone (*b*). Block the medial cutaneous antebrachial nerve by depositing 5 ml of local anesthetic on either side of the cephalic vein, approximately 10 cm proximal to the chestnut (*c*). (C_1 and C_2 are cranial and caudal branches of the medial cutaneous antebrachial nerve.)

As a general rule:
- Joints at the level of the carpi/tarsi distal: use 5-10 ml per joint.
- Joints above the carpi or tarsi: use volumes of 20-50 ml per joint. The largest volume of 50 ml is reserved for the femoropatellar joint.
- Allow 20-30 minutes before assessing the effect.
- Repeat the lameness examination and assess improvement (0%-100%).
- For distal limbs, place an alcohol-soaked wrap over the injection site.

EVALUATING THE RESULTS OF LOCAL ANESTHESIA

The limitations of local anesthesia for the diagnosis of lameness need to be well understood if this method is to be used accurately. Determining which structures have been desensitized by a particular block is sometimes difficult because of variation in nerve supply. Assessing skin sensation does not always reflect the presence of deep pain. Many patients retain skin sensation over the dorsal aspect of the distal limb while deeper structures are adequately anesthetized. Use as many physical parameters as possible to determine the effect of the anesthesia (hoof testers, flexion, and so on). A patient may continue to show lameness even though the unsound area is anesthetized if other sources of lameness are contributing factors. However, there should still be partial improvement or a change in the gait. The lameness does not improve if it is caused by a neurologic or mechanical problem.

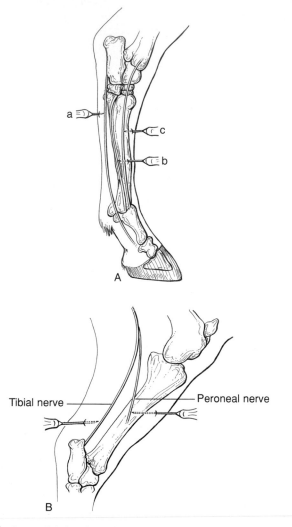

FIGURE 23–3. Sequential sites for perineural anesthesia of the proximal hindlimb.
A, High plantar (*a*), plantar metatarsal (*b*), and dorsal metatarsal (*c*) nerve blocks (22-gauge, 1.5-inch [3.6-cm] needle). Landmarks in the hindlimb are similar to those in the forelimb for the high plantar and plantar metatarsal blocks. Both the medial and lateral plantar nerves should be blocked below the level of the head of the splint bones. Block the dorsal metatarsal nerves with 3 ml of local anesthetic on each side of the long digital extensor tendon in the proximal metatarsus.
B, Tibial and peroneal nerve blocks (20-gauge, 1.5-inch [3.6-cm] needle). Block the tibial nerve by depositing 15 ml of local anesthetic medially between the deep digital flexor tendon and the calcanean tendon, approximately 10 cm proximal to the point of the hock. Deposit the anesthetic beneath the fascial sheath. Block the peroneal nerve laterally with 10 ml of local anesthetic in the groove between the long and lateral digital extensor muscles, approximately 4 cm proximal to the point of the hock.

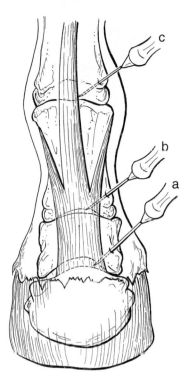

FIGURE 23-4. Intrasynovial anesthesia of the distal limb.
a. **Coffin joint** (20-gauge, 1.5-inch [3.6-cm] needle). Palpate a depression 0.5-1 cm
dorsal to the coronary band either medial or lateral to the common (front limb), long
(hind limb) digital extensor tendon. With the limb in a weight-bearing position, insert a
needle perpendicular to the hoof surface to a depth of 1.5-2.0 cm. Block the joint with
5-8 ml of local anesthetic.
b. **Pastern joint** (20-gauge, 1.5-inch [3.6-cm] needle). Draw a line from the lateral
eminence of the first phalanx to the midline and insert a needle 1 cm distal to this line
and lateral to the common (front limb), long (hind limb) digital extensor tendon. The limb
is in a weight-bearing position, and the needle is parallel to the hoof surface. Block the
joint with 4-6 ml of local anesthetic.
c. **Fetlock joint** (20-gauge, 1.5-inch [3.6-cm] needle). The palmar/plantar pouch is
located between the caudal aspect of the cannon bone and the lateral branch of the
suspensory ligament. With the limb in a standing or flexed position, insert the needle
perpendicular to the limb axis or in a slightly downward direction to a depth of 1.0 cm.
Block the joint with 5-8 ml of local anesthetic. Illustration shows intrasynovial
anesthesia by means of the dorsal approach medial or lateral to the common/long
digital extensor tendon.

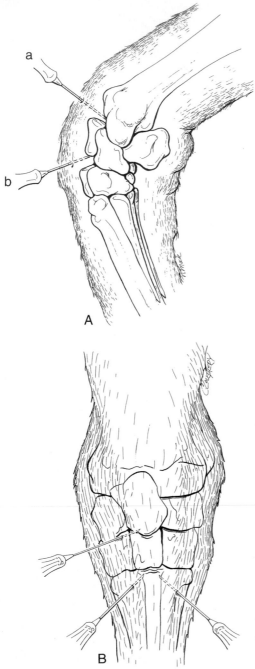

FIGURE 23–5. A, B, Intraarticular anesthesia of the proximal forelimb. **Carpal joints** (20-gauge, 1.5-inch [3.6-cm]). To enter the radiocarpal joint (*a*), locate the depression between the radius and the radial carpal bone with the carpus flexed. Insert the needle medial to the extensor carpi radialis tendon to a depth of 1 cm. Block the joint with 10 ml of local anesthetic. To enter the intercarpal/middle carpal joint (*b*), locate the depression between the radial carpal bone and the third carpal bone. Insert the needle medial to the extensor carpi radialis tendon and block the joint with 10 ml of local anesthetic. The carpometacarpal joint communicates with the intercarpal joint.

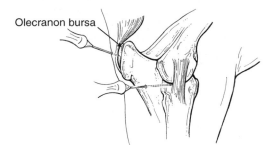

FIGURE 23-6. Elbow joint (20-gauge, 1.5-inch [3.6-cm]). The elbow joint is palpable between the lateral humeral epicondyle and the radial tuberosity. Insert the needle caudal to the lateral collateral ligament in a horizontal direction to a depth of 2-3 cm. Block the joint with 20 ml of local anesthetic.

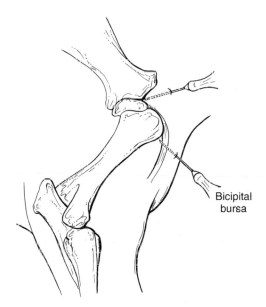

FIGURE 23-7. Scapulohumeral joint (18-gauge, 5-inch [12.5-cm] needle). Palpate a notch between the anterior and posterior portions of the lateral humeral tuberosity (point of the shoulder). Direct the needle in a horizontal and slightly caudomedial direction to a depth of 8-10 cm. Block the joint with 20 ml of local anesthetic.

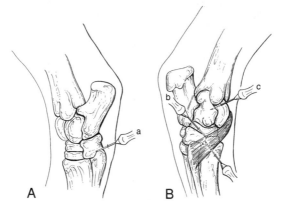

FIGURE 23–8. A, B, Intraarticular anesthesia of the proximal hind limb. **Tarsal joints** (20-gauge, 1.5-inch [3.6-cm] needle). To enter the tarsometatarsal joint (*a*), palpate a small depression proximal to the head of the lateral splint bone. Insert the needle in a horizontal and slightly downward and anterior direction to a depth of 2-3 cm. Block the joint with 4-6 ml of local anesthetic. Enter the distal intertarsal joint (*b*) by inserting a needle distal to the anterior aspect of the cunean tendon on the medial aspect of the hock. Block the joint with 4-6 ml of local anesthetic. Enter the tibiotarsal joint (*c*) on either side of the saphenous vein 2-3 cm below the medial malleolus. Insert the needle to a depth of 1-2 cm and block the joint with 10-15 ml of local anesthetic. The tibiotarsal joint communicates with the proximal intertarsal joint.

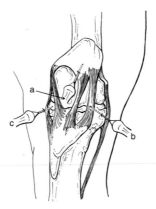

FIGURE 23–9. Stifle joint (18-gauge, 1.5-3-inch [3.6-7.5-cm]) needle). Access the femoropatellar joint by inserting a needle between the middle and medial patellar ligaments approximately 2-3 cm above the palpable proximal tibial crest (*a*). Direct the needle horizontally to a depth of 4-5 cm. Block the joint with 40-50 ml of local anesthetic. Enter the lateral femorotibial joint posterior to the lateral patellar ligament and above the proximal edge of the tibia (*b*). Insert the needle to a depth of 1-2 cm and block the joint with 20-30 ml of local anesthetic. Access the medial femorotibial joint between the medial patellar and medial femorotibial (collateral) ligaments and above the palpable proximal tibia (*c*). Insert the needle horizontally to a depth of 2-3 cm and block the joint with 20-30 ml of local anesthetic.

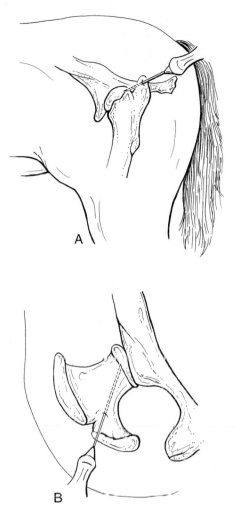

FIGURE 23-10. A, B, Coxofemoral joint (flexible 18-gauge, 5-inch [12.5-cm] needle with stylet). Palpate the greater trochanter and insert a needle 1 cm above the notch present between the anterior and posterior aspects of the trochanter. Thick muscles cover this joint, and the notch is difficult to palpate. Introduce the needle 8-10 cm in a slightly downward and anterior direction. Block the joint with 40 ml of local anesthetic.

Improvement after local anesthesia should be followed with radiography, ultrasonography, and/or nuclear scintigraphy examinations to identify the specific cause for the lameness.

Complications

Infection can be caused by improper skin preparation or concurrent cellulitis. Subcutaneous inflammation and skin sloughing can occur after **perineural anesthesia.** *Use sterile technique and a minimal amount of anesthetic to reduce risk. Rinse the distal limb with alcohol and wrap if multiple injections are performed.*

Joint or tendon sheath infection is a serious sequela to **intrasynovial anesthesia.** Monitor the patient for pain or swelling for 2 weeks after a diagnostic procedure. *Delay the procedure if periarticular cellulitis is present. Do not place a needle through a contaminated wound.* If signs of severe inflammation are present, treat for possible iatrogenic infection and lavage the joint.

Needle breakage is more likely in proximal joints when long, small-gauge needles are used. The needle often is difficult to retrieve if the horse is standing. Use flexible needles (spinal needles) that bend rather than break. Adequate patient restraint minimizes this complication.

> **CAUTION:** Anesthesia of the proximal limb can result in loss of motor function and stumbling. The distal limb should be wrapped to prevent abrasions, and patients should be confined to a stall immediately after the examination.

24 Arthrocentesis and Synovial Fluid Analysis

James A. Orsini and Christine Kreuder

Analysis of the synovial fluid from a joint or tendon sheath can be useful in differentiating diseases that affect these structures. Synovial fluid is an ultrafiltrate of plasma, and pathologic conditions of synovium-bathed structures are reflected in the fluid. Aspiration of synovial fluid from joints and tendon sheaths requires familiarity with the applied anatomy. Patient restraint and strict adherence to aseptic technique are essential for safe arthrocentesis.

Equipment

- Sedative (xylazine hydrochloride and butorphanol tartrate)
- Twitch
- Clippers
- Material for sterile scrub
- Sterile gloves
- Needles (18-22-gauge) and 5-20-ml syringe (not Luer-Lok); see Figs. 23–4 through 23–10 for needle size required for each joint. Needles and syringes should be kept sterile throughout the procedure.
- 25-gauge needle, 3-ml syringe, and 2% local anesthetic if anesthesia of skin is desired
- EDTA and plain Vacutainer tubes*
- Culture material (Port-a-Cul,† blood culture bottles‡)

Procedure

- Clip or shave the site for arthrocentesis. Sites for arthrocentesis are identical to the sites for intraarticular anesthesia in Figs. 23–4 through 23–10.

---

*Vacutainer tubes. Becton-Dickinson Vacutainer Systems, Rutherford, NJ 07070.
†Port-a-Cul culture swab and transport system. Becton-Dickinson Microbiology Systems, Cockeysville, MD 21030.
‡Septi-check, BB blood culture bottle. Roche Diagnostic Systems, Indianapolis, IN 46256.

CAUTION: Do not place the needle through an open or contaminated wound or an area of possible infection. Determination of joint involvement after trauma or infection often requires alternative needle placement if the usual site for joint access is contaminated in any way.

- Sedation is optional. Recommended dosage for adults: 0.3-0.5 mg/kg xylazine with 0.01-0.02 mg/kg butorphanol IV. For neonatal foals: 0.1-0.2 mg/kg diazepam IV **slowly.**
- Place twitch.
- Perform a sterile scrub of the puncture site and any landmarks to be palpated.
- If the joint requires a 20-gauge or larger needle, place a bleb of 2% local anesthetic subcutaneously using a 25-gauge needle.
- Wearing sterile gloves, detach the needle from the syringe and place the needle with a rapid stick through the skin. Care must be taken not to damage the articular cartilage with the needle. Successful needle placement results in synovial fluid at the hub of the needle. Fluid may flow freely (particularly if the joint is distended), or it may have to be aspirated with a syringe. Digital pressure on other aspects of the joint usually increases the flow of fluid from the needle.

Failure to obtain synovial fluid often is caused by placement of the needle within or adjacent to a ligament, cartilage, or synovial lining. Attempt to redirect or rotate the needle without exiting the skin. The needle may also become plugged with tissue during placement. If synovial fluid is not obtained after the needle is redirected, attempt arthrocentesis with a new needle.

- Collect the sample into a plain tube for culture and an EDTA (purple top) Vacutainer tube for cytologic examination. Samples may be transported in the syringe used for collection: remove air and cap with a sterile needle. If the culture sample is not to be processed within 12 hours, place the sample in a blood culture bottle or Port-a-Cul transport system.

SYNOVIAL FLUID ANALYSIS

Color, clarity, volume, and viscosity of fluid collected are parameters immediately assessed. Normal synovial fluid is clear, slightly yellow, and completely free of particulate. Red streaks indicate trauma and bleeding caused by the needle during placement or aspiration. A uniform red or amber tinge may be caused by chronic intraarticular injury. An increase in turbidity or a dark yellow color is caused by inflammation. The presence of particles or purulent material indicates serofibrinous inflammation, which is often associated with infection (septic arthritis or tenosynovitis).

Viscosity is directly related to the amount and quality of hyaluronic acid secreted by the synovial membrane. Depolymerization or dilution of hyaluronate from inflammation causes a decrease in viscosity. Viscosity is assessed subjectively by means of placing a drop of fluid between the thumb and a finger; normal fluid strings out approximately 2-5 cm before breaking. Fluid expressed from a syringe also should form a string approximately 5-7 cm long.

Other important parameters are complete white blood cell count and differential. A slide preparation is made with a drop of the synovial fluid and a drop of Wright stain. The quantity, type, and state of degeneration of the white blood cells are useful for characterizing the inflammation. Total protein level quantifies the

TABLE 24–1. Correlation Between Synovial Fluid Parameters and Intraarticular Disorders

Condition	Appearance	Viscosity	Volume	Total Protein (g/dl)	Nucleated Cells/L	Cytologic Findings	Glucose (mg/dl)
Normal	Light yellow, clear	High	Low	<2.0	<0.4 x 10^9	<20% neutrophils	Equal to blood
Nonseptic synovitis	Yellow, translucent	Low	Generally increased	<3.0	2-10 x 10^9	>75% neutrophils (preserved)	25-50 mg/dl; lower than blood
Septic arthritis	Yellow-green, turbid	Low	Increased	3.0-6.0	30-100 x 10^9	>90% neutrophils (degenerate) with or without intracellular bacteria	<25 mg/dl
Degenerative joint disease (osteoarthritis)	Yellow, clear	Low (variable)	Low	<2.5	0.2-2 x 10^9	10%-30% neutrophils (preserved)	Equal to blood

degree of inflammation. Normal synovial fluid does not clot because it lacks fibrinogen and other clotting factors present during inflammation. Glucose concentration in synovial fluid is compared with serum concentration and may be decreased owing to consumption by inflammatory cells and bacteria. A Gram stain and culture are essential if a septic process is suspected. Negative culture results do not rule out infection; bacteria are isolated in only 50% of samples. Polymerase chain reaction has not been uniformly beneficial to identify pathogens in suspected cases of septic arthritis.

Table 24–1 shows the correlation between synovial fluid parameters and specific equine joint disorders.

Complications

See complications of intrasynovial anesthesia, p. 103.

---

25 Temporomandibular Arthrocentesis

James A. Orsini

Synovial fluid can be obtained from the temporomandibular joint (TMJ) by means of arthrocentesis. Analysis of synovial fluid is useful for determining the pathologic features of disease in this region. Arthrocentesis also can be used to administer intraarticular medications or to perform intrasynovial anesthesia.

NOTE: The following descriptive procedure has not been studied in foals or in young horses that have not reached mature bone growth. Anatomical variations in the growing horse may not correlate directly with the following description to identify the TMJ.

Equipment

- Sedative (IV detomidine hydrochloride)
- Clippers
- Sterile scrub materials (povidone-iodine and alcohol)
- 20-gauge, 1.5-inch (3.8-cm) needles and syringes (3, 6, or 12 ml)
- EDTA and plain Vacutainer tubes
- Culture material

Procedure

- Clip an area bordered by the lateral canthus of the eye and the base of ear and from the facial crest to the zygomatic process of the temporal bone.
- Sedate patient.
- Scrub the area to be injected.
- Maintain aseptic technique.
- Palpate the TMJ by placing one finger on the lateral canthus of the eye and another finger at the base of the ear. With the middle three digits flexed, the third digit marks the lateral portion of the mandible (Fig 25–1).

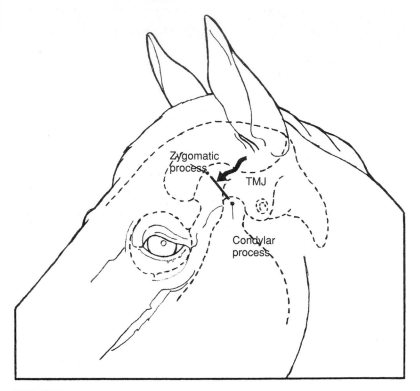

FIGURE 25-1. Location of zygomatic process of the temporal bone. *TMJ,* Temporomandibular joint.

- Palpate the zygomatic process, which is 1-2 cm dorsal to the condylar process of the mandible.
- A soft, depressed region should be palpable midway between the condylar process and 0.5-1.0 cm caudal to the imaginary line between the two bony structures.
- Insert a 20-gauge, 1.5-inch (3.8-cm) needle into the TMJ beginning perpendicular to the skull and directing the needle slightly rostral (approximately 15 degrees). The needle may have to be directed slightly ventral depending on the individual.
- Advance the needle 0.5-1.5 inches (1.6-3.8-cm) into the joint until synovial fluid appears. If bone is encountered, withdraw the needle and redirect it ventrally or dorsally to enter the joint.
- Collect samples into EDTA and red top (no additive) Vacutainer tubes for cytologic examination and culture. If the sample is not to be processed within 12 hours, place it in a blood culture bottle or a Port-a Cul transport system.

Complications
See complications of intrasynovial anesthesia, p. 103.

26 | Endoscopy of the Navicular Bursa

James A. Orsini

Penetrating injuries to the sole of the hoof often result in infectious bursitis because foreign objects tend to be directed toward the concave surface of the coffin bone. *This type of injury is an emergency, and surgical treatment is needed as soon as possible after the injury for the best prognosis.* Endoscopy of the navicular bursa offers an alternative surgical treatment to the traditional "street nail" procedure and results in a better outcome in most cases. The prognosis for puncture wounds resulting in sepsis of the navicular bursa is grave; however, the use of an arthroscope to debride the navicular bursa is the most appropriate treatment.

The technique for evaluation of the navicular bursa is useful for examination of the palmar and plantar surface of the

- Navicular bursa
- Insertions of the navicular suspensory ligaments
- T and impar ligaments
- Navicular bursal synovium (bursa podotrochlearis)
- Dorsal surface of the deep digital flexor tendon
  The technique facilitates the following procedures:
- Navicular bursa lavage
- Pannus debridement
- Synovial resection
- Debridement of lesions of the navicular bone and deep digital flexor tendon

Equipment
- General anesthesia equipment
- Arthroscopy equipment: 4-mm 25- to 30-degree forward oblique arthroscope*
- 18-gauge 3.5-inch needle (1.2 mm × 90 mm)
- EDTA and plain (no additive) Vacutainer tubes
- Culture material (Port-a-Cul, blood culture bottles)

Procedure (Fig. 26–1)
- Administer general anesthesia with patient in lateral recumbency with affected limb uppermost.
- Support limb proximal to metacarpo/metatarsophalangeal joint with the distal limb free.
- Clip or shave the area from the metacarpo/metatarsophalangeal joint 360 degrees to coronary band.
- Clean and debride the sole and point of entry of puncture wound.
- Maintaining aseptic technique, perform a sterile scrub of the puncture and surgical sites on the palmar/plantar aspect of the distal part of the limb:
  - Collect fluid samples for cytologic examination and microbiological cultures, and place the samples in an EDTA (purple top) Vacutainer tube and Port-a-Cul tube

---

*Karl Storz Veterinary Endoscopy-America, Inc; (800) 955-7832.

109

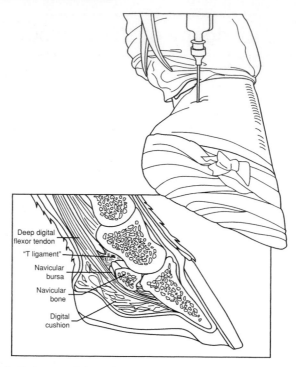

FIGURE 26-1. Endoscopy of the navicular bursa.

- □ Make a 5-mm skin incision proximal to the lateral cartilage ungularis (collateral cartilage) on the abaxial margin of the flexor digitorum profundus tendon (deep digital flexor tendon) axial to the palmar/plantar digital neurovascular bundle.
- □ Direct the arthroscope cannula with a conical obturator through the skin wound and advance it distally and axially dorsal to the deep digital flexor tendon so that it enters the bursa at approximately the midpoint of the phalanx.
- □ After the bursa is entered, withdraw the obturator and replace it with a 4-mm, 25- to 30-degree forward oblique arthroscope.
- ▪ Suture skin portals after the arthroscopic procedure.

Complications

Collateral damage to surrounding soft tissues can occur during insertion of the cannula. This is caused by lack of "hands-on" training and practice with the arthroscope.

REFERENCES

McIlwraith CW: *Diagnostic and surgical arthroscopy in the horse,* Philadelphia, 1990, Lea & Febiger.
Nixon AJ: Endoscopy of the digital flexor tendon sheath in horses, *Vet Surg* 19:255-271, 1990.
Wright IM, Phillips TJ, Walmsley JP: Endoscopy of the navicular bursa: a new technique for the treatment of contaminated and septic bursa, *Eq Vet J* 31:5-11, 1999.

The Eye

27 Corneal Scraping

James A. Orsini

Corneal ulcers often lead to secondary infection. The conjunctival sac normally contains predominately Gram-positive bacteria, along with fungal organisms. These organisms become pathogenic when the normal corneal epithelium is disrupted, such as with corneal ulcers. Scraping the cornea is a useful tool in identifying the appropriate bacterial or fungal microorganisms, which must be managed specifically. This procedure should be performed *before* administration of any local, topical anesthetic, which can inhibit microbial growth.

NOTE: This procedure should *not* be performed if the cornea is perforated or a descemetocele is present.

Equipment
- Kimura platinum spatula (A sterile dulled scalpel blade or blunt end of a scalpel blade also may be used.)
- Sabouraud agar plate
- Blood agar plate
- Blood culture broth
- Glass slides
- Commercial culturettes (pre-moistened), although less desirable, may be used in place of the agar plates
- Gram stain and Wright-Giemsa stain
- Fungal staining agents (Gomori methenamine silver, periodic acid–Schiff)

Procedure
- Scrape the cornea fairly aggressively (after confirming that the eye is not perforated and there is no descemetocele).
- Obtain several samples from both the center and periphery of the lesion.
- Inoculate the first sample into blood and Sabouraud agar plates (a pre-moistened commercial culturette may be used instead of the agar plates) or into a small amount of blood culture broth.
- Use three or four additional samples to make smears on glass slides for cytologic examination.
- Use Gram stain and Wright-Giemsa stain (separately) to identify bacteria.
- For fungal identification, use special stains such as Gomori methenamine silver and periodic acid–Schiff.
- If corneal scraping does not lead to the detection of microorganisms corneal biopsy may be needed.

28 Fluorescein Staining

James A. Orsini, Christine Kreuder, and Nita L. Irby

Fluorescein staining is an important diagnostic aid to identify diseases of the cornea and to determine the patency of the nasolacrimal duct. The most common use of topical fluorescein is to localize corneal ulcers. Defects in the corneal epithelium selectively retain the dye and stain bright green by conversion of absorbed light to fluorescent light. This procedure is indicated in *any* painful eye or whenever a corneal ulcer is suspected or there is a history of direct trauma to the eye.

Equipment
- Fluorescein strip[*]
- 5-ml sterile saline solution in a syringe or collyrium (sterile eye wash)
- Penlight or ophthalmoscope

Procedure
- Insert the fluorescein strip medially between the nictitans and lower lid or place the dry strip in a syringe with sterile saline to create a fresh fluorescein solution that can be sprayed onto the cornea. When the patient blinks, the fluorescein distributes over the cornea. Direct contact of the impregnated fluorescein strip to the cornea causes stain uptake and may be erroneously diagnosed as a corneal defect.
- Gentle flushing with saline solution or collyrium removes any excess stain.
- Using a source of direct light, examine the entire eye for stain uptake. Very deep corneal ulcers may take up stain only along their outermost borders.
- Ultraviolet, cobalt blue light, or a Wood's lamp excite fluorescein, facilitating detection of minute corneal epithelial defects.
- Patency of the nasolacrimal duct is verified if fluorescein dye appears at the nostril within 5 minutes but it can take up to 20 minutes in a normal horse.

---

[*]Fluor-i-strip (fluorescein sodium ophthalmic strip). Ayerst Laboratories, Inc., New York, NY 10017.

29 Nasolacrimal Duct Cannulation

James A. Orsini, Christine Kreuder, and Nita L. Irby

Cannulation of the nasolacrimal duct is indicated whenever obstruction of lacrimal drainage is suspected. Clinical signs often seen with obstruction include epiphora (tearing), staining beneath the eye, and discharge and swelling at the medial canthus. Cannulation is also a valuable method for delivering medications to the eye without having to manipulate the eye or eyelids. This is also a procedure required for dacryocystorhinography, which is used to define a congenital obstruction or acquired inflammatory lesion of the nasolacrimal duct. The duct is easily cannulated at its rostral opening, where it emerges at the mucocutaneous junction on the ventrum of either nostril.

Equipment

- Penlight
- 5F-8F polypropylene catheter* (French conversion: each unit French = 0.33-mm diameter)
- 10- or 12-ml syringe filled with sterile saline solution
- Gauze sponges
- Sterile lubricant†

Procedure

- Reflect the alar fold of the nostril and locate the puncta of the nasolacrimal duct using a light source. The rostral duct opening is easily located on the ventral aspect of the nasal meatus. Some horses have two or more puncta in one nostril and only one is patent, usually the most proximal.
- Swab the inside of the nostril and place the minimally lubricated catheter in the duct. Slide the catheter at least 5 cm proximally.
- To flush the duct, place a finger over the puncta to hold the catheter in place and prevent the saline solution from exiting normograde. Attach the syringe and gently flush the duct retrograde. Patency has been achieved once the saline solution flows from the lacrimal puncta at the medial canthus.
- The catheter may be sutured in place with a butterfly taping technique for routine ophthalmic medication.

---

*Polypropylene catheter. Monoject, Sherwood Medical, St. Louis, MO 63103.
†K-Y lubricating jelly. Johnson and Johnson Products, Inc., New Brunswick, NJ 08903.
H-R lubricating jelly. Carter Products, Division of Carter-Wallace, Inc., New York, NY 10105.

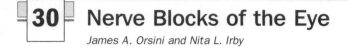

30 Nerve Blocks of the Eye

James A. Orsini and Nita L. Irby

ANATOMY REVIEW

The auriculopalpebral (AP) nerve (the palpebral nerve is one branch of the AP nerve and innervates the eye; the other branch, the auricular nerve, innervates the ear) branches off of the facial nerve (cranial nerve VII) and innervates the orbicularis oculi muscle, which is responsible for blinking. The facial nerve provides motor control of the muscles of the face, and the trigeminal nerve (cranial nerve V) conveys sensory information. The trigeminal nerve has three branches: the maxillary, ophthalmic, and mandibular nerves. The maxillary nerve further branches into the zygomatic nerve, which has sensory innervation to the lateral lower eye. The frontal, lacrimal, and infratrochlear nerves all branch off the ophthalmic nerve. These innervate the central upper eyelid, lateral upper eyelid, and medial canthus, respectively.

AURICULOPALPEBRAL NERVE BLOCK (See chapter 41, Ophthalmology, p. 436)

Auriculopalpebral nerve block affects motor function of the eyelid but does not desensitize the eyelid.

> **NOTE:** The auriculopalpebral nerve block is performed at the base of the ear and any more "distal" block is a palpebral nerve block ; this is an AP block but most described are not.

It is used routinely to examine the eye and to control movement of the eyelid. Branches of the dorsal buccal nerve also may have to be anesthetized along the facial crest to reduce movement of the lower eyelid.

Equipment
- 25-gauge, ⅝-inch (1.6-cm) needle, 5-ml syringe
- 2% Carbocaine (3-5 ml)

Procedure
- Palpate the caudal boarder of the ramus of the mandible and ventral edge of the zygomatic arch.
- A depression is felt, although the nerve itself cannot be palpated.
- Insert the needle into the depression of the temporal region of the zygomatic arch and direct the needle upward and caudal to the highest part of the arch (Fig. 30–1).
- Inject 3-5 ml of 2% Carbocaine (mepivacaine hydrochloride) in a fanlike manner.
- Massage the injection site to disperse the drug along the nerve.

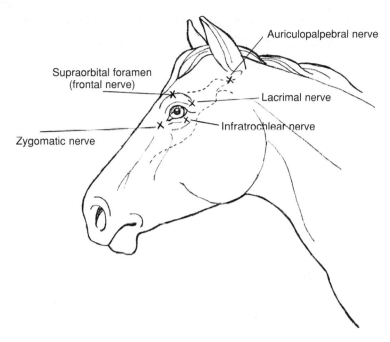

FIGURE 30-1. Nerve blocks of the eye.

FRONTAL NERVE BLOCK: ANESTHESIA OF THE CENTRAL UPPER EYELID (See p. 438)

For anesthetizing the frontal nerve and medial palpebral branch of the palpebral nerves; this block is useful for routine examination of the eye. It is the preferred block for controlling movement of the patient's upper eyelid and affecting sensation.

Equipment
- 25-gauge, ⅝-inch (1.6-cm) needle, 5-ml syringe
- 2% Carbocaine (5 ml)

Procedure
- Palpate the superior rim of the orbit where the supraorbital foramen is located; this foramen is at the midway point on the supraorbital process where it enlarges temporally, directly above the medial canthus.
- Instill 2 ml of 2% Carbocaine through a 1-inch (2.5-cm) needle placed 2 cm (0.75 inch) adjacent to the foramen.

| **NOTE:** It is not necessary to enter the foramen.

- Withdraw the needle while injecting an additional 1 ml of Carbocaine.
- Inject 2 ml into the subcutaneous tissue over the foramen (Fig. 30-1).

ZYGOMATIC NERVE BLOCK: ANESTHESIA OF THE LOWER LATERAL EYELID

Equipment
- 25-gauge, ⅝-inch (1.6-cm) needle, 5-ml syringe
- 2% Carbocaine (2-3 ml)

Procedure
- Place the index finger on ventral rim of the orbit and firmly press against the supraorbital portion of the zygomatic arch.
- Inject medial to index finger along the rim of the orbit into the lower eyelid (see Fig. 30–1).

LACRIMAL NERVE BLOCK: ANESTHESIA OF THE LATERAL UPPER EYELID

Equipment
- 25-gauge, ⅝-inch (1.6-cm) needle, 5-ml syringe
- 2% Carbocaine (2-3 ml)

Procedure
- Inject in a line block medially along the dorsal rim of the orbit, medial to the lateral canthus (see Fig. 30–1).

INFRATROCHLEAR NERVE: ANESTHESIA OF THE MEDIAL CANTHUS

Equipment
- 25-gauge, ⅝-inch (1.6-cm) needle, 5-ml syringe
- 2% Carbocaine (2-3 ml)

Procedure
- Palpate the irregularly shaped notch on the dorsal rim of the orbit near the medial canthus using firm thumb pressure.
- Inject 2-3 ml of Carbocaine deeply and rostrally to the notch (see Fig. 30-1).

31 Subpalpebral/Transpalpebral Catheter Placement

James A. Orsini, Christine Kreuder, and Nita L. Irby

Horses that need frequent or long-term topical administration of an eye medication are candidates for subpalpebral catheters. A catheter is placed through the eyelid, which allows delivery of medication(s) while standing at the patient's side. This system is ideal for difficult individuals that need frequent treatments. If complications do not occur, the catheter may remain in place from several weeks to months.

Equipment
- Sedative (xylazine hydrochloride)
- 2% local anesthetic with 25-gauge, ⅝-inch (1.6-cm) needle, 5-ml syringe
- 12-gauge, 1.5-inch (3.8 cm) needle with hub removed
- Silastic tubing (³⁄₁₀₀-inch [0.75-mm] inner diameter × ¹³⁄₂₀-inch [1.62 mm] outer diameter)* or polyethylene tubing (PE190)[†]
- Feline indwelling catheter (20-gauge) [‡]
- Subpalpebral eye lavage kit[§]
- Injection cap
- White tape
- 2-0 nonabsorbable suture on a straight needle
- Suture scissors

Procedure
- Recommended dose for sedation: 0.3-0.6 mg/kg xylazine IV.
- Anesthetize the auriculopalpebral and supraorbital nerves innervating the upper eyelid (Fig. 31–1).
- Place the lavage system **deep** in the dorsal palpebral fornix to minimize tubing contact with the corneal surface.
- Lift the upper eyelid and insert the 12-gauge needle up through the conjunctiva and skin in the dorsolateral aspect of the lid.
- Insert the Silastic tubing into the lumen of the needle in the same upward direction. Once the tubing exits from the sharp end of the needle, pull the needle out and thread the tubing through the lid until 10 cm of tubing remains below the lid.
- Reinsert the needle up through the conjunctiva and skin in the dorsomedial aspect of the lid, 4 cm medial to the first insertion. Thread the tail end of the tubing through the blunt end of the needle.

---

*Dow Corning Silastic tubing. Bausch & Lomb Surgical, St. Louis, MO 63122.

[†]Intramedic nonradiopaque polyethylene tubing. Clay Adams, Division of Becton-Dickinson and Co., Parsippany, NJ 07054.

[‡]Feline indwelling catheter (20-gauge). Sherwood Medical, 1915 Olive Street, St. Louis, MO 63103; (800) 428-4400.

[§]Subpalpebral eye lavage kit. 12-gauge trocar, 36-inch catheter/Cat. No. 6612; 14-gauge trocar, 18-inch/Cat. No. 6614. Mila International, Inc., 7604 Dixie Highway, Florence, KY 41042; (859) 371-1722, (888) 645-2468.

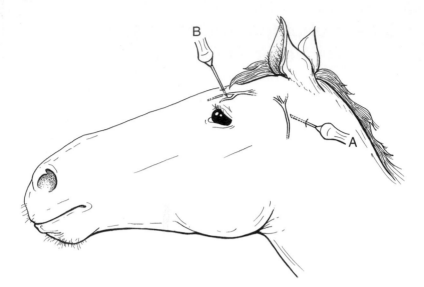

FIGURE 31-1. Needle placement for auriculopalpebral and supraorbital nerve blocks. *A,* Block the auriculopalpebral nerve as it runs along the zygomatic arch with 3-5 ml of local anesthetic. *B,* Block the supraorbital nerve at the ventral rim of the supraorbital fossa with 3-5 ml of local anesthetic.

- Remove the needle from the eyelid and tie several knots in the medial end of the tubing.
- Pull the knotted end of the tubing out of the lid and place a single hole in the tubing with a 25-gauge needle. Place the hole 1-2 cm from the knot so that the eye medication distributes over the eye rather than leaks subcutaneously.

NOTE: *"Two-hole" or more systems are difficult to manage and have an increased incidence of complications.*

- Position the tubing and secure it dorsal to the eyelid in at least two areas on the forehead and near the poll. Place white tape around the tubing and suture the tape to the skin. Secure the tubing to the neck by taping it to a braided mane (Fig. 31-2).
- Insert a feline indwelling catheter (without the needle) into the tubing and attach an injection cap as a portal for drug administration.
- Administer the medication through the injection cap by standing at the withers of the patient. Fill the line with medication until drops are seen spreading over the cornea. Different medications may be mixed in the line. Continuous administration of ophthalmic solution may be delivered by a pressurized fluid bag attached to the mane or a surcingle.

Complications
Corneal ulceration develops if the catheter scratches the cornea. Tubing should be soft and pliable and have no rough edges. *Lift the upper eyelid and check the*

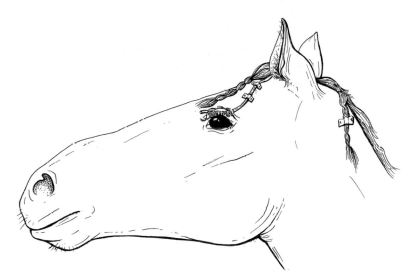

FIGURE 31–2. Placement of a subpalpebral catheter.

position of the catheter several times daily to make sure it has not migrated over the cornea.

A **swollen** and **irritated eyelid** occurs if the catheter migrates into the conjunctiva and medication goes into subcutaneous tissue. Some patients rub their eyes because both the catheter and ocular disease are irritating. *Fly nets or hoods with eye cups prevent trauma to the catheter and the eye.* Use caution when manipulating sharp objects around the eye because sudden movement of even a properly restrained horse can cause puncture of the globe. *Guard the sharp end of the object as much as possible.*

The hole in the Silastic tubing often becomes plugged with fibrin after several days. Retract the tubing from under the eyelid and flush medication through the hole by administering a new dose. If this is unsuccessful, make an additional hole with a 25-gauge needle, taking care not to lacerate the tubing.

Central Nervous System

 32 Cerebrospinal Fluid Collection

James A. Orsini and Christine Kreuder

Cerebrospinal fluid (CSF) analysis is indicated whenever disease of the central nervous system is suspected. Analysis helps determine involvement of the central nervous system (CNS) (as opposed to peripheral neuropathy), and specific changes in the CSF are well correlated with certain infectious diseases. Fluid may be aspirated from two sites: the lumbosacral space and the atlantooccipital space. Collection from the atlantooccipital space must be done under general anesthesia, which may be contraindicated in patients with cerebral swelling.

Equipment
- Twitch and/or sedation (detomidine and butorphanol tartrate)
- Clippers
- Material for sterile scrub
- Sterile gloves
- 2% local anesthetic, 6-ml syringe and 22-gauge, 1.5-inch (3.75-cm) needle
- 15-cm (6-inch) or 20-cm (8-inch), 18-gauge spinal needle for lumbosacral aspirate or 9-cm (3.5-inch), 18-gauge needle for atlantooccipital aspirate* (sterile)
- 12-ml syringe (sterile)
- EDTA and plain Vacutainer tubes†
- Culture‡ or Port-a-Cul§ culture system
- Stool to stand on to reach puncture site
- Styrofoam shipping container with ice packs and appropriate address labels for sample submission by 1- or 2-day delivery to EBI and/or Neogen Corporation (see p. 000)

Procedure
COLLECTION FROM THE LUMBOSACRAL SPACE
- Restrain horse in stocks or perform the lumbosacral aspirate in a stall if there is a concern of an adverse reaction. Sedation is generally not necessary but is

---

*Spinal needles. Becton-Dickinson, Franklin Lakes, NJ 07417.

†Vacutainer tubes. Becton-Dickinson Vacutainer Systems, Rutherford, NJ 07070.

‡Culturette collection and transport system. Becton-Dickinson Microbiology Systems, Cockeysville, MD 21030.

§Port-a-Cul tube. BBL Division of Becton-Dickinson and Company, Cockeysville, MD 21030.

recommended. Recommended dosage: 0.01-0.02 mg/kg detomidine with 0.01-0.02 mg/kg butorphanol IV.
- See Fig. 32–1 for landmarks for the lumbosacral tap.
- Wear sterile gloves and maintain sterility throughout procedure.
- Place a bleb of local anesthetic beneath the skin and 3-5 ml in the deeper muscle layers.
- With the patient standing squarely, insert a 6-inch/8-inch (15-cm/20-cm) spinal needle perpendicular to the midline. The subarachnoid space is approximately 11-15 cm deep to the skin in the average adult. A loss of resistance is often felt as the needle passes into the subarachnoid space and there is often sudden patient movement that varies from tail "tuck" to more violent reactions.
- Remove the trocar from the needle.
- Fluid frequently appears at the needle hub soon after the subarachnoid space has been penetrated. Occlude both jugular veins with digital pressure to increase CNS pressure.
- If the initial sample appears blood contaminated, discard and use another syringe for additional sampling.
- Aspirate fluid with a syringe and place the sample into EDTA and plain Vacutainer tubes and onto a Culturette swab if a culture is indicated.

COLLECTION FROM THE ATLANTOOCCIPITAL SPACE
- Place the patient under general anesthesia to maintain proper position of the head and neck. This spinal tap is performed over the proximal cervical spinal cord and it is therefore possible to traumatize nervous tissue if the head or neck moves.
- Flex the patient's neck so that the head is at a right angle to the neck.
- See Fig. 32–2 for landmarks for the atlantooccipital aspirate.
- Clip area and perform a sterile scrub. Maintain sterility throughout the procedure.
- Wearing sterile gloves, insert the 3.5-inch (8.75-cm) spinal needle to a depth of 5-7 cm. Remove the trocar to determine correct placement in the subarachnoid space.
- Once CSF appears at the needle hub, aspirate the fluid with a syringe or allow the CSF to flow into collection tube.

CEREBROSPINAL FLUID ANALYSIS

CSF is examined grossly for color, clarity, and particulate matter. Normal CSF is clear and colorless. An increase in turbidity or particles occurs with inflammation and infectious diseases. Red streaks in the fluid are caused by contamination during collection, whereas previous hemorrhage in the CNS produces a xanthochromic or yellow-colored sample. Total protein measurement and cytologic examination (including total white blood cell and red blood cell counts) should be performed on every aspirate. Various changes in the cellular content are typical for specific disease processes. See Table 32–1 for correlation between abnormal values and CNS disease. Other parameters to measure are creatine phosphokinase (CPK) level (normally less than 8 IU/dl) and glucose level (normally between 55 and 70 mg/dl). CPK is found in fat and dura, and although the enzyme may be released with neuronal cell damage or degeneration, measurement is generally not a reliable monitor for CNS disease. Glucose levels are lower than normal with inflammation owing to consumption of glucose by white blood cells and bacteria.

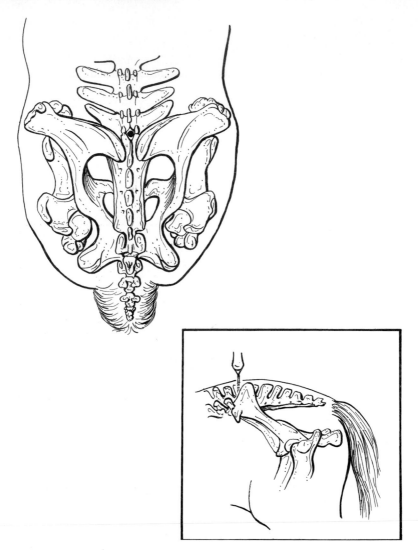

FIGURE 32–1. Needle placement for collection of CSF from the lumbosacral (LS) space. The LS space is generally palpable as a depression caudal to the sixth lumbar spinous process. Palpate the caudal edge of each tuber coxae and draw a line directly to midline to find the depression. This area (*inset*) is often cranial to the prominence of each tuber sacrale. Angle the needle directly perpendicular to the vertebrae.

Complications

Trauma to the spinal cord or brainstem during needle placement, although rare, can cause neurologic impairment. *Minimize patient movement with stocks and/or sedation.*

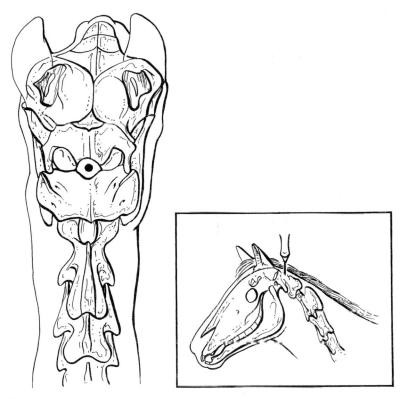

FIGURE 32-2. Needle placement for collection of CSF from the atlantooccipital space. Palpate the cranial borders of the atlas and draw a line directly to midline. The site for puncture *(inset)* is 1-2 cm caudal to this line directly on the midline. Angle the needle perpendicular to the cervical vertebrae.

Infection of the meninges, although very rare, can be fatal; therefore maintain sterile technique.

TABLE 32–1. Correlation of Cerebral Spinal Fluid Parameters and Central Nervous System Disorders

Condition	Appearance*	Total Protein* (mg/dl)	Total Nucleated Cells*/ml	Cytologic Findings
Normal	Clear, colorless	40-90	0-5	All mononuclear cells
Bacterial infection	White-amber to yellow, may be turbid	>100	>50	↑ Neutrophils
Viral infection	Clear-turbid, colorless, amber	100-200	Low normal to increased	Predominantly lymphocytes†
Hemorrhage or trauma	Uniformly red‡ or yellow§	>100	0-variable	Macrophages, erythrophagia and neutrophils
Fungal infection	Clear to yellow	100-200	>100	↑ Neutrophils
Protozoal infection#	Clear to yellow	40-200	0-40	Mixed macrophages, lymphocytes, and neutrophils

*Characteristic finding but may vary.
†May be neutrophilic with severe and/or chronic disease.
‡Recent hemorrhage.
§Past hemorrhage.
#<15% of horses with EPM have abnormal values.

33 Caudal Epidural Catheterization

Michael Tomasic

Placement of a caudal epidural catheter in a horse provides a means of repeat delivery of pharmacologic agents for pain management to the caudal epidural space without having to access that space anew each time. When properly placed, an epidural catheter can be maintained for several days to several weeks. Epidural catheter kits* contain an epidural needle (through which the catheter is inserted), the catheter, and an adapter that provides a standard Luer fitting for syringe or injection-port attachment; the kits are commercially available (Fig. 33–1).

Procedure

- Clip and aseptically prepare the caudal back of the patient, a rectangular area extending from the caudal aspect of the sacrum to the level of the caudal aspect of the third coccygeal vertebra (C_o3) and extending approximately 6 cm on either side of the midline.
- Preferred access to the epidural space is at the level of C_o1-2. Access also is possible at S5-C_o1 or C_o2-3. Inject 2-3 ml of 2% lidocaine or mepivacaine subcutaneously over the insertion site to minimize discomfort associated with insertion of the epidural needle. To facilitate needle insertion, make a 1-2 mm incision through the anesthetized skin on the midline.
- Before placing the epidural needle, pass the catheter through the needle until it is seen at the tip of the needle to confirm catheter position and length.

NOTE: Identify the markings on the catheter at the level of the needle hub or mark with sterile pen as catheter insertion distances are measured from this mark.

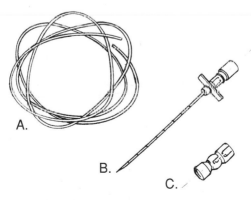

FIGURE 33-1. Contents of Perifix epidural catheter kit. **A,** 20-gauge, blunt tipped polyamide catheter. **B,** 3.5-inch (8.75 cm) Touhy-Schliff epidural needle. **C,** Catheter adapter.

---

*Perifix continuous epidural catheter set, product code CE-18T, B. Braun Medical, Inc., Bethlehem, PA 18017.

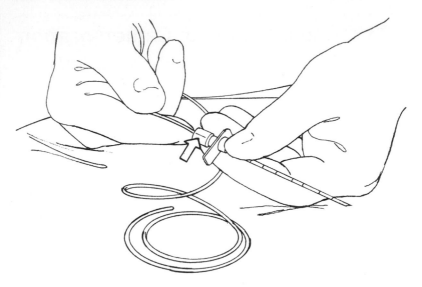

FIGURE 33–2. Identify the catheter mark when catheter is at the needle tip. This mark is used to judge the distance of catheter insertion.

- Advance the epidural needle in a downward direction, with the stylet in place and the bevel of the needle directed cranially, until a loss of resistance to passage is felt, indicating entry into the caudal epidural space. To facilitate advancement of the catheter into the space, the needle may be angled 20-30 degrees caudal to vertical during insertion (Fig. 33–3). Remove the stylet and confirm access to the epidural space using either the **hanging-drop technique** or the **loss of resistance technique.**
- Pass the catheter through the epidural needle (Fig. 33–4). Some initial resistance to catheter passage is felt as the tip of the catheter passes through the end of the needle; thereafter resistance to catheter passage should be minimal. If the catheter does not pass freely or if it advances only a few millimeters beyond the end of the needle, it is *not* in the epidural space. Advance the catheter until the catheter tip is approximately 1-2 cm cranial to the caudal border of S5, that is, just inside the sacral canal.
- While holding the catheter in place, remove the epidural needle. Trim the catheter so the length extending from the skin is approximately 12-20 cm. Secure the catheter adapter onto the free end of the catheter (Fig. 33–5). An injection cap may be added at this time.
- Drug injections can be made at any time.

NOTE: Because of the small diameter and long length of the catheter, considerable resistance to injection of fluids is felt. It is unnecessary and inadvisable to flush any residual drug from the catheter after the injection. Secure the catheter in place using a method that maintains its position, prevents contamination of the entry site, and stops the patient from removing it by rubbing or rolling.

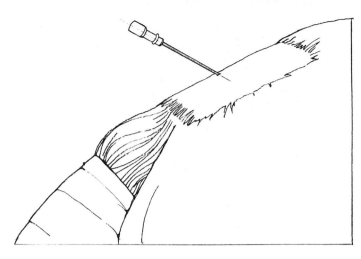

FIGURE 33-3. Insert needle angled slightly back from vertical to facilitate passage of catheter in epidural space.

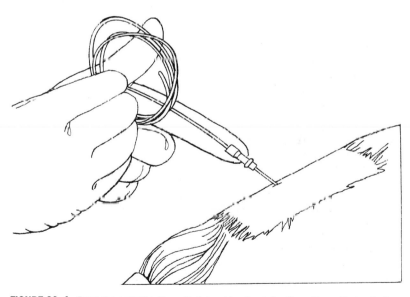

FIGURE 33-4. Pass the catheter through the epidural needle. Once the catheter tip is passed through the needle, resistance to further passage is minimal.

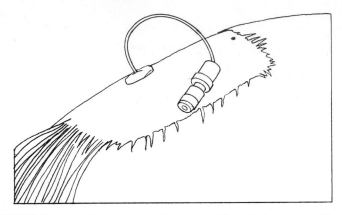

FIGURE 33–5. Excess catheter has been trimmed, and the catheter adapter with injection cap is in place.

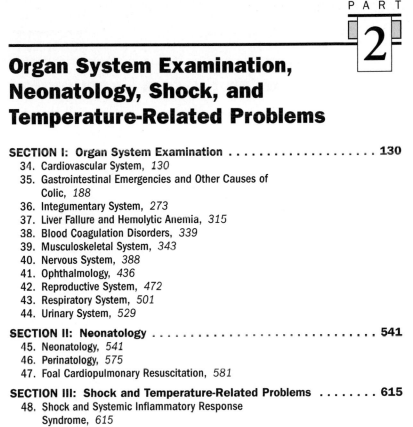

P A R T

Organ System Examination, Neonatology, Shock, and Temperature-Related Problems

Organ System Examination

 34 Cardiovascular System

Virginia B. Reef

PHYSICAL EXAMINATION

A complete cardiovascular examination of a horse includes auscultation of the heart; auscultation of both lung fields; palpation of the precordium; palpation of the arterial pulses; evaluation of the venous system, mucous membranes, and capillary refill time; and an overall assessment of the patient's health. In the emergency setting, the horse usually is distressed, and only a resting examination is indicated. The patient's clinical condition should be assessed as quickly as possible so that the appropriate lifesaving treatment, if needed, can be instituted as soon as possible.

Auscultation of the Heart

Auscultation of the heart is performed from *both* sides of the horse's chest. Heart rate, rhythm, and intensity of heart sounds are evaluated, and any murmurs or transient sounds associated with the cardiac cycle are characterized.

- The normal heart rate is 28-44 beats/min in an adult at rest and may be as high as 80 beats/min in a foal. (Average for an equine neonate is 70 beats/min.)
- The most common normal rhythm in horses is sinus rhythm.
- Second-degree atrioventricular (AV) block is the most common vagally mediated arrhythmia detected in normal horses. It is detected in 15%-18% of horses on a resting electrocardiogram (ECG) and in 44% of horses during 24-hour continuous ECG monitoring.
- Sinus arrhythmia, sinus bradycardia, sinoatrial (SA) block, and SA arrest also occur in normal individuals with high resting vagal tone.
- Identify heart sounds and characterize their timing and intensity. Up to four heart sounds can be auscultated in normal horses (Table 34–1).
- Auscultate the heart over all four valve areas (Fig. 34–1).
- Characterize murmurs by their intensity, timing, duration, quality, point of maximal intensity, and radiation (Table 34–2).
- **Intensity:** The loudness of the murmur and the ability to detect the murmur on palpation of the precordium. The intensity of the murmur, 1/6-6/6, is determined by the quantity and velocity of blood flow through the origin of the murmur, the distance of the murmur from the stethoscope, and the acoustic properties of the interposed tissue.
  - **Grade 1:** The softest audible murmur, detected only after minutes of intense listening

130

TABLE 34–1. Equine Heart Sounds

Sound	Genesis	PMI	Quality
S_1	Early ventricular contraction, abrupt deceleration of blood associated with tensing of the AV valve leaflets and AV valve closure, opening of the semilunar valves, and vibrations associated with ejection of blood into the great vessels	L apex	Loud, high frequency Longer, louder Lower pitch than S_2
S_2	Closure of the semilunar valves, abrupt deceleration of blood in the great vessels, opening of the AV valves	L base	Loud, high frequency Sharper, short Higher pitch than S_1
S_3	Rapid deceleration of blood in the ventricles at the end of the rapid ventricular filling phase; transient AV valve closure may occur	L apex	Soft, low frequency Lower pitch than S_2
S_4	Vibrations associated with blood flow from atria to ventricles during atrial contraction; transient AV valve closure may occur	L base	Soft, low frequency Lower pitch than S_1

PMI, Point of maximal intensity; *AV,* atrioventricular; *L,* left.

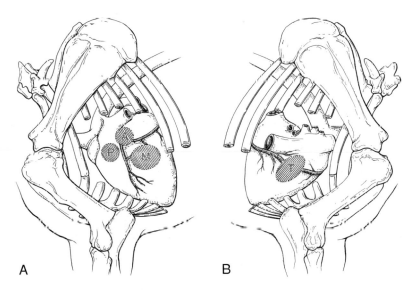

FIGURE 34–1. Cardiac auscultation areas in the horse viewed from the left **(A)** and the right **(B)** side of the thorax. Shaded areas represent the respective valve areas. *P,* Pulmonic valve; *A,* aortic valve; *M,* mitral valve; *T,* tricuspid valve.

- **Grade 2:** A soft murmur that is immediately detected at its point of maximal intensity
- **Grade 3:** A louder, moderate-intensity murmur that is easily heard but lacks a precordial thrill
- **Grade 4:** A loud murmur that has a faint precordial thrill palpable at the point of maximal intensity of the murmur

TABLE 34–2. Characterization of the Common Equine Cardiac Murmurs

Murmur	Intensity (Grade)	Timing	Duration	Quality/ Shape	PMI	Radiation
Physiologic	1-2	S	E, M, L, HS	Low frequency	A, P, Mi, T	
(flow)	1-3	D	E, M, L	Decrescendo	A, P, Mi, T	
MR	2-6	S	HS, PS	Mixed, plateau	Mi A	DCa DCr
MVP	2-6	S	M-L	Crescendo	Mi	DCa
TR	2-6	S	HS, PS	Mixed, plateau	T	DCr, DCa
TVP	2-6	S	M-L	Crescendo	T	
AR	1-6	D	HD	Low frequency, decrescendo musical, decrescendo	A	DCr Apex (left)
PR	1-6	D	HD	Low frequency, musical, decrescendo	P	Apex (right)
VSD	3-6	S	HS, PS	Mixed, plateau	T	P

PMI, Point of maximal intensity; *S*, systolic; *D*, diastolic; *E*, early; *M*, mid; *L*, late; *HS*, holosystolic; *PS*, pansystolic; *HD*, holodiastolic; *A*, aortic valve; *P*, pulmonic valve; *Mi*, mitral valve; *T*, tricuspid valve; *DCa*, dorsocaudal; *DCr*, dorsocranial; *MR*, mitral regurgitation; *MVP*, mitral valve prolapse; *TR*, tricuspid regurgitation; *TVP*, tricuspid valve prolapse; *AR*, aortic regurgitation; *PR*, pulmonic regurgitation; *VSD*, ventricular septal defect.

- □ **Grade 5:** A louder murmur with a strong precordial thrill palpable at the point of maximal intensity of the murmur
- □ **Grade 6:** The loudest possible murmur, with a strong precordial thrill that can be heard when the head of the stethoscope is removed from the chest
- ▪ **Timing:** The phase of the cardiac cycle (systolic, diastolic, or both) that the murmur occupies
- ▪ **Duration:** The length of time the murmur is detectable within each phase of the cardiac cycle
  - □ Early, mid, or late systolic: Occurs in early (immediately after the first heart sound, S_1), mid (midway between S_1 and S_2), or late (immediately before S_2) systole
  - □ Holosystolic: Occurs between S_1 and S_2 but does not encompass these heart sounds
  - □ Pansystolic: Begins at the onset of S_1 and ends at the completion of S_2
  - □ Early, mid, or late diastolic: Occurs in early (between S_2 and S_3), mid (midway between S_2 and S_1), or late (between S_4 and S_1) diastole
  - □ Holodiastolic: Between S_2 and S_1
  - □ Continuous: Through all phases of the cardiac cycle
- ▪ **Quality:** The frequency (high, low, or mixed-pitch) and character (harsh, coarse, rumbling, scratchy, musical, honking, or blowing) of the murmur detected
- ▪ **Shape:** Determined by the phonocardiographic depiction of the intensity of the murmur over time (band- or plateau-shaped, crescendo-decrescendo or diamond-shaped, crescendo, decrescendo, or machinery)

- **Point of maximal intensity**: The point of the thoracic wall (intercostal space or valve area) where the murmur is heard the loudest. This point should correspond to the area of the strongest precordial thrill if a precordial thrill is present.
- **Radiation**: The direction in which the murmur intensity decreases most slowly. The radiation of the murmur usually is from the origin of the murmur in the direction of abnormal blood flow and is also determined by the intensity of the murmur and physical characteristics of the chest.

Auscultation of Other Pulses

- Palpate the precordium over both sides of the chest to detect precordial thrills or abnormal apex beats (accentuated, faint, or displaced).
- Rhythm disturbances are classified as bradyarrhythmias or tachyarrhythmias.
- Evaluate the arterial pulses simultaneously with cardiac auscultation to determine that they are synchronous with every heartbeat.
- Assess the quality of the arterial pulses in the facial or transverse facial artery and in the extremities.
- Evaluate the jugular vein, saphenous vein, and other peripheral veins for distention and pulsations.
- Perform auscultation of both lung fields at rest and, if possible, with the patient breathing into a rebreathing bag. *The rebreathing bag should not be used at all, or should be used with care,* if the horse is in severe respiratory distress.
- Diagnosis of rhythm disturbances is made with an ECG.
- Diagnosis and assessment of the severity of valvular, pericardial, myocardial, or great-vessel disease, are made with an echocardiogram.

ELECTROCARDIOGRAM

Obtain a complete 12-lead ECG whenever possible (Table 34–3, Fig. 34–2). In an emergency, the base-apex lead may be all that is needed to diagnose accurately the rhythm disturbance present in the equine patient. Occasionally, however, because of the extensive Purkinje fiber network present in the equine ventricle, it may be difficult to determine whether the rhythm disturbance detected is ventricular or supraventricular. In these situations at least two different leads are needed to determine the origin of the abnormal depolarization.

- The base-apex lead gives the clinician large, easy to read complexes, and the electrodes usually can be properly applied with minimal resistance from the horse.
- The base-apex lead can be easily obtained in a recumbent horse when obtaining a full 12-lead ECG may be difficult. The electrodes can be applied at the heart base and apex on the same side of the patient if necessary.
- The base-apex lead is the best monitoring lead for radiotelemetry ECG systems, for continuous 24-hour Holter ECG monitoring, and for monitoring cardiac rhythm in critically ill patients, during antiarrhythmic therapy, or during pericardiocentesis.
- Heart rate can be quickly estimated at 25 mm/s paper speed as "Bic pen" × 10.
- Transtelephonic ECG systems have one important disadvantage in an emergency. The clinician transmitting the ECG usually is not able to evaluate the ECG as it is being obtained because he or she does not see the ECG tracing. Instead, the clinician has to wait for the assessment of the person receiving the ECG to

TABLE 34–3. Electrode Placement for Complete 12-Lead Electrocardiogram

Lead I: LA–RA	Left foreleg (left arm) electrode placed just below the point of the elbow on the back of the left forearm. Right foreleg (right arm) electrode placed just below the point of the elbow on the back of the right forearm.
Lead II: LL–LA	Left hindleg (left leg) electrode placed on the loose skin at the left stifle in the region of the patella. Left foreleg (left arm) electrode placed just below the point of the elbow on the back of the left forearm.
Lead III: LL–RA	Left hindleg (left leg) electrode placed on the loose skin at the left stifle in the region of the patella. Right foreleg (right arm) electrode placed just below the point of the elbow on the back of the right forearm.
aV_R: RA–CT	Right foreleg (right arm) electrode placed just below the point of the elbow on the back of the right forearm. The electrical center of the heart or central terminal $\times 3/2$.
aV_L: LA–CT	Left foreleg (left arm) electrode placed just below the point of the elbow on the back of the left forearm. The electrical center of the heart or central terminal $\times 3/2$.
aV_F: LL–CT	Left hindleg (left leg) electrode placed on the loose skin at the left stifle in the region of the patella. The electrical center of the heart or central terminal $\times 3/2$.
CV_6LL: V_1–CT	V_1 electrode placed in the 6th intercostal space on the left side of the thorax along a line parallel to the level of the point of the elbow. The electrical center of the heart (central terminal).
CV_6LU: V_2–CT	V_2 electrode placed in the 6th intercostal space on the left side of the thorax along a line parallel to the level of the point of the shoulder. The electrical center of the heart (central terminal).
V_{10}: V_3–CT	V_3 electrode placed over the dorsal thoracic spine of T7 at the withers. Electrical center of the heart. The dorsal spine of T7 is located on a line encircling the chest in the 6th intercostal space (central terminal).
CV_6RL: V_4–CT	V_4 electrode placed in the 6th intercostal space on the right side of the thorax along a line parallel to the level of the point of the elbow. The electrical center of the heart (central terminal).
CV_6RU: V_5–CT	V_5 electrode placed in the 6th intercostal space on the right side of the thorax along a line parallel to the level of the point of the shoulder. The electrical center of the heart (central terminal).
Base-apex: LA–RA	Left foreleg (left arm) electrode placed in the 6th intercostal space on the left side of the thorax along a line parallel to the level of the point of the elbow. Right foreleg (right arm) electrode placed on the top of the right scapular spine.

select an appropriate treatment. With real-time telemedicine, the clinician can evaluate the ECG with a specialist and be involved in its interpretation.

ARRHYTHMIAS

Cardiac arrhythmias occur commonly in horses and rarely necessitate antiarrhythmic therapy. Certain cardiac arrhythmias, however, can be life threatening and necessitate emergency treatment. Rapid tachyarrhythmias and profound bradyarrhythmias are most likely to necessitate immediate treatment to control the arrhythmia and relieve the signs of cardiovascular collapse.

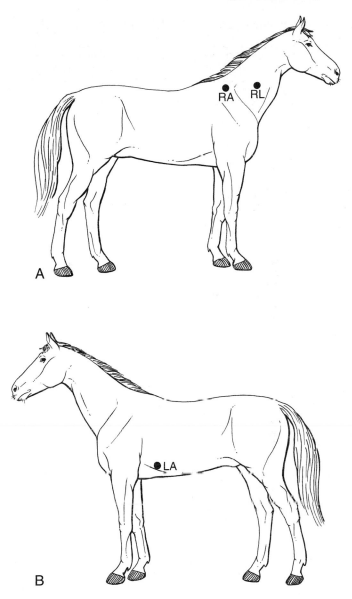

FIGURE 34–2. Sites for lead placement for obtaining a base-apex electrocardiogram (**A** and **B**) and a complete electrocardiogram (*C* and *D*) in a horse. The black circles represent the sites of attachment for the electrodes. **A,** Position of the electrode on the right side of the patient for recording a base-apex electrocardiogram with the electrodes from lead I. *RA,* right foreleg (right arm); *RL,* right hindleg (right leg). **B,** Position of the electrode on the left side of the patient for recording a base-apex electrocardiogram with the electrodes from lead I. *LA,* Left foreleg (left arm).

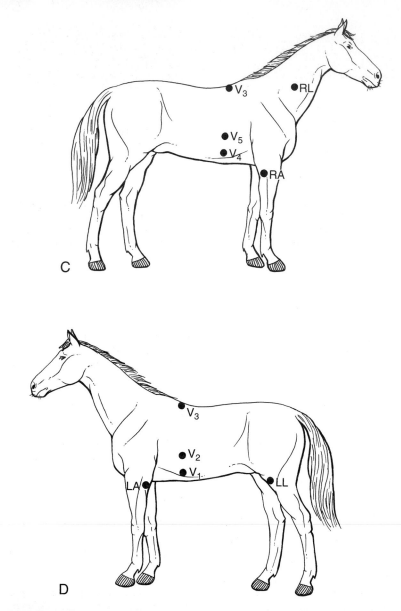

FIGURE 34–2. *Continued.* **C,** Position of the electrode on the right side of the patient for recording a complete electrocardiogram. *RA,* Right foreleg (right arm); *RL,* right hindleg (right leg); V_3, third chest lead (V_{10}); V_4, fourth chest lead (CV_6RL); V_5, fifth chest lead (CV_6RU). **D,** Position of the electrode on the left side of the patient for recording a complete electrocardiogram. *LA,* Left foreleg (left arm); *LL,* left hindleg (left leg); V_1, first chest lead (CV_6LL); V_2, second chest lead (CV_6LU); V_3, third chest lead (V_{10}).

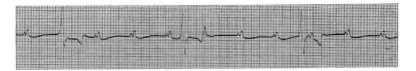

FIGURE 34–3. Base-apex electrocardiogram of a horse with complete heart block. Large, wide QRS complexes are evident and are not associated with the preceding P waves. There is complete atrioventricular dissociation with a rapid, regular atrial rate of 70 beats/min and a slow, regular ventricular rate of 20 beats/min. The PP interval is regular, and the RR interval is regular. This electrocardiogram was recorded at a paper speed of 25 mm/s with a sensitivity of 10 mm = 1 mV.

- An ECG is necessary to confirm the diagnosis of the rhythm disturbance auscultated and to choose the appropriate treatment.
- Perform continuous ECG monitoring on all horses with potentially life-threatening arrhythmias to monitor cardiac rhythm and response to treatment.

Bradyarrhythmias
Complete (Third-Degree) Atrioventricular Block
- Rare
- Usually associated with inflammatory or degenerative changes in the AV node
- Severe exercise intolerance and frequent syncope are common
- Resting heart rate (ventricular rate) usually ≤20 beats/min, with a more rapid, independent atrial rate

AUSCULTATION
- Loud, regular S_1 and S_2
- Slow ventricular rate (≤20 beats/min)
- Rapid, regular independent S_4 (usually ≥60/minute). Occasional *bruit de canon* sounds caused by the summation of S_4 with another heart sound (S_1, S_2, or S_3)

ELECTROCARDIOGRAM
- Rapid atrial rate (more P waves than QRS complexes)
- Regular PP interval
- No evidence of AV conduction, no consistent relation between P waves and QRS complexes (PR intervals of different lengths)
- Abnormal QRS configuration (usually widened and bizarre) unassociated with the preceding P waves (Fig. 34–3)
- The dominant pacemaker is idionodal or idioventricular.
- RR interval usually is regular but is irregular when more than one QRS configuration is present in association with complexes arising from different areas in the ventricle (Fig. 34–4).

TREATMENT
- Should be aggressive when arrhythmia is diagnosed.
- *Vagolytic drugs:* Atropine or glycopyrrolate should be administered IV at a dose of **0.005-0.01 mg/kg** as a bolus. Usually unsuccessful in restoring sinus rhythm;

CARDIOVASCULAR

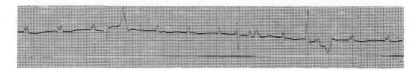

FIGURE 34-4. Lead II electrocardiogram of a horse with complete heart block. Large wide QRS complexes of differing configurations are evident and are not associated with the preceding P waves. There is complete atrioventricular dissociation with a rapid regular atrial rate of 70 beats/min and a slow, irregular ventricular rate of 30 beats/min. The PP interval is regular, and the RR interval is irregular. This electrocardiogram was recorded at a paper speed of 25 mm/s with a sensitivity of 10 mm = 1 mV.

side effects include tachycardia, arrhythmias, decreased gastrointestinal motility, and mydriasis.
- *Corticosteroids:* Dexamethasone is indicated in high doses (**0.05-0.22 mg/kg**) IV (preferable), IM, or PO, in the hope that reversible inflammatory disease is present in the region of the AV node.
  □ *Laminitis* is an undesirable side effect of corticosteroid use in the care of horses. It occurs most frequently after prolonged use of large doses of corticosteroids. Immune suppression and iatrogenic adrenal insufficiency can occur with prolonged use of corticosteroids. Exacerbation or recrudescence of viral and bacterial infections with corticosteroid use also is a potential problem and should be considered in the evaluation of horses with suspected myocarditis.
- *Sympathomimetic drugs* to speed idioventricular rhythm. These drugs should be used with care, or not at all, if other ventricular ectopy is present, because they may exacerbate ventricular arrhythmias.
  □ *Isoproterenol,* **0.05-0.2 μg/kg/min**, is indicated when syncope is present and if no ventricular ectopy is detected. Rapid tachyarrhythmias are an undesirable side effect. *If tachyarrhythmias occur, stop isoproterenol infusion and manage ventricular arrhythmias with lidocaine or propranolol.*
- *Implantation of a cardiac pacemaker.* Definitive management of complete heart block, if no response is seen with corticosteroid therapy. A permanent transvenous pacemaker has been successfully implanted in a horse with complete heart block (Figs. 34-5 and 34-6). Temporary transvenous pacemakers can be tried in the treatment of horses with advanced second-degree or complete AV block until a permanent transvenous pacemaker can be inserted.
  □ Temporary transvenous pacemakers are less successful in capturing the cardiac rhythm because these pacing wires are not anchored in the right ventricle but are free floating. The temporary pacing wires tend to float in the blood within the right ventricular chamber without making consistent contact with the right ventricular free wall. Contact between the pacing wire and the right ventricular free wall is necessary for the electrical impulse to result in ventricular depolarization.

Advanced Second-Degree Atrioventricular Block
- May also be associated with severe exercise intolerance and collapse
- Can be seen with electrolyte imbalances, such as hypercalcemia, digitalis toxicity, and AV nodal disease

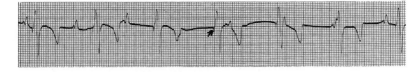

FIGURE 34-5. Base-apex electrocardiogram of a horse with complete heart block treated with a ventricular demand pacemaker and a single pacing electrode in the right ventricle. The pacing spike *(arrow)* initiates the ventricular depolarization at a rate of 50 beats/min. There is a completely independent, slightly faster atrial rate of 60 beats/min and complete atrioventricular dissociation. The QRS complexes appear widened and bizarre. The PP interval is regular, and the RR interval is regular. This electrocardiogram was recorded at a paper speed of 25 mm/s with a sensitivity of 10 mm = 1 mV.

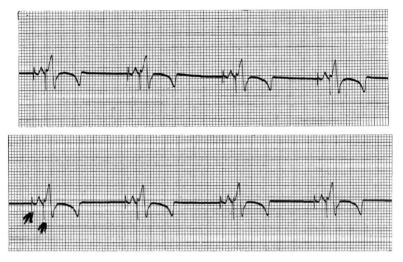

FIGURE 34-6. Continuous base-apex electrocardiogram of a horse with complete heart block treated with a universal pacemaker (DDD) with an atrial pacing electrode in the right atrium and a ventricular pacing electrode in the right ventricle. The pacing spike causes atrial depolarization *(first arrow)*, and the pacing spike causes ventricular depolarization *(second arrow)*. Both the atrial and the ventricular rates are 50 beats/min and are associated with one another. The PP and RR intervals are regular. These atrial electrodes have the ability to sense electrical depolarization of the atria and do not pace the atria if the sinus rate increases, thus allowing the patient to exercise. This electrocardiogram was recorded at a paper speed of 25 mm/s with a sensitivity of 5 mm = 1 mV.

- Should be investigated thoroughly and managed aggressively (see earlier) in the hope of preventing progression of the conduction block to complete AV block

AUSCULTATION
- Regular S_1 and S_2
- Slow to low-normal heart rate (usually 8-24 beats/min)
- S_4 precedes each S_1 and regular S_4 in pauses for each period of second-degree AV block

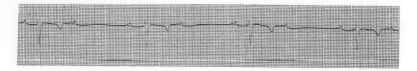

FIGURE 34-7. Base-apex electrocardiogram of a horse with advanced second-degree AV block with 2:1 conduction. Every other P wave is not followed by a QRS complex, but every QRS complex present is preceded by a P wave at a normal PR interval (440 ms). The PP interval is regular, and the RR interval is regular. The atrial rate is slightly increased at 50 beats/minute with a slow ventricular rate of 30 beats/min. This electrocardiogram was recorded at a paper speed of 25 mm/s with a sensitivity of 5 mm = 1 mV.

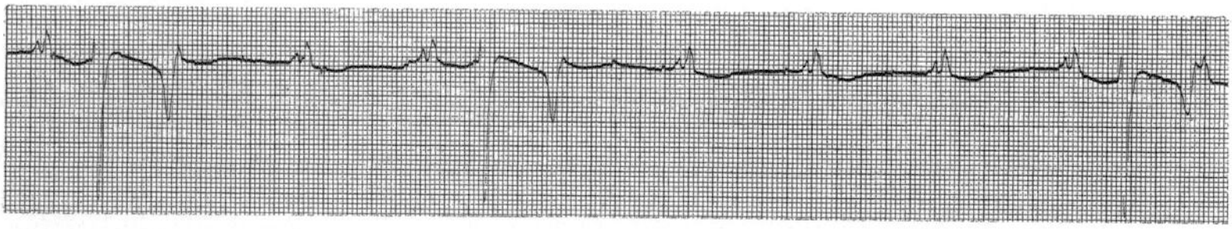

FIGURE 34-8. Base-apex electrocardiogram of a horse with advanced second-degree AV block with variable conduction. Every P wave is not followed by a QRS complex, but every QRS complex present is preceded by a P wave at a normal PR interval (480 ms). The PP interval is regular, and the RR interval is regular. The atrial rate is slightly increased at 60 beats/minute with a slower than normal ventricular rate of 20 beats/min. This electrocardiogram was recorded at a paper speed of 25 mm/s with a sensitivity of 5 mm = 1 mV.

ELECTROCARDIOGRAM
- Rapid atrial rate
- Regular PP interval
- Evidence of AV conduction (PR intervals of similar lengths)
- Normal QRS configuration associated with the preceding P waves (Figs. 34–7 and 34–8)
- RR interval usually is regular, but it may be irregular in some horses (see Fig. 34–8).

Sinus Bradycardia, Sinoatrial Block
- Sinus bradycardia, sinus arrhythmia, and SA block occur in fit horses but are less common than second-degree AV block.

AUSCULTATION
- Regular S_1 and S_2 with a pause in rhythm (SA block) or rhythmic variation of diastolic intervals (sinus bradycardia and sinus arrhythmia)
- Pause in rhythm equal to one diastolic pause or a multiple of the shortest diastolic pause (SA block)
- Slow to low-normal heart rate (usually 20-30 beats/min)
- S_4 precedes each S_1 usually and can be auscultated
- No S_4 in pauses for each period of SA block

ELECTROCARDIOGRAM
- Slow to low-normal atrial rate

- Irregular PP interval
- Evidence of AV conduction
- Normal QRS complex associated with the preceding P waves
- RR interval is rhythmically irregular (sinus bradycardia and sinus arrhythmia) or regularly irregular (SA block), with a diastolic pause equal to the number of beats blocked at the SA node. Usually manifestations of high vagal tone that disappear with exercise or the administration of a vagolytic (**atropine or glycopyrrolate, 0.005-0.01 mg/kg IV**) or sympathomimetic (**isoproterenol, 0.05-0.2 µg/kg per minute**) drug

Sinoatrial Arrest
- An uncommon, vagally mediated arrhythmia in horses

AUSCULTATION
- Regular S_1 and S_2 with a prolonged pause in the rhythm (more than two diastolic periods)
- Slow to low-normal heart rate (usually 20-30 beats/min but may be lower if pathologic)
- S_4 precedes each S_1 and usually can be auscultated
- No S_4 in pauses for period of SA arrest

ELECTROCARDIOGRAM
- Slow to low-normal atrial rate
- Regularly irregular PP interval
- Evidence of AV conduction
- Normal QRS complex associated with the preceding P waves
- RR interval is regularly irregular, with a diastolic pause equal to more than two diastolic periods. Should disappear with exercise or the administration of a vagolytic or sympathomimetic drug.
- Prolonged periods of sinoatrial arrest, profound sinus bradycardia, or high-grade sinoatrial block may indicate sinus node disease. *These horses should be carefully evaluated with exercising ECG, or the response of the horse to vagolytic and sympathomimetic drugs should be determined.* Sinus node disease is rare in horses, but inflammatory and degenerative changes must be considered possible etiologic factors.
- A course of high-dose corticosteroids (*dexamethasone,* **0.05-0.22 mg/kg IV**) should be initiated for patients with life-threatening abnormalities of sinus rhythm in the hope that pacemaker implantation is not necessary.

Sinus Syndrome
- Periods of profound sinus bradycardia and tachycardia have not been reported in horses. Definitive treatment is pacemaker implantation.

Tachyarrhythmias
Atrial Fibrillation
- Occurs frequently in patients and rarely necessitates emergency therapy.
- Most horses have little or no underlying cardiac disease and come to medical attention because of exercise intolerance. Other presenting problems include tachypnea, dyspnea, exercise-induced pulmonary hemorrhage, myopathy, colic,

and congestive heart failure. Atrial fibrillation can be an incidental finding during a routine examination.

- Resting heart rate usually is normal, although the rhythm is irregularly irregular and S_4 cannot be auscultated.
- Intensity of peripheral pulses is irregularly irregular.
- Cardiac output in patients with atrial fibrillation and no significant underlying cardiac disease is normal at rest.

AUSCULTATION
- Heart rate usually is normal (28-44 beats/min), although atrial fibrillation can occur at any heart rate
- Irregularly irregular diastolic periods
- S_4 absent

ELECTROCARDIOGRAM
- Irregularly irregular RR intervals (Fig. 34–9)
- No P waves
- Rapid baseline fibrillation f waves
- Normal QRS complexes
- Patients with little or no underlying cardiac disease are candidates for conversion to sinus rhythm

TREATMENT OF HORSES WITH LITTLE OR NO OTHER UNDERLYING CARDIOVASCULAR DISEASE
PATIENT PREPARATION
- Before beginning quinidine treatment, place an **intravenous catheter** for rapid venous access in case arrhythmias develop.
- Before treatment, ensure adequate whole-body potassium status. This clinicopathologic evaluation should include measurement of a plasma potassium level and fractional excretion of potassium in the urine.
  □ For calculation of fractional excretion, urine and serum samples must be obtained simultaneously. Creatinine and potassium must be measured on both the urine and serum samples, and the fractional excretion of potassium is calculated with the following equation:

$$FE = \frac{Urine\ (K^+)}{Serum\ (K^+)} \times \frac{Serum\ (Cr)}{Urine\ (Cr)} \times 100$$

  □ Normal fractional excretion of potassium is 23.3%-48.1%.

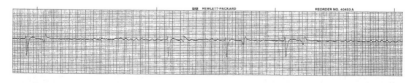

FIGURE 34–9. Base-apex electrocardiogram of a horse with atrial fibrillation. Irregularly irregular RR intervals, absence of P waves, and presence of baseline f waves are evident. The QRS configurations are normal, as is the ventricular rate (30 beats/min). This electrocardiogram was recorded at a paper speed of 25 mm/s with a sensitivity of 5 mm = 1 mV.

- A low fractional excretion of potassium indicates renal potassium conservation and a probable low total body potassium status.
- Red blood cell potassium determination has been investigated by several researchers as a tool for assessing whole-body potassium status, but reports of its reliability vary significantly.
- A *continuous ECG* (Fig. 34–10) should be obtained (easiest with radiotelemetry) throughout the treatment period to monitor cardiac rhythm and conduction times.
- If the arrhythmia is recent, ideally ≤2 weeks, *quinidine gluconate,* **1-2.2 mg/kg**, should be administered IV as a bolus, every 10 minutes to effect, **not to exceed 12 mg/kg total dose.**
  - □ The average half-life of quinidine administered IV in horses is 6.5 hours, with a range of 4-12 hours.
- Successful transvenous electrical defibrillation of horses with atrial fibrillation of very short duration has been reported.
- Successful cardioversion was accomplished under general anesthesia in one horse with a commercial biphasic defibrillator and quinidine gluconate.
- Intravenous flecainide has been successful in the conversion of horses with induced and sustained atrial fibrillation. Concentrations of flecainide in the plasma in horses converted to sinus rhythm from atrial fibrillation was 1303 ± 566 ng/ml.
- If the atrial fibrillation is of more long-standing duration (>2-4 weeks), if there is mild to moderate, but not severe, underlying cardiac disease (mild to moderate tricuspid, mitral, or aortic regurgitation or mild myocardial dysfunction), and if no signs of congestive heart failure are present:
  - □ **Quinidine sulfate** is administered at **22 mg/kg** through a nasogastric tube.
  - □ Quinidine sulfate should be administered through a nasogastric tube q2h until the patient either converts to sinus rhythm, shows adverse reactions or toxic side effects to treatment with quinidine (Box 34–1), or has received four to six treatments at 2-hour intervals (most horses with atrial fibrillation can tolerate only four treatments q2h before exhibiting adverse or toxic side effects).
  - □ Plasma quinidine concentration should be measured 1 hour after the fourth treatment, before every-2-hour dosage is continued, or when the patient exhibits adverse or toxic side effects of treatment. If plasma quinidine concentration cannot be measured, no more than four treatments should be given every 2 hours, before every 6 hour dosage is initiated.

  Therapeutic concentration = 2-5 µg/ml
  Toxic concentration = >5 µg/ml

  - □ Treatment intervals should be increased to every 6 hours if plasma quinidine concentration is ≥4.0 µg/ml.
- Treatment intervals should be increased to every 6 hours until conversion to sinus rhythm, adverse reactions or toxic side effects develop (rare with every-6-hour dosage), or the owner elects to discontinue treatment.
- **Oral digoxin (0.011 mg/kg twice daily)** appears to be helpful in the conversion of some horses that do not convert with quinidine alone. Digoxin should be added on day 2 if conversion has not occurred.

NOTE: Digoxin should not be administered after day 2 without monitoring of serum digoxin concentration (therapeutic concentration, 1-2 ng/ml).

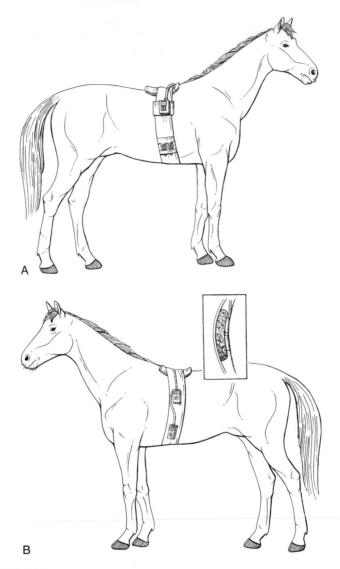

FIGURE 34–10. Contact electrodes in place under a surcingle for obtaining an electrocardiogram by means of radiotelemetry. **A,** Withers pad and the surcingle are in place in the girth area, and the telemetry box is taped to the upper rings of the surcingle just below the withers. **B,** Placement of the grounded electrodes on the left side of the patient under the moistened sponges and held in place by the surcingle. Care must be taken to ensure close contact between the patient's skin and the contact electrodes in the area near the withers as well as in the girth area. The upper grounded electrode (negative electrode) should be placed on the flat portion of the dorsal thorax. The lower grounded electrode (positive electrode) should be placed in the flat portion of the girth area or on the sternum, whichever area ensures better contact.

BOX 34-1. Adverse Reactions and Toxic Side Effects of Quinidine Sulfate and Gluconate Treatment

---

1. Depression

Rx: Occurs in all treated horses, no treatment indicated

2. Paraphimosis

Rx: Occurs in all treated stallions or geldings, no treatment indicated

3. Urticaria, wheals

Rx: Discontinue quinidine; if severe, administer corticosteroids, antihistamines, or both

4. Nasal mucosal swelling

SNORING

Rx: Monitor degree of air flow; discontinue quinidine if there is a significant decrease in air flow through the nares

UPPER RESPIRATORY TRACT OBSTRUCTION

Rx: Discontinue quinidine; sign of quinidine toxicity; if severe, administer corticosteroids, antihistamines, or both; insert nasotracheal tube, preferably, or perform emergency tracheotomy

5. Laminitis

Rx: Discontinue quinidine; administer analgesics and other treatment as needed

6. Neurologic

ATAXIA

Rx: Discontinue quinidine; sign of quinidine toxicity

BIZARRE BEHAVIOR: HALLUCINATIONS?

Rx: Discontinue quinidine; sign of quinidine toxicity

CONVULSIONS

Rx: Discontinue quinidine; sign of quinidine toxicity; administer anticonvulsants as indicated

7. Gastrointestinal

FLATULENCE

Rx: Occurs in many treated horses; treatment not indicated

DIARRHEA

Rx: Usually resolves with discontinuation of drug; discontinue drug administration if diarrhea is severe

COLIC

Rx: Usually resolves with administration of dipyrone; use other analgesics as needed; sign of quinidine toxicity

8. Cardiovascular

TACHYCARDIA: SUPRAVENTRICULAR OR VENTRICULAR—UNIFORM, MULTIFORM, TORSADES DE POINTES

Rx: See Box 34–2, Table 34–4

Continued...

BOX 34-1. Adverse Reactions and Toxic Side Effects of Quinidine
Sulfate and Gluconate Treatment (Cont'd)

PROLONGATION OF THE QRS DURATION (>25% OF PRETREATMENT VALUE)
Rx: Discontinue quinidine; sign of quinidine toxicity

HYPOTENSION
Rx: Discontinue quinidine; administer phenylephrine if needed (see Box 34–2,
Table 34–4)

CONGESTIVE HEART FAILURE
Rx: Discontinue quinidine; administer digoxin if not already given

SUDDEN DEATH
Rx: Cardiopulmonary resuscitation

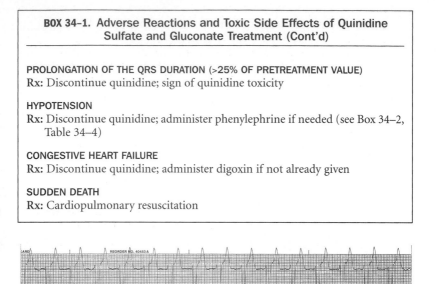

FIGURE 34-11. Base-apex electrocardiogram of the horse in Fig. 34–9 after treatment
with quinidine sulfate and digoxin. This patient has atrial fibrillation with uniform
ventricular tachycardia and digoxin toxicity. Large, wide QRS complexes are ventricular in
origin, P waves are absent, and baseline f waves are evident. This electrocardiogram
was recorded at a paper speed of 25 mm/s with a sensitivity of 5 mm = 1 mV.

Administration of digoxin and quinidine together results in rapid elevations of
serum digoxin concentration and the possible development of digoxin toxicity.
Plasma digoxin concentrations nearly double with concurrent administration of
quinidine sulfate.

Digoxin toxicity manifests as anorexia, depression, colic, or the development
of other cardiac arrhythmias (Fig. 34–11).

- Patients being treated for atrial fibrillation with quinidine should be monitored
  carefully for adverse reactions and signs of quinidine toxicity.
- The detection of any significant adverse reactions or signs of quinidine toxicity
  (see Box 34–1) should prompt discontinuation of quinidine administration and
  may require additional treatment if the induced problem is serious (Box 34–2
  and Fig. 34–12).
- Obtain a plasma sample for determination of plasma quinidine concentration.
  Plasma electrolyte concentrations and a creatinine level also should be determined if the adverse or toxic effects are cardiovascular.

**ELECTROCARDIOGRAPHIC MONITORING FOR QUINIDINE TOXICITY AND
ADVERSE REACTION**
Prolongation of QRS

- Measure the duration of the QRS complex before each planned administration
  of quinidine and compare it with the pretreatment duration.

BOX 34-2. Management of Quinidine-Induced Arrhythmias

Determine whether arrhythmia is supraventricular or ventricular:
- Obtain another electrocardiogram (ECG) lead if unable to determine whether rhythm is supraventricular or ventricular. Look for change in QRS configuration from normal or preceding QRS configuration. Record ECG during entire treatment with radiotelemetry, if possible.
- Measure blood pressure if possible.
- Don't panic!

If arrhythmia is supraventricular:
- If rate is sustained in excess of 100 beats/min, administer **digoxin, 0.0022 mg/kg IV (1 mg/1000 lb) or 0.011 mg/kg PO (5 mg/1000 lb)**.
- If rate is sustained in excess of 150 beats/min or pressures are poor, administer **digoxin, 0.0022 mg/kg IV (1 mg/1000 lb)**. Can repeat dose once in relatively short period of time if necessary. Administer **NaHCO$_3$, 1 mEq/kg IV (450 mEq/1000 lb)**.

If rate still is high or pressures are poor:
- Administer **propranolol, 0.03 mg/kg IV (13.5 mg/1000 lb)**, to slow heart rate.
- Administer **phenylephrine, 0.1-0.2 µg/kg per minute IV to effect**, up to 0.01 mg/kg total dose to improve blood pressure.
- Administer **verapamil, 0.025-0.05 mg/kg IV (11.25-22.5 mg/1000 lb)** every 30 minutes. Can repeat up to 0.2 mg/kg (90 mg/1000 lb) total dose

If arrhythmia is ventricular:
- If wide QRS tachycardia (torsades de pointes) is present, administer **MgSO$_4$, 1-2.5 g/450 kg per minute IV to effect** up to 25 g/1000 lb. Administer in rapid IV drip over 10 minutes or in bolus if necessary.
- If ventricular tachycardia is unstable:
  - Administer **lidocaine hydrochloride, 20-50 µg/kg per minute or 0.25-0.5 mg/kg very slowly IV (225 mg/1000 lb)**. Can repeat in 5-10 minutes.
  - Administer **MgSO$_4$, 1-2.5 g/450 kg per minute IV to effect** up to 25 g/1000 lb. Administer in rapid IV drip over 10 minutes or in bolus if necessary.
  - Administer **procainamide, 1 mg/kg per minute IV (450 mg/min/1000 lb)** to a maximum of 20 mg/kg (9 g/1000 lb).
  - Administer **propafenone, 0.5-1 mg/kg IV (225-450 mg)** in 5% dextrose slowly over 5-8 minutes.
  - Administer **bretylium, 3-5 mg/kg IV (1.35-2.25 g/1000 lb)**. Can repeat up to 10 mg/kg total dose.

- Prolongation of the QRS duration to greater than 25% of the pretreatment QRS duration is an indication of quinidine toxicity (Fig. 34-13).
- Prolongation of the QT interval also occurs.

Rapid Supraventricular Tachycardia
- Occurs in patients being treated for atrial fibrillation with quinidine; associated with a sudden release of vagal tone at the AV node; an idiosyncratic reaction not associated with quinidine toxicity
- Heart rates ≥200 beats/min occasionally occur and are potentially life threatening (Fig. 34-14). Immediate therapy (see Box 34-2) is needed to slow the ventricular response rate and prevent deterioration of the patient's cardiovascular status.
  - Administer **digoxin, 0.0022 mg/kg IV**.
  - Administer **NaHCO$_3$, 1 mEq/kg IV**.
  - If pressures are poor, administer **phenylephrine, 0.1-0.2 µg/kg per minute**.

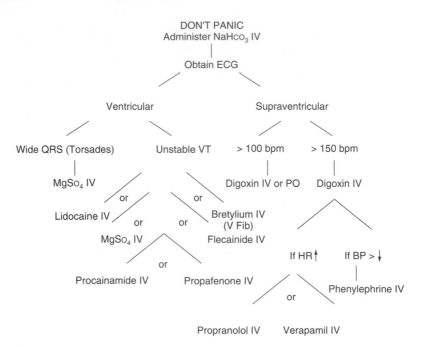

FIGURE 34–12. Decision tree for management of quinidine-induced arrhythmias.

- If heart rate is still high, administer **propranolol, 0.03 mg/kg IV.**
- Associated with decreased cardiac output at rest and may deteriorate into other, more life-threatening ventricular arrhythmias (Fig. 34–15)
- Sustained ventricular response rates ≥100 beats/min (Fig. 34–16) in patients being treated for atrial fibrillation with quinidine should be controlled before quinidine administration is continued, to prevent further deterioration of the cardiac rhythm.

Ventricular Arrhythmias Associated with Quinidine
- If a large number of ventricular premature depolarizations, ventricular tachycardia (Fig. 34–17), or multiform ventricular complexes are detected, quinidine administration should be stopped.
- If the ventricular arrhythmias do not disappear, IV administration of antiarrhythmic drugs should be instituted, usually beginning with **lidocaine, 20-50 μg/kg per minute slowly IV** (see Tables 34–5 and 34–6).
- Ventricular arrhythmias induced by quinidine administration usually are idiosyncratic. These arrhythmias are associated with the proarrhythmic effect of antiarrhythmic drugs and are not associated with quinidine toxicity (see Fig. 34–17).
- Quinidine-induced **torsades de pointes,** a wide ventricular tachycardia (Fig. 34–18), is more likely to occur in hypokalemic patients (Fig. 34–19).

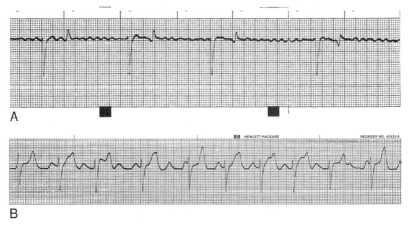

FIGURE 34-13. Base-apex electrocardiograms of a horse with atrial fibrillation **(A)** that was then treated with quinidine sulfate and developed prolongation of the QRS complex **(B)**. Irregularly irregular rhythm with variable RR intervals, no P waves, and baseline f waves are evident in the pretreatment ECG **(A)** with a QRS duration of 100 ms. After treatment with four doses of 22 mg/kg quinidine sulfate, the QRS complexes increased to 140 ms **(B)**, and the ventricular rate increased to 60 beats/min. Large P waves are occurring regularly, buried in many of the QRS and T complexes associated with an atrial tachycardia (atrial rate of 150 beats/min) with block. A quinidine plasma concentration measured at this time was elevated. These electrocardiograms were recorded at a paper speed of 25 mm/s with a sensitivity of 5 mm = 1 mV.

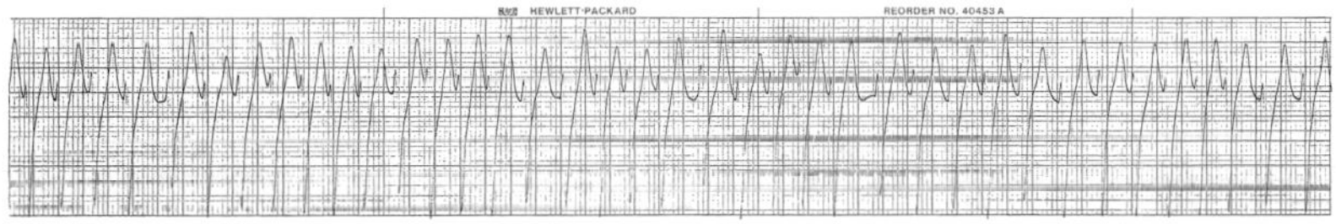

FIGURE 34-14. Base-apex electrocardiogram of a horse with atrial fibrillation that developed a rapid supraventricular tachycardia with a heart rate of 210 beats/min after the second dose of 22 mg/kg quinidine sulfate. RR intervals are slightly irregular, P waves are absent, and the orientation of the QRS complex for the base-apex lead is normal. The T waves are not visible because of the rapid ventricular response rate. This electrocardiogram was recorded at a paper speed of 25 mm/s with a sensitivity of 5 mm = 1 mV.

Therefore, every effort should be made before quinidine treatment to be sure that horses have adequate whole-body potassium status checked.

- **Intravenous MgSO₄** at an infusion rate of **1-2.5 g/450 kg per minute** should be instituted immediately for quinidine-induced torsades de pointes.

Sudden Death
- Probably associated with deterioration of rapid supraventricular or ventricular tachycardia to ventricular fibrillation or cardiac arrest
- Emphasizes the importance of continuous ECG monitoring (see Fig. 34–10) and rapid management of any arrhythmias that do occur

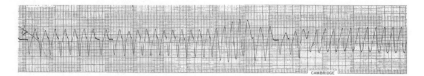

FIGURE 34–15. Base-apex electrocardiogram of a horse with atrial fibrillation and rapid supraventricular tachycardia that developed after two doses of 22 mg/kg quinidine sulfate and then deteriorated into paroxysms of ventricular tachycardia. RR intervals are irregular, P waves are absent, and the orientation of the QRS is normal for a base-apex lead on the left side of the strip. These findings are consistent with rapid supraventricular tachycardia at a heart rate of 240 beats/min in a horse with atrial fibrillation. This rhythm then deteriorates into a paroxysm of wide ventricular tachycardia followed by a couple of normally conducted beats and then a period of more sustained ventricular tachycardia with a heart rate of 270 beats/min. The f waves are not visible because of the rapid ventricular rate. This electrocardiogram was recorded at a paper speed of 25 mm/s with a sensitivity of 2 mm = 1 mV.

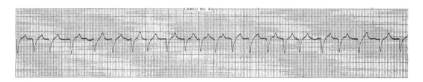

FIGURE 34–16. Base-apex electrocardiogram of a horse with rapid atrial fibrillation and a heart rate of 130 beats/min. RR intervals are irregular, P waves are absent, and the baseline f waves are small. This electrocardiogram was recorded at a paper speed of 25 mm/s with a sensitivity of 2 mm = 1 mV.

Hypotension
- Monitor pulse pressure or blood pressure for quinidine-induced hypotension. Discontinue quinidine administration; if hypotension is severe, administer **phenylephrine at 0.1-0.2 µg/kg per minute to effect.**

Congestive Heart Failure
- Occurs in individuals with severe underlying myocardial dysfunction or compensated congestive heart failure (inappropriate patients for conversion with quinidine)
- Negative inotropic effect of quinidine manifested only at higher drug doses
- Treat with digoxin, **0.0022 mg/kg IV, and furosemide, 1-2 mg/kg IV**, if needed.

Upper Respiratory Tract Obstruction
- Monitor nasal air flow for quinidine-induced upper respiratory tract obstruction secondary to nasal mucosal swelling. If air flow through the external nares decreases, discontinue quinidine administration. Indicative of **quinidine toxicity.**
  □ **Insert a nasotracheal tube** if air flow through the external nares continues to decrease.
  □ If obstruction is severe, administer corticosteroids, antihistamines, or both.
  □ Emergency tracheotomy may be necessary for some patients if a nasotracheal tube is not inserted when a marked decrease in air flow is detected.

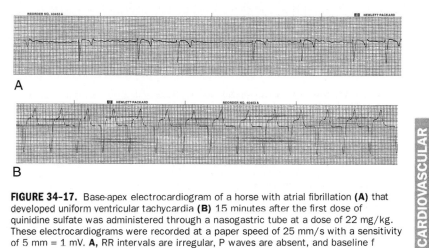

A

B

CARDIOVASCULAR

FIGURE 34-17. Base-apex electrocardiogram of a horse with atrial fibrillation **(A)** that developed uniform ventricular tachycardia **(B)** 15 minutes after the first dose of quinidine sulfate was administered through a nasogastric tube at a dose of 22 mg/kg. These electrocardiograms were recorded at a paper speed of 25 mm/s with a sensitivity of 5 mm = 1 mV. **A,** RR intervals are irregular, P waves are absent, and baseline f waves are present. These findings are characteristic of atrial fibrillation. The resting heart rate is 40 beats/min. **B,** Wide and bizarre QRS complexes with the T wave oriented in the opposite direction to the QRS are consistent with complexes that are ventricular in origin. The ventricular complexes have a uniform configuration, and the heart rate is 90 beats/min. The baseline f waves are barely visible on the electrocardiogram, and no P waves are present.

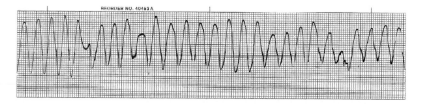

FIGURE 34-18. Base-apex electrocardiogram of a horse with atrial fibrillation that had received two doses of quinidine sulfate (22 mg/kg each) and developed a wide ventricular tachycardia (torsades de pointes). The QRS complexes and T waves twist around the baseline and are difficult to differentiate from one another. The plasma potassium level was normal at this time. This electrocardiogram was recorded at a paper speed of 25 mm/s with a sensitivity of 2 mm = 1 mV.

Urticaria, Wheals
- Discontinue quinidine administration.
- If severe, administer antihistamines and corticosteroids.

Paraphimosis
- Transient in all geldings and stallions
- Disappears with discontinuance of treatment and return of plasma quinidine concentrations to negligible levels. Not necessary to stop quinidine treatment.

Laminitis
- Rare

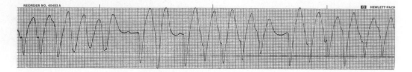

FIGURE 34–19. Base-apex electrocardiogram of a horse with atrial fibrillation that had received six doses of quinidine sulfate (22 mg/kg each) and developed torsades de pointes, which was immediately managed with an intravenous infusion of $MgSO_4$. Widened QRS complexes and T waves are evident, as is twisting of the QRS complexes and T waves around the baseline. This sign is present although the torsades de pointes is resolving. This horse was hypokalemic (2.4 mEq/L) and was receiving an intravenous infusion of $MgSO_4$ at the time of this electrocardiogram. The ventricular rate is 110 beats/min. An occasional f wave is present. The fluids were subsequently spiked with KCl, and the wide QRS tachycardia resolved with magnesium and potassium replacement fluids. This electrocardiogram was recorded at a paper speed of 25 mm/s with a sensitivity of 5 mm = 1 mV.

- If digital pulses are increased, discontinue quinidine administration.
- If patient is uncomfortable, administer analgesics.

Neurologic Signs
- Ataxia, bizarre behavior, seizures
- Indicative of **quinidine toxicity**: Discontinue quinidine treatment.
- Anticonvulsants may be indicated if seizures occur.

Gastrointestinal Signs
- Flatulence is very common: Quinidine administration need not be discontinued.
- Oral ulcerations: Associated with oral administration of the drug, therefore oral administration of quinidine sulfate is contraindicated.
- Diarrhea usually occurs with higher doses of quinidine and usually resolves with discontinuance of quinidine treatment.
- Only one reported case of quinidine-induced diarrhea culturing positive for *Salmonella* organisms
- Colic associated with quinidine toxicity: Discontinue quinidine administration; administer analgesics as needed.

TREATMENT OF HORSES WITH CONGESTIVE HEART FAILURE AND ATRIAL FIBRILLATION
- A small percentage of horses (10%-15%), particularly draft breeds, with atrial fibrillation have severe underlying cardiac disease and present with congestive heart failure.
- The resting heart rates of these individuals are elevated (>60 beats/min) and may exceed 100 beats/min (Fig. 34–20).
- Clinical signs of left-sided heart failure (pulmonary edema, coughing, tachypnea) or right-sided heart failure (generalized venous distention, jugular pulsations, and pectoral, ventral, preputial, or limb peripheral edema) may be present.
- Murmurs of tricuspid or mitral regurgitation usually are present, although patients with severe aortic regurgitation also may have congestive heart failure.
- These patients are *not* candidates for conversion to sinus rhythm with quinidine.

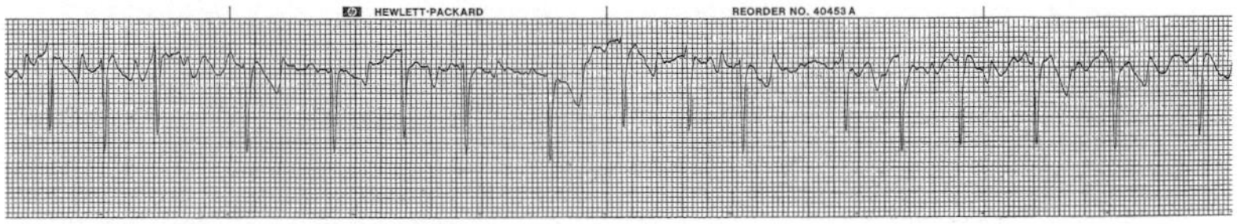

FIGURE 34-20. Base-apex electrocardiogram of a horse with atrial fibrillation and congestive heart failure. Heart rate is rapid (110 beats/min), RR interval is irregular, P waves are absent, and baseline f waves are present. These findings are consistent with atrial fibrillation. This electrocardiogram was recorded at a paper speed of 25 mm/s with a sensitivity of 5 mm = 1 mV.

- Treatment of these horses is directed at slowing the ventricular response rate (heart rate) and supporting the failing myocardium.
  - **Digoxin, 0.0022 mg/kg IV q12h or 0.011 mg/kg PO q12h**, is the drug of choice because of its vagal and positive inotropic effects (Table 34–4).
  - If heart rate is not controlled adequately with digoxin alone, **propranolol, 0.03 mg/kg IV or 0.38-0.78 mg/kg PO q8h**, may be added to further slow the ventricular response rate.
  - **Furosemide (0.5-1.0 mg/kg SQ, IV, or PO)** should be instituted in the treatment of patients with ventral or pulmonary edema.
  - Afterload reducers (vasodilators), such as **hydralazine, 0.5-1.5 mg/kg PO q12h, or enalapril, 0.5 mg/kg PO q24h or q12h**, should be added in the treatment of patients with severe mitral or aortic regurgitation.

Ventricular Tachycardia

- The clinical signs of congestive heart failure become more severe the longer uniform ventricular tachycardia is present and the higher the heart rate.
- Clinical signs of congestive heart failure develop more rapidly in horses with shorter cycle lengths and higher heart rates.
- Clinical signs of low output heart failure also develop more rapidly when the rhythm is multiform rather than uniform.
- Generalized venous distention, jugular pulsations, ventral edema, and pleural effusion develop in patients with sustained uniform ventricular tachycardia at a rate of 120 beats/min.
- Some patients also have pericardial effusion, pulmonary edema, and ascites.
- Syncope has been detected in horses with uniform ventricular tachycardia and a heart rate of ≥150 beats/min.

AUSCULTATION
- Rapid, regular rhythm if uniform; rapid, irregular rhythm if multiform
- Heart sounds are often loud and varying in intensity

ELECTROCARDIOGRAM
- Elevated ventricular rate (usually >60 beats/min) with slower independent atrial rate
- Regular PP interval
- P waves buried in QRS and T complexes (atrioventricular dissociation)
- Regular RR interval (uniform) or irregular RR (multiform) ventricular tachycardia

TABLE 34–4. Drug Therapy for Horses with Myocardial and Valvular Heart Disease and Congestive Heart Failure

Drug	Indication	Dosage
Aspirin	Thrombophlebitis, endocarditis	5-20 mg/kg
Dexamethasone	Myocarditis, arrhythmias	0.05-0.22 mg/kg IV or IM
Digoxin	Congestive heart failure, atrial tachyarrhythmias, control of rapid ventricular response in atrial fibrillation or flutter	0.0022 mg/kg IV q12h (maintenance dose); 0.0044-0.0075 mg/kg IV q12h (loading dose administered for only two doses, rarely used); 0.0022-0.00375 mg/kg IV q12h to control ventricular response rate in atrial fibrillation; 0.011-0.0175 mg/kg PO q12h
Dobutamine	Cardiogenic shock, hypotension, complete atrioventricular block (emergency therapy)	1-5 µg/kg per minute IV
Enalapril	Mitral and aortic regurgitation	0.5 mg/kg PO q12h
Furosemide	Edema	1-2 mg/kg subcutaneous, IM, or IV as needed; 0.5-1 mg/kg PO q12h (maintenance)
Hydralazine	Mitral regurgitation	0.5-1.5 mg/kg PO q12h
Milrinone	Congestive heart failure, low cardiac output	10 µg/kg/min IV; 0.5-1 mg/kg PO q12h

- Abnormal QRS and T-wave configuration unrelated to the preceding P wave. All abnormal QRS complexes and T-waves have same configuration (uniform), or several different QRS complex and T-wave configurations are detected (multiform).
  - □ **Uniform** ventricular tachycardia occurs when the ectopic focus originates from one place in the ventricle and produces only one abnormal QRS and T-wave configuration (Fig. 34–21).
  - □ **Multiform** ventricular tachycardia occurs when the ectopic ventricular complex originates from more than one focus in the ventricle and produces abnormal QRS and T complexes of different orientations (Fig. 34–22). Multiform ventricular complexes are associated with increased electrical inhomogeneity (lacking similarity) and instability and *an increased risk of development of a fatal ventricular rhythm.*
  - □ **R on T,** a QRS complex occurring within the preceding T wave (Fig. 34–23), indicates marked electrical inhomogeneity and instability and increases the risk of development of ventricular fibrillation.
  - □ Wide QRS tachycardia or **torsades de pointes,** in which the QRS and T complexes twist around the baseline (Fig. 34–24), is another ventricular rhythm that can rapidly deteriorate into ventricular fibrillation and cause sudden death.

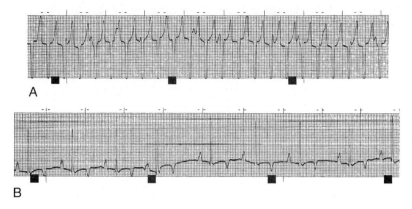

A

B

FIGURE 34–21. Lead II electrocardiogram of a horse with uniform ventricular tachycardia before **(A)** and after **(B)** conversion. **A,** Large, negative QRS complexes with the T wave oriented in the opposite direction, which is an abnormal QRS configuration for lead II in the horse. A rapid, regular ventricular rate of 150 beats/min and slower regular atrial rate of 90 beats/minute are evident. The RR interval and PP interval are regular. The P waves are buried in the QRS and T complexes and are unassociated with the QRS complexes. This electrocardiogram was recorded at a paper speed of 25 mm/s with a sensitivity of 5 mm = 1 mV. **B,** Tall positive QRS complex with a negative T wave deflection after each P wave. The P wave morphology changes from beat to beat, and the PP and RR intervals are not perfectly regular. This electrocardiogram **(B)** shows slight sinus arrhythmia with a wandering pacemaker at a heart rate of 50 beats/min immediately after conversion from sustained uniform ventricular tachycardia. This electrocardiogram was recorded at a paper speed of 25 mm/s with a sensitivity of 10 mm = 1 mV.

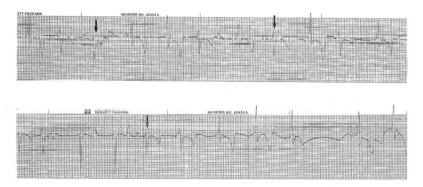

FIGURE 34–22. Continuous base-apex electrocardiogram of a horse with multiform ventricular tachycardia. Multiple configurations of the QRS and T complexes appear widened and bizarre compared with the few normal QRS and T complexes *(arrows)*. The RR intervals are irregular, but the PP intervals are regular. The underlying atrial rate is 60 beats/minute, with a heart rate of 70 beats/min. This electrocardiogram was recorded at a paper speed of 25 mm/s with a sensitivity of 5 mm = 1 mV.

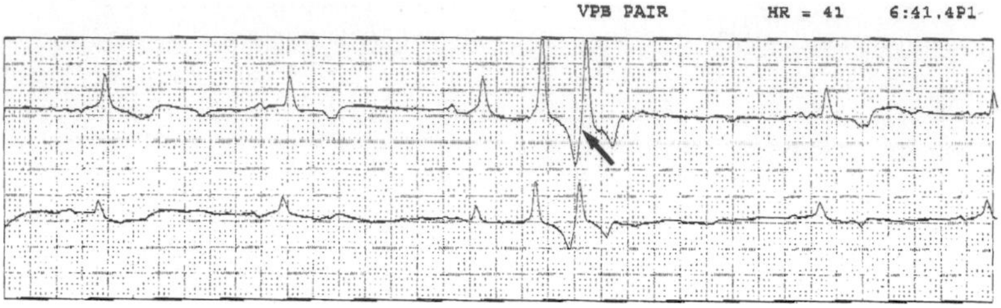

FIGURE 34–23. Base-apex electrocardiogram obtained with a 24-hour Holter recorder for a horse with multiple ventricular premature depolarizations, pairs of ventricular premature depolarizations, and paroxysms of ventricular tachycardia. The R on T occurs with the pair of ventricular premature depolarizations *(arrow)*. The heart rate is 41 beats/min. This electrocardiogram was recorded at a paper speed of 25 mm/s with a sensitivity of 10 mm = 1 mV.

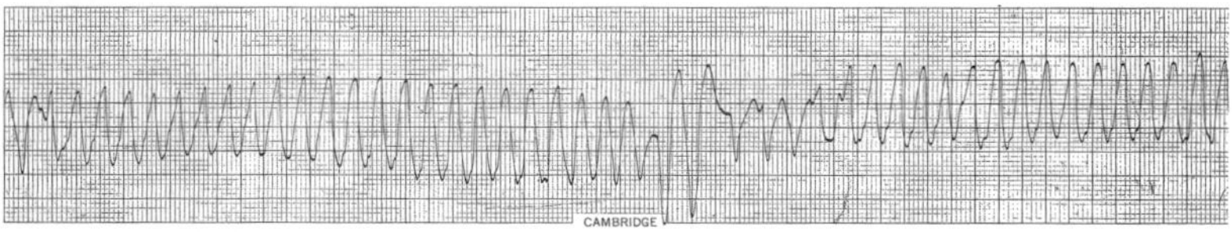

FIGURE 34–24. Base-apex electrocardiogram of a horse with torsades de pointes ventricular tachycardia with a heart rate of 280-300 beats/min. Wide QRS tachycardia and slurring of the distinction between the QRS complex and the T wave are evident, and the electrocardiogram appears to oscillate around the baseline. This electrocardiogram was recorded at a paper speed of 25 mm/s with a sensitivity of 2 mm = 1 mV.

ECHOCARDIOGRAM
- In most horses the only abnormality is that associated with the rhythm disturbance.
- Severe concurrent myocardial dysfunction may be detected in horses with multiform ventricular tachycardia and indicates probable widespread myocardial necrosis (Fig. 34–25).

TREATMENT
- Treatment is indicated if the patient is showing clinical signs at rest attributable to the dysrhythmia, the rate is excessively high, the rhythm is multiform, or R on T complexes are detected (Box 34–3).
- The selection of an appropriate antiarrhythmic agent for a patient with ventricular tachycardia depends on the severity of the arrhythmia, the associated clinical signs, the suspected etiologic factor, and the availability of appropriate antiarrhythmic drugs (Table 34–5).
- Lidocaine (without epinephrine) is readily available and is the most rapidly acting drug.
  - **Lidocaine** must be administered carefully and in small doses **(0.25-0.5 mg/kg slowly as a bolus)** because of the excitement and seizures associated with larger doses. *Diazepam, 0.05 mg/kg IV, may be used to control the excitability or seizures that may result from lidocaine.*

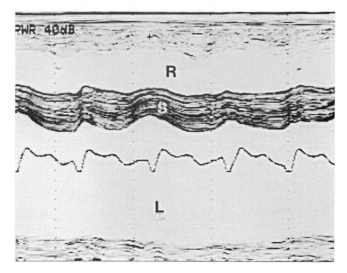

FIGURE 34-25. M-mode echocardiogram of a horse with multiform ventricular tachycardia, severe left ventricular dysfunction, and left-sided congestive heart failure. Lack of systolic thickening of the left ventricular free wall is evident. This echocardiogram was obtained from the right parasternal window in the left ventricular position with a 2.5-MHz sector scanner transducer. An electrocardiogram is superimposed for timing. *R*, Right ventricle; *L*, left ventricle; *S*, interventricular septum.

BOX 34-3. Indications for Urgent Management of Ventricular Tachycardia

Clinical signs of cardiovascular collapse
Rapid heart rate (>120 beats/min)
Multiform ventricular tachycardia
Detection of R on T complex

- Therapeutic plasma concentration is 1.5-5 µg/ml.
- **Quinidine gluconate, 1-2.2 mg/kg IV as a bolus, procainamide, 1 mg/kg per minute IV, propafenone, 0.5-1 mg/kg in 5% dextrose IV, and flecainide, 1-2 mg/kg infused at the rate of 0.2 mg/kg per minute**, are administered more slowly or in graded doses (Table 34-5).
  - All these drugs have negative inotropic effects when administered at high doses but often are very effective in converting ventricular tachycardia in horses.
  - The principal metabolite of procainamide is *N*-acetylprocainamide (NAPA), which is also pharmacologically active. The half-life of procainamide administered intravenously is 3.5 ± 0.6 hours and of NAPA is 6.3 ± 1.5 hours. The therapeutic plasma concentration of procainamide is thought to be 4-10 µg/ml; for NAPA, 7-15 µg/ml; and for procainamide and NAPA together, 10-30 µg/ml.
- Intravenous propafenone, if available, should be reserved for patients with refractory ventricular tachycardia. Therapeutic plasma concentrations appear to be between 0.2 and 3.0 µg/ml in horses.

CARDIOVASCULAR

TABLE 34–5. Antiarrhythmic Therapy

Drug	Indication	Dosage
Atropine or glycopyrrolate	Sinus bradycardia, vagally induced arrhythmias	0.005-0.01 mg/kg IV
Bretylium tosylate	Life-threatening VT, ventricular fibrillation	3-5 mg/kg IV, can repeat up to 10 mg/kg total dose
Dexamethasone	VT, complete atrioventricular block	0.05-0.22 mg/kg IV or IM
Flecainide	Acute AF, ventricular and atrial arrhythmias	1-2 mg/kg infused at the rate of 0.2 mg/kg per minute
Lidocaine*	VT, ventricular arrhythmias	20-50 mg/kg per minute; 0.25 mg/kg (bolus) 0.5 mg/kg very slowly IV to effect, can repeat in 5-10 min
$MgSO_4$	VT	1-2.5 g/450 kg per minute to effect IV, not to exceed 25 g total dose
Phenylephrine HCl	Quinidine toxicosis, arterial hypotension, excessive vasodilatation	0.1-0.2 mg/kg per minute; 0.01 mg/kg to effect
Phenytoin	Digoxin toxicity, atrial arrhythmias	5-10 mg/kg IV first 12 h, then 1-5 mg/kg IM q12h 1.82 mg/kg PO q8h, may increase to 2.27 mg/kg PO q8h after 2-3 days if no drowsiness and to 2.73 mg/kg after 2-3 more days if no drowsiness
Procainamide	VT, AF, ventricular and atrial arrhythmias	1 mg/kg per minute IV, not to exceed 20 mg/kg IV 25-35 mg/kg q8h PO
Propafenone[†]	Refractory VT, AF, ventricular and atrial arrhythmias	0.5-1 mg/kg in 5% dextrose slowly IV to effect over 5-8 min 2 mg/kg PO q8h
Propranolol	Unresponsive VT and SVT	0.03 mg/kg IV 0.38-0.78 mg/kg PO q8h
Quinidine gluconate	VT, AF	0.5-2.2 mg/kg (bolus) q10min to effect; not to exceed 12 mg/kg[†] IV total dose
Quinidine sulfate	AF, VT, atrial and ventricular arrhythmias	22 mg/kg via sulfate nasogastric tube q2h until converted, toxic, or plasma [quinidine] level is 3-5 mg/ml[§]; continue quinidine sulfate q6h until converted or toxic
$NaHCO_3$	Quinidine toxicosis, atrial standstill, hyperkalemia	1 mEq/kg IV; can be repeated
Verapamil	SVT	0.025-0.05 mg/kg IV q30min; can repeat to 0.2 mg/kg total dose

VT, Ventricular tachycardia; *AF,* atrial fibrillation; *SVT,* supraventricular tachycardia.
*Lidocaine without epinephrine for intravenous injection.
[†]Not available for intravenous injection in North America.
[‡]Most horses can tolerate only 12 mg/kg IV total dose if given as 1-2.2 mg/kg q10min.
[§]Not to exceed 6 doses q2h (most horses can tolerate only four doses q2h).

- Intravenous flecainide may be useful for the management of ventricular tachycardia in horses. Therapeutic concentrations for the conversion of atrial fibrillation in horses is 1303 ± 566 ng/ml.

TABLE 34–6. Adverse Effects of Antiarrhythmic Drugs

Drug	Adverse Effect	Cardiovascular Effect
Atropine	Ileus, mydriasis	Tachycardia, arrhythmias
Bretylium tosylate	GI disorder	Hypotension, tachycardia, arrhythmias
Digoxin	Depression, anorexia, colic	SVPD, VPD, SVT, VT
Flecainide	Agitation, prolonged QRS and QT intervals, proarrhythmic effect, neurologic, negative inotrope	
Lidocaine	Excitement, seizures	VT, sudden death
MgSO$_4$	Hypotension	
Quinidine	Depression, paraphimosis, urticaria, wheals, nasal mucosal swelling, laminitis, neurologic disorders, GI	Hypotension, SVT, VT, prolonged QRS and QT intervals, CHF, sudden death, negative inotrope
Phenytoin	Sedation, drowsiness, lip and facial twitching, gait deficits, seizures	Arrhythmias
Procainamide	GI, neurologic disorders similar to effects of quinidine	Hypotension, SVT, VT, prolonged QRS and QT intervals, sudden death, negative inotrope
Propafenone	GI, neurologic disorders similar to effects of quinidine, bronchospasm	CHF, AV block, arrhythmias, negative inotrope
Propranolol	Lethargy, worsening of COPD	Bradycardia, 3° AV block, arrhythmias, CHF, negative inotrope
Verapamil		Hypotension, bradycardia, AV block, asystole, arrhythmias, negative inotrope

GI, Gastrointestinal; *SVPD,* supraventricular premature depolarizations; *VPD,* ventricular premature depolarizations; *SVT,* supraventricular tachycardia; *VT,* ventricular tachycardia; *CHF,* congestive heart failure; *AV,* atrioventricular; *COPD,* chronic obstructive pulmonary disease.

- **Propranolol, 0.03 mg/kg IV,** also has negative inotropic effects and is rarely successful in converting horses with ventricular tachycardia.
  □ Propranolol should be tried, however, in the treatment of patients that do not respond to other antiarrhythmics. Therapeutic plasma concentrations of propranolol may be 20-80 ng/ml in horses.
- **MgSO$_4$, 1-2.5 g/450 kg per minute IV,** often is effective in the management of refractory ventricular tachycardia in horses. It is the drug of choice for quinidine-induced torsades de pointes and has no negative inotropic effects. MgSO$_4$ does cause hypotension, however.
  □ MgSO$_4$ is effective in the treatment of horses that have a normal or low magnesium level but also usually is administered slowly.
  □ **Bretylium tosylate, 3-5 mg/kg IV repeated up to a 10 mg/kg total dose,** should be reserved for patients with severe, life-threatening ventricular tachycardia or ventricular fibrillation.
  □ All antiarrhythmic drugs may have adverse effects and can be proarrhythmic (Table 34–6).

CARDIOPULMONARY RESUSCITATION

Cardiopulmonary resuscitation (CPR) of an adult horse (see p. 000) should be approached according to the same systematic principles applied to CPR of humans and small animals. The major difference is the size of the patient with cardiac arrest. The *ABCD* of CPR reminds the clinician of the order in which cardiopulmonary resuscitation is approached. *A* stands for establishing an airway, *B* for breathing for the patient, *C* for establishing circulation, and *D* for drugs that should be administered.

Establish an Airway

- Easily established with the nasotracheal placement of a smaller endotracheal tube or the orotracheal placement of a larger endotracheal tube.
- If orotracheal or nasotracheal intubation is not possible, emergency tracheotomy can be performed and the endotracheal tube inserted into the trachea through the tracheotomy site.
- The cuff should be inflated and the endotracheal tube attached to a demand valve or anesthetic machine.
- If an endotracheal tube is not available, a 10-foot length of Tygon tubing with a ½-inch (1.25-cm) internal diameter should be inserted nasotracheally and attached to the flow regulator of an E size oxygen cylinder.

Breathe for the Patient

- Four to six breaths/min are reportedly adequate to maintain normal PaO_2 for a horse.
- With a demand valve or large-animal anesthetic machine, the rebreathing bag can be compressed to between 20 and 40 cm water.
- The oxygen flow rate (100% O_2) should be adjusted so that there is moderate expansion of the thorax in 2-3 seconds.
- When Tygon tubing and intranasal oxygen are used, the horse's nose and mouth must be occluded and released alternately.

Establish Circulation in Cardiac Arrest

> An emergency that must be diagnosed and managed as quickly as possible.

- The peripheral arterial pulses should be checked and the heart auscultated to verify cardiac arrest.
- An ECG must be obtained to determine the type of cardiac arrhythmia present in the patient with cardiac arrest.
- **Remember, an airway must be established and breathing initiated for the horse before reestablishment of circulation is begun.**
- The horse should be in lateral recumbency, ideally in right lateral recumbency with the head level or lowered.
- An ECG should be obtained with external or internal cardiac massage to determine the rhythm being generated or initiated during CPR.

External Cardiac Massage

- Forcefully and rapidly compress the horse's chest right behind the horse's elbow with the resuscitator's knee or hands (if the patient is small).
- Initiate at the rate of 60-80 compressions/minute.
- Difficult to perform on adults and rarely successful.
- Monitor the peripheral pulses to determine whether cardiac compressions are adequate.

Internal Cardiac Massage

- Attempt only if external cardiac compression is not successful.
- Internal cardiac massage is associated with a large number of postoperative complications in the horse (pneumothorax, pleuropneumonia, and severe lameness).
- Successful intracardiac compression requires an incision in the fifth intercostal space with retraction of the fifth and sixth ribs or a fifth rib resection and manual compression of the left ventricle.
- Compress the heart 40-60 times/minute.
- Can be performed through an incision in the diaphragm if the patient is undergoing exploratory celiotomy.

Drugs Administered

- Determine the type of cardiac emergency that is being experienced by the equine patient. Further therapeutic intervention depends on whether asystole or ventricular fibrillation is present (Box 34–4).
- Administer drugs into a central vein (cranial vena cava), if possible, or otherwise into the jugular vein as close to the central vein as possible.

Asystole (Fig. 34–26)

- **Epinephrine** should be **administered IV, 10-20 µg/kg per minute or 5-10 ml/500-kg adult, or intratracheally (20-40 µg/kg per minute)**; intracardiac (IC) administration is used as a last resort.
- Periods of asystole must be recognized and intervention begun immediately for treatment of horses to be successful.

Ventricular Fibrillation (Fig. 34–27)

- Epinephrine is unlikely to be successful
- Administer antiarrhythmic drugs with efficacy against ventricular fibrillation (preferable) or refractory sustained ventricular tachycardia.
  □ Administer **bretylium tosylate, 3-5 mg/kg IV**; can repeat up to 10 mg/kg total dose.
- Successful chemical defibrillation of an adult with antiarrhythmic drugs has not been performed.
- Successful electrical defibrillation of one 350-kg horse and several foals has been reported.
- Chemical or electrical defibrillation or both should be attempted, if the necessary drugs and defibrillator are available and the preexisting condition of the patient is not terminal.
- Intravenous fluids should be administered at the rate of 20 ml/kg per hour during resuscitation of a horse to maintain normal or elevated mean circulatory

CARDIOVASCULAR

BOX 34-4. Cardiopulmonary Resuscitation and Treatment of the Horse

ESTABLISH AN AIRWAY
- Nasotracheal placement of an endotracheal tube
- Orotracheal placement of an endotracheal tube

ASYSTOLE
- Initiate external cardiac massage.
- If no heartbeat, inject **epinephrine, 0.3-0.5 mg/kg, 20-40 µg/kg per minute, or 10-20 ml/500 kg** in sterile saline solution **intratracheally** and ventilate vigorously for 4-5 breaths, or inject **0.03-0.05 mg/kg, 10-20 µg/kg per minute, or 5-10 ml/500 kg epinephrine IV**.
- Epinephrine is given by means of intracardiac administration as a last resort and is injected into the left ventricle space.
- Continue CPR, checking the peripheral pulse for effectiveness.
- Establish an IV line and administer lactated Ringer's solution rapidly.
- Reevaluate CPR and ECG findings. If unable to establish a pulse within 2 minutes, open the chest at the 6th intercostal space and begin cardiac massage.

VENTRICULAR FIBRILLATION
- Initiate or continue CPR
- Defibrillate
  - Administer bretylium tosylate IC.
  - Use an electrical defibrillator (direct current) at appropriate W-s/kg. Use adequate amounts of electrode paste on the skin and no alcohol (flammable).
  - Mix **potassium chloride, 1 mEq/kg, with acetylcholine, 6 mg/kg, and inject IC.**

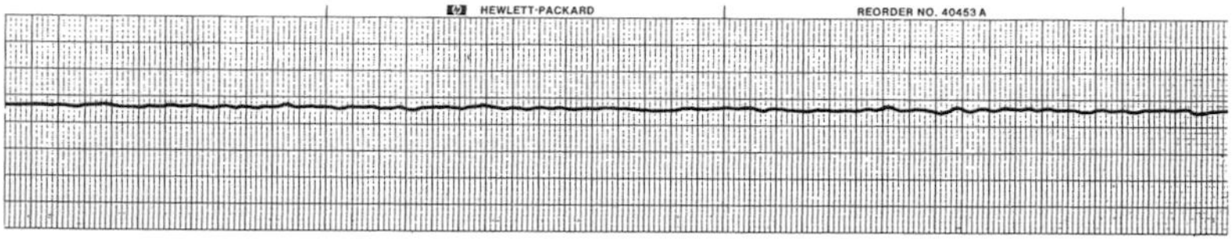

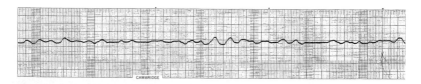

FIGURE 34-26. Base-apex electrocardiogram of a horse with asystole. The ECG recorded line is flat with some baseline undulations and no evidence of atrial or ventricular electrical activity. This electrocardiogram was recorded at a paper speed of 25 mm/s with a sensitivity of 5 mm = 1 mV.

FIGURE 34-27. Base-apex electrocardiogram of a horse with ventricular fibrillation. Baseline fibrillation waves are fine, and there is no evidence of coordinated atrial or ventricular depolarization. This electrocardiogram was recorded at a paper speed of 25 mm/s with a sensitivity of 5 mm = 1 mV.

pressures. Maintaining normal or elevated mean circulatory pressure during CPR increases the probability of a favorable outcome for a dog and is likely also to do so for an equine patient.

Postresuscitation Treatment

- Calcium in the form of **calcium chloride or calcium gluconate (0.1-0.2 mEq/kg slowly IV over 5-10 min)**, *although highly controversial,* may be indicated to increase the force of myocardial contraction and counteract the effects of hypocalcemia and hyperkalemia.
- Once a normal sinus rhythm has been restored, **dobutamine, 1-5 μg/kg per minute IV**, is the drug of choice for maintaining cardiac output and arterial blood pressure.
- The use of $NaHCO_3$ is controversial and is not indicated if circulation is rapidly restored, because large volumes of $NaHCO_3$ can cause hyperosmolality, hypernatremia, hypocalcemia, hypokalemia, and decreases in the affinity of hemoglobin for oxygen.
- Small doses of $NaHCO_3$ may be indicated to manage metabolic acidosis and hyperkalemia in horses that have experienced a prolonged period of cardiac arrest.

ELECTROLYTE DISTURBANCES CAUSING CARDIAC ARRHYTHMIAS
Hyperkalemia

- Most frequently recognized in foals with uroperitoneum but is occasionally seen in adults, primarily those with acute renal failure.
- Also seen in Quarter Horses with hyperkalemic periodic paralysis (HPP).
- Clinical signs include stiffness, muscle weakness, muscle fasciculations, muscle spasm, respiratory stridor, recumbency, and death.
- Death is caused by paralysis of the pharyngeal and laryngeal muscles or by cardiac arrhythmias associated with hyperkalemia.
- Identify individuals predisposed to the development of HPP by testing for HPP-type sodium channel DNA. *Ventricular arrhythmias during exercise are more likely among horses homozygous for HPP.*
- Cardiac arrhythmias may or may not be detected, but an ECG should be obtained for adults or foals with a plasma potassium concentration ≥6 mEq/L.

ELECTROCARDIOGRAM
- Tall, peaked T waves detected with plasma potassium values ≥6.2 mEq/L (Fig. 34–28)
- Progressive slowing of conduction and decreased excitability result in cardiac arrest or ventricular fibrillation.
- Broadening and flattening of the P waves, prolonged PR intervals, and bradycardia develop, conduction slows, and excitability decreases. *Atrial arrest or atrial standstill develops.*
- Atrial and ventricular premature depolarizations and ventricular tachycardia have been reported.
- Widened QRS complexes are further indications of severe (near lethal) hyperkalemia.
- The QT interval is not a reliable indicator of hyperkalemia.

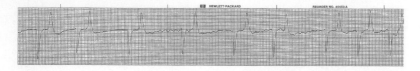

FIGURE 34-28. Base-apex electrocardiogram of a horse with hyperkalemia (plasma K⁺ concentration, 6.6 mEq/L) and a creatinine level of 24 mg/dl. Tall, tented T waves (2.5 mV) are typical of hyperkalemia. This horse also had atrial fibrillation. RR intervals are irregular, P waves are absent, and baseline f waves are present with a heart rate of 50 beats/min. This electrocardiogram was recorded at a paper speed of 25 mm/s with a sensitivity of 5 mm = 1 mV.

TREATMENT

- Uroperitoneum must be managed aggressively as soon as it is diagnosed, because these foals are at high risk of development of cardiac arrhythmias, particularly when they are under general anesthesia during surgical repair of the ruptured bladder, urachus, or ureter.
- Ventricular premature beats, ventricular tachycardia, complete heart block, and atrial standstill have been reported in foals with uroperitoneum.
- **Sodium** deficit should be replaced slowly at the rate of **0.5 mEq/h.**
  - □ 0.45%-0.9% NaCl IV
- **NaHCO₃, 1 mEq/kg, IV** will help drive potassium intracellularly.
- 5%-50% dextrose IV also may be needed to help drive the potassium intracellularly.
- Administer **5% dextrose, 0.5 ml/kg,** and 0.9% saline solution IV.
- If the foregoing measures are unsuccessful, administer **regular insulin, 0.1 IU/kg IV** with **0.5-1 g/kg dextrose IV** to help drive potassium into the cell. Add 5 ml of the foal's blood to the fluid to prevent the insulin from adhering to the fluid administration bag.
- If severe cardiac arrhythmias or atrial standstill is detected, **calcium gluconate, 4 mg/kg,** can be administered slowly (over a 10-minute period) to effect.
  - □ Calcium gluconate should be discontinued if bradycardia occurs after calcium administration.
- Gradual drainage of the uroperitoneum should be performed in conjunction with intravenous fluid replacement therapy, as indicated earlier.
- Surgical correction of the uroperitoneum should be performed after medical stabilization of the foal.

Hyperkalemic Periodic Paralysis

In adult horses with HPP experiencing an acute episode with symptoms such as recumbency, respiratory stridor, or trembling:

- Serum potassium concentration often is greater than 6 mEq/L; draw blood to measure serum potassium concentration.
- Administer
  - □ **0.2-0.4 ml/kg of 23% calcium borogluconate solution IV**
  - □ **6 ml/kg 5% dextrose solution IV or 1 ml/kg 50% dextrose**
  - □ **NaHCO₃, 1-2 mEq/kg IV**
  - □ Insulin may be used as indicated earlier but requires regular monitoring of blood glucose concentration for the following 24 hours.

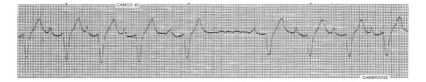

FIGURE 34-29. Base-apex electrocardiogram of a horse with hypokalemia (plasma K+ concentration, 1.4 mEq/L), sinus arrhythmia, and a heart rate of 50 beats/min. Markedly widened QRS and T complexes reflect delayed conduction and abnormal ventricular repolarization. This electrocardiogram was recorded at a paper speed of 25 mm/s with a sensitivity of 5 mm = 1 mV.

TREATMENT
- Feed a diet low in potassium (timothy hay and Bermuda grass hay, no molasses).
- Keep horses in a regular exercise program.
- Kaliuretic diuretics such as **acetazolamide, 2-4 mg/kg PO q6h, or hydrochlorothiazide, 250 mg IM or IV q6h**, have been useful in reducing the frequency and severity of clinical signs but are expensive.
- Do not use affected horses for breeding because the mode of inheritance is autosomal dominant.

Hypokalemia
- Common among horses with heat exhaustion with hypochloremia, hypocalcemia, and metabolic alkalosis
- Also occurs in patients with severe diarrhea

ELECTROCARDIOGRAM
- Prolongation of the QT interval is an indication of hypokalemia.
- Supraventricular and ventricular arrhythmias occur:
  □ Atrial tachycardia with block (Fig. 34-29) and junctional tachycardia are common supraventricular arrhythmias among patients with hypokalemia.
  □ Ventricular tachycardia, torsades de pointes, and ventricular fibrillation can occur with severe hypokalemia.

TREATMENT
- Replace calculated potassium deficit slowly IV, adding **KCl, 20-40 mEq/L;** *do not* exceed a rate of **0.5 mEq/kg per hour.** Serum potassium concentration should be monitored during treatment.
- Administer **KCl, 0.1 g/kg PO** if the gastrointestinal tract is patent.
- Correct other electrolyte abnormalities, if present, and do not cause diuresis with excessive intravenous fluids unless the patient has volume contraction.

Hypomagnesemia
- Magnesium deficiency usually is associated with hypokalemia or hypocalcemia.

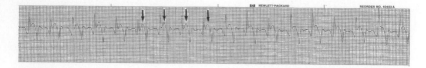

FIGURE 34-30. Lead II electrocardiogram of a horse with severe hypomagnesemia (Mg^{2+} concentration, 0.7 mg/dl), hyperkalemia (K^+ concentration, 6.2 mEq/L), and azotemia (creatinine concentration, 6.0 mg/dl). Rapid, regular rhythm with a ventricular rate of 100 beats/min. The QRS complexes are normal for lead II, but the P waves are buried in the QT complex *(arrows),* suggesting junctional tachycardia. The T waves are large ($\geq$1 mV and spiked). This electrocardiogram was recorded at a paper speed of 25 mm/s with a sensitivity of 10 mm = 1 mV.

ELECTROCARDIOGRAM

- Serious ventricular arrhythmias are most likely in patients with significant hypomagnesemia, but supraventricular tachycardia (Fig. 34–30) and atrial fibrillation also occur in patients with severe hypomagnesemia.
- PR interval prolonged, QRS complex widened, ST segment depressed, and T wave peaked

TREATMENT

- Administer **$MgSO_4$, 1-2.5 g/450 kg per minute IV** at a rate **not to** exceed **25 g/450 kg**, and follow it with **oral $MgSO_4$ supplementation (0.2-1 g/kg).**

Hypocalcemia

- Hypocalcemic tetany, lactation tetany, transport tetany, and eclampsia are uncommon in horses.
- When associated with lactation, hypocalcemia often occurs after peak lactation, approximately 60-100 days postpartum.
- Occasionally occurs after prolonged or strenuous exercise, especially in hot weather, in prolonged transport, or in horses with diarrhea.
- Occurs among horses fed a diet low or deficient in calcium. Magnesium also may be deficient in the diet, which can lead to multiple cases of hypocalcemia on a farm.
- Occurs among horses with cantharidin (blister beetle) toxicosis.
- Hypoalbuminemia reduces the total serum concentration of calcium and of protein-bound calcium *but not of ionized calcium.*
- To measure serum calcium more accurately in patients with hypoalbuminemia if ionized calcium cannot be measured:

    Corrected calcium = Measured calcium (mg/dl) − Albumin (g/dl) + 3.5

- Alkalosis reduces the concentration of ionized calcium in the blood. Two different clinical syndromes occur among horses with moderate to severe hypocalcemia:
    - Horses with a low serum calcium level (5-8 mg/dl) and low serum magnesium level: Tachycardia, synchronous diaphragmatic flutter, laryngospasm with loud, labored breathing, trismus, protrusion of the nictitans, dysphagia, abdominal pain, goose-stepping or stiff hindlimb gait, and ataxia may be present. Rhabdomyolysis, convulsions, coma, and death may ensue.

□ Horses with an even lower serum calcium concentration (<5 mg/dl) and normal serum magnesium concentration: Flaccid paralysis, mydriasis, stupor, and recumbency are usually present.

ELECTROCARDIOGRAM
- ECG abnormalities other than tachycardia are rare.
- Atrial or ventricular premature beats or ventricular tachycardia is occasionally detected.
- Cardiac arrest or ventricular standstill may occur.
- Q_0T_c interval inversely correlated with ionized plasma calcium concentration

TREATMENT
- **Intravenous** infusion of **calcium gluconate, 4 mg/kg slowly** (over a 10-minute period) to effect
- Analyze the horse's ration and ensure an adequate calcium to phosphorus ratio (1.3-2:1) and adequate magnesium in the diet.

Hypercalcemia

- Occurs among horses with chronic renal failure, lymphosarcoma, paraneoplastic syndromes, and hypervitaminosis D and after ingestion of *Cestrum diurnum*
  □ *Cestrum diurnum* contains 1,25-dihydroxycholecalciferol and may induce hypervitaminosis D.
  □ Hyperphosphatemia occurs and is an early and reliable indicator of vitamin D intoxication.
- Results in soft-tissue mineralization and mineralization of the heart and blood vessels, especially aorta, pulmonary artery, coronary arteries, and endocardium.

ELECTROCARDIOGRAM
- Initially heart rate slows, and sinus arrhythmia and partial AV block are detected.
- Tachycardia and extrasystoles are a common finding.
- Atrial and ventricular tachycardia may occur.
- Q_0T_c interval inversely correlates with ionized plasma calcium concentration.
- Cardiac arrest, ventricular fibrillation, or ventricular standstill is a lethal event.

TREATMENT
- Search for the underlying cause of hypercalcemia and remove or control it if possible.
  □ Discontinue all exogenous supplements containing calcium, phosphorus, and vitamin D, and remove horses from *Cestrum diurnum*–infected pasture.
- Emergency treatment is indicated in the care of patients with cardiac disease, severe renal decompensation, and systemic disease with hypercalcemia in the 15-20 mg/dl range.
  □ Administer 0.9% NaCl IV to expand the extracellular fluid volume and increase the glomerular filtration rate. **Potassium, 20 mEq/L, and magnesium, 10 g/L, not to exceed 25-30 g** over 30 minutes, supplementation of the intravenous fluids should be administered more slowly or be added to oral fluids.

□ Begin diuretic therapy with a calciuric diuretic such as **furosemide, 1-2 mg/kg q12h** and keep intravenous fluid maintenance levels at 5 ml/kg per hour (or at least equal to urine output).

□ Administration of corticosteroids may reduce calcium concentrations and decrease the likelihood of soft-tissue and cardiac mineralization by decreasing calcium loss from bone, decreasing intestinal calcium absorption, and increasing renal excretion of calcium. (Steroid-responsive forms of hypercalcemia include lymphoma, lymphosarcoma, leukemia, multiple myeloma, thymoma, vitamin D toxicity, granulomatous disease, and hyperadrenocorticism.)

□ Treatment with salmon calcitonin may be indicated if severe, prolonged hypercalcemia is present.

CONGESTIVE HEART FAILURE

Congestive heart failure has a multitude of causes in horses, both congenital and acquired. Most patients with congestive heart failure have acquired cardiac disease: valvular heart disease, myocardial disease, or both. Severe cardiac arrhythmia, primarily ventricular tachycardia, also causes clinical signs of congestive heart failure. Severe congenital cardiac disease is an uncommon cause of congestive heart failure in horses. Congestive heart failure in these individuals may develop slowly over a prolonged period or suddenly and necessitate emergency intervention.

- Horses with severe primary myocardial disease, acute onset of severe valvular heart disease (mitral or aortic, Box 34–5), or multifocal ventricular tachycardia are most likely to have clinical signs of acute, left-sided heart failure and need emergency treatment.

Clinical Signs of Acute, Left-Sided Heart Failure

- Anxiety, tachypnea, dyspnea, tachycardia, coughing, foamy nasal discharge, expectoration of a foamy fluid, lethargy, and exercise intolerance.
  - □ Diagnosis often is missed because of the subtlety of clinical signs in many horses.

BOX 34-5. Clinical Signs and Physical Examination Findings in Horses with Acute Mitral or Aortic Regurgitation

---

- **Tachycardia:** Heart rate usually ≥60 beats/min
  - □ Irregular rhythm present or absent: Usually atrial fibrillation but may have atrial or ventricular premature contractions or both
  - □ Loud third heart sound
- **Tachypnea:** Respiratory rate usually ≥24 breaths/min with increased respiratory effort, flared nostrils, and prolonged recovery after exercise
- **Coughing:** At rest or during or after exercise
- **Expectoration** of foamy fluid may or may not occur
- **Exercise intolerance** or poor performance
- **Syncope:** Rare
- **Harsh** inspiratory and expiratory vesicular sounds
- **Crackles** or moist sounds: Rare

- □ Rupture of mitral valve chordae tendineae is the most likely cause of acute fulminant pulmonary edema in individuals with primary valvular heart disease.
- □ Patients with bacterial endocarditis also may have acute left- or right-sided heart failure because of rapid destruction of the valve apparatus by the vegetative lesion. The most common site of endocarditis in the horse is the mitral valve; next is the aortic valve. Patients also may have fever, weight loss, and "shifting" leg lameness. Systemic septic emboli frequently occur.
- □ Acute severe myocarditis with severe left ventricular dysfunction is the most common cause of frank pulmonary edema in horses with primary myocardial disease. Many of these horses have a history of fever (often a suspected equine herpesvirus, other viral, or influenza infection) in the weeks or months preceding the signs of cardiac disease.
- □ Most horses with multifocal ventricular tachycardia and acute severe pulmonary edema also have severe myocardial disease.
- Weakness or syncope may occur, particularly with multifocal or rapid unifocal ventricular tachycardia.
  - □ Patients with ventricular tachycardia also have frequent jugular pulses.
- Arterial pulses usually are weak, and extremities may be cool.
- Cyanosis at rest is rarely detected but occasionally is induced by exercise.

AUSCULTATION
- Coarse breath sounds over the entire lung field in most patients. Occasional horses also have crackles or moist sounds detected in the perihilar or ventral lung field. However, moist sounds are infrequently detected in horses with left-sided congestive heart failure because the edema is primarily interstitial.
- The abnormal lung sounds are most frequently detected when the patient is taking deep breaths in a rebreathing bag.
- Horses easily become distressed when breathing in a rebreathing bag or with breath holding, often cough, may expectorate foamy fluid, and have a prolonged recovery time to resting respiratory rate.
- Cardiac murmurs usually are heard if severe valvular, congenital, or myocardial disease is the cause of the congestive heart failure. Loud (grade 3/6-6/6), coarse, band-shaped, holosystolic, or pansystolic murmurs of mitral regurgitation are detected in most patients with acute, left-sided heart failure.
  - □ Murmurs associated with ruptured mitral chordae tendineae usually are loud and honking initially. These murmurs often decrease in intensity with time.
  - □ Most horses also have slightly quieter murmurs of tricuspid regurgitation.
  - □ Some patients with bacterial endocarditis do not have a murmur.
  - □ A small number of patients also have holodiastolic decrescendo murmurs of aortic regurgitation.
  - □ Murmurs associated with a congenital defect, such as a ventricular septal defect, are infrequently detected.
- The cardiac rhythm usually is rapid and regular, unless multifocal ventricular tachycardia is the underlying cause of the congestive heart failure.
  - □ Atrial fibrillation is more common among horses with chronic valvular regurgitation.
  - □ Ventricular premature depolarizations or paroxysms of ventricular tachycardia may be present in horses with bacterial endocarditis of the mitral or aortic leaflets.

- Loud S_3 may be heard in association with ventricular volume overload.

TREATMENT
- Emergency management of pulmonary edema should be instituted as soon as possible and should include **furosemide, 1-2 mg/kg IV**, and intranasal oxygen. Drugs to reduce anxiety should be administered if needed. If the heart rate exceeds 120 beats/min, ventricular tachycardia should be suspected.

Additional Diagnostics
- ECG to establish the underlying cardiac rhythm.
- Echocardiography to evaluate myocardial function (Fig. 34–31), determine the severity of underlying congenital or valvular heart disease (Figs. 34–32 and 34–33), and look for evidence of pulmonary hypertension (Fig. 34–34).
  □ A dilated pulmonary artery is compatible with significant pulmonary hypertension and the possibility of impending pulmonary artery rupture (see Fig. 34–34).
- Cardiac isoenzyme levels of creatine kinase (CK) and lactate dehydrogenase (LDH) should be measured by means of protein electrophoresis to determine whether myocardial injury and necrosis have occurred. Elevated cardiac isoenzyme levels are a good indicator of myocardial cell damage; however, normal laboratory values do not exclude myocardial insult.
- Cardiac troponin I[1] is a more sensitive and specific indicator of myocardial cell damage. Normal values for horses are similar to those in humans and small animals (<0.1 ng/ml).

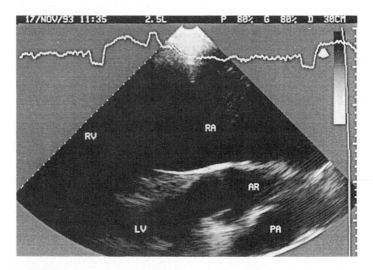

FIGURE 34–31. Long axis two-dimensional echocardiogram of a horse with right ventricular cardiomyopathy, syncope, and congestive heart failure. Evident are the markedly enlarged right atrium *(RA)* and right ventricle *(RV)* and the small pulmonary artery *(PA)* associated with severe pulmonary hypoperfusion. This echocardiogram was obtained from the right parasternal window in the left ventricular outflow tract position with a 2.5-MHz sector scanner transducer. The electrocardiogram is superimposed for timing. *AR,* aortic root; *LV,* left ventricle.

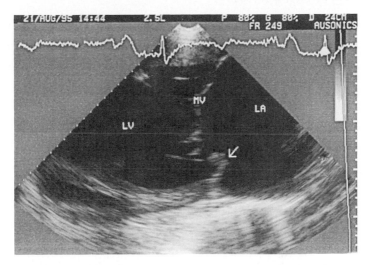

FIGURE 34-32. Long axis two-dimensional echocardiogram of a horse with ruptured chordae tendineae of the mitral valve *(arrow)* and acute left-sided congestive heart failure. This echocardiogram was obtained from the left parasternal window in the mitral valve position with a 2.5-MHz sector scanner transducer. An electrocardiogram is superimposed for timing. *MV,* Mitral valve; *LA,* left atrium; *LV,* left ventricle.

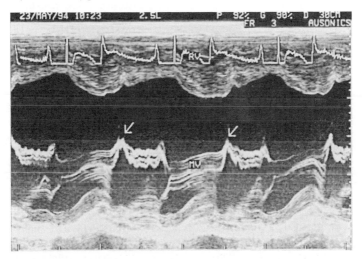

FIGURE 34-33. M-mode echocardiogram of a horse with acute, severe aortic regurgitation. Marked separation between the mitral valve E point *(arrows)* and the interventricular septum is associated with marked left ventricular volume overload and dilatation of the left ventricular outflow tract. The septal leaflet of the mitral valve has high-frequency vibrations caused by turbulence in the left ventricular outflow tract associated with the regurgitant jet. This echocardiogram was obtained from the right parasternal window with a 2.5-MHz sector scanner transducer. An electrocardiogram is superimposed for timing. *MV,* Mitral valve.

CARDIOVASCULAR

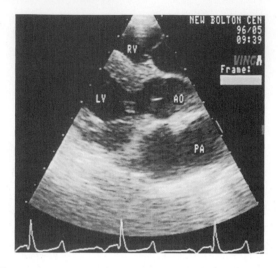

FIGURE 34–34. Long axis two-dimensional echocardiogram of a horse with ruptured chordae tendineae of the mitral valve and acute left-sided congestive heart failure. The small diameter of the aortic root *(AO)* and the larger diameter of the pulmonary artery *(PA)* are consistent with severe pulmonary hypertension. This echocardiogram was obtained from the right parasternal window in the left ventricular outflow tract position with a 2.5-MHz annular array transducer. An electrocardiogram is superimposed for timing. *RV,* Right ventricle; *LV,* left ventricle.

- A chemistry profile, complete blood cell count, and measurement of total protein content and fibrinogen should be obtained to ascertain whether there is underlying disease and to evaluate the severity of any renal compromise (usually prerenal azotemia).
- If ventricular tachycardia is the cause of acute congestive heart failure, antiarrhythmic therapy should be instituted as soon as possible. Selection of the appropriate antiarrhythmic drug depends on the severity of the arrhythmia and the associated clinical signs (see earlier).
- If sinus tachycardia, supraventricular tachycardia, or atrial fibrillation is present, positive inotropic support should be instituted immediately and consist of either **digoxin, 0.0022 mg/kg IV, or dobutamine, 1-5 µg/kg per minute IV.**
- Modify the dose of digoxin (increase dosing intervals to once daily or decrease dose) if prerenal azotemia is present.
- After an initial clinical response, oral therapy with **digoxin, 0.011 mg/kg, and furosemide, 0.5-1 mg/kg,** can be instituted.
- Afterload reducers (vasodilators), such as **hydralazine, 0.5-1.5 mg/kg PO q12h,** or angiotensin-converting enzyme (ACE) inhibitors**, 0.5 mg/kg enalapril PO q12h,** if needed, should be administered to patients with severe mitral or aortic regurgitation to improve cardiac output and reduce myocardial work.
- If the horse has bacterial endocarditis, broad-spectrum bactericidal intravenous antimicrobial therapy (both Gram-positive and Gram-negative coverage) should be instituted after several blood cultures are obtained.

Right-Sided Congestive Failure

Patients with long-standing congenital, valvular, or myocardial disease that gradually leads to congestive heart failure frequently have little in the way of clinical signs referable to the respiratory system. These horses usually have clinical signs of right-sided congestive heart failure and rarely need emergency treatment.

Clinical Signs
- May have tachypnea at rest, an occasional cough, prolonged recovery times to resting respiratory rate after exercise, and biventricular failure or a large pleural effusion associated with right-sided heart failure.
- The veterinarian usually is consulted because the horse has preputial, pectoral, or ventral edema.
- Generalized venous distention and jugular pulsations usually are present.
- Syncope may be present in patients with severe right-sided congestive heart failure and decreased pulmonary blood flow.

AUSCULTATION
- Coarse vesicular sounds at rest or with a rebreathing bag; crackles or moist sounds are rarely detected.
- Dullness may be detected in the cranioventral lung field on auscultation or percussion associated with pleural effusion.
- In rare instances, the heart may sound muffled because of a small pericardial effusion.
- Murmurs of mitral and tricuspid valvular regurgitation are frequently detected.
- Some affected horses also have murmurs of aortic regurgitation or a ventricular septal defect (or another, usually complex, congenital defect).
- The heart rate usually is elevated and irregularly irregular with atrial fibrillation.
- Patients with uniform ventricular tachycardia and congestive heart failure usually have a more rapid (>120 beats/min) and regular rhythm but have similar clinical signs.
- These patients should be treated with antiarrhythmic drugs to correct ventricular tachycardia (see earlier section, p. 153).
- A loud S_3 may be associated with ventricular volume overload.

Treatment
- Treatment with furosemide, positive inotropic drugs (usually digoxin), and vasodilators (hydralazine or ACE inhibitors) as indicated earlier should be started. Intravenous administration can be selected initially if the signs of congestive heart failure are severe, but most patients respond well to oral therapy. Clinical improvement is noticed within 24 hours (see Table 34–4).
- Serum or plasma samples should be obtained for measurement of digoxin concentration after several days of oral therapy to see whether adjustments in dosage are necessary.
  - Peak (sample obtained 1-2 hours after oral digoxin administration) and trough digoxin concentrations should be measured and should fall within the therapeutic range of 1-2 ng/ml.
  - Digoxin toxicity has been reported in horses with digoxin concentrations >2 ng/ml.

- Clinical improvement within several days usually occurs with this treatment regimen. However, because of the severity of the underlying cardiac disease in most horses with clinical signs of congestive heart failure, the improvement usually is of short duration (2-6 months).
- Digoxin has a narrow therapeutic to toxic range; therefore the patient should be monitored for any signs of digoxin toxicity.
- Anorexia, lethargy, colic, and the development of other cardiac arrhythmias have been reported among individuals with digoxin toxicity.
- Hypokalemia potentiates the toxic effects of digoxin, yet digoxin toxicity can cause extracellular hyperkalemia by interfering with the Na-K pump; therefore careful monitoring of potassium status is important.
- Ectopic foci, usually atrial, develop with relatively small doses of digoxin in hypokalemic patients.
- The administration of digoxin should be discontinued in the treatment of all horses when digoxin toxicity is suspected. A blood sample should be obtained for measurement of serum or plasma digoxin, potassium, and creatinine concentrations.
  - *Oral potassium* **supplementation, 40 g/450 kg PO**, if the patient is hypokalemic may be adequate if the clinical signs associated with digoxin toxicity are mild.
  - *Intravenous potassium,* **40 mEq/L**, may be administered slowly in intravenous fluids to the hypokalemic patient if life-threatening arrhythmias are present.
  - *Lidocaine,* **20-50 µg/kg per minute**, is indicated for the management of ventricular arrhythmias associated with digoxin toxicity.
  - *Phenytoin,* **5-10 mg/kg IV** for the first 12 hours, then **1-5 mg/kg IM q12h or 1.82 mg/kg PO q12h**, may be indicated in the management of supraventricular arrhythmias associated with digoxin toxicity. *Side effects* of phenytoin include a mild tranquilizing effect. Overdosing can lead to lip and facial twitching, gait deficits, and seizures. Do not use in conjunction with other medications, particularly trimethoprim-sulfamethoxazole.
  - Administer cardiac glycoside-specific antibodies or their Fab fragment (Digibind). These agents bind excess circulating digoxin and prevent further development of digoxin toxicity. This treatment should be reserved for patients with life-threatening digoxin toxicity and is very expensive. In humans with digoxin toxicity and hyperkalemia, this treatment almost always results in a reversal of digoxin-induced cardiac arrhythmias.
- Chronic administration of high doses of furosemide can lead to hypokalemic metabolic alkalosis.
  - Plasma potassium should be regularly monitored (weekly).
  - Feed the horse high-quality hay, such as alfalfa, that is rich in potassium.
  - Oral potassium supplementation should be considered, in addition to feeding high-quality hay. KCl salt is not very palatable and must be gradually introduced into the horse's grain (1 tablespoon per feeding with gradual increases if the horse consumes up to 1 ounce q12h).
- Patients with bacterial endocarditis involving the pulmonic or tricuspid valve may have severe pneumonia or pulmonary thrombosis secondary to septic emboli. Tricuspid valve endocarditis has frequently been associated with septic thrombophlebitis of the jugular vein.

PERICARDITIS, PERICARDIAL EFFUSION

Pericarditis is uncommon among horses, but it usually manifests in an emergency with clinical signs of cardiovascular collapse. Concurrent or historical respiratory tract disease is present in approximately 50% of patients with pericarditis.

- Many patients with pericarditis exhibit signs of discomfort that are initially interpreted as abdominal pain; they are therefore *usually referred for colic.*
- Physical examination findings at presentation include depression; tachycardia; generalized venous distention; pectoral, ventral, and preputial edema; and muffled heart sounds. Fever, lethargy, anorexia, jugular pulsations, weak arterial pulses, pericardial friction rubs, tachypnea, dullness in the cranioventral thorax, and weight loss also may be detected.
  - Arrhythmias are infrequently detected, usually are atrial if present, and indicate the presence of concurrent myocarditis.
  - Patients with pericarditis, particularly those with septic pericarditis, may have mild anemia, neutrophilic leukocytosis, hyperproteinemia, and hyperfibrinogenemia.

Cardiac tamponade can occur when fluid accumulates rapidly within the pericardial sac, impedes ventricular filling, and causes a rapid decrease in cardiac output. The three determinants of the development of cardiac tamponade are the distensibility of the pericardial sac, the rate at which fluid accumulation occurs within the pericardial sac, and the amount of fluid present within the pericardial sac.

- Cardiac tamponade should be suspected in any horse with increasing venous pressure, tachycardia, muffled heart sounds, decreasing arterial blood pressure, and pulsus paradoxus.
  - Pulsus paradoxus is an inspiratory reduction in arterial blood pressure >10 mm Hg.
- Central venous pressures of up to 43 cm water (normal central venous pressure, 10-15 cm water) have been reported in patients with cardiac tamponade, large pericardial effusions, or constrictive pericarditis.
- Right atrial, right ventricular, and pulmonary arterial end-diastolic pressures may be increased in horses with cardiac tamponade.

Echocardiography is the diagnostic modality of choice for the assessment of the amount of pericardial fluid, its character, and the degree of cardiac compromise. Fibrinous effusive pericarditis is most common in horses. The volume of fluid associated with pericarditis ranges from none detectable to >14 L (Fig. 34–35). Fluid within the pericardial sac usually is anechoic to slightly hypoechoic in horses with septic or idiopathic pericarditis. Sheets of fibrin with frondlike projections usually are imaged on the epicardial and pericardial surfaces. Compartmentalization of this fluid can occur, and walled-off areas develop in the pericardial sac. Concurrent pleural effusion often is present. Effusive pericarditis without fibrin is most common in patients with congestive heart failure, not in patients with primary pericardial disease. Hemopericardium has been detected in several horses that have sustained thoracic trauma and in one foal with penetration of the right ventricular free wall by a broken and dislodged intravenous catheter. Blood within the pericardial sac looks like echogenic swirling fluid.

- Excessive motion (swinging) of the right ventricular free wall is detected echocardiographically in patients with pericardial effusion (Fig. 34–36).

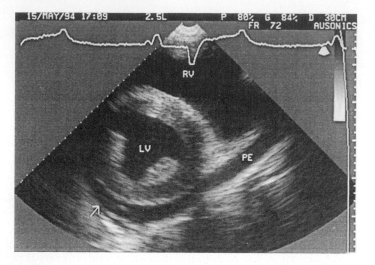

FIGURE 34–35. Short axis two-dimensional echocardiogram of a horse with pericarditis. The arrow points to some fibrin within the pericardial sac. This echocardiogram was obtained from the right parasternal window in the left ventricular position with a 2.5-MHz sector scanner transducer. An electrocardiogram is superimposed for timing. *LV,* Left ventricle; *RV,* right ventricle; *PE,* pericardial effusion.

- Diastolic collapse of the right ventricular free wall occurs as the amount of pericardial fluid begins to increase. It is first pictured in the right ventricular outflow tract because this area is easiest to compress.
- Early echocardiographic signs of cardiac tamponade include an inspiratory increase in the dimension of the right ventricle, an inspiratory decrease in the internal diameter of the left ventricle, and collapse of the right atrium during systole (right atrial inversion).
  - □ Right atrial inversion (Fig. 34–37) becomes more severe as hemodynamically significant cardiac tamponade develops.
  - □ Doppler-detected increased tricuspid and decreased mitral inflow during exhalation are other indications of developing cardiac tamponade.
- ECG reveals small-amplitude P, QRS, and T complexes caused by damping of the electrical impulse by the surrounding pericardial fluid (Fig. 34–38).
- Electrical alternans, a cyclical variation in the size of the QRS complexes, has been found in horses with pericardial effusion but is infrequently seen (Fig. 34–39). Electrical alternans is believed to be caused by the swinging motion of the heart in the pericardial fluid.
- A globoid cardiac silhouette is detected during thoracic radiography. This sign usually is accompanied by opacification of the ventral thorax due to concurrent pleural effusion. However, this radiographic appearance cannot be definitively differentiated from other forms of cardiac enlargement, and good-quality lateral thoracic radiographs cannot be obtained with portable radiographic equipment, except in evaluation of foals.

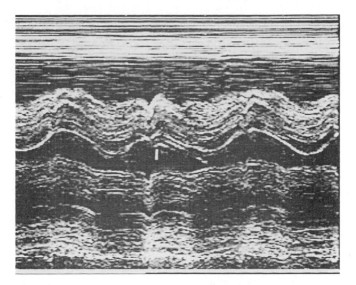

FIGURE 34–36. M-mode echocardiogram of a horse with idiopathic pericarditis and a fibrinous pericardial effusion demonstrating the swinging pattern of right ventricular free wall motion. The slight increase in right ventricular diameter is associated with inspiration *(I)*. This echocardiogram was obtained from the right parasternal window in the left ventricular position with a 2.5-MHz sector scanner transducer.

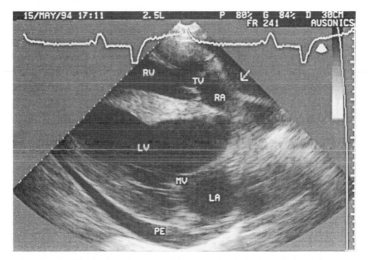

FIGURE 34–37. Two-dimensional echocardiogram of a horse with pericarditis shows inversion of the right atrium *(arrow)*. This echocardiogram was obtained from the right parasternal window in the mitral valve position with a 2.5-MHz sector scanner transducer. An electrocardiogram is superimposed for timing. *RA,* Right atrium; *TV,* tricuspid valve; *RV,* right ventricle; *LV,* left ventricle; *MV,* mitral valve; *LA,* left atrium; *PE,* pericardial effusion.

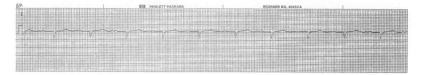

FIGURE 34–38. Base-apex electrocardiogram of a horse with pericarditis shows damping of the P, QRS, and T waves from the pericardial effusion. Tachycardia is present (60 beats/min) and is a common finding in horses with pericarditis. The PP interval and RR interval are regular. This electrocardiogram was recorded at a paper speed of 25 mm/s with a sensitivity of 10 mm = 1 mV.

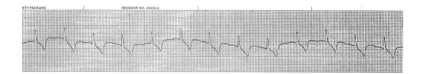

FIGURE 34–39. Base-apex electrocardiogram shows electrical alternans in a horse with pericardial effusion. The slight variation in the amplitude of the QRS complexes from 0.6 mV to 0.8 mV is evident. The amplitude of the P, QRS, and T complexes is damped. This electrocardiogram was recorded at a paper speed of 25 mm/s with a sensitivity of 10 mm = 1 mV.

Treatment

- Pericardiocentesis is the diagnostic and therapeutic tool of choice for horses with pericarditis, as long as there is enough pericardial fluid to perform this procedure safely.
- Echocardiography should be used to reliably select a site for pericardiocentesis and placement of an indwelling tube, if considerable volumes of pericardial fluid are imaged.
- In most patients with pericarditis, the ideal site is the left fifth intercostal space, above the level of the lateral thoracic vein and below a line level with the point of the shoulder (over the left ventricular free wall and below the left atrium and atrioventricular groove).
  - □ Lacerations of the left atrium, coronary vessels, or right ventricle are avoided if this site is chosen for pericardiocentesis.
- ECG monitoring (base-apex as rhythm strip is preferable) should be performed during pericardiocentesis to monitor the patient for the development of arrhythmias induced by the procedure (Fig. 34–40).
- Place an intravenous catheter before pericardiocentesis is begun, for rapid venous access in case arrhythmias do develop.
  - □ If a large number of ventricular premature depolarizations, ventricular tachycardia, or multiform ventricular complexes are detected, stop advancement of the pericardiocentesis catheter.
  - □ If the ventricular arrhythmias do not disappear, institute intravenous administration of antiarrhythmic drugs or withdraw the pericardiocentesis catheter, depending on the severity of the arrhythmias detected. The catheter can be repositioned once the arrhythmia has resolved.

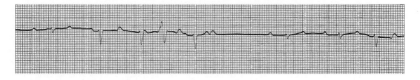

FIGURE 34-40. Lead II electrocardiogram obtained during pericardiocentesis of a horse with pericarditis. A paroxysm of ventricular premature depolarizations is evident. There are two different configurations of ventricular premature complexes in the paroxysm. The amplitude of the P, QRS, and T complexes is very damped. This electrocardiogram was recorded at a paper speed of 25 mm/s with a sensitivity of 10 mm – 1 mV.

- Insert a large-bore (28F-32F) Argyle catheter containing a trocar as an indwelling tube if there is a large volume of pericardial fluid or if cardiac tamponade is present.
  - This tube can be used for both sample collection and pericardial drainage and lavage.
  - Smaller-bore (12F-24F) Argyle catheters containing a trocar can be used if the volume of fluid within the pericardial sac is small.
- Submit the sample obtained for culture and sensitivity testing, cytologic evaluation, and viral isolation, if possible (Table 34–7).
  - Streptococcal organisms are most frequently isolated from horses with pericarditis, but *Actinobacillus equuli* also has been isolated from adults and foals with pericarditis.
  - Perform thoracocentesis if pleural effusion is present. Obtain a transtracheal aspirate if pulmonary disease is suspected. Request culture and sensitivity testing of both these fluids; they may yield the etiologic agent responsible for the concurrent pericarditis.
- Lavage of the pericardial sac after drainage of the pericardial fluid markedly improves the prognosis for patients with pericarditis. Lavage the pericardial sac with 2 L or more of warm sterile 0.9% saline solution.
  - Infuse the lavage fluid and leave it in the pericardial sac for 0.5-1 hour. Drain the fluid and instill 1-2 L of sterile 0.9% saline solution with 10-20 × 10⁶ IU sodium penicillin per liter or 1 g gentamicin per liter.
  - Leave this infusate in the pericardial sac for the next 12 hours.
  - Repeat drainage, lavage, drainage, and instillation of sterile fluid until ≤0.5 L of pericardial fluid is retrieved at the time of the initial drainage or the pericardial catheter falls out and fluid does not reaccumulate.
- Administer broad-spectrum systemic antibiotics.
  - Continue use of systemic and intrapericardial antimicrobial agents until results of the cytologic examination and culture and sensitivity testing have ruled out a bacterial cause of pericarditis.
  - Although systemic concentrations of antibiotics are reached in the pericardial fluid with the administration of systemic antimicrobials alone, the use of intrapericardial antimicrobials increases threefold the concentrations of antimicrobials in the pericardial fluid. This local increase in antimicrobial concentration is helpful because of the fibrinous nature of pericarditis in horses and the rapid inactivation of many antimicrobial agents by fibrin.

TABLE 34–7. Causes of Pericardial Effusions in Horses

Type of Effusion	Cause	Cytologic Finding	Culture Result	Treatment
Blood	Neoplasia	Neoplastic cells (usually red blood cells and lymphocytes)	No growth	Drainage and corticosteroid therapy (symptomatic only)
	Left atrial rupture (rare)	Blood	No growth	Intravenous fluids
	Aortic root rupture	Blood	No growth	Intravenous fluids
Trauma		Blood	No growth unless penetrating wound of the pericardium	Drainage if cardiac tamponade; intravenous fluid support
	Iatrogenic injury (intravenous or cardiac catheterization or cardiac puncture)	Blood	No growth unless iatrogenic contamination	Drainage if cardiac tamponade; intravenous fluid support
Transudate	Congestive heart failure		No growth	
	Hypoproteinemia		No growth	
Exudate	Idiopathic pericarditis	Lymphocytes, plasma cells, and red blood cells in large numbers	No growth, seroconversion to viral diseases possible	Drainage and lavage with sterile saline solution and instillation of broad-spectrum antibiotics, systemic broad-spectrum antibiotics until cytologic and culture results are negative for bacterial infection, then systemic corticosteroids
	Septic pericarditis	Neutrophils	±Positive culture (*Streptococcus* or *Pasteurella* organisms)	Drainage and lavage with sterile saline solution and instillation of broad-spectrum antibiotics, systemic broad-spectrum antibiotics until the results of culture and sensitivity tests are available, minimum 4 weeks of antimicrobials

□ Long-term (4-6 weeks) of systemic antimicrobial therapy is indicated in the care of horses with septic pericarditis.
- Patients with pericarditis should initially be given a guarded to cautiously optimistic prognosis, until response to treatment with pericardial drainage and lavage is detected, at which time the prognosis usually can be changed to good for both life and performance.
- Corticosteroids (**dexamethasone, 0.045-0.09 mg/kg IV q24h** for 3 days followed by a tapering dose) are indicated in the treatment of horses with idiopathic pericarditis (often lymphocytic plasmacytic), once a bacterial cause has been definitively excluded.
- Therapy for septic or idiopathic pericarditis should continue for several weeks after the patient is afebrile, the condition is clinically normal, and the pericardial effusion has resolved. During this time the patient should be stall rested and handwalked, with subsequent turnout in a small paddock for an additional month.
- Echocardiographic reevaluation is indicated at that time to determine whether the horse is ready to return to work.
- Intravenous fluids may be needed if the creatinine level is elevated, to prevent or control renal failure.

IONOPHORE TOXICITY

Horses are uniquely sensitive to the cardiotoxic effects of several of the ionophores (monensin, salinomycin, and lasalocid). The median lethal dose (LD_{50}) of these ionophores in horses is much lower than that in other domestic species. The ionophores are primarily cardiotoxic, although other signs of systemic toxicity may be detected in exposed individuals. Horses of any age or breed or either sex can be exposed to ionophore-contaminated feed. The contamination can come from feed accidentally contaminated at the feed mill or from accidental feeding of or exposure to ionophore-containing steer or poultry feed.

- Feed samples should be obtained for toxicologic analysis if ionophore exposure is suspected.
- Gastrointestinal samples from any horse that has experienced sudden death should be similarly analyzed.

Clinical Signs
- Sudden death often is the first indication of exposure to high doses of ionophores.
- Fever, depression, lethargy, restlessness, exercise intolerance, and profuse sweating are some of the signs first noticed by the owners or trainers of affected horses.
- Anorexia, poor appetite, and feed refusal are common because ionophore-contaminated feed is less palatable.
- Muscle weakness, trembling, and ataxia often occur.
- Affected horses may be polyuric and become oliguric or anuric.
- Diarrhea, colic, or ileus has frequently been reported.
- Muddy or injected mucous membranes and thready arterial pulses may be detected initially.
- Cardiac arrhythmias may develop at any time after ionophore exposure but are most likely in the first few days to weeks after exposure.

- Generalized venous distention, jugular pulses, ventral edema, and murmurs of mitral or tricuspid regurgitation may develop weeks to months after ionophore exposure.
- Recumbency may occur without heart failure.

Diagnosis and Prognosis

- Echocardiography is the diagnostic modality of choice in situations of suspected or known ionophore exposure, to determine the severity of the myocardial injury in exposed horses.
  - Patients with normal left ventricular function and normal fractional shortening (30%-40%) have an excellent prognosis for life and performance.
  - Patients with slightly depressed fractional shortening have a good prognosis for life and a fair-to-good prognosis for performance. They should be able to perform successfully in lower levels of athletic work.
  - The detection of a fractional shortening <20% in exposed horses is a grave prognostic sign. Affected horses with a fractional shortening of >10% but <20% may survive monensin exposure but have persistent left ventricular dysfunction and exercise intolerance.
  - Horses with a fractional shortening of ≤10% do not survive monensin exposure and are usually dead 24-48 hours after the echocardiographic examination (Fig. 34–41).
- ECG abnormalities can be detected in horses recently exposed to ionophores but are not good prognostic indicators of the severity of the myocardial injury.

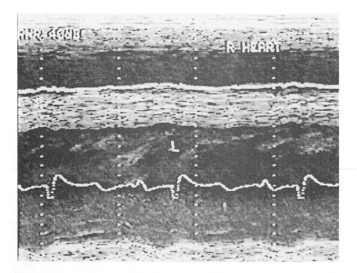

FIGURE 34–41. M-mode echocardiogram of a horse with monensin toxicosis. Minimal thickening of the left ventricular free wall and interventricular septum in systole are evident. This echocardiogram was obtained from the right parasternal window in the left ventricular position with a 2.5-MHz sector scanner transducer. An electrocardiogram is superimposed for timing. *L,* Left ventricle.

- Axis shifts, ST-segment depression, T-wave changes, atrial and ventricular premature beats, atrial fibrillation, ventricular tachycardia, and a variety of bradyarrhythmias have been found in horses exposed to ionophores (Fig. 34-42).
- Most horses exposed to ionophores in the field situation, however, do not have cardiac arrhythmias.
- Elevations in the cardiac isoenzymes of CK and LDH have been reported in some outbreaks of monensin toxicity, but elevations were only slight or were not found in other field outbreaks. Elevations in the level of cardiac troponin 1 should be detected in horses exposed to ionophores, because cardiac troponin 1 is a sensitive and specific indicator of myocardial cell damage.
  - Elevation in levels of the cardiac isoenzymes of CK or LDH and the magnitude of elevation have not been useful prognostic indicators of survival or the severity of permanent myocardial injury.
- Other clinicopathologic abnormalities that have been reported include elevations in hematocrit, total plasma protein concentration, osmolality, total bilirubin level, and serum levels of blood urea nitrogen, creatinine, aspartate aminotransferase, and alkaline phosphatase, and decreases in serum level of calcium and plasma level of potassium.
  - The presence of none of these abnormal clinicopathologic abnormalities, however, confirms the diagnosis of monensin or other ionophore exposure.

Treatment
- Remove all suspected contaminated feed.
- Administer activated charcoal or mineral oil to decrease further absorption of recently ingested feed.
- Administer large doses of vitamin E as soon as possible after exposure in an attempt to stabilize cell membranes and control peroxidation-mediated cell injury.
- Provide appropriate supportive care (Box 34-6).
- Keep exposed horses at stall rest for a minimum of 2 months.
- **Digoxin** is **contraindicated** in the management of acute monensin exposure because monensin and digoxin have an additive effect, causing calcium to flood into the myocardial cell. The use of digoxin in a patient recently exposed to monensin can result in further overload of the intracellular calcium sequestration mechanisms and increase the amount and severity of myocardial cell injury and cell death.

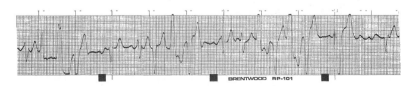

FIGURE 34-42. Lead II electrocardiogram of a horse with monensin toxicosis and multifocal ventricular tachycardia. Markedly different QRS complexes are evident, and some are occurring in rapid succession. The ventricular rate is 110 beats/min. This electrocardiogram was recorded at a paper speed of 25 mm/s with a sensitivity of 5 mm = 1 mV.

BOX 34-6. Approach to the Horse with Potential Ionophore Exposure

- Perform complete physical and cardiovascular examinations.
- Treat affected horses with antiarrhythmics as needed to control life-threatening arrhythmias.
- Pass a nasogastric tube and administer activated charcoal or mineral oil in attempt to prevent further absorption of the ionophore.
- Administer vitamin E or vitamin E with selenium as soon as possible.
- Keep exposed horses at stall rest and minimize stress.
- Do not administer digoxin, which is contraindicated if exposure is recent.
- Perform echocardiography:
  □ Evaluate myocardial function carefully, looking for myocardial hypokinesis, dyskinesis, or akinesis.
  □ Evaluate the myocardium for heterogeneity of muscle echogenicity (tissue characterization).
- Obtain blood for measurement of cardiac troponin I, isoenzymes of creatine kinase (isoenzyme of creatine kinase with muscle and brain subunits), and lactate dehydrogenase (LDH_1 and LDH_2 or hydroxybutyrate dehydrogenase).
- Obtain an electrocardiogram, including 24-hour continuous ECG, if possible.

□ Monensin is a sodium-selective ionophore that makes the myocardial cell membrane more permeable to sodium. The sodium influx into the cell is followed by a calcium influx.

□ Digoxin inhibits the Na^+-K^+-ATPase pump. This influx of sodium is followed by an influx of calcium.

AORTIC ROOT RUPTURE

Aortic root rupture in horses most frequently results in sudden death associated with massive hemorrhage into the thoracic cavity. If the aortic rupture is intracardiac rather than extrapericardial, the affected horse survives for a variable time. The longevity depends on the extent of the aortic rupture, the severity of the intracardiac shunt, the chamber or structure into which the rupture occurred, the severity of the resultant cardiac (ventricular) arrhythmias, the patient's myocardial function, and the presence or absence of other cardiac disease. Several horses with aortic rupture have lived for a year or more after the initial event.

- Affected horses usually are male, primarily stallions, 10 years or older.

Clinical Signs at Time of Rupture

- Distress (which usually is interpreted initially as colic), tachycardia (usually with rapid regular heart rates ≥120 beats/min), jugular distention, and jugular pulsations.
- The rapid regular heart rate and jugular pulsations suggest a rhythm of ventricular tachycardia.

Physical Examination Findings

- Bounding arterial pulses, loud continuous murmur with its point of maximal intensity in the right fourth intercostal space, and a loud S_3.
  □ Systolic murmurs of tricuspid regurgitation have been reported in horses with aortic root rupture.

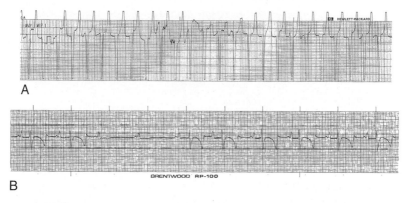

FIGURE 34–43. Lead aVf electrocardiograms of a horse with aortic root rupture and an aortic-cardiac fistula. Uniform ventricular tachycardia **(A)** is present at a ventricular rate of 160 beats/min, which is successfully converted to sinus rhythm with second-degree atrioventricular (AV) block **(B)** after treatment with quinidine gluconate, lidocaine, MgSO$_4$, and procainamide. The horse converted to sinus rhythm and a ventricular rate of 60 beats/min with the procainamide infusion. This electrocardiogram was recorded at a paper speed of 25 mm/s with a sensitivity of 5 mm – 1 mV.

- Auscultation of the abdomen usually reveals normal gastrointestinal sounds. A rectal examination yields normal findings.

Diagnosis
- ECG usually exhibits uniform ventricular tachycardia (Fig. 34–43) with a heart rate of 120-250 beats/min (higher heart rates are possible but have not been recorded among horses with aortic root rupture).
- Echocardiographic examination depicts the rupture in the aortic root at the right aortic sinus or right sinus of Valsalva (Fig. 34–44).
  - Aneurysmal dilatation and rupture of the right sinus of Valsalva (Fig. 34–45) are detected in approximately one half of affected horses, whereas in the other horses, no preexisting aortic root disease is detected.
  - The aortic root can dissect apically, down the interventricular septum (Fig. 34–46) with subsequent endocardial rupture into the right or left ventricle (most frequent), or rupture into the right atrium, tricuspid valve, or right ventricle.
  - Generalized cardiomegaly is common, and pulmonary artery dilatation is imaged in approximately one half of patients with aortocardiac fistulas from aortic root rupture.
  - Aortic ruptures into the pericardial sac occur but are uncommon and are not localized to the right aortic sinus.
  - Pulsed wave, continuous wave, and color flow Doppler echocardiography and contrast echocardiography can be used to detect the intracardiac shunt flow and to attempt to semiquantify the severity of this shunt.

Treatment
- Correct the uniform ventricular tachycardia, as indicated earlier, if the heart rate exceeds 120 beats/min, the patient has clinical signs of cardiovascular collapse,

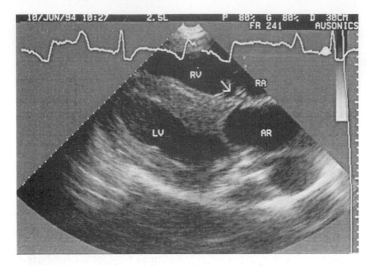

FIGURE 34–44. Two-dimensional echocardiogram of a horse with aortic root rupture and the presence of an aortic-cardiac fistula (same horse as in Fig. 34–43). The defect is evident in the right side of the aorta *(arrow)* just under the septal leaflet of the tricuspid valve. This echocardiogram was obtained from the right parasternal window just cranial to the left ventricular outflow tract view with a 2.5-MHz sector scanner transducer. *RA,* Right atrium; *RV,* right ventricle; *LV,* left ventricle; *AR,* aortic root.

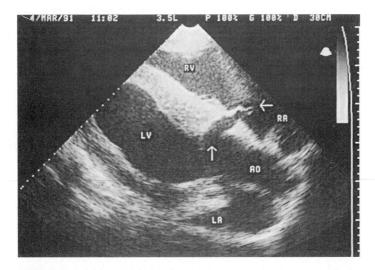

FIGURE 34–45. Two-dimensional echocardiogram of a horse with a ruptured sinus of Valsalva aneurysm. The communication *(vertical arrow)* between the aortic root *(AO)* and the right atrium *(RA)* is evident. Torn aneurysmal tissue *(horizontal arrow)* is floating in the right atrium. This echocardiogram was obtained with a 3.5-MHz sector scanner transducer from the right parasternal window slightly cranial to the left ventricular outflow tract view. *RV,* Right ventricle; *LV,* left ventricle; *LA,* left atrium.

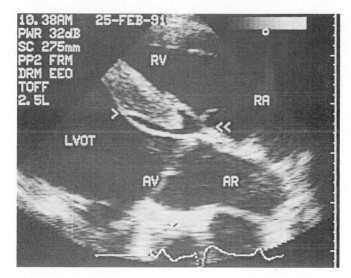

FIGURE 34-46. Two-dimensional echocardiogram of a horse with a ruptured sinus of Valsalva aneurysm and subendocardial dissection of blood down the interventricular septum (same horse as in Fig. 34–45). Dissection of blood down the left (primarily) *(arrowhead)* and right side of the interventricular septum is evident. The aortic-cardiac fistula is between the right aortic sinus (see Fig. 34–45) and the right atrium *(double arrowhead)*. This echocardiogram was obtained with a 2.5-MHz sector scanner transducer from the right parasternal window in the left ventricular outflow tract view. *RA,* Right atrium; *RV,* right ventricle; *LVOT,* left ventricular outflow tract; *AV,* aortic valves; *AR,* aortic root. An electrocardiogram is superimposed for timing.

the rhythm is multiform (not reported), or an R on T is detected in the ECG (not reported).

- Afterload reduction (**enalapril, 0.5 mg/kg PO q12h, or hydralazine, 0.5-1.5 mg/kg PO q12h**) is indicated to help decrease the severity of the intracardiac shunt.
- Diuretics and positive inotropic drugs may be indicated if the horse has congestive heart failure.

Prognosis

- Affected individuals have a *grave* prognosis for life and should not be used for performance, even if the clinical condition or echocardiographic findings improve. These horses are always at increased risk of sudden death.

REFERENCES

Corley KT, Furr MO: Cardiopulmonary resuscitation in newborn foals, *Compend Contin Ed Pract Vet* 22:957-966, 2000.

Ellis EJ, Ravis WR, Malloy M et al: Pharmacokinetics and pharmacodynamics of procainamide in horses after intravenous administration, *J Vet Pharmacol Ther* 17:265-270, 1994.

McGuirk SM, Muir WW: Diagnosis and treatment of cardiac arrhythmias, *Vet Clin North Am Equine Pract* 1:353-370, 1985.

Muir WW: Anesthetic complications and cardiopulmonary resuscitation in the horse. In Muir WW, Hubbell JAE: *Equine anesthesia: monitoring and emergency therapy,* St. Louis, 1991, Mosby–Year Book.

Muir WW, Bednarski RM: Equine cardiopulmonary resuscitation: part II, *Compend Contin Educ Pract Vet* 5:S287-S295, 1983.

Muir WW, McGuirk SM: Pharmacology and pharmacokinetics of drugs used to treat cardiac disease in horses, *Vet Clin North Am [Equine Pract]* 1:335-352, 1985.

Muir WW, Reed SM, McGuirk SM: Treatment of atrial fibrillation in horses by intravenous administration of quinidine, *J Am Vet Med Assoc* 197:1607-1610, 1990.

Ohmura H, Nukada T, Mizuno Y et al: Safe and efficacious dosage of flecainide acetate for treating equine atrial fibrillation, *J Vet Med Sci* 62:711-715, 2000.

Reef VB: Echocardiographic examination in the horse: the basics, *Compend Contin Educ Pract Vet* 12:1312-1320, 1990.

Reef VB: Echocardiographic evaluation of ventricular septal defects in horses, *Equine Vet J Suppl* 19:86-96, 1995.

Reef VB: Heart murmurs in horses: determining their significance with echocardiography, *Equine Vet J Suppl* 19:71-80, 1995.

Reef VB, Bain FT, Spencer PA: Severe mitral regurgitation in horses: clinical, echocardiographic, and pathologic findings, *Equine Vet J* 30:18-27, 1998.

Reef VB, Reimer JM, Spencer PA: Treatment of equine atrial fibrillation: new perspectives, *J Vet Intern Med* 9:57-67, 1995.

Worth LT, Reef VB: Pericarditis in horses: 18 cases (1986-1995), *J Am Vet Med Assoc* 212: 248-253, 1998.

---

35 Gastrointestinal Emergencies and Other Causes of Colic

■ A. CLASSIFICATION AND PATHOPHYSIOLOGY OF COLIC

P. O. Eric Mueller and James N. Moore

A variety of enteric diseases can result in the manifestation of abdominal pain (**colic**) in horses. Abnormalities of the equine gastrointestinal tract are broadly classified as physical or functional obstructions. With a *nonstrangulating physical obstruction,* the mesenteric blood supply is intact but the bowel lumen is occluded. This can be caused by either intraluminal masses or reduction of the lumen by intramural thickening or extramural compression. *Strangulating obstruction* implies both luminal occlusion and reduction or occlusion of the mesenteric blood supply. *Incarceration of the intestine* through internal or external hernias, intussusception, or a greater than 180-degree twist of a segment of intestine on its mesentery can result in strangulating obstruction. *Functional obstruction,* referred to as adynamic or paralytic ileus, can be idiopathic, results from inflammatory disease (e.g., duodenitis/proximal jejunitis and colitis), or is caused by serosal irritation due to surgical manipulation.

Intestinal obstruction prevents the aboral movement of gastrointestinal contents and results in distention of the intestine. As the distention increases, venous drainage from the intestinal wall is impaired, and the mucosa becomes congested and edematous. *If the obstruction persists for a prolonged time (>24 hours), significant compromise of intestinal vascular integrity can result in mucosal ischemia.* With progressive distention, gastric, cecal, or colonic rupture can result. In strangulating obstruction, these events are combined with rapid tissue hypoxia and ischemia of the affected segment and lead to necrosis and transmural leakage of bacteria and endotoxin. Cardiovascular deterioration rapidly follows transperitoneal absorption of endotoxin, resulting in hypovolemia and endotoxic shock.

DIAGNOSIS
Early History
- Previous episode of colic, duration of colic, recent changes in management (feed, water, deworming, medication, exercise routine), breeding, pregnancy

Recent History
- Degree and change in pain (looking at flank, pawing, kicking at abdomen, rolling), last defecation, sweating, treatment, and response to treatment

Physical Examination
Assess the following parameters immediately and completely during initial examination of the patient with a history of acute abdominal pain:

- Attitude
- Abdominal shape (distention)
- Body temperature, pulse, and respiratory rate (TPR)
- Skin turgor, mucous membrane moisture and color, and capillary refill time (CRT)
- Abdominal auscultation and percussion
- Nasogastric intubation (quantity and characteristics of fluid)
- Rectal examination

The *physical examination* starts with observation of external appearance and attitude. Abdominal distention is generally a sign of large-intestinal disease, but it can occur with severe small-intestinal distention. Multiple abrasions, particularly around the periorbital area, indicate that the patient recently experienced severe abdominal pain. Recent enlargement of an umbilical or abdominal hernia or the scrotum can indicate intestinal incarceration with obstruction or strangulation. Assess the degree of pain with the patient in a quiet environment.

Signs of Abdominal Pain in Order of Severity—Less Severe to Most Severe
- Lying down for excessive periods
- Inappetence
- Restlessness
- Quivering of the upper lip
- Turning of the head toward the flank
- Repeated stretching as if to urinate
- Kicking with the hind feet at the abdomen

- Crouching as if wanting to lie down
- Sweating
- Dropping to the ground and rolling

Severe, unrelenting pain may require analgesics before examination (Table 35–1).

Consider previous treatment by the owner or trainer when assessing the amount of abdominal pain present. Depression with mild to moderate abdominal pain and fever may indicate an inflammatory condition (enteritis or colitis). In the absence of extreme muscle exertion, suspect inflammatory disease (enteritis, colitis, peritonitis) as the cause of abdominal pain accompanied by fever. Loud "fluid and bubbling" sounds can be heard on abdominal auscultation in some patients with impending colitis. Ultrasound examination can be helpful in delineating enteritis (distended small intestine with increased motility) from strangulating obstruction (distended small intestine with no motility).

Tachycardia and tachypnea can serve as indicators of abdominal pain, cardiovascular shock, and endotoxemia.

Skin turgor, mucous membrane moisture and color, and CRT can aid in assessment of dehydration resulting from intestinal dysfunction. Mucous membrane moisture and color change from moist and pale pink to dry and red with a decrease in circulating blood volume. With the onset of shock and endotoxemia, mucous membrane color can progress to reddish-blue or purple (cyanosis).

Auscultate for *intestinal borborygmi* in all abdominal quadrants. Pain and inflammation related to the gastrointestinal tract result in decreased borborygmi. Increased borborygmi can be present early with enteritis or colitis, only to progress to ileus and cessation of the sounds as the bowel becomes progressively inflamed and distended. Increased borborygmi are present early in patients with obstruction, but intestinal sounds decrease as the obstruction becomes complete. Simultaneous auscultation and percussion may reveal high-pitched sounds (pinging) due to cecal (right flank) or colonic (left flank) tympany. A sound similar to an ocean wave can be heard in some patients with sand impaction; if sand is suspected, perform auscultation of the ventral abdomen for 5 minutes.

TABLE 35–1. Analgesics and Relative Efficacy for Control of Acute Abdominal Pain

Analgesic	Trade Name	Dosage	Efficacy
Flunixin meglumine	Banamine	0.25-1.1 mg/kg IV or IM	Excellent
Detomidine hydrochloride	Dormosedan	5-40 µg/kg IV or IM*	Excellent
Xylazine hydrochloride	Rompun	0.2-1.1 mg/kg IV or IM*,†	Good
Butorphanol tartrate	Torbugesic	0.02-0.08 mg/kg IV or IM†,§	Good
Ketoprofen	Ketofen	1.1-2.2 mg/kg IV or IM	Good
Meperidine hydrochloride	Demerol	1.1-2.2 mg/kg IV or IM*,§	Good
Morphine sulfate		0.3-0.66 mg/kg IV§,#	Good
Pentazocine	Talwin	0.3-0.6 mg/kg IV§	Poor
Chloral hydrate		30-60 mg/kg IV titrated	Poor
Dipyrone	Novin	10-22 mg/kg IV or IM	Poor
Phenylbutazone	Butazolidin	2.2-4.4 mg/kg IV	Poor

*Intravenous administration can cause severe hypotension.
†Repeated administration can compromise cardiac output and colonic motility.
‡Doses in upper range can cause ataxia.
§A controlled substance.
#Use only with xylazine (0.66-1.1 mg/kg IV) to avoid central nervous system excitement.

Apply nasogastric intubation *immediately* when a patient demonstrates abdominal pain. Gastric decompression is essential to determine whether gastric distention is present and to provide relief to patients with primary or secondary gastric distention. Nasogastric reflux can be caused by small-intestinal obstruction or secondary ileus from large-intestinal disease. Horses with anterior enteritis characteristically have large volumes of reflux (10-20 L). Blood-tinged, foul-smelling reflux fluid may indicate small-intestinal strangulating obstruction or severe anterior enteritis. *If small-intestinal obstruction or enteritis is suspected, it is essential to leave the tube in place to prevent spontaneous gastric rupture and subsequent death!*

A careful *rectal examination* is important when examining a horse that has abdominal pain. Before beginning the examination, note the amount and consistency of fecal material in the rectum. Absence of fecal material or the presence of dry, fibrin- and mucus-covered feces is abnormal and suggests delayed intestinal transit. Fetid, watery fecal material often is seen in horses with colitis. Examine in a consistent, systematic manner to minimize missing a lesion. Intraabdominal structures palpable in a normal horse (Fig. 35–1), starting in the left cranial abdominal quadrant and progressing clockwise, are as follows:

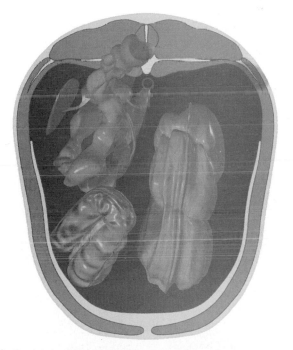

FIGURE 35-1. Caudal view of a standing horse shows the abdominal structures palpable in normal patients during a rectal examination. Beginning in the left dorsal abdominal quadrant and progressing in a clockwise direction, palpable structures include the caudal border of the spleen, nephrosplenic ligament, caudal pole of the left kidney, small colon containing fecal balls, root of the mesentery, cecal base and ventral taenia, portions of the left ventral and dorsal colon, and the pelvic flexure.

Palpable Intraabdominal Structures
- Caudal border of the spleen
- Nephrosplenic (renosplenic) ligament
- Caudal pole of the left kidney
- Mesenteric root
- Ventral cecal band (no tension)
- Cecal base (empty)
- Small colon containing distinct fecal balls
- Pelvic flexure

The small intestine is not palpable unless an underlying abnormality exists. Determination of the presence of bowel distention of any form is important in formulating a tentative diagnosis.

Abnormal Rectal Examination Findings
- Cecal distention
- Gas- or ingesta-distended small intestine (Fig. 35–2), large colon (Fig. 35–3), or small colon
- Marked intramural or mesenteric edema
- Bowel malposition (see Fig. 35–3)
- Herniation

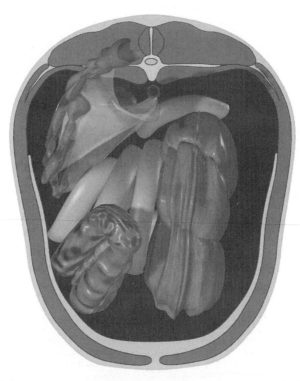

FIGURE 35-2. Caudal view of a standing horse shows severe small-intestinal distention. Multiple loops of gas- and fluid-distended small intestine are palpable.

- Impaction
- Intussusception
- Intraabdominal mass, abscess, or hematoma
- Enterolithiasis
- Volvulus of the mesenteric root

Always examine the internal inguinal rings, urethra, and bladder (male) and reproductive tract and bladder (female). Sequential rectal examinations often are helpful in determining the rate and severity of disease and the need for surgical intervention.

Ultrasonography (see Chapter 40, p. 388)

Response to Analgesics

The degree of pain demonstrated by a horse with gastrointestinal disease is variable and depends on the characteristic pain threshold of the individual horse and

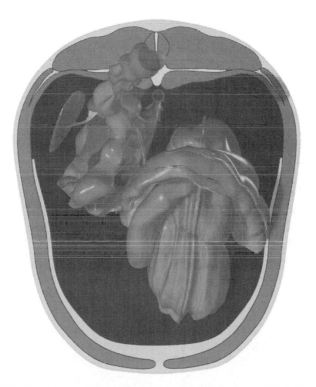

FIGURE 35–3. Caudal view of a standing horse reveals right dorsal displacement of the large colon. The left ventral and dorsal colon are displaced lateral to the cecum. The colon and associated taenia are palpated immediately cranial to the pelvic canal, coursing from the right caudal abdomen, transversely across the abdomen, and then continuing out of the examiner's reach toward the left cranial abdomen.

the severity of disease present. In general, the greater the pain, the more severe is the disease. In the later stages of disease abdominal pain may be replaced by marked depression and cardiovascular deterioration as a result of bowel necrosis and systemic endotoxemia. Pain control is accomplished with gastric decompression through a nasogastric tube and administration of peripherally and centrally acting analgesics (see Table 35–1). Assessment of a patient's response to analgesics is helpful in determining the severity of disease and likelihood of successfully treating the patient with medical management. *Horses demonstrating unrelenting pain not responsive to analgesics need immediate surgical exploration or euthanasia.*

Clinicopathologic Evaluation

- Packed cell volume (PCV)
- Total plasma protein (TPP)
- Complete blood count (CBC)
- Blood gases
- Electrolyte determination

PCV and TPP

Hypovolemia secondary to intestinal dysfunction results in dehydration. The PCV-TPP is the most accurate measurement to support a clinical assessment of dehydration in most patients with abdominal pain.

	PCV (%)*	TPP (g/dl)
Mild dehydration	45-50	7.5-8.0
Moderate dehydration	50-60	8.0-9.0
Severe dehydration	≥60	≥9.0

Marked increases in PCV without corresponding increases or decreases in TPP may indicate protein loss into the intestinal lumen or peritoneal cavity or sympathetic and endotoxin-induced splenic contraction.

CBC

Most simple or strangulating obstructions do not cause a significant change in the white blood cell (WBC) count until the terminal stages of diseases. Acute inflammatory diseases (enteritis, colitis), however, often cause leukopenia (<4000 cells/µl). Marked leukopenia (<1000 cells/µl) also occurs with fulminant septic peritonitis secondary to acute bowel rupture. Mature neutrophilia and high TPP and fibrinogen levels may indicate chronic peritonitis secondary to abdominal abscessation.

Blood Gases

Acidemia with advanced hypovolemic shock may be seen. Evaluation of blood gases is important for appropriate management of severe acid-base abnormalities, especially in patients who need general anesthesia and surgical treatment. Patients with simple colon displacements may have an insignificant base excess, whereas patients with strangulating obstruction usually have an obvious base deficit.

---

*These values are not relevant to nursing foals, which generally have lower PCV and protein values.

Electrolytes

Measurement of serum electrolytes rarely is helpful in making a diagnosis. A rare exception is acute abdominal pain caused by hypocalcemia and ileus (synchronous diaphragmatic flutter may be present). Electrolyte determinations are vital for appropriate management before, during, and after surgical treatment. Hyponatremia and hypochloremia may suggest impending colitis.

Abdominocentesis

Abdominocentesis (see p. 83) is a useful diagnostic tool for assessment of intestinal compromise. It is performed with an 18-gauge, sterile hypodermic needle or a blunt cannula (teat cannula or canine female urinary catheter). Collect fluid in a sterile tube containing EDTA for cytologic analysis of the fluid and into a second sterile tube without additives for culture and sensitivity, if indicated. Fluid analysis includes specific gravity and protein determinations and cell types, numbers, and morphology (see Table 19–1). Ultrasonography with a 7.5-MHz transducer may be useful in locating peritoneal fluid. *Caution in performing abdominocentesis on foals; needle perforation of the bowel can cause adhesions, and using the teat cannula method can result in herniation of omentum unless performed in the most caudal part of the abdomen.*

Normal peritoneal fluid is odorless, nonturbid, and clear to pale yellow. The nucleated cell count should be less than 3000-5000/μl, with a total protein concentration less than 2.5 g/dl. With early, simple obstruction of the small or large intestine, peritoneal fluid characteristically remains normal. With strangulating obstruction or severe intestinal inflammation, the peritoneal fluid can become serosanguineous with increases in nucleated cell count and total protein concentration.

Dark, turbid fluid with the smell of ingesta, increased nucleated cell counts, and increased protein concentration, signifies bowel necrosis and leakage. The presence of plant material and intracellular bacteria indicates bowel rupture (see Color Plate 14). *(If this material has been collected by needle aspiration, it should be repeated with a teat cannula before the diagnosis of ruptured viscus is made.)*

The presence of blood-tinged fluid indicates splenic puncture, intraabdominal or iatrogenic hemorrhage, or intestinal necrosis.

With splenic puncture, the PCV of the fluid is greater than the peripheral PCV, and the fluid contains large numbers of small lymphocytes. Fluid from intraabdominal hemorrhage reveals a PCV less than that of peripheral blood, erythrocytophagia, and few to no platelets.

NOTE: The absence of gross or cytologic abnormalities in the peritoneal fluid does not exclude the presence of compromised intestine.

Some strangulating lesions, such as intussusception, external hernia, and epiploic foramen incarceration may not demonstrate abnormalities in the peritoneal fluid owing to sequestration of the fluid in the omentum, intussuscipiens, or hernial sac.

If sand impaction is suspected or if marked cecal or colonic distention is present, abdominocentesis should be performed only to confirm suspected bowel rupture.

If physical examination reveals other findings consistent with a surgical lesion and referral for surgery is considered, abdominocentesis should not be performed in the field because of risk to the patient and the examiner.

MEDICAL VERSUS SURGICAL MANAGEMENT

Considerations in determining the need for exploratory surgery (Box 35–1):

- Pain
- Response to analgesic therapy
- Cardiovascular status
- Rectal examination findings
- Quantity of gastric reflux
- Abdominocentesis results

A history of abdominal pain often requires reassessment of these parameters over time. A change in one or more clinical criteria may determine the need for surgical or medical management. Manifestation of pain and the response to analgesic therapy are the most valuable measurements in assessing the need for surgical intervention. *Patients demonstrating unrelenting pain, or recurrent pain after administration of analgesics, are considered surgical candidates.*

  Rectal examination is the next most valuable criterion for surgery. Demonstration of pain concurrent with abnormal rectal examination findings is a strong indicator. Failure of medical therapy, systemic cardiovascular deterioration, and/or changes in peritoneal fluid results supporting intestinal degeneration, are additional justification for surgical intervention.

TREATMENT

Treatment of horses demonstrating acute abdominal pain is directed at:

- Pain relief
- Stabilization of cardiovascular and metabolic status
- Minimizing the deleterious effects of endotoxemia
- Establishing a patent and functional intestine. This can be accomplished with one or more of the following therapeutic modalities:
  - Analgesic therapy (see Table 35–1)
  - Fluid therapy and cardiovascular support
  - Laxatives and cathartics
  - Antiendotoxin therapy
  - Therapy for ischemia-reperfusion injury

BOX 35-1. Indications for Exploratory Celiotomy in Horses Demonstrating Acute Abdominal Pain

Severe, unrelenting abdominal pain[*]
Refractory to analgesics[*]
Increased heart rate[†]
Large quantities of gastric reflux[†]
Absence of borborygmi[†]
Abnormal rectal examination[†]
Serosanguineous abdominal fluid with increased total protein and nucleated cell count[†]

---

[*]These parameters alone are indications for emergency exploratory celiotomy.
[†]These parameters are not sole indications for emergency exploratory celiotomy but must be evaluated in view of other clinical findings.

- Antimicrobial therapy
- Nutritional support
- Surgical intervention

Analgesic Therapy

Pain relief is accomplished by means of gastric decompression with a nasogastric tube and administration of peripherally and centrally acting analgesics (see Table 35–1). Perform gastric decompression (see p. 81) (approximately every 2 hours) using an indwelling nasogastric tube; it may be necessary to prevent distention, which can potentially lead to pain, gastric rupture, and death. Patients being referred for possible exploratory surgery should have an *indwelling nasogastric tube* in place during transport to the referral facility.

Fluid Therapy and Cardiovascular Support

Intravenous administration of polyionic, balanced electrolyte solutions is necessary to maintain intravascular fluid volume. Administration of hypertonic saline solution (5% or 7% NaCl, 1-2 L, IV) improves systemic blood pressure and cardiac output. *Hypertonic saline solution may be administered initially but* **must** *be followed by adequate fluid replacement with balanced crystalloid solutions (ideally within 1 hour after administration of hypertonic saline solution).* Monitor hydration status with clinical assessment and measurement of PCV and TPP. Monitor blood gas values and serum electrolyte levels and adjust the intravenous solutions to correct deficits.

If the plasma protein concentration is less than 4.5 g/dl and the patient is dehydrated, administer plasma (2-10 L, IV, slowly) or a synthetic colloid (hetastarch) to maintain plasma oncotic pressure and avoid inducing pulmonary edema during rehydration with intravenous fluids.

Laxatives

Laxatives are used to increase gastrointestinal water content, soften ingesta, facilitate intestinal transit, and manage impaction of the cecum and large and small colons. *For maximal effect, oral and intravenous fluids should be administered concurrently.* Do not administer laxatives orally to patients with nasogastric reflux.

Commonly Used Laxatives

- Mineral oil (6-8 L/500 kg body weight) can be administered to facilitate passage after the impaction begins to resolve; however, mineral oil is not useful for penetrating or hydrating the primary impaction.
- Magnesium sulfate (Epsom salts, 500 g diluted in warm water per 500 kg body weight, daily). Do not use longer than 3 days or to treat patients with decreased renal function to avoid enteritis and possible magnesium intoxication. *Preferred for large-colon impactions.*
- Psyllium hydrophilic mucilloid (Metamucil, 400 g/500 kg body weight q6-12h) until the impaction resolves. *Especially useful for sand impaction.*
- Dioctyl sodium sulfosuccinate (DSS, 10-20 mg/kg up to two doses, 48 hours apart). *Can cause mild abdominal pain and diarrhea.*

Antiendotoxin Therapy

Antiserum (500-1000 ml) directed against the Gram-negative core antigens of endotoxin (Endoserum, Immvac, Columbia, MO) can be administered intravenously diluted in balanced electrolyte solution. Significant amounts of endotoxin have been reported in Endoserum. Endoserum should be warmed to room temperature and administered slowly to avoid undesired side effects, such as tachycardia and muscle fasciculations. Hyperimmune plasma directed against the J-5 mutant strain of *Escherichia coli* (Polymune-J, San Luis Obispo, CA, or Foalimmune, Lake Immunogenics Inc., Ontario, NY) or normal *equine plasma* (2-10 L) administered intravenously *slowly* can be equally as or more beneficial than supplying protein, fibronectin, complement, antithrombin III, and other inhibitors of hypercoagulability. Polymyxin B (Bedford Laboratories, Bedford, OH), 2000-6000 IU/kg, IV, q12h for 24-48 hours, binds and neutralizes circulating endotoxin and may be beneficial in the management of systemic endotoxemia.

Therapy for Ischemia-Reperfusion Injury

If ischemia is suspected, dimethyl sulfoxide (DMSO), a hydroxyl radical scavenger, can be administered intravenously (100 mg/kg q8-12h) diluted to a 10% solution in a balanced electrolyte solution. Efficacy has not been verified. Kinetic studies support *q12h* use at the antiinflammatory dose.

Antimicrobials

- Antimicrobial agents are not routinely administered to patients that demonstrate acute abdominal pain unless an underlying infectious agent is suspected. Broad-spectrum antimicrobials are indicated if the patient has sepsis and neutropenia (<2000 cells/μl) to minimize bacteremia and organ colonization by enteric organisms and if the patient is undergoing exploratory celiotomy.
- Penicillin (22,000-44,000 IU/kg IV q6h or IM q12h) often is administered to patients with duodenitis or proximal jejunitis. The suspected agent is *Clostridium perfringens* type A.

Nutritional Support

Horses demonstrating abdominal pain should have hay and grain withheld for 12-18 hours. If they do not have gastric reflux, they should be allowed free-choice water and should have access to trace mineral salt. A patient that responds to initial treatment should be gradually returned to a normal diet over 24-48 hours (moist bran and alfalfa pellet mash, grazing grass, hay, then grain). Patients being referred for possible exploratory surgery *should not be fed* during transport to the referral facility.

Surgical Intervention

Candidates for exploratory celiotomy (see Box 35–1) have the following signs:

- Unrelenting pain
- Recurrent pain after administration of analgesics

- Systemic cardiovascular deterioration
- Changes in peritoneal fluid results indicating intestinal degeneration
- Failure of medical therapy

Ventral midline celiotomy is the surgical approach of choice. Specific treatments are discussed with each gastrointestinal disorder.

B. DISORDERS OF THE MOUTH AND SALIVATION (PTYALISM) AND EQUINE DENTISTRY
David Foster

GENERAL

- The nomenclature used for the mouth is a mixture of classic, archaic, and modern systems. A consistent, coherent nomenclature improves communication between veterinarians and assists in maintaining records. Most veterinarians use the Triadan nomenclature system (see Fig. 17–3) because it is specific and understandable.
- No oral examination is complete unless a full mouth speculum is used to see and safely palpate the horse's mouth.
- Only *severe* oral problems prevent a horse from eating.
- Drooling or quidding should alert the clinician to an oral emergency.

NOTE: Rabies *must* be considered in a differential diagnosis and other, neurologic diseases such as botulism and tetanus.

- Vaccination history, physical examination, gloves, and eye protection are essential for performing an oral examination.
- Examine the ventral aspects of the tongue and the caudal buccal tissues, which are frequently overlooked.
- Fractured teeth may have exposed pulp tissue that requires vital pulpotomy. This procedure needs specialized equipment not commonly available in the field. Removing the tooth is an alternative but is complicated by the loss of exposed crown secondary to the fracture.

EMERGENCY CARE: DENTAL-ORAL

- Most emergencies are traumatic.
- Lacerations are cleaned, anesthetized, debrided, and apposed with absorbable suture material such as polydioxanone (PDS, Ethicon, Somerville, NJ).
- Supportive treatment decreases healing time: antiinflammatory drugs (phenylbutazone or flunixin meglumine), antibiotics, and oral flushes with 1% chlorhexidine diacetate (Nolvasan) in water q12h.
- Lacerations of the tongue are occasionally seen. These can be transverse lacerations caused by inappropriate use of a bit, linear lesions produced by instruments during routine dental care, wounds caused by mandibular tooth fragments, incomplete shedding of the mandibular premolars, sharp edges of the lingual aspect of the mandibular cheek teeth, or wounds that occur when horses bite their tongues while racing and jumping.

GI

NOTE: An infected deep laceration of the tongue causes severe pain and presents with the chief complaint of difficulty eating, drooling, quidding, and depression.

- Rabies should be considered in the differential diagnosis and precautions taken to protect the examining clinician and assistants.
- Sedation is needed to completely evaluate lacerations and injuries involving the mouth.
- Fresh lacerations are primarily repaired and older wounds are best left to heal by secondary intention.

Injury to the Incisor Teeth

Self-inflicted injury to the deciduous incisors is common in young horses. Avulsions of the juvenile teeth occur when the teeth are "caught" on a relatively immovable object such as a stall guard, webbing, feed tub, or bucket. The individual panics and pulls back with partial avulsion of the incisor teeth. The injuries may not be noticed for hours or even days.

Presentation
- Juvenile teeth displaced rostrally
- Torn mucosal border
- Contaminated exposed root area of the affected teeth

First Priority
Consider the viability of the permanent incisors originating below the deciduous teeth. Aggressive debridement and repositioning of the deciduous teeth can injure the developing permanent teeth. The delicate tooth buds frequently are injured by the sharp, apical edges of the unstable, partially avulsed deciduous teeth.

- Remove the unstable juvenile teeth.
- Debride the wound edges.
- Allow the wound to heal by secondary intention.

Often the permanent teeth develop and erupt without problems. Young horses missing several deciduous incisors rarely have difficulties, whereas the loss of permanent incisors over many years causes significant incisor malalignment requiring dental care to maintain incisor balance.

External trauma to the deciduous incisors caused by kicks, collisions, and falls is treated as described for self-inflicted injury. Generally, these injuries almost always result in injury to the permanent teeth. Gentle debridement of the wound and anatomic replacement and stabilization of the teeth with stainless steel wire may correct incomplete or minor avulsion of the teeth.

If the avulsion involves permanent incisors, a more aggressive attempt to "rescue" these teeth is needed. Debridement of the contaminated wound followed by repositioning and stabilization of the area with cerclage wire can reclaim some of the teeth.

NOTE: It is important to determine whether the permanent incisors are fractured and if so, remove the fractured ends and evaluate the remaining apical portion of the tooth for viability.

PRACTICE TIP: Geriatric horses with newly fractured incisors: often they have a history of a sleep disorder and have fallen on their muzzle after "passing out."

ACUTE SALIVATION (PTYALISM)

Thomas J. Divers

Acute salivation (ptyalism/sialorrhea) can be caused by the inability to swallow normally produced saliva (i.e., choke) (see p. 202, and the Botulism section, Chapter 40, p. 400). This condition can be caused by neurologic disturbances (see p. 388) or by excessive production of saliva. A thorough physical examination and history are necessary to differentiate local causes from a focal manifestation of a generalized disease to arrive at an accurate diagnosis. *The most common causes of excessive salivation are red clover poisoning and choke in adults. In foals the cause is usually gastric and esophageal ulceration* (see p. 209-211).

The cause of salivation can be found in the mouth and diagnosed with oral examination in some cases. Evaluate the entire oral cavity looking for a laceration, ulcerations, vesicular disease, foreign body, abscess of tooth root or soft tissue, a fractured tooth (see p. 200), injury to the palate, or evidence of chemical injury. Sedation (detomidine with butorphanol) and the *careful* use of an equine mouth speculum may be needed to improve examination of the mouth. *Without proper sedation, the mouth speculum becomes a dangerous weapon to the examiner if the patient "throws" its head.* Excessive biting on the speculum also can result in fracture of a tooth.

Localized Causes

- The most common equine foreign body is a wooden stick large enough to become lodged between the upper arcade of teeth or a smaller stick penetrating the soft tissue of the pharyngeal cavity or soft palate.
- Evaluate the tongue for blisters, ulceration, or cellulitis.
- Burrs or grass awns can become stuck in the mouth and cause salivation. This may be a farm problem.
- Patients that have licked mercury blister compounds are prone to severe oral erosions.
- Most vesicles are idiopathic, but consider vesicular stomatitis, which appears most commonly in New Mexico and Colorado every 3 to 7 years. Immune-mediated pemphigus vesicular formation in the oral cavity occurs but is rare.
- *Actinobacillus lignieresii* infection can cause wooden tongue in horses.
- Consider also sialadenitis (inflammation of a salivary gland), fractured teeth, or fractured bones of the mouth and stylohyoid.
- Primary pharyngitis or epiglottiditis, retropharyngeal lymphadenopathy, guttural pouch empyema, pharyngeal edema, and choke are other frequent causes of ptyalism.

Diagnosis

Ancillary diagnostic tests include radiography, ultrasonography, and endoscopy of the mouth and pharyngeal area. Ultrasonography may define an area that can be aspirated for cytologic examination and culture. Observe carefully from a distance whether the ability to prehend, masticate, and swallow is retained. In some cases, a complete oral examination with the horse under anesthesia may be necessary before a cause can be determined.

Treatment

Treatments may include:

- Removal of foreign bodies
- Tooth extraction
- Antibiotic therapy for infectious causes
- Intravenous fluids
- Nonsteroidal antiinflammatory drugs (NSAIDs)
- Other symptomatic treatment:
  - 2% potassium permanganate as a mouth disinfectant
  - Furacin-prednisolone spray for pharyngeal edema and inflammation. Penicillin is often the initial antibiotic choice because many commensal oral organisms are sensitive to penicillin. Some patients may need a tracheotomy if laryngeal-pharyngeal swelling is compromising the airway. Regarding fluid therapy, it is important to remember that in the horse, the anion of highest concentration in saliva is chloride and that there is a relatively low concentration of bicarbonate. When a horse has an acid-base disturbance primarily from salivary loss, hypochloremic metabolic alkalosis usually is expected. Therefore fluid therapy consisting of 0.9% sodium chloride and 20 mEq/L KCl is used.

Systemic Causes

Slaframine toxicity (slobber syndrome; see Chapter 53), caused by the ingestion of red clover (hay or more commonly pasture) that has been infected with the fungus Rhizoctonia leguminicola, *can cause excessive salivation.* The clinical signs usually resolve within 48-96 hours after withdrawal from the affected forage; death is rare.

Other toxicities include organophosphates and carbamates, mercury, monensin, NSAID toxicity, acorn, oleander, potato, and cantharidin (blister beetle). An index of suspicion regarding potential exposure to toxins or chemical irritants that may have been ingested is necessary.

Other systemic diseases that can cause salivation include *botulism, equine protozoal myelitis,* leukoencephalomalacia, and renal or liver disease.

▧ C. DISORDERS OF THE ESOPHAGUS

P. O. Eric Mueller and James N. Moore

The most common clinical problem affecting the esophagus of a horse is obstruction of the lumen (choke). This disorder occurs either as a single acute episode or as a chronic, intermittent problem. In either case, these conditions are emergencies. If the condition recurs, diverticulum or stricture should be considered a possible cause.

ESOPHAGEAL OBSTRUCTION

Esophageal obstruction, most often acute, results from obstruction of the esophageal lumen with food, wood chips, or bedding. These problems occur among horses with ravenous eating habits, especially older horses being fed pelleted feed. *The most common clinical signs are excessive salivation, retching, coughing with saliva, and food dripping from the nostrils.* In most instances, enlargement of the esophagus can be palpated over the trachea if the obstruction is in the cervical region and is of recent origin. Over time, swelling and muscle spasm in this region make it difficult to delineate the mass. The likelihood that the obstruction is in the cervical portion of the esophagus increases if the patient retches immediately after attempting to swallow. There is a 10- to 12-second delay between the swallow and the onset of retching if the obstruction is in the distal esophagus.

Diagnosis and Medical Management of Choke

Confirm the diagnosis with endoscopy or by passing a nasogastric tube and encountering an obstruction in the esophagus. The initial aim of treatment is to reduce the patient's level of anxiety and allow the esophageal muscles to relax.

Tranquilize the patient with acepromazine and provide further sedation with *xylazine or detomidine. Withhold water and feed until an esophageal obstruction can be safely ruled out.*

If choke is suspected, advise owners to remove hay and water immediately. These conservative treatments frequently are sufficient to relax the esophagus and allow the obstruction to pass on its own within 4-6 hours.

Oxytocin 0.11-0.22 IU/kg body weight, IV q6h may help resolve the obstruction by decreasing esophageal smooth-muscle tone. Oxytocin administration may be associated with transient abdominal discomfort, sweating, and muscle tremors. *Oxytocin should not be administered to pregnant mares* because of the abortifacient properties.

To reduce the likelihood of aspiration pneumonia, administer one dose (0.02 mg/kg IV) of atropine to decrease salivation. *Do not repeat the atropine treatment owing to the side effects of this drug on the gastrointestinal tract!*

If this treatment is unsuccessful in relieving choke in 4-6 hours, administer further treatment, including gentle lavage. *With the patient sedated with xylazine or detomidine, causing the patient to lower its head, pass a stomach tube to the proximal limit of the obstruction;* gently instill a small volume of water through the tube and against the obstructing mass. Gently massage the obstructed area while the mass is advanced with the end of the stomach tube. This process may have to be repeated several times to help break up the obstruction.

CAREFUL MANIPULATION IS ESSENTIAL TO AVOID ESOPHAGEAL INJURY AND SECONDARY STRICTURE OR ESOPHAGEAL PERFORATION.

Intravenous fluids are an important supportive treatment in prolonged cases of choke to prevent dehydration and worsening of the esophageal obstruction.

If more aggressive lavage is needed, a warmed, cuffed endotracheal tube passed intranasally *into the esophagus* provides the security of an inflatable cuff and prevents aspiration of water during lavage of the esophagus. Warming the tube before passage facilitates passage by making it more flexible. Fluid can then be pumped through the endotracheal tube or through a small-diameter stomach tube that has been passed inside the larger endotracheal tube. The lavage solution is most commonly warm water.

An alternative procedure is to pass the endotracheal tube into the trachea and inflate the cuff before flushing the esophagus. If the obstruction cannot be cleared or if the patient becomes unmanageable under sedation, general anesthesia, with the head positioned down, is required for more aggressive lavage.

Prophylactic antimicrobial agents are indicated for all choke cases because of the risk of aspiration pneumonia. A broad-spectrum combination of antibiotics usually is administered for 5-7 days (e.g., procaine penicillin G, 22,000 IU/kg IM q12h initially or trimethoprim-sulfamethoxazole, 20-30 mg/kg PO q12h after the obstruction is relieved). If aspiration is known to have occurred, copious lavage is performed. If respiratory signs develop or crackles are present on auscultation or thoracic ultrasonography, indicating abnormalities of the pleura, add metronidazole (15-25 mg/kg PO q8h).

Once the obstruction is resolved, initially offer the patient only water, because esophageal dilation after obstruction increases the likelihood of reimpaction for 48 hours. Advise the owner to withhold feed for 48 hours or if that is impractical, to allow small amounts of a soft diet to prevent recurrence of the obstruction. Endoscopic examination after the obstruction is relieved allows evaluation of the esophageal mucosa and provides information concerning the likelihood of secondary complications (e.g., reobstruction, stricture, and perforation).

Surgical Treatment

If all attempts to dislodge the obstruction are unsuccessful, surgical intervention is indicated. Although several procedures are used to manage strictures, diverticula, tumors, and other rare causes of obstruction, cervical esophagotomy is the only emergency procedure.

Cervical esophagotomy is performed with the horse under local or general anesthesia. The decision depends on the temperament of the patient, the type of obstruction, cost, and the surgeon's preference. Make an incision either on the midline or ventral to the left jugular vein over the obstruction. Once the obstructed portion of the esophagus can be identified, attempt extraluminal massage and manual breakdown of the mass before entering the esophagus. If these maneuvers are unsuccessful, make a longitudinal incision distal to the obstruction on the ventral or ventrolateral aspect of the esophagus (see p. 88). These sites are used to aid in ventral drainage if the incision is left open to heal by secondary intention or if dehiscence of the primary incision occurs. A 2- to 3-cm incision is made in the muscular layer of the esophagus, and the mucosa is grasped with a forceps and incised. A sponge forceps is used to remove the obstructing mass.

A stomach tube is passed normograde and retrograde to ensure a patent lumen. For suturing of the esophagus, a simple continuous 3-0 monofilament PDS or polypropylene suture is placed in the mucosa and submucosa with the knots in the lumen of the esophagus. Close the muscular layer of the esophagus using an interrupted pattern of absorbable material. Position a suction drain adjacent to the esophagus and close the subcutaneous tissues. The suction drain remains in place for 48 hours, all food is withheld, and fluids are administered intravenously. Feed the patient a slurry of pelleted feed for 8-10 days, beginning on postoperative day 5.

An alternative is to use a second esophagotomy distal to the site of the obstruction to feed the patient a gruel and water mixture through an indwelling stomach tube sutured in place. This tube can be used for 10 days to allow the sutured proximal esophagotomy time to heal by primary intention. If dehiscence occurs, a traction diverticulum can develop but is usually associated with few complications.

If necrotic tissue is debrided at the obstruction site, a stomach tube is recommended. Suture the tube in place and feed the individual a gruel and water mixture through it for 10 days. The stoma is left to heal by secondary intention after tube removal.

Prognosis and Complications

The prognosis for survival with simple esophageal obstruction is excellent. The prognosis is favorable for horses with pulsion diverticula but poor if strictures occur that necessitate resection and anastomosis of the esophagus. Aspiration pneumonia is a serious sequela, to be recognized early and managed aggressively. Use ultrasonography to determine the severity of aspiration pneumonia. The incidence of these complications is directly related to the time to resolution of the primary obstruction. Treat the patient aggressively with particular care to avoid possible iatrogenic complications. Choke in miniature horse foals is relatively common and has a guarded prognosis.

ESOPHAGEAL PERFORATION

Causes for esophageal perforation (rupture) include

- Chronic obstruction
- Swallowed perforating foreign body
- Penetrating external wounds
- Repeated, traumatic nasogastric intubation
- Extension of infection from surrounding tissues

Clinical signs vary from a fistula draining saliva and feed material with open perforation to severe cervical swelling, cellulitis, abscessation, and subcutaneous emphysema with closed esophageal perforation. Dyspnea may develop and necessitate emergency tracheotomy.

Confirm the diagnosis with endoscopy, radiography, or contrast radiography. Small perforations may be difficult to detect with endoscopy. Survey radiographs may reveal subcutaneous emphysema, and positive-contrast studies may demonstrate leakage of aqueous medium into the surrounding tissues.

Treatment

- Acute (6-12 h) perforations can be debrided and closed primarily if sufficient viable esophageal tissue is present.
- Maintain affected horses with nothing by mouth for 48-72 hours after surgery to allow time for mucosal healing and to minimize postoperative fistula formation.
- Administer broad-spectrum antimicrobial therapy. Antimicrobial combinations commonly used include
  - Na^+/K^+ penicillin, 22,000-44,000 IU/kg IV q6h, and aminoglycosides: gentamicin, 6.6 mg/kg IV q24h or amikacin, 19.8 mg/kg IV q24h
  - Metronidazole, 15-25 mg/kg PO q6h, for anaerobes
- Intravenous, balanced, polyionic fluids to correct electrolyte and acid-base abnormalities *or if aminoglycosides are being administered to preserve sufficient renal perfusion.*
- NSAIDs
- Tetanus prophylaxis

If primary closure is not possible, adequate ventral drainage is established to minimize extension of the cellulitis along fascial planes, which could result in septic mediastinitis and pleuritis.

Nutritional supplementation through an esophagostomy and indwelling nasogastric tube placement distal to the site of perforation, or total parenteral nutrition (TPN), may be needed during the convalescent period.

Prognosis and Complications

The prognosis for acute esophageal perforation is fair if prompt, aggressive therapy is instituted and primary closure of the defect is possible. In chronic cases, the prognosis is guarded because of the high probability of secondary complications such as esophageal stricture, reobstruction, and septic mediastinitis or pleuritis.

▓ D. DISORDERS OF THE STOMACH

P. O. Eric Mueller, James N. Moore, and Thomas J. Divers

ACUTE GASTRIC DILATION

Primary gastric dilation is believed to be associated with the ingestion of highly fermentable feed, such as grass clippings or excessive amounts of corn or other grain. Secondary gastric dilation occurs when fluid from the small intestine accumulates in the stomach because of ileus, obstruction of the small-intestinal lumen, strangulation obstruction involving the small intestine, or severe inflammation of the small intestine. In one study of 50 horses with gastric rupture, horses drinking water from a bucket, stream, or pond were at greater risk of gastric rupture than were those with access to an automatic waterer.

- Horses exhibit signs of severe pain and increased heart and respiratory rates due to pain and diaphragmatic pressure.
- If the dilation is primary, the mucous membranes are pale, and on rectal examination the spleen can be palpated displaced caudally by the enlarged stomach. If the dilation is secondary to a problem involving the small intestine, the patient may exhibit signs of toxicity, the peritoneal fluid may reflect intraabdominal ischemia (discoloration with erythrocytes, increased WBC, count and protein concentration), and several loops of distended small intestine may be palpable on rectal examination.
- In some cases spontaneous regurgitation may occur immediately before the stomach ruptures along its greater curvature.

Treatment

For acute abdominal pain, the primary goal is to relieve intragastric pressure by passing a medium- or large-bore stomach tube. *Lidocaine may be needed to relax the cardiac sphincter, and it may be necessary to create a "siphon" effect to ensure that all excess fluid is removed from the stomach.* Once emergency care is given, perform a complete physical examination to determine the cause. In primary dilation, the patient should remain pain-free once the pressure is relieved. If the dilation is secondary to a small-intestinal problem, relief is transient. If the stomach ruptures, the patient immediately appears comfortable, but then rapid deterioration occurs as the result of endotoxic and cardiovascular shock. Ingesta are evident in the peritoneal fluid, and the serosa of the intestines is roughened on rectal examination. Euthanasia is recommended.

Prognosis

The prognosis for primary dilation is excellent, provided intragastric pressure is rapidly relieved. The prognosis for secondary gastric dilation depends on the underlying disease and the duration of the condition before treatment is started.

GASTRIC IMPACTION

Occurs infrequently. The most common causes are

- Grain overload
- Dry, impacted ingesta
- Squamous cell carcinoma of the stomach

If the impaction is associated with causes other than squamous cell carcinoma, the patient may show signs of moderate to severe pain. Most often these patients do not show evidence of systemic toxicity unless the grain overload has progressed, resulting in signs of acute laminitis. Horses with impacted ingesta in the stomach may be in uncontrollable pain, which necessitates immediate exploratory surgery. The diagnosis in these cases is made at surgery.

Treatment

At surgery, administer 2-3 L of water through a 3-inch (7.5-cm) intraabdominal needle placed through the gastric wall. Redirect the end of the needle, infiltrating different areas of the mass with gentle massage of the impaction. Postoperative care includes lavage of the stomach and drainage through a large-bore gastric tube.

Prognosis

Guarded.

EMERGENCY GRAIN OVERLOAD

Clinicians often are called in an emergency to examine and treat a horse that has accidentally ingested an excessive quantity of grain (either commercially prepared concentrate or a cereal grain hay such as barley). If the patient has no clinical signs at examination, the following treatment is recommended:

- Pass a gastric tube and check for gastric reflux; if there is no reflux, administer by means of *gravity flow* (funnel) 1 lb (450 g) Epsom salts ($MgSO_4$) or 1 lb (450 g) activated charcoal mixed in 1 gallon (3.8 L) warm water (per 500-kg adult).
- 0.3 mg/kg flunixin meglumine IV or IM q8h for 48 hours
- 0.5 mg/kg doxylamine succinate SQ q6h for 24h (other favored antihistamines may be substituted)
- Remove all feed for 24 hours

Prognosis

Should be excellent if the treatment is given before any clinical signs develop.

SYMPTOMATIC GRAIN OVERLOAD

The clinical signs most frequently seen are colic, marked abdominal distention, severe lameness (laminitis), trembling, sweating, polypnea, and, less frequently, diarrhea. Clinical findings include bright red to purple membranes, tachycardia, absence of intestinal sounds (some pings may be heard on simultaneous auscultation and percussion of the abdomen), gastric reflux, and colonic distention with tight bands palpated at rectal examination.

CBC usually reveals severe polycythemia, neutropenia with a left shift, and vacuolization of neutrophils (toxic changes).

Treatment

- Intravenous fluid therapy. Hypertonic saline solution initially, but this must be followed within 1-2 hours by administration of a polyionic fluid at 2-4 L/h for the adult; 23% calcium borogluconate, 500 ml, can be administered but must be diluted with several liters of polyionic fluids. Add KCl, 20-40 mEq, to each liter of fluid after urination is documented.
- Administer plasma if possible (2-4 L for an adult). Hyperimmune plasma containing antibodies against endotoxin is preferred but not essential.
- Administer flunixin meglumine 1 mg/kg IV initially and 0.3 mg/kg q8h after signs of colic are no longer evident.
- Pass a nasogastric tube and leave it in place to relieve gastric distention. If there is no gastric reflux, administer ½ lb (225 g) of charcoal in ½ gallon (1.9 L) warm water (per 500-kg adult) by means of *gravity flow.*
  □ Polymyxin B 2000-6000 IU/kg IV q12h for 1-2 days can be used, if renal function is normal, to bind circulating endotoxin.
- Pentoxifylline (8.4 mg/kg PO q8h) may be administered if there is no gastric reflux. Pentoxifylline can inhibit cytokine production. Pentoxifylline also can be given intravenously (see Chapter 52, p. 000).
- Remove feed, bed heavily, apply pads to the feet, or perform a combination of these maneuvers.
- Adminster aggressive and early therapy for laminitis if signs of founder are present (see p. 368).
- If there is a marked cecal distention, perform trocarization and infuse 10×10^6 units of penicillin into the cecum.
- Administer lidocaine 1.3 mg/kg by slow bolus and follow it with 0.05 mg/kg per minute continuous infusion if severe ileus and abdominal distention are present.

Prognosis

The prognosis if there are marked clinical signs is poor. *If severe abdominal pain and significant abdominal distention are present, affected patients usually die within 24-48 hours with even the most aggressive therapy.*

If signs of laminitis occur before signs of the existence of intestinal disease abate, the prognosis is very grave.

GASTRIC ULCERS (ADULTS)

Although affected patients often have no signs, ulcers can be a cause of colic in both young and older horses. The cause is unknown but is believed related to physiologic stress, prolonged acidity, reflux of bile acids, high grain to low pasture diet, exercise-induced ischemia, and acid reflux or administration of NSAIDs.

In adults, ulcers cause signs ranging from severe acute pain to chronic intermittent low-grade colic, poor appetite, and poor body condition. Gastric ulcers in adults most commonly involve the squamous epithelial mucosa adjacent to the margo plicatus, although ulcers in the antrum and pylorus are being diagnosed with increasing frequency. Ulcers may be especially implicated as the cause of colic if signs develop after eating. Affected horses may roll or may remain standing and continually paw. The diagnosis is confirmed with the finding of ulcers at gastroscopy (after feed is withheld for 6-8 hours) and lack of other abnormalities affecting the gastrointestinal tract, response to established treatment with histamine type 2 (H_2) receptor antagonists or proton pump blocker (omeprazole), within 72 hours, and healing of ulcers.

Treatment

Clinical disease believed to be caused by ulcers responds to ranitidine (6.6 mg/kg PO q8h) or other H_2 or proton pump blockers within 24-72 hours with improvement in ulcer appearance in 75% of cases. *If there is no clinical response within 72 hours after H_2-receptor antagonist treatment at the recommended dose, suspect another cause of the pain.* Stop training and feed a risk-free feed most useful to stimulate eating (e.g., grass). The controversy regarding the onset of action of omeprazole is questionable and therefore many clinicians begin treatment with ranitidine in "colicky" horses. If there is a rapid response, then switch to omeprazole because of the convenience and effectiveness of the medication. If the ulcers are believed to be a result of NSAID treatment, therapy should be as follows:

- Omeprazole (GastroGard) 4 mg/kg PO once a day
- Misoprostol 2.5 µg/kg q8-12h
- Sucralfate (Carafate) 8 g/500 kg q8-12h

Prognosis

The prognosis for adults is good to excellent with treatment. Recurrence may occur in individuals that continue to race or train.

GASTRIC ULCERS IN FOALS

Gastric ulcers are common in foals and can cause pain, disruption with nursing, and general loss of body condition. Gastric ulceration is caused by an imbalance between ulcerogenic and protective factors in the stomachs of foals. Many physiologic stress factors can lead to this imbalance, including a recent episode of diarrhea (the highest risk factor), and the use of NSAIDs in the care of foals.

Diagnosis

COMMON CLINICAL SIGNS

- Grinding of teeth (bruxism/odontoprisis)
- Excessive salivation (ptyalism)
- Rolling on the back, particularly after nursing

ANCILLARY TESTS

The signs are so commonly characteristic of gastric ulceration that ancillary tests usually are unnecessary. However, gastroscopy may be used to confirm a diagnosis of gastric ulceration. Older foals (>60 days) commonly have severe lesions on the lesser curvature (nonglandular portion) of the stomach. In younger foals or in those with ulcers associated with NSAID administration, lesions can be more severe in the glandular area. *Occult fecal blood tests are not indicated, because a negative result does not exclude gastric ulceration.*

Treatment
- Administer either H$_2$-receptor antagonists *or* proton-pump blockers in combination with sucralfate, as follows. *In severe cases, it is best to administer initial therapy intravenously.*
  □ **H$_2$ Antagonists**
    Ranitidine: 1.5 mg/kg IV q8h or 6.6 mg/kg PO q8h (recommended)
    Famotidine: 0.5-1.0 mg/kg IV q24h or 3-4 mg/kg PO q24h
    Cimetidine: 6.6 mg/kg IV or 20 mg/kg PO q8h
  □ There should be a response to H$_2$-receptor antagonist therapy in 3-5 days. If not, other possibilities include duodenal outflow abnormality (especially in older foals) and inadequate therapy.
  □ **Proton-pump blocker**
    Omeprazole (GastroGard): 1-4 mg/kg PO q24h.
  □ **Sucralfate**
    1-2 g (or 2-4 g for large foals) PO q6h. **This may not be effective for nonglandular ulcers.**

NOTE: Because sucralfate is in gel form and decreases absorption of concurrently administered drugs, do not administer sucralfate at the same time as oral H$_2$-receptor antagonists. Administer sucralfate simultaneously with intravenous H$_2$-receptor blockers.

- Pain can be managed with xylazine or butorphanol. Do not use NSAIDs because they can promote gastric ulceration. If repeated doses of xylazine or butorphanol fail to control pain, an antacid "cocktail" (approximately 0.5 L of bismuth subsalicylate [Pepto-Bismol] or simethicone [Mylanta] mixed with 0.5 L of warm water, 100 ml of alumina and magnesia [Maalox-TC] liquid, 4 sucralfate [Carafate] tablets dissolved, and 1 cup [240 ml] activated charcoal) may provide immediate relief from pain. This should be administered through a soft nasogastric tube after sedation.
- Supportive therapy must be initiated to correct or to decrease the predisposing factors. For example, if the foal has diarrhea, fluid therapy would likely be indicated. If there is clinical evidence of severe gastroesophageal reflux (marked salivation or obvious distention of the esophagus) or the esophagus is found at gastroscopic examination to be severely eroded, bethanechol, 0.03 mg/kg SC q8h, should be administered until the signs improve.
- Misoprostol: 2 mg/kg PO q12h should be administered if gastric ulcers are believed to be caused by NSAIDs.

Prognosis
If the predisposing cause can be corrected and the foal responds to treatment within 3-5 days, the prognosis is good for a return to full function. Duodenal stric-

ture is a serious complication that would prevent a favorable prognosis. Foals with salivation and odontoprisis generally have some outflow obstruction. If this persists, a barium study is indicated. *Perforations can occur, although most do so without noticeable characteristic signs of gastric ulceration.*

Prevention

Minimize the risk factors. Control diarrhea promptly and minimize the use of NSAIDs, especially if the foal is dehydrated. Administer prophylactic treatment to moderately or severely ill foals or stressed foals (those receiving frequent treatments) with oral sucralfate, an acid-inhibiting drug, or both. There is a general impression among equine neonatologists that sucralfate is effective in preventing ulcers in stressed foals, although this has not been documented. Recumbent foals receiving critical care often are not treated with H_2-receptor or proton pump blockers because the gastric pH may already be elevated. Once the foal begins to stand, H_2-receptor blockers should be used.

> **NOTE:** If the history or condition of the foal suggests that the problem may not be acute, pass a nasogastric tube after sedation. If there is a large volume of gastric reflux fluid, the foal should undergo further diagnostic testing (barium radiographs) to rule out duodenal stricture.

DUODENAL OR GASTRIC PERFORATION

Duodenal or gastric perforation usually occurs in foals younger than 8 weeks. Risk factors include the use of NSAIDs and stresses on the foal, including diarrhea. Many cases occur with minimal warning signs of gastric ulceration.

Diagnosis
COMMON CLINICAL SIGNS
Foals often are found acutely depressed or "colicky" with a tight abdomen, increased heart and respiratory rates, and a high fever, but they may continue to nurse. Often diarrhea accompanies duodenal perforation; the diarrhea is present either before the perforation or as a consequence of endotoxemia.

ANCILLARY TESTS
- Ultrasonography: large amounts of flocculent fluid are seen
- Abdominocentesis: performed to confirm septic peritonitis

Treatment
Euthanasia except for those patients with a small perforation that may be found at exploratory surgery and sealed by the omentum.

Prevention
NSAIDs should be administered to young foals only when absolutely necessary, as in the management of endotoxemia, *especially to foals with diarrhea.* If an NSAID has been administered to a foal, initiate treatment with omeprazole 2-4 mg/kg PO once a day. Do not rely on sucralfate alone to prevent ulcers if NSAIDs are being used. Carprofen 1.4 mg/kg PO q12-24h may be the safest NSAID to use when more long-term therapy for skeletal disorders is required.

■ E. DISORDERS OF THE SMALL INTESTINE THAT CAUSE COLIC

P. O. Eric Mueller and James N. Moore

INTUSSUSCEPTION

Small-intestinal intussusception usually occurs in younger horses and involves an invagination of a segment of bowel (**intussusceptum**) and mesentery into the lumen of an adjacent distal segment of bowel (**intussuscipiens**). Continued peristalsis draws more bowel and its mesentery into the intussuscipiens, causing venous congestion, edema, infarction, and necrosis of the involved segment. Small-intestinal obstruction and strangulation result. Intussusception results from alterations in intestinal motility.

Predisposing factors

- Enteritis
- Maladjustment of septic foals in intensive care units
- Abrupt dietary changes
- Heavy ascarid *(Parascaris equorum)* or tapeworm *(Anoplocephala perfoliata)* infestation
- Anthelmintic treatment
- Intestinal anastomosis in most cases; no specific factor is identified. Jejunojejunal and jejunoileal intussusception is more common in foals, whereas ileocecal intussusception is more common in adults.

Diagnosis

- Clinical signs of jejunojejunal and ileocecal intussusception vary with the degree and duration of the condition.
- Most commonly, intussusception leads to complete intestinal obstruction and strangulation of the intussusceptum, causing an acute onset of unrelenting abdominal pain.
- Nasogastric reflux develops, and progressive dehydration and hypovolemia rapidly follow.
- Rectal examination reveals loops of distended small intestine, and occasionally the intussusception can be palpated. With ileocecal intussusception, a turgid segment of bowel may be palpable within the cecum.
- Increased peritoneal protein concentration and nucleated cell count reflect devitalization of the affected bowel. Changes in the peritoneal fluid, however, may not accurately reflect the degree of intestinal compromise owing to isolation of the devitalized intussusceptum within the intussuscipiens.
- In foals, the intussusception usually is identified with ultrasound.

Chronic ileocecal intussusception with partial obstruction causes intermittent or continuous abdominal pain, weight loss, poor general physical condition, and varying degrees of anorexia and depression. This can continue for weeks to months but eventually leads to an acute episode of severe abdominal pain corresponding to complete obstruction of the intestine.

Treatment

INITIAL THERAPY IS SUPPORTIVE

- Gastric decompression

- Balanced polyionic intravenous fluids (e.g., lactated Ringer's solution)
- Analgesics (e.g., xylazine, butorphanol tartrate, or flunixin meglumine)
- Monitoring of physiologic and clinical parameters (pain, nasogastric reflux, heart rate, mucous membranes, hematocrit, PCV/TPP, borborygmi)
- Surgical exploration is indicated if intussusception is suspected

EXPLORATORY SURGERY
- Ventral midline exploratory celiotomy
- Manual reduction of the intussusception
- Resection and anastomosis of the affected intestine

Some intussusceptions cannot be reduced because of the length of bowel involved, venous congestion, and edema. These cases necessitate en bloc resection and anastomosis. Even if the intestinal segment appears viable, consider resection and anastomosis because of the possibility of mucosal necrosis, serosal inflammation, and postoperative adhesion formation.

Prognosis
- Good with early diagnosis and surgical repair. Poor if the intussusception is advanced and irreducible owing to the likelihood of ileus, peritonitis, and postoperative adhesion formation.

VOLVULUS

Volvulus is the rotation of a segment of intestine around the long axis of its mesentery. Although most cases are not accompanied by a predisposing lesion, adhesions, infarction, intestinal incarceration, pedunculated lipoma, and mesodiverticular bands can lead to volvulus. Abrupt dietary changes and verminous arteritis also have been implicated. The length and segment of the intestine involved are variable. The ileum is frequently included because of its fixed attachment at the ileocecal junction.

Diagnosis
- Acute onset of progressive, moderate to severe, continuous pain that may initially respond to analgesics. Analgesic effectiveness rapidly decreases as the disease progresses.
- Rapid, progressive cardiovascular deterioration occurs as evidenced by poor peripheral perfusion (rapid, weak pulse, hyperemic or cyanotic mucous membranes, and a prolonged CRT).
- Hypovolemia and hemoconcentration develop rapidly. *Nasogastric reflux often is present, but decompression may not provide pain relief as it does in simple obstruction.*
- Rectal examination usually reveals moderate to severe small-intestinal distention (see Fig 35–2) and occasionally a tight mesenteric root. Mild tension on the mesentery may elicit a pain response.
- Lack of palpable small-intestinal distention *does not rule out* the possibility of a strangulating lesion, because the distended intestine may be beyond the reach of the examiner.
- Abdominocentesis may yield normal or serosanguineous fluid with increased peritoneal protein concentration (>3.0 g/dl) and nucleated cell count (>10,000 cells/µl). The devitalized portion of intestine may be isolated from the peritoneal cavity (e.g., within the omental bursa), and results of peritoneal fluid analysis therefore may not accurately reflect the degree of intestinal change.

- Abdominal ultrasonography reveals dilated, nonmotile small intestine.

Treatment

INITIAL THERAPY IS SUPPORTIVE
- Gastric decompression
- Balanced polyionic intravenous fluids (e.g., lactated Ringer's solution) with plasma
- Analgesics (e.g., xylazine, butorphanol tartrate, and/or flunixin meglumine)
- Monitoring of physiologic and clinical parameters (pain, nasogastric reflux, heart rate, mucous membranes, hematocrit, PCV/TPP, borborygmi)
- Surgical exploration if volvulus is suspected

EXPLORATORY SURGERY
- Ventral midline exploratory celiotomy
- Identification of the strangulated portion of intestine
- Determination of the direction of rotation of the affected segment by means of palpation of the mesentery
- After correction, evaluate intestinal viability and perform resection and anastomosis if needed

Prognosis

- Depends on the duration of illness and amount of intestine involved in the volvulus. Prognosis is good with early detection and rapid treatment. For patients with long-standing strangulation, postoperative peritonitis, ileus, and adhesion formation are common sequelae. When resection of more than 50% of the small intestine is needed, there is a high incidence of postoperative complications (malabsorption, weight loss, and liver damage).

HERNIATION

Herniation of the small intestine is classified as internal or external. *Internal hernias* occur within the abdominal cavity and do not involve a hernial sac. Examples are displacement of the small intestine through the epiploic foramen, mesenteric defects, and rents in the gastrosplenic and broad ligaments. *External hernias* extend outside the limits of the abdominal cavity and include inguinal, umbilical, ventral abdominal, and diaphragmatic hernias.

Epiploic Foramen Herniation

The epiploic foramen is a potential opening, approximately 4 to 6 cm in length, that separates the omental bursa from the peritoneal cavity. It is bounded dorsally by the caudate lobe of the liver and caudal vena cava and ventrally by the right lobe of the pancreas and the portal vein. It is limited cranially by the hepatoduodenal ligament and caudally by the junction of the pancreas and mesoduodenum. Adults (older than 8 years) are predisposed to epiploic foramen entrapment owing to enlargement of this space caused by atrophy of the right caudate lobe of the liver. Herniation through the foramen can occur as right to left (from the lateral side) or as left to right (from the medial side) displacement.

Diagnosis

- Acute onset of moderate to severe pain that may initially be responsive to analgesics. The effectiveness of analgesics decreases as the disease progresses.
- Rapid cardiovascular deterioration occurs, and hypovolemia and hemoconcentration develop rapidly.
- Nasogastric reflux is present, but decompression may not provide pain relief.
- Rectal examination reveals moderate to severe small-intestinal distention (see Fig 35–2).
- Some horses may have mild signs of pain with no nasogastric reflux or palpable intestinal distention. The lack of palpable small-intestinal distention does not rule out a strangulating lesion, because the distended intestine may be beyond the reach of the examiner. Ultrasonography generally reveals distended nonmotile bowel.
- Abdominocentesis is useful in determining the severity of the lesion and the need for surgical intervention. Peritoneal fluid analysis may reveal normal or serosanguineous fluid with increased protein concentration (>3.0 g/dl) and nucleated cell count (>10,000 cells/μl). The devitalized portion of intestine within the omental bursa may be isolated from the rest of the peritoneal cavity. Therefore, fluid obtained at abdominocentesis may not accurately reflect the severity of intestinal compromise.

Treatment

INITIAL THERAPY IS SUPPORTIVE

- Gastric decompression
- Balanced polyionic intravenous fluids (e.g., lactated Ringer's solution)
- Analgesics (e.g., xylazine with or without butorphanol tartrate or flunixin meglumine)
- Monitoring of physiologic and clinical parameters (pain, nasogastric reflux, heart rate, mucous membranes, hematocrit, PCV/TPP, borborygmi)
- Surgical intervention if epiploic entrapment is suspected

EXPLORATORY SURGERY

- Frequently needed to confirm the diagnosis
- Ventral midline exploratory celiotomy
- Decompression of the bowel, careful manual dilation of the foramen, and reduction of the hernia
- Traumatic dilation of the foramen can result in life-threatening rupture of the caudal vena cava or portal vein
- Evaluate intestinal viability and perform resection and anastomosis if necessary

Prognosis

- Depends on the duration of illness, the length of intestine requiring resection, and difficulty encountered reducing the hernia.

Gastrosplenic Ligament Incarceration

Incarceration of the small intestine through the gastrosplenic ligament is uncommon. Anatomically, the ligament attaches the greater curvature of the stomach to the hilum of the spleen and continues ventrally with the greater omentum. Defects in the ligament are generally acquired as the result of trauma. The distal jejunum and ileum are most commonly involved, herniation occurring in a caudal to cranial direction.

Diagnosis

Clinical signs are similar to those of epiploic foramen herniation:

- Acute onset of severe abdominal pain, nasogastric reflux, small-intestinal distention at rectal examination, and rapid systemic deterioration.
- Distended small intestine may not be palpable early in the disease because of the cranial location in the abdomen.
- Abdominocentesis may yield normal to serosanguineous fluid with an increased total protein and nucleated cell count. The severity of the signs depends on the location, duration, and extent of the lesion.
- Exploratory celiotomy is frequently needed for a definitive diagnosis.

Treatment

INITIAL THERAPY IS SUPPORTIVE

- Gastric decompression
- Balanced polyionic intravenous fluids (e.g., lactated Ringer's solution)
- Analgesics (e.g., xylazine with or without butorphanol tartrate or flunixin meglumine)
- Monitoring of physiologic and clinical parameters (pain, nasogastric reflux, heart rate, mucous membranes, hematocrit, PCV/TPP, borborygmi)
- Surgical intervention if strangulating obstruction is suspected

EXPLORATORY SURGERY

- Ventral midline exploratory celiotomy
- Reduction of the hernia
- The ligament is relatively avascular, and digital enlargement of the rent facilitates reduction of the incarceration with minimal risk of life-threatening hemorrhage
- Resection and anastomosis of devitalized bowel
- The defect in the ligament is not closed

Prognosis

- Depends on the duration of illness and length of intestine resected (see epiploic foramen herniation).

Mesenteric Defects

Defects or rents in the mesentery, broad ligaments, or greater omentum produce a potential space for intestinal incarceration or strangulation. Mesenteric defects most often occur in the small-intestinal mesentery and less commonly in the large- and small-colonic mesentery. Defects commonly are acquired as a result of blunt abdominal trauma or surgical manipulation of bowel and mesentery. A segment of intestine may pass through the defect and become incarcerated or strangulated. A mesodiverticular band, a congenital remnant of a vitelline artery and its associated mesentery, extends from one side of the mesentery to the antimesenteric border of the jejunum or ileum and is a common site of incarceration. This tissue normally atrophies during the first trimester. Failure to atrophy results in formation of a triangulated mesenteric sac. A loop of intestine can become incarcerated in the sac; the result is mesenteric rupture, herniation, and strangulation.

Diagnosis

Clinical signs are similar to those of volvulus:

- Acute onset of abdominal pain
- Nasogastric reflux with small-intestinal distention at rectal examination
- Systemic cardiovascular deterioration
- Abdominocentesis reveals normal to serosanguineous fluid with increased protein concentration and nucleated cell count. The severity of the signs depends on the location, duration, and severity of the lesion

Treatment

INITIAL THERAPY IS SUPPORTIVE

- Gastric decompression
- Balanced polyionic intravenous fluids (e.g., lactated Ringer's solution)
- Analgesics (e.g., xylazine with or without butorphanol tartrate or flunixin meglumine)
- Monitoring of physiologic and clinical parameters (pain, nasogastric reflux, heart rate, mucous membranes, hematocrit, PCV/TPP, borborygmi)
- Surgical intervention if a strangulating obstruction is suspected

EXPLORATORY SURGERY

- Needed for definitive diagnosis
- Ventral midline exploratory celiotomy
- Reduction of the hernia
- The hernial ring may require manual dilation to reduce the hernia.
- Closure of the mesenteric defect
- Resection and anastomosis of devitalized bowel
- Defects near the root of the mesentery are difficult to close because of limited exposure

Prognosis

- Depends on the duration of illness and the length of intestine that needs resection. The prognosis is poor if difficulty is encountered reducing the hernia and closing the defect.

Inguinal Hernia

Acquired inguinal hernias in stallions are associated with breeding or strenuous exercise and cause acute abdominal pain. A sudden increase in intraabdominal pressure or an enlarged internal inguinal ring may predispose to inguinal hernia. Inguinal hernias are commonly unilateral and occur frequently among Standardbred, Saddlebred, and Tennessee Walking horses. Inguinal herniation and evisceration occur as a sequela to castration.

Congenital inguinal hernias in foals usually close spontaneously as the foal matures and only occasionally cause intestinal problems, e.g., if the hernia cannot be reduced or if it is very large. Scrotal herniation may require surgical correction when the bowel ruptures through the parietal tunic.

Diagnosis

Acquired inguinal and scrotal herniation in a stallion can produce acute intestinal obstruction that necessitates emergency surgical intervention. Incarcerated bowel is strangulated; hypovolemic and endotoxic shock occur and cause systemic cardiovascular deterioration. The hernia is usually indirect and unilateral, the incarcerated intestinal segment descending through the vaginal ring and contained within the tunica vaginalis.

Affected horses have a rapid onset of moderate to severe abdominal pain. Palpation of the scrotum may reveal a firm, swollen, cold testicle on the affected side, but early scrotal swelling may be absent. A swollen and slightly turgid tail of the epididymis may be palpated in early cases owing to passive congestion. The loop of herniated small bowel may be palpable per rectum passing through the internal inguinal ring.

The signs of strangulating obstruction—tachycardia, dehydration, endotoxemia, and cardiovascular deterioration—develop with time. Abdominocentesis reveals fluid with an increased total protein level and nucleated cell count. Peritoneal fluid analysis may not accurately reflect the severity of intestinal compromise because of sequestration of fluid within the scrotum.

Herniation and rupture of the vaginal tunic in newborn foals can cause mild pain and depression, local edema, and subsequent abscessation.

Treatment

INITIAL THERAPY IS SUPPORTIVE

- Gastric decompression
- Balanced polyionic intravenous fluids (e.g., lactated Ringer's solution)
- Analgesics (e.g., xylazine with or without butorphanol tartrate or flunixin meglumine)
- Monitoring of physiologic and clinical parameters (pain, nasogastric reflux, heart rate, mucous membranes, hematocrit, PCV/TPP, borborygmi)
- Surgical intervention if inguinal or scrotal herniation is suspected

EXPLORATORY SURGERY

- Ventral midline exploratory celiotomy
- Inguinal incision to achieve adequate surgical exposure and reduction
- Reduction, resection, and anastomosis of the affected bowel
- Unilateral castration and inguinal herniorrhaphy usually required

Inguinal herniation in newborn colts may be contained in the vaginal tunic or may rupture through the tunic and lie subcutaneously. Those within the vaginal tunic may be manually reduced and generally correct spontaneously. Those that rupture through the tunic or those that are large and cannot be reduced require surgical repair through inguinal and scrotal incisions.

Prognosis

- Good if reduction and repair are performed within hours of herniation, before strangulation occurs. The prognosis worsens with increasing duration before correction. The prognosis for breeding soundness is good if only one testicle is involved.

Diaphragmatic Hernia

Diaphragmatic hernia can be congenital or acquired and is an unusual cause of abdominal pain in horses. Most often it results from strenuous exercise, a hard fall, hitting something while running, or being hit by a car. Pregnant or periparturient mares also are at risk.

Diagnosis

Clinical signs of diaphragmatic hernia include abdominal pain, tachypnea, and dyspnea. The severity of signs depends on the size of the hernia opening and degree of visceral herniation. The presence of viscera within the thoracic cavity may reduce the intensity of lung sounds and cause dullness to percussion. Radiography or ultrasonography (Fig. 35–4) is helpful in finding fluid or ingesta-filled loops of intestine in the thoracic cavity. Blood gas measurement may indicate respiratory compromise and hypoxemia. *Thoracocentesis* and *abdominocentesis* may yield blood-tinged fluid with an increased total protein level and nucleated cell count, which are evidence of the presence of devitalized bowel. Exploratory celiotomy often is necessary for a definitive diagnosis.

Treatment

INITIAL THERAPY IS SUPPORTIVE
- Gastric decompression
- Balanced polyionic intravenous fluids (e.g., lactated Ringer's solution)
- Analgesics (e.g., xylazine with or without butorphanol tartrate or flunixin meglumine)
- Supplemental oxygen therapy if necessary
- Monitoring of physiologic and clinical parameters (pain, nasogastric reflux, heart rate, mucous membranes, hematocrit, PCV/TPP, borborygmi)

EXPLORATORY SURGERY
- Ventral midline exploratory celiotomy
- Reduction, resection, and anastomosis of the affected bowel

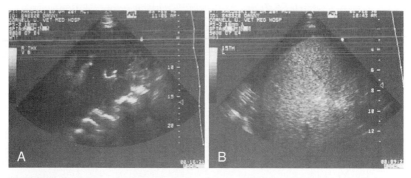

FIGURE 35–4. A, Ultrasound scan of the thorax of a 20-year-old gelding with mild pain, sternal edema, and thoracic effusion. The 5-MHz scan reveals multiple loops of small intestine (*white reflections*) in the thoracic cavity and an unusually well-defined posterior vena cava. To the left of the screen is fluid and fibrin. **B,** Ultrasound scan of the same patient shows the liver in the thoracic cavity.

- Closure of the diaphragmatic defect by suturing or use of a synthetic mesh (Marlex, Proplast)

Prognosis
- Guarded to poor because of difficult surgical exposure and a high incidence of postoperative complications, septic pleuritis, implant failure, and hernia recurrence. The prognosis is better in young horses as a result of the improved surgical exposure.

PEDUNCULATED LIPOMA

Pedunculated lipoma is a common cause of small-intestinal strangulation or obstruction in horses older than 10 years. Lipomas attach to the mesentery by a fibrovascular stalk of variable length. They are frequently incidental findings at exploratory surgery or necropsy. These masses have the potential to incarcerate a segment of small intestine and produce strangulating obstruction.

Diagnosis

Pedunculated lipoma should be considered in the differential diagnosis when a horse older than 10 years has signs of small-intestinal obstruction.

CLINICAL SIGNS
- Acute abdominal pain
- Hemoconcentration
- Decreased borborygmi
- Nasogastric reflux usually is present but may be absent early in the disease.
- Multiple loops of small intestine are palpable at rectal examination (see Fig 35–2), and increases in peritoneal total protein concentration and nucleated cell count reflect the degree of intestinal compromise.

Treatment
INITIAL THERAPY IS SUPPORTIVE
- Gastric decompression
- Balanced polyionic intravenous fluids (e.g., lactated Ringer's solution)
- Analgesics (e.g., xylazine with or without butorphanol tartrate or flunixin meglumine)
- Monitoring of physiologic and clinical parameters (pain, nasogastric reflux, heart rate, mucous membranes, hematocrit, PCV/TPP, borborygmi)
- Surgical intervention if a strangulating obstruction is suspected

EXPLORATORY SURGERY
- Ventral midline exploratory celiotomy
- Ligation and transection of lipoma
- Resection and anastomosis of the affected bowel
- Remove any lipomas found at surgery to minimize recurrence

Prognosis
- Favorable with early diagnosis and prompt treatment. If devitalized bowel cannot be resected or if peritonitis is severe, the prognosis is guarded to poor.

ILEAL IMPACTION

The ileum is the most common site of small-intestinal intraluminal impaction. The incidence varies with geographic location. This condition is more common in Europe and the southeastern United States. The cause is unknown. An association with fine, high-roughage forage and coastal Bermuda hay has been implicated. Ingesta accumulate in the ileum, causing obstruction. Spasmodic contraction and absorption of water from the ileal lumen exacerbates the impaction. Mesenteric vascular thrombotic disease, tapeworm infestation *(A. perfoliata),* and ascarid impaction *(P. equorum)* are less common causes. Ileal hypertrophy should be considered in older horses with a history of chronic colic.

Diagnosis

Clinical signs are variable and depend on the duration of the impaction:

- Moderate to severe abdominal pain due to focal intestinal distention and spasmodic contraction around the impaction. Affected horses usually have a transient response to analgesics.
- Rectal palpation reveals multiple loops of moderately to severely distended small intestine (see Fig 35–2). Early examination may reveal 5- to 8-cm-diameter, firm, smooth-surfaced ileum originating at the cecal base and coursing from the right of the midline obliquely downward and to the left side.
- Nasogastric reflux may be absent in the early stages. During the 8-10 hours after the initial episode of colic, small-intestinal and gastric distention develops and results in recurrence of signs of pain and progressive dehydration.
- Gastric decompression often provides temporary pain relief. Borborygmi diminish or disappear, and intestinal distention without motility is seen at ultrasound examination.
- CBC, electrolytes, blood gases, and findings at abdominocentesis frequently are within normal limits.
- Hemoconcentration and increased total peritoneal protein level and nucleated cell count may occur with long-standing impaction.

Treatment

INITIAL THERAPY IS SUPPORTIVE

- Gastric decompression
- Balanced polyionic intravenous fluids (e.g., lactated Ringer's solution)
- Analgesics (e.g., xylazine with or without butorphanol tartrate or flunixin meglumine)
- Monitoring of physiologic and clinical parameters (pain, nasogastric reflux, heart rate, mucous membranes, PCV/TPP, borborygmi)
- The impaction may resolve with medical therapy; more commonly surgical intervention is needed.

EXPLORATORY SURGERY

- Ventral midline exploratory celiotomy
- Reduction of the obstruction by extraluminal massage
- Mixing of the impaction with jejunal fluid or infusion of the impaction with sterile saline solution or sodium carboxymethylcellulose with or without 2% lidocaine to facilitate reduction

- With marked mural edema and congestion, jejunal enterotomy facilitates emptying of the ileal contents without excessive manipulation of the bowel.
- Resection and anastomosis (ileocecostomy or jejunocecostomy) may be needed if additional problems exist, e.g., ileal hypertrophy or mesenteric vascular thrombotic disease.

Prognosis
- Good if no further problems exist (e.g., ileal hypertrophy), and guarded if ileocecostomy or jejunocecostomy is needed because of postoperative ileus and the high incidence of intraabdominal adhesions.

ASCARID IMPACTION

Heavy ascarid *(P. equorum)* infestation can lead to intraluminal obstruction in foals, weanlings, and yearlings. Affected horses have a history of a poor parasite control program leading to heavy infestation with ascarids. *Impaction commonly follows use of one of the highly effective anthelmintics, piperazine, pyrantel, or organophosphates,* tranquilizers, or general anesthetics. Ivermectin, although highly effective, has a relatively slow onset of action and therefore is not commonly implicated in the development of ascarid impaction. Intestinal rupture, peritonitis, and intussusception are possible sequelae. Foals develop an immunity to the parasite by 6 months to 1 year of age. Consequently, this condition is uncommon in adults.

Diagnosis

Clinical signs depend on the duration and degree of small-intestinal obstruction and include unthriftiness, poor hair coat, and mild to severe abdominal pain. Nasogastric reflux usually is present and may contain ascarids. Rectal examination reveals multiple loops of distended small intestine. The diagnosis is based on signalment, history, and the presence of signs of small-intestinal obstruction.

Treatment
PARTIAL OBSTRUCTION OF THE INTESTINE WITH ASCARIDS
- Intestinal lubricants (e.g., mineral oil)
- Balanced polyionic intravenous fluids (e.g., lactated Ringer's solution)
- Analgesics (e.g., xylazine with or without butorphanol tartrate or flunixin meglumine)
- Low-efficacy or slow-onset anthelmintics (fenbendazole, ivermectin) are preferred to prevent future recurrence.

VENTRAL MIDLINE EXPLORATORY SURGERY TO RELIEVE THE OBSTRUCTION
- With complete obstruction, or if medical therapy is unsuccessful
- Multiple enterotomies may be needed to remove the ascarids

Prognosis
- Good if medical treatment is successful. Guarded if surgery and multiple enterotomies are performed because of the high occurrence of intraabdominal adhesions.

DUODENITIS AND PROXIMAL JEJUNITIS

Duodenitis and proximal jejunitis are characterized by transmural inflammation, edema, and hemorrhage in the duodenum and proximal jejunum. The stomach and proximal small intestine are moderately distended with fluid, whereas the distal jejunum and ileum usually are flaccid. Histologic lesions include hyperemia and edema of the mucosa and submucosa, villous epithelial degeneration and sloughing, neutrophil infiltration, hemorrhage in the muscular layer, and fibrinopurulent exudation on the serosa. The cause of this extensive intestinal damage is unknown. *C. perfringens* is a presumed etiologic agent and frequently can be cultured from the gastric reflux.

Proximal small-intestinal distention, gastric reflux, dehydration, and hypovolemic and endotoxic shock result from the intestinal damage. The inflammation and damage can alter intestinal motility, causing adynamic ileus.

Diagnosis

CLINICAL SIGNS
- Acute abdominal pain
- *Large volumes of nasogastric reflux fluid* (red to greenish-brown)
- Absent borborygmi
- Tachycardia
- Dehydration
- Slight increase in body temperature (38.6°C-39.1°C [101.5°F-102.4°F])
- Hyperemic mucous membranes
- Increased hematocrit
- Moderate to severe small-intestinal distention on rectal examination. However, early in the disease, small-intestinal distention may be absent.
- Distended proximal small intestine with thickened wall and mild to moderate motility at ultrasound examination

CLINICAL LABORATORY FINDINGS
- Increased PCV and TPP (hemoconcentration)
- Increased creatinine concentration indicating prerenal or renal azotemia
- Increased peritoneal total protein concentration
- Mild to moderate increase in nucleated cell count (5000 to 25,000 cells/ml)
- Hypokalemia
- Sometimes metabolic acidosis
- CBC may reveal a normal, increased (neutrophilia due to inflammation), or decreased (neutropenia and left shift due to endotoxemia and consumption) WBC count
- Gram stain of the gastric reflux fluid shows a large number of large gram-positive rods (Fig. 35–5)

The clinical findings can be confused with those of strangulating or nonstrangulating obstruction. *After nasogastric decompression, abdominal pain usually subsides and is replaced by depression in patients with duodenitis and proximal jejunitis.* The presence of abdominal pain with serosanguineous abdominal fluid supports the diagnosis of strangulating obstruction, but serosanguineous abdominal fluid can be present with proximal enteritis.

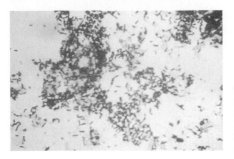

FIGURE 35-5. Gram stain of gastric fluid from a horse with proximal duodenitis-jejunitis that demonstrates many large gram-positive rods (compatible with *Clostridium perfringens*).

Treatment

- Voluminous gastrointestinal reflux is produced for 1-7 days, requiring gastric decompression through an indwelling nasogastric tube every 2 hours to prevent distention, pain, and gastric rupture.
- Food and oral medication are withheld until small-intestinal borborygmi return.
- Intravenous administration of a balanced crystalloid solution to maintain intravascular fluid volume.
- Monitoring of blood gases and serum electrolytes (Na^+, K^+, Cl^-, HCO_3^-, Ca^{2+}) daily and adjustment of the intravenous solution to correct any deficiencies.
- Low-dose flunixin meglumine, 0.25 mg/kg IV q8h, to reduce the adverse effects of arachidonic acid metabolites (thromboxane A_2 and prostaglandins).
- Antiserum (Endoserum) directed against gram-negative core antigens (endotoxin) administered intravenously diluted in a balanced electrolyte solution. Hyperimmune plasma directed against the J-5 mutant strain of *E. coli* (Polymune-J or Foalimmune) or normal *equine plasma* (2-10 L) administered intravenously *slowly* may be equally beneficial, supplying protein, fibronectin, complement, antithrombin III, and other inhibitors of hypercoagulability.
- Heparin 100 U/kg SQ q12h may decrease the incidence of laminitis.
- 10% DMSO solution can be administered intravenously (100 mg/kg q8h or q12h).
- Na^+ or K^+ penicillin (22,000-44,000 IU/kg IV q6h) or procaine penicillin (22,000-44,000 IU/kg IM q12h) for *C. perfringens*, as the suggested etiologic pathogen.
- Motility modifiers can be useful in reducing gastric reflux and may decrease the cost of treatment and complications associated with frequent passage of the nasogastric tube.
- Recommendations: 2% lidocaine, slow intravenous bolus, 1.3 mg/kg (approximately 20 ml/450-kg adult) followed by 0.05 mg/kg per minute infusion, or cisapride, 0.1-0.2 mg/kg IV q8h, 0.3 mg/kg PO q8h.
- Monitor serum creatinine concentration and urine output after fluid therapy because secondary renal failure is common.
- Laminitis is a common complication. The feet should be monitored and treatment incorporated in the medical therapy, including:
  □ Heavily bed the stall with shavings or sand
  □ Removing shoes, trim and balance feet, apply styrofoam support to the feet
  □ Apply lower limb support bandages

- □ Phenylbutazone (2.2-4.4 mg/kg PO or IV q12h)
- □ Acepromazine (0.02 mg/kg IM q8h) for its vasodilatory properties
- □ Nitroglycerin cream, 1-inch (2.5-cm) strip q24h over palmar (posterior) digital arteries
- With prolonged (>7 days) nasogastric reflux, bowel decompression or intestinal bypass through a standing right flank laparotomy or ventral midline celiotomy can be used to augment medical therapy.
- Some surgeons, particularly in the U.K., believe immediate exploratory laparotomy and decompression results in a more rapid recovery.

Prognosis

- With aggressive medical management, the disease resolves in most cases. Sequelae that adversely affect the prognosis include laminitis, renal failure, intraabdominal adhesion formation, pharyngeal or esophageal injury, and gastric rupture. Patients with red gastric reflux fluid appear to be more prone to complications than are horses without such reflux.

NONSTRANGULATING INFARCTION

Nonstrangulating infarction is an inadequate blood supply (necrosis due to loss of blood supply) of the intestine without a strangulating lesion. Postmortem examination commonly reveals the cause to be thrombus formation at the cranial mesenteric artery from damage by migration of the fourth and fifth stages of *Strongylus vulgaris* larvae. It is hypothesized that infarction is the result of hypoxia induced by vasospasm.

Diagnosis

A poor parasite control program may predispose horses to nonstrangulating ischemia and infarction. The disease also occurs in horses regularly treated with anthelmintics. Clinical signs of variable severity range from depression to moderately severe abdominal pain:

- Heart rate, respiratory rate, and body temperature may be normal or increased, and hyperemic mucous membranes suggest endotoxemia or inflammation due to migrating parasites.
- Rectal examination findings may be normal or include distended small intestine.
- Pain, tremitus, or thickening is commonly evident on palpation of the mesenteric root.
- Auscultation of the abdomen may reveal normal, increased, or decreased borborygmi.
- Gastric reflux may be present owing to functional obstruction of the intestinal segment.
- PCV, TPP, and creatinine level may be increased because of dehydration.
- Peripheral blood examination may reveal a normal, decreased (neutropenia with a left shift due to endotoxemia), or increased (neutrophilia due to inflammation) WBC count.
- TPP may be increased owing to chronic inflammation caused by parasites or decreased as a result of protein loss through damaged intestinal mucosa.
- Abdominal fluid is normal or contains an increased amount of total protein (>3.0 mg/dl), and the WBC count is as high as 200,000/µl.

Treatment

- Balanced crystalloid intravenous fluids to correct dehydration and enhance reperfusion of the affected intestinal segments
- Maintenance of gastric decompression
- Broad-spectrum antimicrobial drugs (K^+ penicillin, 22,000 IU/kg IV q6h; gentamicin, 2.2 mg/kg IV q8h or 6.6 mg/kg IV q24h if peritonitis is present)
- Flunixin meglumine, 0.25 mg/kg IV q8h, to reduce thromboxane production and increase mesenteric perfusion
- 10% DMSO solution, 100 mg/kg IV q8-12h to decrease superoxide radical injury during reperfusion
- Aspirin (20 mg/kg PO every other day) and heparin (40-100 IU/kg IV or SQ q6-12h) to diminish and/or prevent thrombosis. Monitor the hematocrit closely for red blood cell (RBC) agglutination and declining hematocrit secondary to heparin administration
- Exploratory surgery for patients unresponsive to medical therapy

Prognosis

- Poor for patients that need surgery for intestinal resection. Ischemia not obvious at the time of exploratory surgery may progress to infarction. Ileus and adhesions are common postoperative complications. Large segments of affected intestine may be too extensive for resection. Identification and resection of diseased small or large intestinal segments sometimes is successful with fluorescein dye, Doppler ultrasonography, or surface oximetry to determine intestinal viability.

■ F. DISORDERS OF THE LARGE INTESTINE THAT CAUSE COLIC

P. O. Eric Mueller and James N. Moore

CECAL IMPACTION

Inflammatory bowel disease frequently predisposes the colon, especially the small colon, to impaction and may be associated with positive fecal cultures for *Salmonella* organisms. In many cases, a predisposing factor is never identified.

Cecal impaction occurs as the result of other diseases, especially those associated with endotoxemia, surgery, or chronic pain, owing to septic metritis, infectious arthritis, fractures, and corneal disease.

Diagnosis

CLINICAL FINDINGS

- Anorexia
- Reduced fecal output
- Mild to severe abdominal pain

NOTE: Occasionally there are few prodromal signs, such as only slight depression.

- Abdominal distention may be present but is often absent. With severe impaction, abdominal auscultation reveals a right-sided "cecal ping."

- Heart rate varies with the severity of pain, and mucous membranes usually are pink and tacky.
- Nasogastric reflux is unusual unless cecal dysfunction results in ileus of the small intestine.
- PCV, plasma protein, and creatinine levels are increased as a consequence of dehydration. In cases of cecal perforation, peritoneal total protein concentration and nucleated cell count are increased.
- *The diagnosis is confirmed at rectal examination; the ventral cecal taenia is tight and displaced ventrally and medially.* Dry ingesta are palpable in the body and base of the cecum, and moderate amounts of gas fill the base. The cecal distention can make the dorsal and medial cecal taeniae readily palpable and leave the left colon and small colon empty.

Treatment

MEDICAL MANAGEMENT OF MILD TO MODERATE CECAL IMPACTION

- Give nothing by mouth except water if there is no gastric reflux
- Administer three times the daily maintenance requirement of fluid (balanced crystalloid solutions with 20 mEq/L KCl) intravenously and water orally to rehydrate the impaction: 6-8 L of water/500 kg q2h through an indwelling nasogastric tube.
- Administer laxatives to facilitate rehydration of impacted material (see Laxatives, p. 197)
- Reintroduce feed slowly to avoid recurrence
- Feed grass, water-soaked pellets, and bran mashes for the first 24-48 hours

CONDITIONS NEEDING SURGICAL MANAGEMENT

- Uncontrollable pain
- Severe impaction (extremely tight medial cecal band)
- Unsuccessful medical therapy
- Characteristics of peritoneal fluid suggesting cecal compromise
- The surgical options through ventral midline celiotomy include
  - Extraluminal massage
  - Typhlotomy and evacuation
  - Partial or complete typhlectomy
  - Cecocolic anastomosis
  - Ileocolic anastomosis
  - Jejunocolic anastomosis
- Jejunocolic or ileocolic anastomosis is considered superior to cecocolic anastomosis because it has fewer long-term sequelae. Complete typhlectomy through a right paralumbar laparotomy is difficult, and fecal contamination of the abdomen is a complication

Prognosis

- Good for patients with mild to moderate cecal impaction without underlying cecal dysfunction. Severe cecal impaction necessitating surgical treatment is complicated by peritonitis, adhesions, perforation, and death. The prognosis for severe impaction is guarded.

CECAL PERFORATION

The site is generally the medial or caudal surface of the base owing to excessive tension on the cecal wall as a result of severe impaction. Perforation also is associated with late gestation and parturition. The pathogenesis remains unknown; tapeworm *(A. perfoliata)* infestation is implicated.

Diagnosis

Signs of cardiovascular shock secondary to septic peritonitis. The rate of deterioration is directly related to the degree of peritoneal contamination. Rectal examination reveals enlargement of the cecum with emphysema and roughening of the serosa of the cecal base. The peritoneal fluid, obtained with a teat cannula, has an increased or a decreased nucleated cell count and increased total protein concentration; degenerative WBCs and intracellular and extracellular bacteria and plant material are present.

Treatment: Symptomatic Only

- Balanced, polyionic, intravenous fluids
- Broad-spectrum antimicrobial agents
- Flunixin meglumine

Prognosis

- Poor. Grave if fecal contamination occurs, owing to septic peritonitis and endotoxic shock.

LARGE-COLON IMPACTION

Large-colon impaction occurs at two sites of narrowing, the pelvic flexure and the transverse colon. At these locations, retropulsive contractions (propagation in an oral direction) retain ingesta for microbial digestion. These contractile patterns can contribute to impaction.

Predisposing Factors

- Poor dentition
- Ingestion of coarse roughage
- Inadequate fluid intake
- Stress associated with transportation
- Intense exercise resulting in hypomotility
- Inadequate water intake
- Excessive fluid loss through sweating

Diagnosis

CLINICAL FINDINGS

- Anorexia
- Abdominal distention
- Decreased fecal output
- Mild, initially intermittent, to severe abdominal pain
- Heart rate varying with the degree of pain; pink and tacky mucous membranes
- Nasogastric reflux uncommon unless ileus of the small intestine or compression of loops of small intestine occurs
- PCV, TPP, and creatinine concentration increased when clinical dehydration is present
- With complete luminal obstruction, marked abdominal distention

- Rectal examination reveals impacted ingesta with varying degrees of distention of the pelvic flexure and ventral colon; in severe cases, the colon is palpable in the pelvic canal
- Impaction in the transverse colon is not palpable

In chronic, severe cases, distention of the colonic wall can cause pressure necrosis of the bowel wall and peritonitis. The peritoneal fluid TPP level and nucleated cell count reflect intestinal compromise. Abdominal pain usually is severe and unrelenting, and signs of toxemia (hyperemia, cyanotic mucous membranes, or both), tachycardia, and tachypnea are apparent.

Treatment
- Withhold food to prevent continued accumulation of ingesta.
- Allow access to water if there is no nasogastric reflux.
- Provide medical management:
  - Patients with mild impaction respond to administration of water and mineral oil or magnesium sulfate (preferred) and electrolytes through a nasogastric tube.
  - Intravenous fluids (4-5 L/h per 450 kg) and laxative therapy are needed for moderate to severe colon impaction.
  - Analgesics as needed.
- Surgical decision based on
  - Unsuccessful medical management
  - Unrelenting abdominal pain
  - Rectal examination that reveals large colon displacement
  - Endotoxemia, cardiovascular deterioration
  - Changes in peritoneal fluid indicating intestinal compromise
- Ventral midline exploratory celiotomy:
  - Extent of impaction
  - Other abnormalities: colon displacement, enterolith
  - Pelvic flexure enterotomy
  - Lavage of lumen of colon to evacuate ingesta

Prognosis
- Good for medical management of mild to moderately severe large-colon impaction. Fair to good for surgical correction of severe impaction, unless necrosis of the intestinal wall or colonic devitalization results in intestinal perforation.

SAND IMPACTION
Ingestion of sand while grazing or eating hay on closely grazed pastures in areas with sandy soil may result in sand impaction. The ingested sand settles in the large colon, where it accumulates and eventually results in a nonstrangulating obstruction.

Diagnosis
CLINICAL SIGNS
- Similar to those of large-colon impaction; the signs of pain are frequently acute.

- Auscultation of the cranial ventral abdomen, when performed for 4-5 minutes, may reveal a sound similar to an ocean wave.
- Sand may be palpated at rectal examination and found in feces placed in water; the ingesta float in water, and the sand settles to the bottom of the container.
- The impaction is commonly palpable at rectal examination in the pelvic flexure or cecum, whereas impaction in the right dorsal (most common) or transverse colon is not palpable.
- Abdominocentesis, if performed, should be done with *extreme caution* to avoid enterocentesis due to the location of the sand-filled colon on the ventral abdominal floor.
- The irritating effect of the sand on the colonic mucosa can cause diarrhea.
- Under the weight of the sand, degeneration and necrosis of the bowel wall can result in endotoxemia and peritonitis.

Treatment

MEDICAL MANAGEMENT
- Frequently responds to early administration of fluids and laxatives (mineral oil) Psyllium hydrophilic mucilloid (Metamucil) is the most effective laxative: 400 g/500 kg q6h until the impaction resolves. Once in contact with cold water, the mucilloid forms a gel that can be difficult to pump through a nasogastric tube; therefore, the tube must be in place and the mixture administered immediately. The gel lubricates and binds with the sand, moving it distally and relieving the obstruction.
- Continue psyllium treatment at 400 g/500 kg once a day for 7 days to remove residual sand. Alternating psyllium and mineral oil may prevent obstruction associated with retrograde movement of sand and psyllium.

SURGICAL MANAGEMENT
- Ventral midline exploratory celiotomy for patients that do not respond to medical treatment or have other abnormalities, such as colonic displacement.
- Remove sand through a pelvic flexure enterotomy.
- Sand can cause extensive damage to the colonic wall, such as postoperative ileus, bowel wall degeneration, and peritonitis.

PREVENTIVE MANAGEMENT
- Do not overgraze pastures.
- Provide a hay supplement when needed, and do not place feed on the ground.
- Add prophylactic psyllium treatment to feed to remove sand from the colon.
- Consider administering psyllium, 400 g/500 kg once a day for 7 days, for preventive treatment every 4-12 months, depending on sand exposure.
- Consider using flavored or soluble psyllium, which may be more palatable than unflavored forms.

Prognosis
- Good for mild to moderately severe sand impaction. The surgical prognosis for severe sand impaction is good unless necrosis or devitalization of the intestinal wall results in rupture of the colon.

CECOCOLIC INTUSSUSCEPTION

Cecocolic intussusception is an unusual cause of intestinal obstruction that results from invagination of the apex of the cecum through the cecocolic orifice into the right ventral colon. The entire cecum can invaginate into the colon and become strangulated. The cause is unknown, although conditions causing aberrant intestinal motility, such as parasite infestation, diet changes, impaction, mural lesions, and the presence of motility-altering drugs, have been implicated. Cecocolic intussusception is more common among horses younger than 3 years.

Diagnosis

Patients with strangulating intussusception may present with signs of acute, severe abdominal pain. In contrast, affected horses with chronic nonstrangulating intussusception may have mild to moderate abdominal pain, depression, weight loss, and scant, soft feces. The intussusception is frequently palpable per rectum as a large mass in the right caudal abdomen; if the ileum is involved, distended small intestine is palpable. The presence of a firm mass palpable in the cecal base or the right ventral colon is confirmatory. Abdominocentesis reveals increases in peritoneal total protein and nucleated cell count. These changes may not be evident until late in the disease because the cecum is sequestered within the ventral colon. Failure to respond to medical therapy leads to exploratory surgery and a definitive diagnosis.

Treatment

- Ventral midline exploratory celiotomy.
- Reducing the intussusception is difficult because of mural edema and adhesions between the serosal surfaces.
- If extraluminal reduction is successful, cecal viability is assessed, and if required, complete or partial typhlectomy performed.
- Reduction and resection of the devitalized portion of cecum can be performed through an enterotomy in the right ventral colon if extraluminal reduction is impossible.

Prognosis

- Fair if the apex of the cecum is involved and extraluminal reduction is possible; poor if reduction requires enterotomy or the entire cecum is involved, because of the risk of septic peritonitis.

LARGE-COLON DISPLACEMENT

The left ventral and dorsal colons are freely movable, allowing for intestinal displacement and volvulus. The cause is unknown, alterations in colonic motility, excessive gas production, rolling secondary to abdominal pain, dietary changes, excessive concentrate intake, grazing lush pastures, and parasite infestation have been implicated. Generally, no etiologic factor is identified.

Right dorsal displacement of the colon is displacement of the left colon lateral to the cecum between the cecum and the right body wall (see Fig 35–3). The pelvic flexure commonly moves lateral to the cecum, in a cranial to caudal direction, and rests at the sternum. Displacement may be accompanied by a variable degree of volvulus.

Left dorsal displacement of the colon is a displacement of the left colon to a position between the dorsal body wall and the nephrosplenic (renosplenic) ligament. It is unknown whether the colon passes through the nephrosplenic space from a cranial to caudal direction or migrates dorsally, lateral to the spleen.

GI

Diagnosis

CLINICAL SIGNS

- Abdominal pain and abdominal distention, the severity of which depends on the duration and amount of colonic tympany. The signs generally develop rapidly and are more severe than with impaction because of tension on the mesentery and greater colonic tympany.
- The displacement may place pressure on the duodenum and cause nasogastric reflux.
- Peritoneal fluid usually is normal in the early stages of displacement; increases in peritoneal total protein and nucleated cell count occur with chronic displacement.
- *Right dorsal displacement* is characterized at rectal palpation by mild to severe gas distention of the cecum, colon, or both with large-colon taeniae palpable lateral to the cecum or horizontally crossing the pelvic inlet (see Fig 35–3). In some cases, GGT and direct bilirubin may be markedly increased due to biliary obstruction. It is unusual for other GI displacements to cause these changes. Additionally, ultrasound examination of the mid to lower right abdomen may reveal distended vessels within the displaced right colon.
- *Left dorsal displacement* is characterized at rectal palpation by mild to severe gas distention of the cecum, colon, or both with palpable large-colon taeniae coursing cranially and to the left, dorsal to the nephrosplenic ligament. Signs of pain are elicited when the nephrosplenic area is palpated and the spleen is rotated caudally, away from the left body wall owing to tension on the ligament. Several loops of moderately distended small intestine may be palpable if the small intestine is secondarily involved. Decompression of the stomach and cecum provides temporary pain relief.

Treatment

RIGHT DORSAL DISPLACEMENT

- Ventral midline exploratory celiotomy
- Examination of the colon for volvulus and correction of the displacement
- Enterotomy is unnecessary unless the colon is secondarily impacted

LEFT DORSAL DISPLACEMENT: NONSURGICAL CORRECTION (Fig. 35–6)

- General anesthesia with the patient positioned in right lateral recumbency. Hobbles are placed on the hindlimbs, and the patient is positioned in dorsal recumbency.
- The hindlimbs are lifted to raise the hind end of the patient off the ground; the abdomen is vigorously balloted.
- The large colon falls cranially and to the right.
- The patient is then rolled 360 degrees back to right lateral recumbency and allowed to recover.
- Rectal palpation is performed to assess the position of the colon with the patient in lateral recumbency or after recovery.
- If unsuccessful, the procedure may be repeated several times; it is reported to be 70%-90% successful in patients with a stable cardiovascular system and without severe colonic distention or devitalization.
- An additional nonsurgical method is to administer phenylephrine 8-16 mg/450 kg in 1 L of 0.9% sodium chloride slowly IV over 15 minutes to contract the spleen, to provide light exercise for 5-10 minutes, and to perform a rectal examination. This is the preferred initial treatment in most cases!

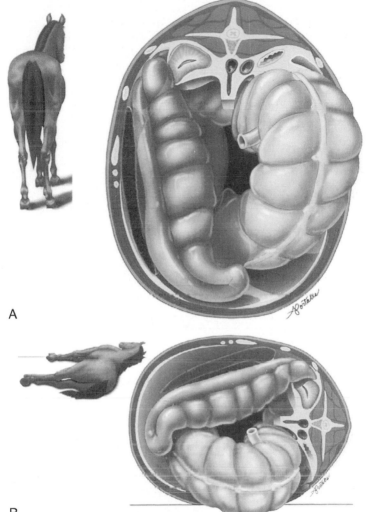

FIGURE 35-6. Nonsurgical correction of a left dorsal displacement of the large colon. **A,** Caudal view of the standing horse with the left ventral and dorsal colons entrapped over the nephrosplenic ligament. **B,** The patient is anesthetized and placed in right lateral recumbency.

NOTE: Do not use the phenylephrine method to treat severely volume-depleted patients or those with cardiovascular instability.

POTENTIAL COMPLICATIONS OF NONSURGICAL CORRECTION (ROLLING)

- Worsening or recurrence of displacement
- Iatrogenic colonic or cecal volvulus
- Cecal or colonic rupture

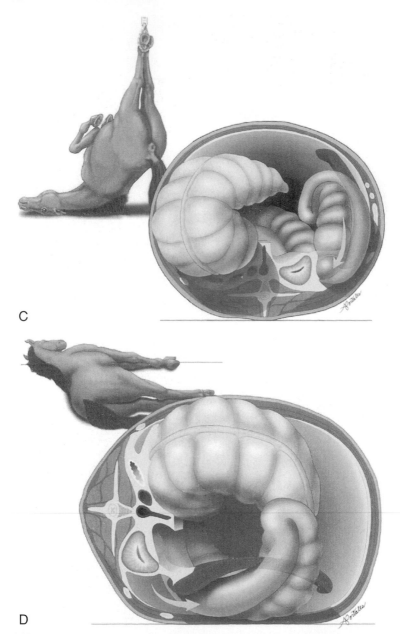

C

D

FIGURE 35–6. *(Continued)* **C,** Hobbles are placed on the hind limbs, and the patient is positioned in dorsal recumbency. The hind limbs are lifted to raise the hind end off the ground. The large colon falls cranially, laterally, and to the right *(arrow)*. **D,** The patient is then positioned in left lateral recumbency. This allows the colon to continue to fall ventrally and laterally to the spleen *(arrow)*.

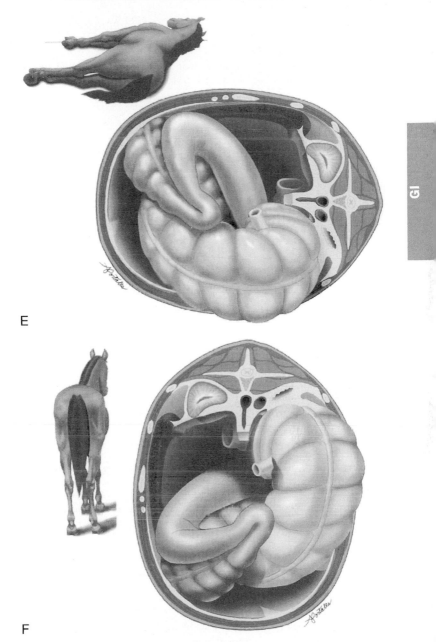

E

F

FIGURE 35-6. *(Continued)* **E,** The 360-degree rotation is completed by rolling the individual into sternal recumbency (*not shown*) and then back to right lateral recumbency. The colon comes to rest in a position medial to the spleen. **F,** The patient is allowed to recover. If the procedure is successful, the colon assumes a position ventral and medial to the spleen. Rectal palpation is performed to assess the position of the colon.

GI

LEFT DORSAL DISPLACEMENT

Surgical correction is performed when

- Colonic distention is severe
- Evidence of intestinal devitalization is found during peritoneal fluid analysis
- Increased risk is present for colonic or cecal rupture and resulting fatal peritonitis

Prognosis

- Good to excellent for complete recovery. The incidence of adhesions and laminitis with large-colon displacement is low.

LARGE-COLON VOLVULUS

Large-colon volvulus is rotation of the ventral and dorsal colons on their long axes and frequently includes the cecum. With the horse in dorsal recumbency, the colon usually is seen to twist in a counterclockwise direction (Fig 35–7). The large colon and cecum can rotate on the vertical axis of the mesentery (volvulus). Rotation of 360 degrees causes the colon to lie in an apparently normal position with the mesenteric root occluded. Large-colon volvulus is one of the *most severe* acute abdominal emergencies among horses; it can be fatal. The cause is unknown, but hypomotility due to dietary changes, electrolyte imbalances, and stress can predispose the colon to excessive gas accumulation and volvulus. There is a *higher incidence of colonic volvulus* among *periparturient mares.* Large-colon volvulus recurs in 20%-30% of cases of colic.

Diagnosis

- Colonic volvulus (>180 degrees) causes an acute onset of *severe* abdominal distention and continuous abdominal pain only mildly responsive to or refractory to analgesic therapy. Xylazine or detomidine alone or in combination with butorphanol provides transient pain relief.
- Tachycardia, tachypnea, and blanched or congested mucous membranes usually are present.
- Respiratory acidosis can develop if colonic distention impairs normal respiratory function.
- Serosanguineous peritoneal fluid with an increased total protein concentration and nucleated cell count reflect the presence of intestinal ischemia and necrosis.
- Rectal palpation reveals severe colonic distention, frequently accompanied by mural and mesenteric edema due to venous congestion. Taeniae traversing the abdomen may be palpable, *but a complete rectal examination is frequently impossible because of the marked colonic distention.*
- Rotations (twists) >180 degrees may manifest as moderate pain only and slow deterioration.

Treatment

- Successful treatment requires *early diagnosis* and *emergency surgical correction.*
- Ventral midline exploratory celiotomy.
- Decompression and enterotomy often are necessary to facilitate correction.
- Affected bowel typically appears bluish-gray initially and becomes red to black after reperfusion.
- Nonviable colon requires resection or humane destruction of the horse.

GI

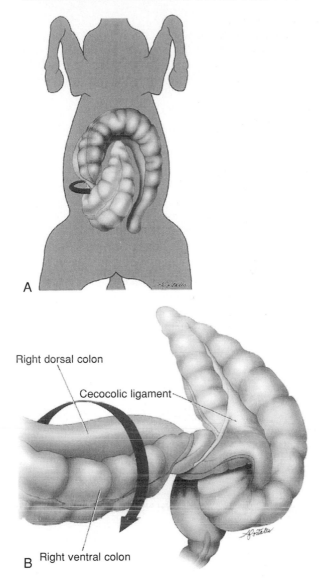

FIGURE 35-7. Large-colon volvulus. **A,** Ventral view of a horse in dorsal recumbency with 360-degree counterclockwise *(arrow)* volvulus of the large colon. **B,** Right lateral view of a patient in dorsal recumbency with 180-degree counterclockwise *(arrow)* volvulus of the large colon.

- 95% of the ascending colon may be resected without adversely affecting colonic function.
- Plasma, DMSO, and heparin may be useful in attenuating "reperfusion injury."

Prevention of Recurrence

Colopexy, or suturing the lateral taenia of the left colon to the abdominal wall, is performed by some surgeons to reduce the risk of recurrence. Tearing of the adhesion, suture failure, and colonic rupture are reported complications. Elective colonic resection is performed to minimize the likelihood of recurrence; this procedure is preferred for performance athletes.

Prognosis

- Depends on early diagnosis and surgical intervention. Intestinal ischemia and necrosis rapidly progress to hypovolemia, endotoxemia, peritonitis, and irreversible shock. Therefore the prognosis is poor unless surgery is performed within a few hours of the onset of clinical signs. In some patients, postoperative absorptive dysfunction, diarrhea, and protein-losing enteropathy occur and may be short-lived or permanent.

ATRESIA COLI

Atresia coli is congenital absence or closure of a portion of the intestine. It manifests in three forms:

- Membrane atresia: a tissue diaphragm occludes the bowel lumen
- Cord atresia: a fibrous cord connects the noncommunicating ends of the bowel
- Blind-end atresia: the *most common type*, in which there is no connection or mesentery between the noncommunicating ends of bowel

Atresia coli results from ischemia of the affected segment during development; the condition is believed to be hereditary. *Lethal white foal disease* is an autosomal recessive pigmentary disorder in which *newborn paint foals* have albinism coupled with congenital defects of the intestinal tract, most commonly atresia coli. These defects are not compatible with life.

Diagnosis

Abdominal pain in the newborn during the first 12-24 hours of life and lack of meconium stool are the first signs. Digital palpation of the rectum reveals mucus and no meconium. Abdominal radiography may reveal an enlarged segment of colon with no obvious obstruction; contrast radiography is needed to confirm the diagnosis. Abdominal distention and pain are indications for surgical exploration. Meconium impaction is the primary condition to rule out (see Disorders of the Small Colon and Rectum).

Treatment

- Surgical correction is the only treatment.
- Ventral midline exploratory celiotomy.
- The distance and size disparity between the affected bowel segments make anastomosis difficult.
- The aboral segment often is too small for end-to-end anastomosis. Side-to-side anastomosis may be needed but often is not possible because of the excessive distance between the proximal and distal intestinal segments; therefore euthanasia is necessary.

Prognosis

- Guarded owing to the difficult technical aspects of performing the anastomosis in this part of the intestine.

NONSTRANGULATING INFARCTION
See Disorders of the Small Intestine (p. 212).

ULCERATIVE COLITIS (NSAID TOXICITY)
See Chapter 53.

▓ G. DISORDERS OF THE SMALL COLON AND RECTUM
P. O. Eric Mueller and James N. Moore

SMALL-COLON IMPACTION AND FOREIGN BODY OBSTRUCTION
Dehydration of fecal matter can cause impaction of the small colon and a foreign body or an enterolith (see Enterolithiasis) can cause an obstruction. Complete obstruction causes severe abdominal pain. Tympany and secondary ileus of the proximal small and large colons are secondary to the obstruction. The diagnosis is confirmed at rectal examination with palpation of the impaction or gas-distended loops of small colon. The small colon is identified on rectal examination by its characteristic single, wide band on the anti-mesenteric surface.

Foreign-body impaction occurs more commonly among horses younger than 4 years, because they are curious. For example, they eat portions of hay nets, rubber fencing, bits of rope, and string. *Small colon impaction is common among miniature horses.* Impaction is frequently accompanied by inflammatory bowel disease, such as salmonellosis.

Treatment
MEDICAL TREATMENT
- Analgesics
- Large volumes of balanced, polyionic intravenous fluid
- 6-8 L of water q2h through an indwelling nasogastric tube if no gastric reflux is recovered
- Warm water enemas to soften the fecal material

| **CAUTION:** Use extreme care to prevent rectal perforation during administration of enemas.

SURGICAL TREATMENT
- Needed with unrelenting pain, severe gas distention, or failure of medical treatment
- Ventral midline exploratory celiotomy
- Enemas and extraluminal massage of the small colon to break down the impaction
- Enterotomy to remove a foreign body or enterolith
- Pelvic flexure enterotomy and evacuation of large-colon ingesta
- Patients with small-colon impaction frequently have culture results positive for *Salmonella* organisms. The condition of these horses can become toxic with secondary laminitis, peritonitis, and adhesions. The role of *Salmonella* infection in the development of the impaction is unknown

Prognosis

- Fair to good for patients with foreign body obstruction or simple impaction of the small colon. Guarded if the culture result for *Salmonella* organisms is positive. *Rectal examination of horses with small-colon impaction presents great risk of perforation.*

ENTEROLITHIASIS

Enteroliths are concretions of magnesium and ammonium phosphate crystals deposited around a nidus, frequently a piece of wire, stone, or nail. There may be one or multiple concretions, and they do not cause a clinical problem until they become lodged in the transverse or small colon. The *specific geographic distribution* of the condition (California, Florida, Indiana) has led to speculation that undetermined constituents of the soil and water in these areas may be inciting causes. Enterolithiasis is most commonly seen in middle-aged horses (5-10 years of age), and the condition is overrepresented in Arabians and miniature horses.

Diagnosis

- Affected horses may have a history of *chronic weight loss* and recurring acute bouts of mild to moderate abdominal pain *or* acute, severe abdominal distention and pain with no history of colic.
- The obstruction most commonly is at the proximal small colon or transverse colon. Smaller enteroliths are located distally in the small colon. When the obstruction is complete, pain is severe and distention of the colon is marked.
- Heart and respiratory rates are increased, and mucous membranes are pink.
- Rectal examination reveals colonic and cecal distention.
- Peritoneal fluid is generally normal unless the wall of the colon is compromised.
- *Abdominal radiography* may confirm the diagnosis of enterolithiasis, but in the field, imaging can be performed only on miniature horses.
- Patients with chronic enterolithiasis often have gastric ulcers, which can confound the diagnosis.

Treatment

- Central midline exploratory celiotomy.
- Decompression of the distended colon and cecum.
- Removal of small, freely movable enteroliths through a pelvic flexure enterotomy.
- Removal of large enteroliths in the transverse colon and proximal small colon through a large-colon enterotomy at the diaphragmatic flexure.
- If an enterolith has a *polyhedral* shape, multiple enteroliths are present.

Prognosis

- Good; the survival rate is 65%-90%.

MECONIUM IMPACTION

A common cause of acute pain in newborn foals is retention of meconium in the small colon and rectum. It occurs more frequently in males, weak newborns after a dystocia, and foals born at more than 340 days of gestation.

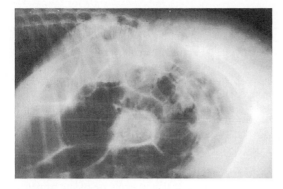

FIGURE 35-8. Radiograph demonstrates the abdomen of a 2-day-old foal with meconium impaction of the colon causing severe gaseous distention. Surgery was needed to correct the problem.

GI

Clinical Signs
- Acute abdominal pain during the first 24 hours after foaling
- Tachycardia
- Repeated attempts to defecate
- Rolling
- Abnormal stance
- Swishing the tail
- Abdominal tympany if obstruction of the small colon is complete (Fig. 35–8)
- The foal appears transiently normal for short periods and nurses. The diagnosis often is confirmed with digital palpation of meconium impaction in the distal small colon and rectum

Treatment
- Enemas with warm, soapy water delivered by means of gravity flow through a soft rubber tube
- Acetylcysteine enema (see p. 570)
- Intravenous, balanced polyionic fluids
- Mineral oil
- Sedatives as needed
- Ventral midline exploratory celiotomy for refractory patients and for those with proximal impaction (see Fig. 35–8), accompanied by enemas and extraluminal massage of the affected colon
- Small-colon enterotomy rarely is necessary.

NOTE: Repeated enemas or enemas with caustic solutions result in rectal edema and irritation and a syndrome that mimics meconium impaction. The condition of foals receiving several enemas often becomes very toxic.

Prognosis
- Excellent.

MESOCOLIC RUPTURE
Mesocolic rupture affects mares during parturition and results in tearing of the mesentery of the small colon. The condition is complicated by prolapse of the rectum, bladder, uterus, vagina, small intestine, or a combination of these organs. Multiparous mares older than 11 years are at greatest risk.

Clinical signs of abdominal pain develop during the first 24 hours postpartum and are complicated by intraabdominal hemorrhage and peritonitis. The mare's clinical condition deteriorates rapidly if the blood supply to the small colon is compromised or the intestine is entrapped in the mesocolic rent. Rectal examination reveals impaction or tympany of the small colon.

Treatment
- Ventral midline exploratory celiotomy
- Resection and anastomosis of the affected small colon
- Colostomy if the tear involves the mesorectum

Prognosis
- Poor because of ischemia of the small colon, difficult surgical exposure, and complications associated with the colostomy, such as prolapse of the proximal small colon through the colostomy stoma and adhesions.

RECTAL TEAR

A complication of performing a rectal examination is the risk of rectal tear. The incidence is highest among young, nervous, anxious patients; older horses with a weakened rectal wall, such as those with small-colon impactions; and patients that strain during rectal examination. The incidence is higher among Arabians than it is among other breeds, presumably because of the size of Arabians. Stallions and geldings are at greater risk than are mares. The tears occur at the 10-12 o'clock position 25-30 cm from the anus. The tear is longitudinal and hypothesized to occur where blood vessels penetrate the intestinal wall. Rectal tears are classified as follows:

- Grade I: Mucosa or submucosa
- Grade II: Muscular layer only
- Grade III: Mucosa, submucosa, and muscular layers without serosal penetration, including mesorectum
- Grade IV: Tears involving all layers and extending into the peritoneal cavity

NOTE: Grades III and IV are life-threatening with cellulitis, abscessation, and acute septic peritonitis as sequelae. The diagnosis is confirmed with careful examination of the tear after the patient is sedated and the rectum evacuated. Intraluminal lidocaine gel or epidural anesthesia facilitates rectal examination.

Treatment
- Immediately begin administration of broad-spectrum antimicrobial agents.
- Provide intravenous, balanced polyionic fluids.
- Administer NSAIDs.

GRADE I TEARS
- Managed conservatively unless the tear can be easily sutured with 2-0 or 0 poly-dioxanone (PDS, Ethicon) in a simple continuous pattern. These tears heal with minimal or no complications.

GRADE II TEARS
- Because of the lack of frank blood in the lumen of the rectum, grade II tears frequently are not diagnosed at the time of injury. They are identified weeks later when a perirectal fistula or abscess develops.

GRADE III OR IV TEARS

- Atropine to reduce peristalsis
- Packing of the rectal lumen from the anus to cranial to the tear
- Colostomy to divert feces from the site and prevent peritoneal contamination

NOTE: Grade IV tears necessitate a colostomy. For grade III tears, colostomy is recommended (Fig. 35–9).

- Loop colostomy is performed with the patient under general anesthesia or under sedation and local anesthesia. The colostomy exits through the left flank.
- An alternative is to oversew the proximal end of the distal small colon; the distal end of the proximal small colon exits from the flank as a diverting colostomy.
- If the patient is placed under general anesthesia, large-colon enterotomy is performed to reduce fecal bulk exiting from the colostomy.
- A rectal liner (Rectal Ring, Regal Plastic Co., Detroit Lakes, MN) is used in the management of grade III tears to bypass the tear and avoid colostomy.
- Grades III and IV tears heal by secondary intention; the loop colostomy is reversed after the tear heals.

Prognosis

- Excellent for grades I and II rectal tears. Guarded for grade III tears. Guarded to poor for grade IV tears.

RECTAL PROLAPSE

Rectal prolapse is caused by straining due to constipation, obstipation, dystocia, colitis, urethral obstruction, or foreign body impaction of the distal small colon or rectum. In some cases no known predisposing cause can be identified. The condition occurs more commonly in mares and is classified according to severity as follows:

- **Type I** prolapse involves only the rectal mucosal and submucosa and appears as a large circular anal swelling.
- **Type II** involves the entire rectal wall and is called "complete" prolapse; the ventral portion of prolapsed tissue is thicker than the dorsal portion.
- **Type III** includes invaginated peritoneal rectum or small colon and is difficult to differentiate from type II prolapse.
- **Type IV** involves intussuscepted peritoneal rectum or small colon beyond the anus. A palpable invagination adjacent to the intussuscepted intestine differentiates type IV from type III prolapse.

Treatment

TYPE I OR TYPE II PROLAPSE

- Reduce the edema in the tissues with topical application of glycerin or dextrose and apply petroleum jelly (Vaseline).
- Reduce the prolapse under epidural anesthesia.
- Tranquilize the patient unless contraindicated.
- Place a purse-string suture in the anus.
- Administer stool softeners, such as mineral oil.
- Perform submucosal resection if medical treatment is unsuccessful.

TYPE III OR IV PROLAPSE

- Perform celiotomy to reduce the intussusception.

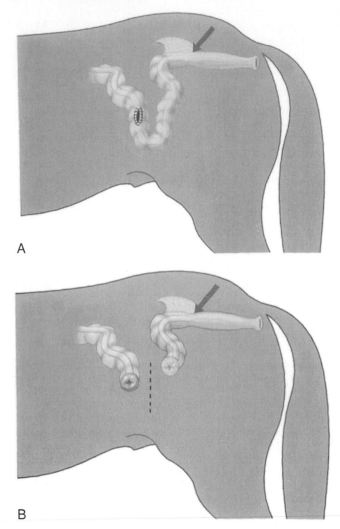

FIGURE 35-9. Colostomy technique. **A,** Loop colostomy. **B,** Diverting colostomy positioned in the left flank. *Arrows* indicate the location of the rectal tear. Loop colostomy is performed at the initial flank incision. The diverting colostomy is performed with a separate incision cranial to the initial flank incision *(dashed line).*

- Perform colostomy for type IV prolapse because of compromise of the blood supply to the affected bowel.

Prognosis
- Good for types I and II prolapse. Guarded to poor for types III and IV.

■ H. COLIC IN THE LATE-TERM PREGNANT MARE

P. O. Eric Mueller and James N. Moore

Colic in a mare during the last trimester of pregnancy often is a diagnostic challenge. Gastrointestinal disorders must be ruled out with careful clinical examination, but the large, gravid uterus often prevents a complete rectal examination. The effect of the colic episode on the fetus is always of concern, because abortion can result in substantial emotional and financial loss. The overall post-colic abortion rate among mares is between 16% and 18%. Endotoxemia and intraoperative hypoxia or hypotension during colic surgery in the last 60 days of gestation have been associated with a higher incidence of abortion. Causes of colic in late-term pregnant mares not associated with the gastrointestinal tract include

- Abortion and premature parturition
- Uterine torsion
- Hydrallantois
- Ruptured prepubic tendon

Pregnant mares with colic and endotoxemia during the first 2 months of pregnancy may benefit from treatment with progestin supplementation, altrenogest 22-44 mg PO q24h for a 450-kg adult or injectable progesterone 150-300 mg/450-kg adult IM q24h for 100-200 days of pregnancy. The adverse effects of chronic endotoxemia in late pregnancy may be prevented by administering NSAIDs.

ABORTION AND PREMATURE PARTURITION

Mares may have signs of mild to moderate abdominal pain and minimal udder development. Vaginal examination reveals loss of the cervical plug and relaxation of the cervix. This finding alone does not indicate impending abortion because similar findings occur in many normal mares days or weeks before delivery. Rectal examination often reveals the fetus to be positioned within the birth canal.

Treatment

Treatment is supportive and directed at an uncomplicated delivery and postpartum care of the mare. Postmortem examination of the aborted fetus and placenta may determine the cause of the abortion, such as equine herpesvirus 1 (see abortion evaluation, Chapter 42, p. 497). The mare should be isolated until the results of the examination are available.

UTERINE TORSION

Uterine torsion can be a cause of colic in late-term pregnant mares. It usually occurs between 8 months of gestation and term. Unlike the case of cows, in which the torsion is most often diagnosed at term, mares affected near term usually are not in labor when clinical signs are first evident. Also unlike the disorder in cows, torsion in mares usually is cranial to the cervix and vagina, thereby minimizing the benefit of a vaginal examination in making the diagnosis. The degree of torsion ranges from 180 to 540 degrees and occurs in either direction with equal frequency. Uterine rupture can occur as the result of torsion and is an uncommon complication.

Diagnosis

Mild to moderate intermittent abdominal pain is the most consistent sign; however, some mares may demonstrate severe, unrelenting pain. A mild increase in heart and respiratory rates also may be present. Diagnosis is made with the signalment, history, and findings at rectal examination. Rectal palpation of the broad ligaments reveals the ligaments to be tight as they cross the caudal abdomen below and above the cervix. Palpation of the dorsal-most ligament, and occasionally the body of the uterus, indicates the direction of the torsion. In *clockwise torsion*, as viewed from behind, the *left broad ligament is pulled tight over the uterus and courses to the right in a horizontal to oblique direction*. In counterclockwise torsion, the opposite is true.

Treatment

Early recognition and intervention are imperative for a successful outcome for both the mare and the foal. The optimal method of correction depends on the condition of the mare and fetus and the stage of gestation.

NONSURGICAL CORRECTION: ROLLING
See Fig. 42–2.

SURGICAL CORRECTION (PREFERRED)
FLANK CELIOTOMY
- Provides the *least stress* for the foal and mare; can be performed during any stage of gestation.
- Performed with the standing mare under sedation (xylazine or detomidine with or without butorphanol) and local anesthetic infiltration along the proposed incision site.
- Controversy exists as to the preferred side of entry relative to the direction of the torsion. Many surgeons prefer to enter the abdomen from the side to which the torsion is directed (e.g., right flank for clockwise torsion).
- If the abdomen is entered from the side to which the torsion is directed, the surgeon's hand is passed ventrally to the uterus, and the uterus is lifted and rotated upward to correct the torsion.
- If the abdomen is entered on the side opposite that to which the torsion is directed (e.g., right flank for counterclockwise torsion), the surgeon's hand passes dorsally to the uterus, and the uterus is pulled toward the surgeon to correct the torsion.
- Correction can be facilitated by means of grasping the limbs of the fetus through the wall of the uterus and *gently* "rocking" the uterus to gain enough momentum for complete rotation and final correction.
- An alternative is to enter both sides simultaneously.

VENTRAL MIDLINE CELIOTOMY
Ventral midline celiotomy provides the best exposure for assessment and manipulation of the gravid uterus. Indications for ventral midline celiotomy include *uterine rupture, uterine tearing,* and *uterine devitalization.* This approach also allows identification and correction of concurrent intestinal disorders. It can be performed during any stage of gestation.

- Standard ventral midline celiotomy.
- If hysterotomy is indicated, the ventral midline approach provides the best surgical exposure.
- Ventral midline celiotomy *should be reserved for cases not amenable to nonsurgical correction or flank celiotomy* because of the associated risks of general anesthesia to the mare and foal.

Prognosis
- Good to excellent for complete recovery and future breeding soundness of the mare with uterine torsion. Fetal viability depends on the duration and degree of torsion. The abortion rate after uterine torsion is reported to be between 30% and 40%.

UTERINE RUPTURE

Uterine rupture can be a complication of manipulation during dystocia or during apparently normal foaling. It also can be a sequela to *uterine torsion* or hydrallantois. The tear usually occurs at the dorsal aspect of the uterus (see Chapter 42, p. 485).

Diagnosis and Treatment
Suspect uterine rupture in any mare demonstrating postpartum abdominal pain. Large ruptures may result in significant blood loss and produce signs of hemorrhagic shock. Diagnosis is confirmed at vaginal and uterine examination. *If a uterine tear is suspected, irrigating solutions should not be infused into the uterus.*

- Broad-spectrum antimicrobial agents
- Balanced, polyionic intravenous fluids
- Plasma or synthetic colloids
- NSAIDs
- Peritoneal drainage
- Allow small tears to heal by secondary intention. Close large tears primarily; general anesthesia and ventral midline celiotomy are necessary

Prognosis
- Depends on the size of the tear, duration before recognition and treatment, degree of peritoneal contamination, and nature of the intrauterine contents. Good for small tears recognized early and poor for large tears with an emphysematous fetus and gross peritoneal contamination.

HYDRALLANTOIS

See Chapter 42, p. 486.

RUPTURED PREPUBIC TENDON

The prepubic tendon is a strong, thick, fibrous structure that attaches to the cranial border of the pelvis and provides attachment for the rectus abdominis, oblique abdominis, gracilis, and pectineus muscles. It forms the medial borders of the external inguinal rings. Hydrallantois, twins, or fetal giants may predispose to prepubic tendon rupture.

Diagnosis

Must be differentiated from ventral hernia, which also occurs most frequently in late-term pregnant mares. Ventral hernia may respond favorably to surgical repair; the prognosis is poor, however, for prepubic tendon rupture.

CLINICAL SIGNS

- Severe, progressive, ventral abdominal swelling and edema with the *pelvis tilted cranially and ventrally. The mammary gland also assumes a more cranioventral position.*
- Mild to moderate abdominal pain usually is apparent, and the *mare is reluctant to walk.* In contrast, mares with a *ventral hernia are not reluctant to walk, and the pelvis and mammary gland are in a normal position.*
- Identification of the defect by means of external palpation may be difficult because of excessive edema formation.
- *Rectal examination and ultrasonography* are helpful in differentiating prepubic tendon rupture from ventral herniation.

Treatment

- In mares near term, early induction of parturition and *assisted foaling* may be required.
- *Exploratory celiotomy* and cesarean section should be performed immediately on mares that demonstrate intractable pain or systemic deterioration or in which a concurrent incarcerating intestinal lesion is suspected.
- Stabilized mares should be confined to stall rest, placed in abdominal support bandages, and administered NSAIDs.
- *Low-bulk, pelleted feed* should be fed to decrease the volume of ingesta.
- These mares may foal normally; however, they should be *observed closely* and assisted with foaling if necessary.

Prognosis

- Stabilized mares not in pain may successfully raise a foal but should not be used for breeding. The likelihood of long-term survival is poor.

ABDOMINAL PAIN AFTER FOALING

- This is very common in mares and is usually mild and associated with bruising of the pelvic canal and secondary ileus.
- More serious conditions, such as small colon impaction, large colon volvulus, ruptured uterus, cecum and/or bladder must be ruled out by clinical, laboratory and ultrasound examination and surgically corrected if necessary. Medical therapy alone may be appropriate for small colon impaction and occasionally small dorsal tears of the uterus and/or bladder.

▓ I. PERITONITIS

P. O. Eric Mueller and James N. Moore

Peritonitis, inflammation of the peritoneal cavity, is classified according to:

- Origin: primary or secondary
- Onset: peracute, acute, or chronic

- Extent of involvement: diffuse or localized
- Presence of bacteria: septic or nonseptic

Peritonitis usually is acute, diffuse, and secondary to gastrointestinal compromise or infectious disease. Severity depends on the etiologic agent, virulence of the organism, host defenses, extent and site of involvement, recognition of problems, and treatment. Generally the aboral sites, cecum to small colon, contain more bacteria and anaerobes and therefore are associated with more severe disease. The organisms frequently cultured are enteric aerobes *(E. coli, Actinobacillus* organisms, *Streptococcus equi* and *Streptococcus zooepidemicus* and *Rhodococcus* organisms*)* and anaerobes *(Bacteroides, Peptostreptococcus, Clostridium,* and in rare cases, *Fusobacterium* organisms).*

Causes

- Idiopathic
- Perforation of the gastrointestinal or genitourinary tract
- Infectious disease (actinobacillus)
- Trauma
- Iatrogenic after abdominal surgery

Diagnosis

Clinical signs depend on the etiologic agent and the extent and duration of disease. *Local* peritonitis has minimal systemic signs; *diffuse* peritonitis has signs of endotoxemia and septicemia, abdominal pain, pyrexia, anorexia, weight loss, and diarrhea.

Peracute peritonitis due to intestinal rupture causes severe signs of endotoxemia, depression, and rapid cardiovascular deterioration; severe abdominal pain, sweating, muscle fasciculations, tachycardia, red to purple mucous membranes with increased capillary refill time; dehydration; and depression.

In acute diffuse peritonitis, death occurs 4-24 hours after the primary insult. Fever and abdominal pain may not occur and depend on the stage of endotoxic shock. Ileus and gastric reflux may develop as the result of peritoneal and serosal inflammation. Rectal examination may yield normal findings or dry, emphysematous, "gritty" serosa and peritoneum and distention of the large and small intestine due to ileus

Affected horses with localized, subacute to chronic peritonitis have signs of depression, anorexia, weight loss, intermittent fever, ventral edema, intermittent abdominal pain, and mild dehydration

CLINICAL LABORATORY FINDINGS

- Increased PCV
- Increased (hemoconcentration) or decreased (protein loss into the peritoneal cavity) TPP concentration
- Hyperfibrinogenemia
- Increased creatinine concentration: prerenal or renal azotemia
- Metabolic acidosis

RESULTS OF CBC IN THE PRESENCE OF SEVERE ENDOTOXEMIA

- Marked leukopenia: neutropenia and left shift due to endotoxemia and consumption in peracute and acute peritonitis

- Leukocytosis: neutrophilia due to inflammation and hyperfibrinogenemia in chronic peritonitis

PERITONEAL FLUID ANALYSIS
- Collect peritoneal fluid in an EDTA tube for cytologic examination, measurement of total protein, and WBC count. Collect samples for bacterial culture in a sterile tube.
- Increased total protein concentration and nucleated cell count: 20,000-400,000/μl.
- Cytologic examination: free or phagocytized bacteria in leukocytes.
- Perform Gram stain for initial evaluation and selection of antimicrobial agents while awaiting culture and susceptibility results.

Treatment
Prompt and aggressive treatment is needed.

- Management of the primary disease
- Pain relief
- Reversal of endotoxic and hypovolemic shock
- Correction of metabolic and electrolyte abnormalities
- Correction of dehydration
- Correction of hypoproteinemia
- Broad-spectrum antimicrobial therapy
- Intravenous administration of a balanced electrolyte solution to maintain intravascular fluid volume
- Hypertonic saline solution (7% NaCl, 1 to 2 L IV) improves systemic blood pressure and cardiac output. Hypertonic saline solution administered initially must be followed by adequate fluid replacement with a balanced crystalloid solution.
- A TPP concentration >4.5 g/dl necessitates administration of plasma, 2 to 10 L IV slowly, to maintain plasma oncotic pressure and minimize pulmonary edema during rehydration with intravenous fluids.
- Antiserum (Endoserum) against gram-negative core antigens (endotoxin) administered intravenously diluted in a balanced electrolyte solution. Hyperimmune plasma directed against the J-5 mutant strain of *E. coli* (Polymune-J, Foalimmune) or normal *equine plasma* (2-10 L) administered intravenously, *slowly*, may be equally beneficial for supplying protein, fibronectin, complement, antithrombin III, and other inhibitors of hypercoagulability.
- Flunixin meglumine, 0.66-1.1 mg/kg IV q12h, or low-dose, 0.25 mg/kg IV q8h, to reduce the adverse effects of arachidonic acid metabolites. These drugs should be used with *caution* in the care of hypovolemic, hypoproteinemic patients to avoid gastrointestinal and renal toxicity.
- Monitor blood gas and serum electrolyte levels and correct deficiencies.
- Start antimicrobial therapy immediately after a peritoneal fluid sample has been obtained for culture and susceptibility. Antimicrobial combinations commonly used include
  - Na^+/K^+ penicillin, 22,000-44,000 IU/kg IV q6h, and/or
  - Aminoglycosides: gentamicin, 2.2 mg/kg IV q8h or 6.6 mg/kg IV q24h, or amikacin, 6.6 mg/kg q8h or 19.8 mg/kg IV q24h
  - Metronidazole, 15-25 mg/kg PO, or suppository q6h for anaerobes

- Duration of antimicrobial therapy depends on the
  - Severity of the peritonitis
  - Etiologic agent
  - Response to treatment
  - Complications: thrombophlebitis, abdominal abscessation
- Use clinical signs and sequential evaluation of clinicopathologic parameters and peritoneal fluid to assess response to treatment. Generalized septic peritonitis may necessitate 1-6 months of antimicrobial therapy.
- After stabilization, perform surgical intervention to correct the primary problem and reduce peritoneal contamination by abdominal drainage, peritoneal lavage, and peritoneal dialysis.

Prognosis

- Depends on the severity and duration of the disease, the primary etiologic agent, and complications, which include intraabdominal adhesion formation, laminitis, and endotoxic shock. Fair to good in mild, acute, diffuse peritonitis if prompt, aggressive management of the underlying problem is successful or if it is unknown. A poor prognosis if there is significant abdominal contamination or intestinal perforation.

J. ACUTE DIARRHEA
Thomas J. Divers

Fever, colic, and *diarrhea* are the clinical signs caused by enteritis in horses. In many cases, colic precedes the diarrhea and may be severe. This is particularly true in young foals. Adult diarrhea is almost always a result of colonic dysfunction, therefore the terms *colitis* and *diarrhea* are often used synonymously. In foals, diarrhea is most severe with small-intestinal dysfunction. This section is divided into descriptions of adult, weanling-yearling, and foal problems due to age differences, although some of the etiologic agents, such as *Salmonella* organisms, can affect all age groups.

DIARRHEAL DISEASE IN ADULTS

Acute colitis is almost always an emergency in adults. Salmonellosis, Potomac horse fever (PHF), and drug-induced colitis (antibiotics, NSAID toxicity) are the most common causes. Approximately 30% of cases go undiagnosed (idiopathic). Affected individuals may present with *colic, fever, or both before the onset of diarrhea.* Take the rectal temperature of patients with abdominal pain before giving NSAIDS! Make a presumptive diagnosis of acute colitis in the presence of fever with fluidlike bowel sounds (the sound of fluid rushing through pipes).

Causes
SALMONELLA INFECTION AND POTOMAC HORSE FEVER
Many patients with PHF have fever, depression, and anorexia without diarrhea. *PHF is a common cause of fever in endemic areas during the summer months.* Bloody diarrhea may be more common with *Salmonella* infection but occurs with other

TABLE 35–2. Comparison of Epidemiologic Features of Salmonellosis and Potomac Horse Fever

Feature	Salmonella	PHF
Stress factors	+	–
Seasonal	– (may be some increase during spring)	+ (June to November in northeast, mid-Atlantic, and north central United States)
Age	All	Mostly adults
Epidemic	Occasionally	Occasionally
Endemic in area of farm or track	+	+
Hospital associated	+	–

etiologic agents. Although the clinical signs of salmonellosis and PHF *(Ehrlichia risticii)* are *indistinguishable*, the epidemiology has some important differences (Table 35–2).

➤ Fewer than 20% of horses infected with *Neorickettsia risticii* infection experience diarrhea. Even without diarrhea, this infection should be a differential diagnosis for fever or laminitis of unknown origin during the endemic season.

ANTIBIOTIC-INDUCED DIARRHEA

The history is important in determining the likelihood of the presence of antibiotic-induced diarrhea. The diarrhea generally occurs 2-6 days after starting antibiotic treatment (although some cases occur 1-2 days after stopping the treatment). The condition is believed to result from pathogenic *Clostridium difficile* or *C. perfringens* overgrowth or their inflammatory and secretory effects on the colon. A decrease in roughage consumption can predispose a horse to enteric clostridiosis. All antimicrobial drugs, especially those given orally, have the potential for causing diarrhea. The following are the most commonly implicated drugs:

- Oral trimethoprim-sulfamethoxazole: Mostly if the horse has been stressed, transported, or is recovering from surgery
- *Erythromycin: Patients older than 6 months*
➤ - Also can occur in mares when their foals are being treated with erythromycin
- Tetracycline: Intravenous tetracycline *rarely* causes diarrhea in horses and has received an undeserved bad reputation. Nevertheless, it should be considered a possible cause, especially in stressed patients. Doxycycline given orally may occasionally cause diarrhea.
- Penicillin: Administered orally and occasionally after parenteral
- Ceftiofur: Occasionally after parenteral administration
- Enrofloxacin: Occasionally after parenteral or oral administration

NSAID TOXICITY

NSAID toxicity can occur from excessive administration of oral or parenteral phenylbutazone, flunixin meglumine, or ketoprofen. Phenylbutazone is believed to be more damaging to the gastrointestinal tract than are the other two.

➤ *Affected horses generally have hypoproteinemia early in the disease and usually have plasma protein levels less than 4.5 g/dl (adults) before the diarrhea.* The protein level is lower in foals. *The very low protein level at the onset or before the diarrhea occurs does not confirm but is highly suggestive of the diagnosis of NSAID toxicity.* Colic may be more common with NSAID toxicity than with other forms of colitis.

CYATHOSTOMIASIS

Acute diarrhea associated with encysted cyathostomes can occur in yearlings or adults. Affected individuals are generally thin before the onset of diarrhea and have a questionable history regarding proper parasite control. The onset of clinical signs is most common in October through April. The history is important in making a tentative diagnosis of cyathostomiasis diarrhea. Fever and leukopenia may be absent. Fecal examination for parasites may not be useful because the encysted larvae are the problem. A rectal biopsy should be performed; the presence of eosinophils or the finding of an encysted larva supports the disease. Adult small strongyles may be found in the manure or on the rectal sleeve after examination in a small percentage of cases.

COLITIS X

Colitis X is an all-encompassing term for acute colitis, endotoxemia, and ana-phylaxis. *There are multiple causes!* Segmental edema of the colon is characteristic. Stress or a change in feed may precede the acute disease. The syndrome has occurred on a few occasions in horses recently (2-5 days) introduced to winter grazing.

Acute collapse and signs of shock are characteristic, although some individuals have a more prolonged course. Severe pain, mild abdominal distention, and fever are common. There may be severe diarrhea, mild "cow flop" manure, or no manure passed. The colon may be palpated to be edematous at rectal examination, and in a few cases blood is found in the manure. Sometimes the affected horses may improve initially with treatment but within a few days die suddenly. Necropsy reveals severe edema (sometimes hemorrhage) of the colon, cecum, or both. The lesions may be segmental.

Fecal specimens should be submitted for *Salmonella* and *Clostridium* culture and *Clostridium* toxin assay. Clinical pathologic data are typical of those found in many patients with endotoxemia and colitis (leukopenia, left shift, toxic-appearing neutrophils, thrombocytopenia, hyponatremia, hypochloremia, hypocalcemia, and acidosis).

General Diagnostic Tests for Acute Adult Colitis

▶ Routine hematology, including CBC, chemistry panel (hypochloremia and hyponatremia with azotemia are the most common findings early in all colitis diseases).

▶ *Hyperkalemia is a clue that the azotemia may be more than prerenal in origin.*

- PHF titer >1:640 on most fluorescent antibody tests establishes the diagnosis if the patient is unvaccinated; >1:2560 *often* confirms the diagnosis if the patient has been vaccinated, although some vaccinated horses may have higher titers and not have infection. (Some horses with PHF have lower titers early in the course of the disease.)
- Polymerase chain reaction (PCR) for PHF: Place an EDTA blood sample on ice, and ship it express mail to Cornell Diagnostic Laboratory or another laboratory that performs the test on a daily basis. PCR should be used in addition to indirect fluorescent antibody assay to confirm the diagnosis of PHF. That some patients have negative results of blood PCR suggests the organism may have moved from the circulating monocyte to the colon.
- Fecal culture is used to support a diagnosis of *Salmonella*. Repeated samples (5-10 g) are required. If the sample cannot be submitted immediately to a

reference laboratory, place fecal specimen in a cup (not refrigerated) or place feces (10%) in a whirl pack of Selenite or Ames transport media for storage. If you do your own culturing, it is best to perform direct culture on selective media. Place some feces in enrichment (Selenite F) medium for later plating. Results of *Salmonella* cultures are most often positive as the manure firms. Fecal cultures also can be tested for *Salmonella* with PCR. Cornell Diagnostic Laboratory, Ithaca, NY 14853; (607) 253-3900 or Diagnostic and Biologic Technologies, Inc., San Antonio, TX 78258; (800) 336-3060; Fax (210) 496-2517.

- *C. difficile* infection is believed to be one of the main causes of antibiotic-induced colitis. The role of *C. perfringens* is unconfirmed, but this organism may cause diarrhea in some adult horses. Feces should be submitted for *Clostridium* culture and toxin assay for *C. difficile* toxin A and B and *C. perfringens* enterotoxin. *C. difficile* and its toxins are not found in healthy adults or in adults with colic. *C. perfringens* and even its enterotoxin are found in rare instances in individuals that are colicky but do not have diarrhea. If *C. perfringens* appears in large numbers on the Gram stain and if the patient has hemorrhagic diarrhea, a β_2 toxin assay should be requested. Cary-Blair Transport Media, Meridian Diagnostics, Cincinnati, OH 45244 should be used for *Clostridium* culture. Frozen feces shipped overnight is recommended for toxin assay, although the toxin, unlike the organism, is viable under aerobic conditions for days. Send samples to Diagnostic Laboratory, New York State College of Veterinary Medicine, Cornell University, Box 786, Upper Tower Road, Ithaca, NY 14851; (607) 253-3333. For anaerobic culture and toxin assay when specific media are not available, at least 50 ml should be transported overnight to an appropriate laboratory. A Gram stain on the feces often is helpful, and with clostridiosis, there are a majority of uniformly large Gram-positive organisms. If *C. difficile* is the etiologic agent, many of the organisms may have spores.
- It is *not* routinely recommended to perform an abdominocentesis unless peritonitis is suspected (see Table 19–1). The peritoneal fluid of patients with severe colitis often has an increase in protein. This finding rarely affects treatment, but the abdominocentesis procedure increases the subcutaneous abdominal edema associated with hypoproteinemia. Stallions with ventral edema may experience severe cellulitis of the scrotum.
- It is also *not* routine to perform rectal examinations on individuals with acute colitis unless the patient is colicky or has abdominal distention. Tenesmus and rectal prolapse may result.

Treatment
MANAGEMENT OF ABDOMINAL PAIN ASSOCIATED WITH ACUTE COLITIS
Pass a nasogastric tube, and perform a rectal examination and abdominocentesis to aid in ruling out an obstructive disease in individuals *with persistent pain.* Ultrasound examination can be important in separating obstruction from ileus. (Small-bowel distention may be found with both disorders, but some loops are *amotile* with obstruction. With colitis, the colon wall may appear thick and edematous, and the contents may have a more fluidlike appearance as opposed to a more normal gaslike appearance.) If in addition to the history and laboratory findings, the information suggests colitis, the abdominal pain is most likely a result of ileus, fluid distention of the bowel, edema of the bowel, stretching of the mesentery, mucosal ulcerations, or infarction of the bowel.

Intravenous calcium therapy may be useful in relieving the ileus in some cases. Lidocaine (2%) can be given intravenously, 1.3 mg/kg as a slow bolus, followed by

0.05 mg/kg per minute as a continuous infusion. For patients with colitis that are in tremendous pain and have a *large* ping over the base of the cecum, decompress the cecum (see cecal trocharization procedure, p. 87). Two liters to 4 L per adult of hydroxyethyl starch (hetastarch) or plasma with 1 L of hypertonic saline solution and DMSO 1 g/kg IV can be administered to reduce colonic edema. If no other treatment is effective in relieving the pain or improving motility and fecal output, and pain is believed associated with colonic edema and pooling of fluid in the bowel and ileus, a single treatment with dexamethasone (0.5 mg/kg) or mannitol 1 g/kg IV may diminish the ultrasound evidence of colonic edema and relieve the abdominal pain.

Administer flunixin meglumine, 0.3 mg/kg IV q8h, for endotoxemia. A larger dose, 1.0 mg/kg IV, can be administered once or twice for severe abdominal pain. Flunixin should not be used at the higher dose if NSAID toxicity is a likely diagnosis. Xylazine, detomidine, or butorphanol can be used on a short-term basis to control pain. If a long-term effect is needed and flunixin cannot be administered, chloral hydrate may be administered, as a sedative, to effect. Fentanyl patches (2 × 100 µg/h) can be used for patients with persistent pain due to right dorsal colitis.

GENERAL MANAGEMENT OF COLITIS, REGARDLESS OF THE CAUSE
FLUID THERAPY
- *Lactated Ringer's* and Plasmalyte are preferred in most cases. In patients with severe colitis, replace *at least* one-half the plasma volume in the first 6-8 hours.
- Administer *hypertonic saline solution*, 2-4 ml/kg IV, if severe hypotensive shock is suspected or as a means of cardiovascular support until intravenous fluids can be started and maintained uninterrupted. Hypertonic saline solution can also be given for prognostic purposes to patients with azotemic and hyperkalemic colitis to determine importance of the colitis. Patients that void a large volume of urine after receiving hypertonic saline solution rarely have life-threatening renal failure.
- *Hetastarch*: up to 10 ml/kg can and should be given along with crystalloids early in the management of severe colitis while plasma is thawing. During crystalloid therapy, hetastarch and plasma should be used to maintain oncotic pressure greater than 16 mm Hg.
- *Plasma*, 2 L minimum, has many advantages beside providing specific antiendotoxic antibodies. Plasma contains fibronectin, antithrombin III, and other beneficial proteins.

NOTE: Plasma with antibodies against lipopolysaccharide is recommended. It is preferred that commercially available hyperimmune serum not be used because of the adverse effects associated with endotoxin in the product. Heparin should be added to plasma to equal a dose of 40 U/kg q8h.

- *Bicarbonate* is rarely indicated initially unless the venous pH is unusually low (<7.1). Always add potassium to the fluids (20-40 mEq/L) as soon as it becomes apparent that the patient is urinating.

LOW-DOSE FLUNIXIN MEGLUMINE
- 0.25 mg/kg q8h initially; continue until signs of toxemia, fever, leukopenia, and so forth have resolved. Do not administer at higher dosages unless the patient has severe abdominal pain.

ACTIVATED CHARCOAL (COMMERCIAL GRADE)
- 0.5 kg/500-kg horse PO; check for gastric reflux first. Other oral antidiarrhea medications have been used but have not been useful in the treatment of adults with infectious colitis. A smectite clay product* may be effective in the management of clostridial diarrhea.

PENTOXIFYLLINE
- 8.4 mg/kg IV (the oral tablets can be dissolved in saline solution and filtered through a 0.5-μm pore filter for intravenous administration). Pentoxifylline decreases cytokine production in vitro after endotoxin challenge and may make RBCs more deformable. The effect in vivo is unknown.

POLYMYXIN B
- Administered at 1000-6000 U/kg IV, polymyxin B may diminish the harmful effects of the endotoxin. A noticeable clinical response in patients has not been consistently seen.

NITROGLYCERINE CREAM
- Should be applied to the posterior pastern area for 2 days.

OMEPRAZOLE
- Omeprazole is used by many veterinarians in supportive therapy for adult equine colitis. Generally omeprazole is given to individuals that are not eating well or in performance horses or if results of a gastroscopic examination confirm the presence of gastric ulcer. A review of adult horses that died or were humanely destroyed because of severe colitis showed that moderate to severe gastric ulceration was uncommon in untreated horses.

SPECIFIC MANAGEMENT OF ADULT COLITIS
ANTIBIOTICS FOR ADULT SALMONELLOSIS
- Antibiotic therapy has not been shown to be of benefit in the management of *Salmonella* infection in *adults*; however, most veterinarians prefer to administer antibiotics for salmonellosis in adults. Enrofloxacin 5 mg/kg IV q24h is recommended.

RISKS ASSOCIATED WITH ANTIBIOTIC USE
- Fungal colitis and pneumonia occur occasionally with broad-spectrum antibiotics, including ceftiofur
- Nephrotoxicity if aminoglycosides are used
- *Do not use aminoglycosides to treat patients with diarrhea unless intravenous fluids are being administered, urination is documented, and creatinine concentration is monitored.*

POTOMAC HORSE FEVER
- Tetracycline, 6.6 mg/kg IV diluted 1 part tetracycline and 3 parts saline solution q12h for 3-5 days. *The sooner in the course of the disease tetracycline is administered, the better is the response.*

---

*Bio-sponge. Platinum Performance Inc., Buelton, CA 93427; (805) 688-6510, (800) 553-2400.

NSAID TOXICITY
- Plasma, 4-8 L
- Sucralfate, 6-8 g/adult q6-12h
- Misoprostol (Cytotec), 2-4 µg/kg PO q12h. Mild diarrhea and an increase in rectal temperature have been seen after administration in a few horses.
- Do not use in pregnant mares or dispense if owners or handlers are or may be pregnant!
- Many horses with NSAID toxicity have colic without diarrhea. The history, results of clinical examination, and finding of low total serum protein concentration support a tentative diagnosis. Treatment is plasma and polyionic fluids, sucralfate, misoprostol, and feeding a low-residue diet (no hay) with slow introduction of up to ½ cup (120 ml) dietary linseed oil added twice daily.
- Use analgesics only if pain is persistent or severe.
- Dipyrone, xylazine, butorphanol, lidocaine, or fentanyl patch can be used.

ANTIBIOTIC INDUCED DIARRHEA
- Metronidazole, 15 mg/kg q6-8h PO. Look for clinical improvement within 3 days or discontinue treatment.
- Chloramphenicol, 44 mg/kg PO q6-8 h is a second choice.
- Probiotics or yogurt may be of some help but the efficacy has not been demonstrated. Smectite may have a greater number of positive effects because it binds bacterial toxins before they attach.

CYATHOSTOMIASIS
- Moxidectin (American Cyanamid), 400-500 µg/kg PO once, and fenbendazole, 10 mg/kg daily for 5 days

ADDITIONAL MANAGEMENT OF ALL CAUSES OF COLITIS
- Unless the patient is in pain, offer free-choice water *with* and *without* electrolytes, including NaCl (15 g), dextrose (15 g), either anhydrous dextrose or 30 ml 50% dextrose, baking soda (12 g), and KCl (10 g per gallon [3.8 L] of water).
- Feed grass hay without grain or with grain in small amounts.
- Place a wrap on the tail and use petroleum jelly on the perineal-scrotal area to protect from the effects of diarrhea.

CAUTION: If tail wraps are used, be sure they are not too tight; do not use Vetwrap.

- Monitor closely for signs of laminitis. Some clinicians routinely use frog pads as a prophylactic treatment. Topical nitroglycerin cream over palmar (posterior) digital arteries can be used for 1-3 days if there is chemical or laboratory evidence of toxemia.
- Take measures to prevent exposure of other horses (through contact with feces or feces-contaminated equipment or personnel) until a diagnosis is confirmed. The ideal disinfection of stalls for either *Salmonella* organisms or *C. difficile* is not known. Removal of organic debris and repeated application of diluted bleach (1:10 down to 1:2 may be required).
- Use care in placing the jugular catheter because patients with colitis are at risk for thrombophlebitis. Use a Mila catheter (Mila International, Inc., Covington, KY 41011) for patients with colitis and other conditions that are likely to receive

large volumes of intravenous fluids for several days or are at high risk of thrombosis, such as those with a rapid drop in protein concentration, severe hemoconcentration, or marked leukopenia with toxic changes.

- Obtain samples from the transverse facial sinus (see procedure on p. 3), and save the jugular veins for catheter placement.

Prognosis

The most difficult patients to treat are those that continue to have pain or are in a very toxic condition and produce scant, watery manure in the first 24 hours; *the prognosis is poor*. The prognosis for horses with diarrhea caused by NSAIDs also is poor. The prognosis for all patients with colitis is affected by appetite; those that continue to eat have a better outcome.

Degree of hemoconcentration: patients with a PCV of 60%-65% or more have a poor prognosis, as do those with purple mucous membranes. These patients may recover from colitis but seem to have a higher incidence of failure to gain weight, laminitis, and renal failure.

Laminitis: Guarded to poor prognosis with ongoing colitis. If the patient is to be a performance horse and it develops laminitis associated with colitis, marked *improvement in the laminitis within 3 days of treatment must be seen or the prognosis for returning to performance is poor*.

Renal failure: Fair prognosis if polyuria occurs with fluid therapy; otherwise grave. Most individuals with acute colitis are azotemic, often having serum creatinine concentrations of 3.0-7.0 mg/dl. Most have a rapid decline in serum creatinine concentration to normal range within 24-36 hours; this finding suggests that the azotemia is mostly prerenal. Suspect acute renal failure if the patient does not urinate after administration of several liters of polyionic fluids or 1 L of hypertonic saline solution and if the plasma potassium concentration is more than 5.5 mg/dl.

NOTE: Plasma and serum potassium concentrations may be falsely elevated if the plasma and serum are not separated from the RBCs for several hours.

CANTHARIDIN INTOXICATION (BLISTER BEETLE POISONING)

Cantharidin is the toxic principle found in male and inseminated female blister beetles (*Epicauta* species). Three-striped blister beetles (Fig. 35–10) are most often associated with the toxicity. The beetles feed on alfalfa in middle to late summer and can be incorporated into *alfalfa hay* during processing, especially when cutting and crimping are performed simultaneously. Ingestion of the beetles or the toxin (released when the beetles are crushed) causes direct damage to the *oral mucous membranes and the gastrointestinal mucosa*. Once absorbed from the gastrointestinal tract, the toxin is rapidly excreted by the kidneys, damaging the *renal parenchyma* as well as the mucosa of the lower urinary tract in the process. Direct *myocardial* damage can occur with cantharidin intoxication. *As few as 5-10 beetles are lethal.*

Diagnosis

Clinical manifestations are not specific and vary with the amount of toxin ingested. The signs are associated with shock, gastrointestinal and urinary tract irritation, renal insufficiency, myocardial failure, and *hypocalcemia* within hours to days after ingestion of contaminated alfalfa hay (rarely pellets).

CLINICAL SIGNS AND FINDINGS

- Increased heart and respiratory rates

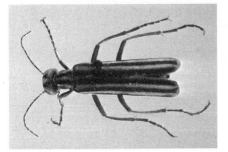

FIGURE 35–10. Three-striped blister beetle. (Courtesy of Dave Schmidt, Texas A & M University.)

GI

- Elevated temperature
- Abdominal pain (most common)
- Anorexia
- Depression
- Sweating
- Oral irritation: Salivation, playing in water
- Frequent attempts to urinate
- Diarrhea: Blood uncommon
- Cold extremities
- *Synchronous diaphragmatic flutter (thumps)*
- Stiff gait*
- Hematuria, hemoglobinuria, or both
- Sudden death
- Neurologic signs
- Cantharidin can be isolated from urine or stomach contents. However, concentrations decrease dramatically within 3 days of ingestion. It may be necessary to submit several hundred milliliters of fluid to identify it. One or more pints of urine can be submitted to the Diagnostic Laboratory at Texas A & M University, College Station, Texas 77843. Postmortem samples of gastric contents and kidneys should be submitted

Treatment
- Remove the toxin.
- Evacuate the gastrointestinal tract.
  - Mineral oil in repeated doses serves as a laxative and binds the lipid-soluble toxin. *Mineral oil should be administered prophylactically to all possibly poisoned horses.*
- Diuresis: Begin as early as feasible to increase toxin excretion. Administer furosemide, 0.25-1.0 mg/kg IV *only* after adequate rehydration.

SUPPORTIVE CARE
- Fluid therapy as indicated by serum electrolyte determination, urine production, and serum creatinine.
  - If synchronous diaphragmatic flutter occurs, to the first day's replacement fluids add calcium borogluconate, 24 mg calcium per kilogram body weight

---

*Indicative of hypocalcemia.

(for an adult, ~500 ml Ca borogluconate diluted in several liters of fluid with magnesium sulfate, 25 mg/kg body weight, 0.05 ml/kg of a 50% $MgSO_4$ solution).

☐ *Administer slowly* intravenously, not subcutaneously.
☐ Monitor cardiac rhythm; discontinue administration if cardiac irregularities develop or worsen.

- Analgesics: Flunixin meglumine, 1.1 mg/kg IM.
- Corticosteroids: Dexamethasone, 0.25 mg/kg IV bolus, occasionally used.
- Broad-spectrum antibiotics: Ceftiofur, *not* aminoglycosides or sulfonamides.
- If renal failure is present, determine whether the failure is oliguric (see Chapter 44, p. 531).

Prognosis

- Guarded in most cases. If a lethal dose has been ingested, no treatment reverses the effects. Heart rate, respiratory rate, and serum creatinine concentration should be monitored for patients that survive several days; increases indicate deterioration. An increase in the cardiac and gastrointestinal enzyme creatine kinase MB is an unfavorable finding.

Prevention

The beetles feed in middle to late summer; therefore alfalfa harvested before June is less likely to be contaminated.

NOTE: Know where the alfalfa is harvested. Instruct owners who grow their own alfalfa to inspect their fields before cultivation and avoid harvesting in areas with insect swarms. An alternative is to treat fields with malathion before cutting, but appropriate withdrawal times should be observed. The toxicity of cantharidin does not decrease with storage, and the pelleting process does not denature it.

K. DIARRHEA IN NURSING FOALS

T. Douglas Byars and Thomas J. Divers

NECROTIZING ENTEROCOLITIS

Necrotizing enterocolitis is a common cause of *colic* and *diarrhea* (sometimes hemorrhagic) in young foals, usually within the first week and sometimes within the first day of life. It is believed caused by the anaerobic organisms: *C. perfringens* (most commonly type A or C), *C. difficile*, or *Bacteroides fragilis*. Diarrhea caused by *C. perfringens* type A or *C. difficile* may be a farm problem. *C. perfringens* type C may affect only one foal on a farm, often with no recognizable predisposing factors. Orphan and maladjusted foals fed large volumes of colostrum and milk replacer seem to be at increased risk.

Clinical Signs

- Colic often precedes the diarrhea by a few hours and can be severe.
- Mild to moderate abdominal distention generally precedes the diarrhea.
- There may be some reflux after passage of a soft nasogastric tube, but more commonly reflux is absent or minimal.
- *Fever* usually is present!

- The diarrhea is bloody in some cases of *C. perfringens* infection.

Diagnosis

Diagnosis is based on the clinical findings, history of fever, leukopenia, low serum sodium and chloride concentrations, and fluid-like bowel sounds. Rule out other causes of colic. *The most common causes of colic in young foals are enteritis and meconium impaction.* Ultrasound examination of the ventral abdomen is helpful in differentiating strangulating lesions from enteritis as a cause of abdominal pain. A 6.0- to 7.5-MHz probe (with standoff) is ideal; however, standard 5.0-MHz reproductive probes are adequate. With enteritis, the small-intestinal wall is more hypoechoic and thickened than normal (Fig. 35–11), and motility may be increased. With strangulating lesions, motility usually is absent. The ultrasound examination should be performed with the foal standing if possible.

Radiographic examination of a foal can be performed with 85 kV(p) and 20 mA with rare earth screen cassettes. This examination is useful in differentiating colic and enteritis from surgical conditions such as intussusception. The presence of diffuse gas distention of the small intestine is supportive of enteritis (Fig. 35–12). With surgical conditions of the small intestine, gas distention generally is less diffuse; instead, a few distinct inverted U loops of bowel are seen (Fig. 35–13).

Perform abdominocentesis only if a strangulating lesion is suspected and only after ultrasound examination has shown a discrete fluid pocket. Indiscriminate abdominocentesis in foals is fraught with complications: Hypodermic needles frequently puncture the bowel lumen in foals, and the perforation can cause peritonitis and adhesions. Teat cannulas can cause herniation of omentum at the site of centesis, however, omental herniation can be minimized by aspirating in the more caudal portion of the abdomen.

Fecal cultures should be performed for identification of *Clostridium* organisms (Port-a-Cul anaerobic tube, Becton-Dickinson, Cockeysville, MD 21030) and toxin assay (place feces in a fecal cup). The specimens should be *taken to the laboratory immediately or shipped overnight on ice. A Gram stain of the feces is beneficial in the diagnosis if there are an abundant number of large gram-positive rods.* Blood cultures should be submitted because many of the foals have blood culture results positive for *C. perfringens* or other enteric organisms.

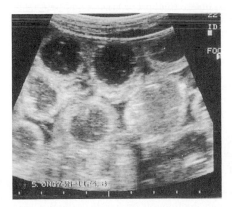

FIGURE 35–11. Ultrasound scan shows the abdomen of a 1-day-old foal with *Clostridium perfringens* diarrhea. Thickening of the bowel wall is evident.

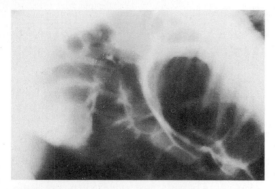

FIGURE 35-12. Radiograph demonstrates the abdomen of a 1-week-old foal with gaseous distention of the intestinal tract. The foal had diarrhea within 4 hours after the radiograph was obtained.

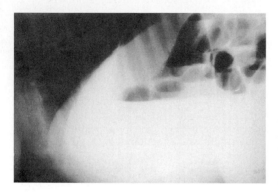

FIGURE 35-13. Radiograph shows the abdomen of a 2-week-old foal with abdominal pain. Intussusception was found at exploratory celiotomy.

Treatment

- Control pain in colicky foals to minimize injury. *Begin with dipyrone, 3-5 ml IV, or butorphanol, 4-6 mg IM or IV. If the pain is not controlled, administer xylazine or flunixin meglumine.* Foals with colic, ileus, and severe or progressive "gaseous" abdominal distention that are unresponsive to appropriate medical treatment, and are believed *not* to have an obstructive disorder, can be given neostigmine, 0.2-0.4 mg SQ q1hr, with a short-acting anesthetic in an attempt to evacuate the gas. Lidocaine IV can also be used.
- Intravenous fluids: lactated Ringer's solution. Add KCl (20 mEq/L) if the foal is hypokalemic or if sodium bicarbonate and dextrose have been administered and the foal is urinating. Additional potassium is generally needed by foals with diarrhea for more than 2 days or foals receiving large volumes of intravenous fluids. If the foal appears weak, add 100 g dextrose per liter unless the Dextrostix result indicates normal blood glucose. If the blood glucose level is normal, add 50 g/L. *Continuous administration of intravenous fluids is seldom practical because the mare often is in the way and the foal may be colicky. An alternative is to give foals 1 to 2 L of fluids by bolus over 20 to 30 minutes two to six times a day, depending on the clinical condition of the foal.*
- Plasma: 2 L administered intravenously. Preferably the plasma should have antibodies against endotoxin, although the lipopolysaccharide antibodies may

not be as important as some naturally occurring factors in plasma, such as antithrombin III.

- If the foal is in hypotensive shock and plasma and polyionic fluids do not improve the condition (determined with blood pressure monitoring or clinical impressions, such as poor capillary refill, severe and persistent tachycardia, no urine production, and cold extremities), administer dobutamine (5-10 µg/kg per minute) in a slow intravenous drip with or without norepinephrine, 0.5-1.0 µg/kg per minute. If this does not improve the blood pressure, methylene blue, 5-8.8 mg/kg IV, can be administered slowly.
- Antibiotics: penicillin, 44,000 IU/kg IV q6h; amikacin,* 18 mg/kg q24h (loading dose, 22 mg/kg); and metronidazole, 15 mg/kg PO two or three times a day for 3-5 days.
- Gastric ulcer prophylaxis:
  □ Sucralfate, 2 g PO q6h
  □ Ranitidine, 1.5 mg/kg IV q8h. Once the pain subsides, these drugs can be given by mouth. Omeprazole 2 mg/kg once a day.
  □ Allow the foal to nurse unless abdominal distention is evident.
  □ Lactaid, yogurt and Pepto-Bismol administered orally via catheter tip syringe 4-6 times a day is supportive.
  □ Intranasal oxygen should be used if there is abdominal distention.

Prognosis

- Initially guarded, because intestinal necrosis can progress rapidly, but if the foal survives the first 2 days of the enteritis, the prognosis usually improves dramatically. Cachexia can become a problem if the foal does not improve within 3 days, and parenteral nutrition may be needed.
- Farm problems can be epidemic! Cleaning the mare's udder and legs before foaling and prophylactic administration of metronidazole, 10 mg/kg q12h every 2-5 days appears successful in approximately 30% of farm outbreaks. Administration of ovine clostridium C & D antitoxin orally (30 ml) is of unproven efficacy. In some outbreaks, the only way to stop the morbidity is to move the foaling unit outside.

FOAL SALMONELLOSIS

Clinical Findings

- Fever (usually >39.4°C or 103°F), depression, tachycardia, tachypnea, and variable diarrhea.
- The diarrhea can be scant, profuse, or bloody; tenesmus may be present.
- Clinical findings more often result from the bacteremia and endotoxemia rather than from intestinal fluid and electrolyte loss.
- The sclera often is injected, and a green discoloration of the iris may be found (presumably a result of septicemia-induced uveitis).
- Lameness can be caused by septic arthritis or physitis.
- Rales, which are caused by hematogenous pneumonia, may be heard at thoracic auscultation.

---

*Administer amikacin only after urine production has been documented. Administer metronidazole only if the feces have a large number of Gram-positive rods on Gram stain. There are other contagious causes of diarrhea in young foals, generally viral, that do not resolve with metronidazole therapy.

- Serosal salmonellosis can result in pleuritis or peritonitis.
- Stupor or seizure may be a result of meningitis or severe electrolyte abnormalities, such as hyponatremia.
- Subcutaneous abscesses may form.
- Horses are susceptible to salmonellosis at any age, and outbreaks are not uncommon among nursing to weanling foals. In many cases of salmonellosis in nursing foals, it is presumed that the mare is the source of the infection. *It is unusual to find clinical signs in both the mare and the foal, although both are usually feces-positive for* Salmonella *organisms.*

Diagnosis

Blood can be collected in a BBL Vacutainer tube (Becton-Dickinson, Cockeysville, MD 21030) for blood culture. *To reduce the cost of submitting every blood culture tube to the laboratory, the specimen can be incubated or left at room temperature for 24-48 hours; broth that becomes turbid should be submitted for culture.* Feces can be obtained by means of digital examination (be careful not to initiate severe tenesmus); the fecal sample should be placed in Ames transport medium for aerobic culture* (10% feces). Aerobic organisms that may be significant in foals with diarrhea include all *Salmonella* organisms, some *E. coli, Aeromonas hydrophila, Yersinia enterocolitica,* and *Campylobacter, Streptococcus,* and *Pseudomonas* organisms. *Salmonella*-selective medium and selenite enrichment medium should both be used for fecal cultures. CBC usually reveals neutropenia with a left shift, toxic changes in the neutrophils, and a high-normal to increased fibrinogen value. A low platelet count suggests a secondary coagulopathy, disseminated intravascular coagulation (DIC). "Fluidy" feces may be collected by passing a small rubber tube.

ELECTROLYTES AND CHEMISTRIES

Acidosis, hypochloremia, hyponatremia, and azotemia are the most common findings. If the azotemia is caused in part by intrinsic renal failure, the potassium level may be high. If the diarrhea has been present for more than 24 hours and renal function is normal, especially if bicarbonate-dextrose has been administered, *life-threatening hypokalemia could be present.*

Treatment

The emphasis is on fluid therapy, antibiotics, and good nursing care.

FLUID THERAPY

- Any balanced electrolyte product is acceptable, but a polyionic fluid is preferred over normal saline solution, which is an acidifying fluid. Use hypertonic saline solution only if polyionic fluids are unsuccessful in correcting clinically apparent or measurable hypotension.

NOTE: If hyponatremia is severe (<115 mEq/L), administer 1-2 ml/kg hypertonic saline solution as a bolus at 30-minute intervals until serum sodium concentration is 125-130 mEq/L but *no higher.*

NOTE: Severe hyponatremia can cause seizures.

---

*Use Campy Thio transport medium for *Campylobacter.*

- Potassium chloride (20 mEq/L) should be added to the fluids once urination is documented or if the plasma potassium concentration is less than 3.5 mEq/L!
- If the foal remains severely depressed and acidotic in spite of polyionic fluid therapy, administer isotonic sodium bicarbonate (1.25% solution or 12.5 g baking soda per liter sterile water). If sodium bicarbonate therapy is used, add additional KCl (20-40 mEq/L).
- One liter or preferably more liters of equine plasma with antibodies against lipopolysaccharide should be administered. The plasma is helpful not only in combating endotoxemia and DIC but also in improving the cardiodynamic effect gained from the administration of polyionic fluids.

ANTIBIOTIC THERAPY
- Ticarcillin–clavulanic acid, 44 mg/kg IV q6h, and amikacin,* 18 mg/kg IV q24h, or ceftiofur, 5 mg/kg IV q8h, and amikacin are appropriate antimicrobial treatment for salmonellosis in foals. *The use of effective antibiotics administered at high doses early in the disease is extremely important.*

ANTIULCER PROPHYLAXIS AND THERAPY
- Ranitidine, 1.5 mg/kg IV or 6.6 mg/kg PO q8h; famotidine, 0.7 mg/kg IV q24h or 2.8 mg/kg PO q24h; or omeprazole (GastroGard), 2-4 mg/kg PO q24h.
- Sucralfate, 2 g PO q6h, preferably 30-60 minutes before the administration of the preceding antiulcer medications.

ADDITIONAL THERAPY
- *If, and only if,* the foal has clinical or laboratory findings that suggest life-threatening endotoxemia, administer 0.25 mg/kg of flunixin meglumine after fluid therapy has been initiated.
- Carprofen, 1.5 mg/kg PO q24h, can be used to manage septic arthritis and is believed to be less ulcerogenic than flunixin meglumine.

NURSING CARE
- *Examine joints to detect early evidence of septic arthritis or physitis and monitor for lameness.*
- Place a plastic bag on the base of the tail using Elasticon, *wrapped loosely,* with a separate strip extending dorsally over the midsacral area. *Do not use Vetwrap or apply the Elasticon too tightly.* Clean the perineal area and apply petroleum jelly.
- If the foal is colicky, administer dipyrone (5-10 ml IV), butorphanol (4-6 mg IM/IV), xylazine (0.6-1.0 mg/kg IV or IM), ketoprofen, or flunixin. Limit the number of times these drugs are administered! Lidocaine can also be used.
- Apply a topical ophthalmic corticosteroid and atropine (1%) to the eye four to six times daily if uveitis is apparent and *if there is no corneal ulcer.*
- Do not separate the mare and foal. It is probable that the mare is already feces culture–positive for *Salmonella,* and the stress of separation could be detrimental to both.

---

*Do not administer the amikacin at the loading dose of 22 mg/kg until the foal has been observed to urinate a normal amount.

ROTAVIRUS DIARRHEA

Rotavirus (group A) is the most common infectious cause of diarrhea. As a rule, several foals in a barn are affected over several days. *The diarrhea is watery, yellow to yellowish-green, and has a characteristic pungent smell.* Onset of infection and clinical disease varies from a couple of days to several weeks. Individual foals may be several months of age. Affected foals are frequently seen to be depressed and not nursing normally before diarrhea is noticed. After the diarrhea begins, the foal's attitude may become more alert and the foal may nurse more vigorously. If dehydration or severe acidosis (bicarbonate level <18 mEq/L) develops, the foal becomes more depressed. Mild abdominal pain may be noted early in the disease; signs of pain (odontoprisis/bruxism, rolling, and ptyalism) later in the course of the diarrhea suggest gastric ulcer.

Diagnosis

- The history, age, and clinical findings are important in making a clinical diagnosis.
- Collect feces in a cup and submit the sample to a laboratory for enzyme-linked immunosorbent assay (ELISA) for the viral antigen. (Foals that have had the disease for several days may have negative test results.)
- Monitor CBC and electrolytes if the foal becomes depressed or if the diarrhea has been present for several days. Immature neutrophils and toxic changes within the neutrophils are not characteristic of rotavirus infection and suggest a more severe disease (e.g., necrotizing enterocolitis or salmonellosis). Hypochloremia, hyponatremia, hypokalemia, and acidosis may develop, and these indicate a need for fluid therapy.
- *Foal heat diarrhea is common among 7- to 12-day-old foals and should be considered a differential diagnosis for diarrhea in the case of a bright and alert foal of this age.*

Treatment

In general, treatment may not be needed if the foal is bright and alert and has normal electrolyte levels and an immunoglobulin G level >800 mg/dl (in foals younger than 10 days of age).

- Bismuth subsalicylate, 1-2 oz (30-60 ml) q6h through a dose syringe, may be of some medical value.
- If the foal is depressed and not nursing, administer 500-750 ml of warm electrolyte solution through a nasogastric tube. Examine the tube for gastric reflux and administer the electrolyte solution only by gravity flow (funnel). Commercial electrolyte replacers with only glucose, glycine, Na, K, and Cl, such as Resorb and Ion-aid, are preferred. These should be mixed so they are nearly isotonic (300 mmol/L).
- If the foal is still colicky, markedly depressed, or has significant electrolyte abnormalities, administer intravenous fluid therapy, 20 ml/kg of lactated Ringer's solution with 20 mEq/L KCl or another balanced electrolyte solution two to four times daily, depending on the severity of the diarrhea and the clinical condition of the foal.
- Administer antiulcer medication (see p. 210) to all foals that need intravenous therapy or repeated administration of oral fluids. Provide electrolyte fluids and free water.

■ Lactose tablets may be administered several times per day.

Measures to Prevent Spread of Disease

■ Isolate all affected foals.
■ Enter the patient's stall last during daily treatment or cleaning and instruct all personnel to do the same.
■ Place a foot bath with a newer generation of quaternary ammonium or hypochlorite outside the stall and wear boots and coveralls when entering the stall.
■ Wash hands with disinfectant soaps.
■ Keep pets and birds away from the stall.

| **NOTE:** Other unidentified infectious viral diarrheal diseases in foals are likely.

■ Consider prophylactic vaccination of mares to provide partial protection to foals, decrease the incidence of disease, and attenuate the clinical signs in nursing foals.

CRYPTOSPORIDIA

Cryptosporidium parvum–associated diarrhea occurs in catabolic foals being treated for other illnesses. *C. parvum* also can cause diarrhea in older nursing foals and sometimes appears without identifiable stress factors. In severe cases, electrolyte abnormalities and volume depletion can cause death. The diagnosis can be made when results of a fecal flotation test performed with a saturated sugar solution show several 4.5- to 5.5-μm-diameter oocysts. Submit a fresh sample and a sample in 10% formalin to a parasitology laboratory for confirmation because experience is helpful in the microscopic identification of the oocyst.[*]

Treatment

Treatment is generally supportive. Fluid and electrolyte replacement therapy and ulcer prophylaxis are as discussed for rotavirus diarrhea. Paromomycin, 100 mg/kg, administered PO q24h for 5 days, can be given, but efficacy is unproved in the treatment of foals. A concentrated hypochlorite solution is reported to be the disinfectant of choice. The organism can be killed with steam heat. Cleaning the stall is very important, because reinfection can occur. Most transmission is from foal to foal and not from the mare.

Hand washing should be adhered to strictly because the zoonotic potential is real.

ENTEROTOXIGENIC *ESCHERICHIA COLI*

E. coli (both pili- and enterotoxin-positive) can cause diarrhea in young foals (usually 2-3 weeks of age). Documented cases are rare, and the infection commonly affects one foal on a farm.

---

[*]*Eimeria* and *Giardia* organisms may be found in the feces of foals and adults, but there is no proof that they are pathogenic to horses.

Clinical Signs

- Watery diarrhea
- Moderate to severe depression
- Acidosis
- No fever in most instances
- Signs of gastric ulceration in a large number of cases

Diagnosis

Submit feces for rotavirus detection (ELISA), electron microscopic examination, aerobic cultures, and parasite examination for *Cryptosporidia* organisms. A heavy growth of mucoid *E. coli* should be submitted to a laboratory that can test the organism for adhesion and enterotoxin.

Treatment

- Similar to treatment for other causes of foal diarrhea.
- Intravenous fluids (lactated Ringer's solution supplemented with KCl and plasma in early stages).
- If the foal becomes severely acidotic, depressed, and stops nursing, administer isotonic bicarbonate (1.25% solution or 12 g mixed in 1 L sterile water) with 20-40 mEq/L of KCl IV.
- Administer prophylactic antiulcer medication (see p. 210).
- Give affected foals a broad-spectrum antibiotic (e.g., ceftiofur, 2.2-6.6 mg/kg IV q12h).

FETAL DIARRHEA

In utero diarrhea in the newborn foal with obvious staining of the amnionic fluid at birth is not unusual. Affected foals are depressed, may have signs of sepsis, and are at high risk of aspiration pneumonia from the meconium-stained amnionic fluid. Fecal cultures do not show a uniform pathogen. Foals with obvious sepsis should have their blood cultured.

Treatment

- Suction the trachea to remove the meconium fluid.
- Suction should only be for short intervals, 10-15 seconds at a time, to prevent iatrogenic hypoxemia.
- Administer broad-spectrum antibiotics (as for *Salmonella*, see p. 265).
- Administer polyionic fluids and plasma.
- If respiratory signs develop or worsen 24-48 hours after birth and aspiration of meconium amnionic fluid has occurred, administer dexamethasone, 0.1-0.25 mg/kg, or hydrocortisone at 2 mg/kg/IV to reduce the chemical pneumonitis. A lower-dose therapy should be continued for 2-3 days if there is improvement from the initial treatment.

■ L. DIARRHEA IN WEANLINGS AND YEARLINGS

Thomas J. Divers

RHODOCOCCUS EQUI

Rhodococcus equi causes diarrhea in foals 3 weeks of age up to yearlings. The diarrheal syndrome may or may not be associated with *R. equi* pneumonia in younger foals (<4 months of age). Septic physitis or arthritis may accompany the diarrhea, and abdominal abscessation also occurs in affected foals.

Diagnosis

Diagnosis can be difficult! If there are a large number of *R. equi* organisms, such as more than 10^5 per gram of feces or more than 100 colonies per plate from a swab of feces taken from the affected foal, and other known causes are ruled out a tentative diagnosis of *R. equi* diarrhea can be made. Additional documentation of the organism as the pathogen can be based on the presence of specific antigens associated with virulence (85-kbp plasmid and associated 15- to 17-kd antigens). Serologic testing is probably of little or no positive predictive value in the diagnosis of *R. equi* diarrhea. A negative result may help rule out the disease.

Treatment

- Administer erythromycin stearate, phosphate, or estolate, 25 mg/kg q8h PO, and rifampin, 5 mg/kg q12h PO. If there is evidence of systemic involvement (e.g., septic physitis), azithromycin, 10 mg/kg q24h PO for 5 days followed by a regimen of every-other-day (EOD) or every-third-day (ETD) treatment for an extended period may be used as a substitute for erythromycin.
- Administer intravenous fluids (e.g., lactated Ringer's solution), with 20 mEq/L KCl to replace the fluid and electrolyte loss.
- Administer plasma (2-4 L), with antibody directed against endotoxin, to valuable foals or foals with severe hypoalbuminemia. This therapy improves the efficacy of the polyionic fluids and may provide additional protection against endotoxemia.
- Administer medication to prevent or manage gastric ulceration (see p. 210).
- Apply a topical corticosteroid ophthalmic ointment and 1% atropine ointment to the eyes if *nonulcerative* uveitis is evident. This is most commonly detected by a green discoloration of the iris.

Prognosis

- Variable. Guarded to poor if arthritis, physitis, or abdominal abscessation is present. Otherwise, fair to good with appropriate treatment. Foals that have weight loss preceding the diarrhea have a more guarded and often grave prognosis if mesenteric abscessation is present.

ANTIBIOTIC-INDUCED DIARRHEA

Antibiotic-induced diarrhea is most commonly associated with oral administration of trimethoprim-sulfamethoxazole products or *erythromycin*. Nursing foals generally tolerate erythromycin well, but weanlings and older horses occasionally have severe "gaseous" colic, diarrhea, and toxemia associated with its administration. *Most cases of antibiotic-induced diarrhea occur 2-6 days after administration of the drug is begun.* The condition does not seem to be related to the brand or preparation of erythromycin or trimethoprim-sulfamethoxazole used.

Clinical Signs

- Colic usually precedes the diarrhea with moderate to severe gaseous distention of the bowel and abdomen.
- Signs and findings of toxemia (scleral injection, tachycardia, cold extremities) can be severe!
- The diarrhea often is fetid but may not be different from that of salmonellosis.

Laboratory Findings

- Clinical pathologic findings are nonspecific and often include elevations of PCV, blood urea nitrogen, and creatinine.
- Serum sodium and chloride values are decreased, and the bicarbonate value may be low depending on the severity of the disease.
- The neutrophil count may be decreased or increased, but toxic changes can be seen in the neutrophils.
- Submit fecal samples for *Salmonella* and *Rhodococcus* culture and for *C. difficile* and *C. perfringens* culture and toxin assay (see p. 261). Despite the suspicion that *C. difficile* or *C. perfringens* often is involved in antibiotic-induced diarrhea, this organism or toxin in the feces of affected individuals is found only sporadically.

Treatment

- Control abdominal pain with dipyrone, 22 mg/kg IV, and butorphanol, 0.05 mg/kg IM or IV, administered after xylazine, 0.5-1.0 mg/kg. Limit the number of times these drugs are used.
- Administer intravenous fluids: *Any polyionic fluid is adequate. Volume is the most important consideration*; add KCl at 20 mEq/L unless
  □ Oliguria is present
  □ Creatinine concentration is >5 mg/dl
  □ Potassium concentration is >5.0 mEq/L.
  □ Bicarbonate is generally not needed and is administered if the foal is very depressed or the bicarbonate concentration is <16 mEq/L. Isotonic sodium bicarbonate can be prepared by mixing 12.5 g of baking soda in 1 L of sterile water; 20-40 mEq KCl usually is added to each L of bicarbonate. If 0.9% NaCl is used, it can cause acidosis. Hypertonic NaCl (4 ml/kg) can be administered in a single dose if severe hypotension is present.
- Administer plasma, 1-2 L IV, to improve hemodynamics and alleviate the effect of endotoxin-derived mediators of septic shock. More than 2 L may be needed for severe hypoalbuminemia and edema.
- Administer flunixin meglumine, 0.25 mg/kg, if there are clinical signs or laboratory findings suggestive of severe endotoxemia.
- Administer sucralfate, 2-4 g q6h, to foals receiving NSAIDs and weanling foals with severe diarrhea.
- Administer antiulcer medication (see p. 210).
- Administer metronidazole, 15 mg/kg PO q8h. Recommended only for antibiotic-induced colitis. If no improvement occurs within 3 days, discontinue the treatment.

SALMONELLOSIS

Weanlings with salmonellosis are treated the same way as foals with salmonellosis (see p. 263). *Yearlings* are treated as adults (see pp. 254 and 263), except enrofloxacin is more frequently used.

Lawsonia Intracellularis

Lawsonia intracellularis infection is a chronic cause of diarrhea and weight loss in 4- to 10-month-old foals. This should be considered in the differential diagnosis of weanling diarrhea when there is clinical evidence of chronic disease.

Diagnosis

- Fecal PCR (sensitivity is not high) or serologic testing (Purdue or University of Minnesota) may be helpful.

Treatment

- Tetracycline 6.6 mg/kg q24h IV, erythromycin 25 mg/kg q8h PO, or azithromycin 10 mg/kg q24h PO for 5 days followed by every-other-day treatment for 2 weeks. Supportive therapy, including plasma and good quality, easily digestible food (complete feed), is very important.

Acute Strongyle Migration

Acute strongyle migration causes fever, diarrhea, and colic in young foals when large numbers of L4 larvae penetrate the bowel wall. Diagnosis is difficult because results of fecal examination may be negative. Rule out other causes of diarrhea and fever, a history of heavy parasite exposure, and response to treatment with ivermectin.

| **CAUTION:** Do not use moxidectin to treat young foals!

Potomac Horse Fever

In areas known to harbor *E. risticii*, weanlings with fever or diarrhea should be tested serologically (immunofluorescence assay) and with PCR (EDTA sample) for PHF. The disease is believed rare in weanlings.

Treatment

- See p. 256.

REFERENCES

General
Mair T, Divers T, Ducharme N: *Manual of equine gastroenterology,* London, 2002, WB Saunders.

Colic
Baxter G: The steps in assessing a colicky horse, *Vet Med* 87:1012-1018, 1992.
Spurlock S, Ward M: Fluid therapy for acute abdominal disease. In White N, editor: *The equine acute abdomen,* Philadelphia, 1990, Lea & Febiger.
Steckel R: Diagnosis and management of acute abdominal pain (colic). In Auer J, editor: *Equine surgery,* Philadelphia, 1992, WB Saunders.
White N: Examination and diagnosis of the acute abdomen. In White N, editor: *The equine acute abdomen,* Philadelphia, 1990, Lea & Febiger.
White N, Moore J: Treatment of endotoxemia. In White N, editor: *The equine acute abdomen,* Philadelphia, 1990, Lea & Febiger.

Mouth and Salivation
Hintz HF: Mold, mycotoxins and mycotoxicosis, *Vet Clin North Am Equine Pract* 6:419-431, 1990.
Kim L, Morley PS, McCluskey BJ et al: Oral vesicular lesions in horses without evidence of vesicular stomatitis virus infection, *J Am Vet Med Assoc* 216:1399-1404, 2000.
Turnquist SE et al: Foxtail-induced ulcerative stomatitis outbreak in a Missouri stable, *J Vet Diagn Invest* 13:238-240, 2001.

Esophagus
Whitehair KJ et al: Esophageal obstruction in horses, *Compend Contin Educ Pract Vet* 12:91-96, 1990.

Stomach

Murray MJ: Endoscopic appearance of gastric lesions in foals: 94 cases (1987-1988), *J Am Vet Med Assoc* 195:1135-1141, 1989.

Murray MJ: Gastric ulceration in horses: 91 cases (1987-1990), *J Am Vet Med Assoc* 201:117-120, 1992.

Murray MJ, Nout YS, Ward DL: Endoscopic findings of the gastric antrum and pylorus in horses: 162 cases (1996-2000), *J Vet Intern Med* 15:401-406, 2001.

Sanchez LC, Lester GD, Merritt AM: Intragastric pH in critically ill neonatal foals and the effects of ranitidine, *J Am Vet Med Assoc* 218:907-911, 2001.

Small Intestine

Doran R, Allen D, Orsini J: Small intestine. In Auer J, editor: *Equine surgery,* Philadelphia, 1992, WB Saunders.

Hance S et al: Intra-abdominal hernias in horses, *Compend Contin Educ Pract Vet* 13:293-298, 1991.

Mueller P, Parks A, Baxter G: Small intestinal diseases of horses: diagnosis and surgical intervention, *Vet Med* 87:1030-1036, 1992.

Large Intestine

Gaughan E, Hackett R: Cecocolic intussusception in horses: 11 cases (1979-1989), *J Am Vet Med Assoc* 197:1373, 1990.

Harrison I: Equine large intestinal volvulus: a review of 124 cases, *Vet Surg* 17:77-81, 1988.

Kalsbeek H: Further experiences with non-surgical correction of nephrosplenic entrapment of the left colon in the horse, *Equine Vet J* 21:442-443, 1989.

Ross M, Hanson R: Large intestine. In Auer J, editor: *Equine surgery,* Philadelphia, 1992, WB Saunders.

Small Colon and Rectum

Murray R, Green E, Constantinescu G: Equine enterolithiasis, *Compend Contin Educ Pract Vet* 14:1104-1112, 1992.

Ruggles A, Ross MW: Medical and surgical management of small colon impaction in horses: 28 cases (1984-1989), *J Am Vet Med Assoc* 199:1762-1766, 1991.

Colic in the Late-term Pregnant Mare

Boening KJ, Leendertse IP: Review of 115 cases of colic in the pregnant mare, *Equine Vet J* 25:518-521, 1993.

Santschi EM et al: Types of colic and frequency of postcolic abortion in pregnant mares: 105 cases (1984-1988), *J Am Vet Med Assoc* 199:374-377, 1991.

Peritonitis

Hawkins J et al: Peritonitis in horses: 67 cases (1985-1990). *J Am Vet Med Assoc* 203:284-288, 1993.

Diarrheal Diseases

Durando MM, Mackay RJ, Stalley LA: Effects of polymyxin B and *Salmonella typhimurium* antiserum on horses given endotoxin intravenously, *Am J Vet Res* 55:921-927, 1994.

Vaverud V, and others: *Clostridium difficile* associated with acute colitis in mares when their foals are treated with erythromycin and rifampicin for *Rhodococcus equi* pneumonia, *Equine Vet J* 30:482-488, 1998.

Weese JS: Clostridial colitis in adult horses and foals: a prospective study. In *Proceedings of the 47th annual convention of the American Association of Equine Practitioners,* 2001.

Cantharidin Intoxication

Schmitz DG: Cantharidin toxicosis in horses, *J Vet Intern Med* 3:208-215, 1989.

Diarrhea in Nursing Foals

Cohen ND, Snowden K: Cryptosporidial diarrhea in foals. In *Proceedings of the 13th annual veterinary medical forum of the American College of Veterinary Internal Medicine,* 1995.

Dwyer RM: Control and prevention of foal diarrhea outbreaks. In *Proceedings of the 47th annual convention of the American Association of Equine Practitioners*, 2001.

Lester GD: Infectious diarrhea in foals. In *Proceedings of the 47th annual convention of the American Association of Equine Practitioners*, 2001.

Diarrhea in Weanlings and Yearlings

Lavoie JP, Drolet R, Parsons D: Equine proliferative enteropathy: a cause of weight loss, colic, diarrhea, and hypoproteinemia in foals on three breeding farms in Canada, *Equine Vet J* 32:418-425, 2000.

Netherwood T, Wood JL, Townsend HG: Foal diarrhea between 1991 and 1994 in the United Kingdom associated with *Clostridium perfringens, rotavirus, Strongyloides westeri*, and *Cryptosporidium* spp, *Epidemiol Infect* 117:375-383, 1996.

Nordman P, Kersledjian JJ, Ronco L: Therapy of *Rhodococcus equi* disseminated infections, *Antimicrob Agents Chemother* 36:1244-1248, 1992.

36 Integumentary System

■ A. WOUND HEALING AND WOUND MANAGEMENT

Ted S. Stashak

THE SKIN

Anatomy

- The skin is one of the largest and most important organ systems.
- It is derived from two embryonic germ layers
  - □ Epidermis from ectoderm has the ability to regenerate.
  - □ Dermis (corium) from mesoderm cannot completely regenerate.
- The primary function is to protect and maintain homeostasis of the underlying structures.

EPIDERMIS

- Epidermis is made up of five stratified squamous cell layers (Fig. 36-1).
- Nourishment is by diffusion of fluids from the capillary beds in the dermis
- Stratum basale (base layer) has two nucleated cell types:
  - □ Keratinocytes constantly reproduce and push upward toward the surface to replace cells that have sloughed off the surface.
  - □ Melanocytes are responsible for producing the melanin that gives hair and skin their color.
- Stratum spinosum (prickle-cell layer): Cells in this layer are nucleated and become activated to reproduce when the outer epidermal layers are stripped off.
- Stratum granulosum (granular cell layer): Composed of cells that are in the process of dying with nuclei that are shrinking and undergoing chromatolysis.
- Stratum lucidum (clear cell layer): Composed of nonnucleated keratinized cells and is only present in hairless areas of the body.
- Stratum corneum (horny cell layer): Composed of fully keratinized dead cells that are constantly being shed from the surface as scales. This layer forms a

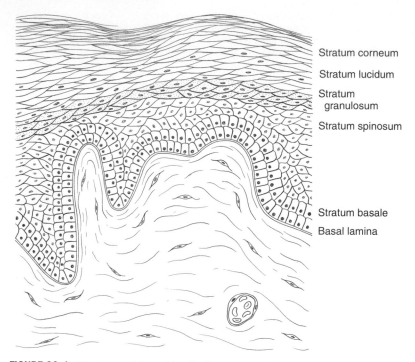

Stratum corneum

Stratum lucidum

Stratum granulosum

Stratum spinosum

Stratum basale

Basal lamina

FIGURE 36-1. The layers of the epidermis. The stratum spinosum and stratum basale are collectively referred to as the stratum germinativum. (From Stashak TS: Wound healing. In Jenning PB, editor: *The practice of large animal surgery,* Philadelphia, 1984, WB Saunders.)

barrier that protects the underlying tissue from irritation, invasion of bacteria and noxious substances, and fluid and electrolyte losses.

DERMIS
- Papillary layer, lies below the epidermis
- Reticular layer, extends from the papillary layer down to the subcutaneous tissue.
- Contains a rich supply of blood vessels, lymphatics, hair follicles, sebaceous and apocrine sweat glands, and sensory nerve endings (Fig. 36–2)
- Fiber types: Collagenous, reticular, and elastic
- Cell types: Fibroblasts, histiocytes, and mast cells

WOUND HEALING
Phases
- Inflammation
- Debridement
- Repair
- Maturation

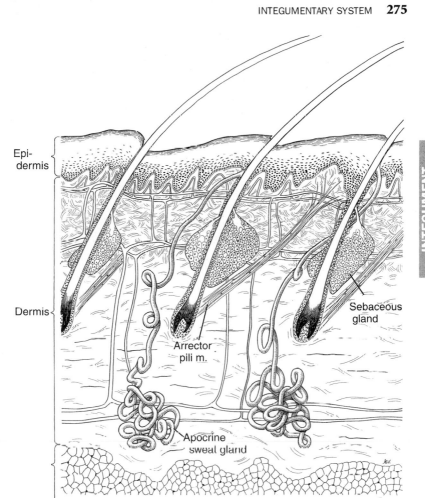

Epi-
dermis {

Dermis {

Sebaceous
gland

Arrector
pili m.

Apocrine
sweat gland

Subcutaneous fatty tissue

FIGURE 36-2. The anatomy of the skin.

INFLAMMATORY PHASE

- Acute response affected by the severity of the injury.
- Characterized by a vascular and cellular response that protects the body against excessive blood loss and invasion of foreign substances.
- Fibrocellular clot that develops maintains internal hemostasis and forms a scaffold for repair. Dehydrates superficially to form a scab, which acts like a bandage to protect the wound from external contamination.
- Factors affecting duration:
    - Degree of trauma
    - Nature of injury
    - Foreign substances (foreign bodies)

   □ Infection
- *Treatment with nonsteroidal antiinflammatory drugs (NSAIDs), proper cleansing, and debridement of the wound and selection of appropriate antibiotics can influence the duration.*

DEBRIDEMENT PHASE
- Neutrophils and monocytes chemotactically stimulated by leukotaxine and a lymph node–promoting factor that migrate into the wound and begin the cleanup process.
- Primary functions of neutrophil
  - □ Ingestion of microorganisms by phagocytosis
  - □ Lysosomal enzymes contribute to the inflammatory response
  - □ Aid the mononuclear cells in further breakdown of dead tissues
- Monocytes
  - □ Become macrophages on entering the wound
  - □ Phagocytize dead tissues and debris
- Important functions of monocyte
  - □ Produce many growth factors
  - □ *Attract fibroblasts into the wound* and may stimulate them to undergo maturation for collagen synthesis
- Duration depends on amount of devitalized tissue, the degree of contamination, and whether infection develops.
- Clinicians have the most influence on this phase. Consequently proper *surgical debridement and wound lavage, good hemostasis, and adequate drainage can greatly hasten wound healing.*

REPAIR PHASE
EPITHELIALIZATION
- Basal cells of the epidermis begin to separate, duplicate, and migrate toward areas of cell deficit.
- Epithelial cells migrate under the scab and detach it by secreting proteolytic enzymes.
- Epithelial cells continue to migrate on the surface of a wound until like cells are contacted.
- The scab falls off when epithelialization is complete.
- Basal cells begin to reproduce to restore the normal thickness of the epidermis.
- Important factors that arrest epithelialization include:
  - □ Infection
  - □ Excessive production of granulation tissue
  - □ Repeated dressing changes
  - □ Extreme hypothermia
  - □ Desiccation of the wound surface
  - □ Reduction in oxygen tension
- Epithelialization can be accelerated by the application of certain growth factors and topical antimicrobial agents (e.g., triple antibiotic ointment) and by the use of semiocclusive dressings (e.g., Telfa).

FIBROPLASIA
- Fibroblasts advance along the previously formed fibrin lattice within the clot and begin secreting the ground substance.

- Collagen is synthesized by the fibroblasts predominantly from hydroxyproline and hydroxylysine.
- Immature tropocollagen fibrils bind together to form a mature collagen fiber.
- As collagen increases, the ground substance decreases, and wound strength improves with maturity.

GRANULATION TISSUE

- Result of proliferating capillaries that form vascular loops.
- Vascular loops grow behind the fibroblasts and form multiple anastomoses.
- Lymphatics develop at a slower rate.
- *Granulation tissue* formation in an open wound is beneficial.
  - Provides a surface for epithelial cells to migrate over
  - Is resistant to infection
  - The process of wound contraction is centered around its development
  - Carries the fibroblast responsible for collagen formation
- *Healing of wounds in the distal extremities of horses is rapid and excessive, tending toward abnormal repair, which can result in exuberant granulation tissue formation.*

WOUND CONTRACTION

- Wound contraction is a process whereby an open skin wound reduces in size by centripetal movement of the full thickness skin toward the wound's center (Fig 36–3).
- It is independent of epithelialization.
- Modified fibroblasts called *myofibroblasts cause contractile properties of skin.* These are found in granulation tissue adjacent to the wound.

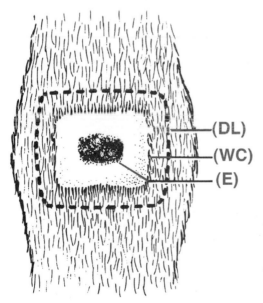

FIGURE 36–3. Illustration of wound contraction. The dashed line *(DL)* indicates the original size of the wound. *(WC)* indicates the extent of the wound contraction and *(E)* represents the extent of epithelialization.

INTEGUMENT

- This works best where the skin is relatively loose. In these areas, wound contraction usually is sufficient to bring about complete closure of the wound with minimal scar formation.
- Where skin is under tension, a wider scar forms.
- Contraction stops when:
  □ Contact inhibition of like cells occurs
  □ Tension of surrounding skin equilibrates with pulling forces of contraction
  □ Exuberant granulation tissue impedes the wound's ability to contract
  □ Full thickness skin grafts are applied to the wound before the fifth day of healing
  □ Carbon dioxide (CO_2) laser excision or debridement of a wound reduces myofibroblast function and numbers, resulting in delayed wound contraction

MATURATION PHASE
- Characterized by a reduction in fibroblast numbers with an equilibration of collagen production and collagen lysis. Functionally oriented collagen fibers begin to predominate as nonfunctional ones are dissolved. Despite the reduction in fibroblasts, blood vessels, and collagen fibrils, the tensile strength of the wound increases.
- Wound tensile strength results from:
  □ Alignment of collagen along lines of tension, collagen cross-linking
  □ Formation of more collagen contact bundles

NOTE: Skin grafts may be useful in wounds that exceed epithelialization and wound contraction.

SELECTED FACTORS THAT AFFECT WOUND HEALING
Anemia and Blood Loss
- Normovolemic anemia unrelated to malnutrition or chronic disease does not appear to affect wound healing until the packed cell volume (PCV) drops below 12%.
- Hypovolemic anemia due to blood loss with vasoconstriction can impair wound healing. Reduced oxygen tension renders the wound more susceptible to infection by altering phagocytic mechanisms.
- Wound healing should progress normally if the following are corrected:
  □ Anemia with PCV <12%
  □ Chronic infection
  □ Malnutrition
  □ Hypovolemia

Malnutrition and Protein Deficiency
WOUND HEALING
- Impaired with mild to moderate short- or long-term protein-energy malnutrition
- The direction in which the patient is moving metabolically (positive or negative) at the time of injury or surgery is very important.
- Hypoproteinemia adversely affects wound healing by impairing the following:
  □ Fibroplasia
  □ Neoangiogenesis
  □ Wound remodeling
  □ Wound tensile strength

- *Plasma protein concentration <6 g/dl results in markedly retarded healing.*
- Impairment in wound healing is easily reversed with adequate nutrition.

RECOMMENDATIONS
- Offer balanced nutrition in sufficient amounts before elective surgery and/or after wounding and emergency surgery.
- Feeding DL-methionine to protein-deficient patients reverses the retardation in wound healing. DL-Methionine converts to cysteine, which serves as an important cofactor in collagen synthesis and disulfide cross-linking as collagen matures.
- Generally vitamin deficiencies are not a problem. Exception: When the patient is chronically debilitated and undernourished, consider vitamin supplementation.

Nonsteroidal Antiinflammatory Drugs
- Because inflammation is a part of the wound-healing process, it is logical that antiinflammatory drugs such as phenylbutazone, aspirin, indomethacin, and flunixin meglumine would affect wound healing.
- These drugs are useful because they:
  - Diminish pain from inflammation
  - Improve overall well-being
  - Encourage ambulation, resulting in improved circulation
  - Reduce the adverse effect of endotoxins on wound healing
- *Recommendation: Administer the lowest dosage for the desired effect.*

Corticosteroids
- Administer in moderate to large amounts within the first 5 days after injury; these drugs markedly retard wound healing.
- Retard healing by stabilizing the lysosomal membrane, preventing release of enzymes responsible for initiating the inflammatory response.
- They also suppress:
  - Fibroplasia
  - Ground substance formation
  - Collagen formation
  - Capillary proliferation
  - Granulation tissue formation
- They also retard:
  - Wound contraction
  - Gain in tensile strength
  - Epithelialization

| **NOTE:** Corticosteroids have little effect when given 5 days after wounding.

Trauma
- Excessive trauma within the wound or from other sites (e.g., multiple lacerations or fractures):
  - Prolongs the early phase of healing
  - Decreases the gain in tensile strength
  - Makes the wound more susceptible to infection
  - Results in excessive scar production
- Delay in wound tensile strength is seen as long as 15 days after trauma

- Delay in gain of wound tensile strength is proportional to the degree of trauma
- *Tissue trauma can be reduced by:*
  - Debriding the wound completely
  - Reducing surgery time
  - Using isotonic or iso-osmolar lavage solutions
  - Maintaining hemostasis
  - Reducing fluid accumulation in tissues
  - Apposing tissues with the proper tension with nonreactive suture material
  - Administering systemic antibiotics and NSAIDs
  - If there is excessive blood loss, administering intravenous fluids improves capillary perfusion

Infection

- Wound infection is defined as the presence of replicating microorganisms within a wound with subsequent host injury. Whether infection develops or not depends on the following:
  - Dose of microorganisms
  - Virulence
  - Local and systemic factors
- Wound infection results when the number of organisms reaches a concentration of 10^6 organisms per gram of tissue or 10^6 organisms per milliliter of fluid.
- Virulence factors include:
  - Secretion of adhesions (causes adherence of host cells)
  - Formation of cell capsules, which protect against phagocytosis
  - Formation of a biofilm, which assures bacterial replication
  - Release of enzymes and toxins
- Contaminated wounds with lesser concentrations of organisms can become infected when:
  - Foreign bodies are present
  - Excessive necrotic tissue is left in the wound
  - Hematoma develops
  - Local tissue defenses are impaired (burn patients or immunosuppressed patients)
  - The vascular supply is altered
- Wounds contaminated with dirt have a higher risk of infection due to specific infection-potentiating fractions (IPFs) in the organic components and inorganic fractions. These IPFs:
  - Decrease the effect of white blood cells (WBCs)
  - Decrease humoral factors
  - Neutralize antibodies
  - As few as 100 organisms can cause infection
- Wounds contaminated with feces are highly susceptible to infection. Feces can contain as many as 10^{11} organisms per gram.

HOW INFECTION DELAYS HEALING

- Infection mechanically separates the wound edges with exudate
- It releases endotoxins, which inhibit growth factors and collagen production
- It reduces the vascular supply (a result of mechanical pressure and a tendency to form microthrombi in small vessels adjacent to the wound)
- It increases cellular responses with prolongation of the inflammatory and debridement phases of wound healing

- Bacteria also produce proteolytic enzymes that digest collagen
- *Bacterial injury results in cellular and vascular responses typical of inflammation*

NOTE: Wound infection rates develop in approximately 5% of equine surgical patients overall and nearly 2.5% of the patients undergoing clean elective procedures. These rates are similar to those reported in humans.

METHODS TO REDUCE INFECTION IN ELECTIVE SURGERY
- Reduce the depth of anesthesia. Excessive depth of anesthesia leads to reduced tissue perfusion, which results in reduced oxygen tension, acidosis, and impaired resistance to infection.
- Reduce the length of anesthesia. Prolonged anesthesia:
  □ Impairs the alveolar macrophage function
  □ Depresses neutrophil function and migration, chemotaxis of WBCs, and phagocytosis
  □ Increases wound infection rates 5% for each minute after 60 minutes of anesthesia
- *Do not clip the hair before surgery. Clipping the hair before induction of anesthesia has been shown to increase the infection rate.*
- Limit use of electrocautery. Excessive electrocautery can double infection rates.
- Decrease surgery time. Wound infection rates double after 90 minutes of surgery and nearly triple when surgery lasts more than 120 minutes.
  The use of propofol increases infection rates 3.8 times in clean wounds.
- Use aseptic technique.
- Meticulous hemostasis.
- Eliminate dead space and use suction drains if necessary.
- Select nonreactive sutures.
- Use proper suturing techniques.
- Antimicrobials are generally not needed if the patient is in good health and has adequate immune status, for short, clean procedures (<90 minutes), and in a clean environment.
- Antimicrobial agents generally are needed in cases of tissue ischemia and for surgery longer than 90 minutes.
  □ Administer less than 2 hours before surgery. IV is more predictable. Continue for 12 to 24 hours.
- Perioperative antibiotics administered within 2 hours of surgery and for 24 hours after surgery have a 2.2% infection rate compared to patients not receiving antibiotics who have a 4.4% infection rate. Patients receiving antibiotics longer than 24 hours postoperatively have a 6.3% infection rate compared to patients given postoperative antibiotics who only have an 8.2% infection rate.

METHODS TO REDUCE INFECTION IN A TRAUMATIC WOUND
- Proper wound preparation.
- Clipping the hair and shaving the area with a guarded razor. Be sure the wound is protected from contamination from hair clipping, dust, and dander.
- Copious lavage with sufficient pressure (at least 7 psi).
- Thorough debridement.
- Administration of the systemic antimicrobial agent(s) that has broad-spectrum coverage.
- Choose the agent on the basis of culture and sensitivity when applicable.
- Pulse dosing improves antibiotic penetration.
- Parenteral route recommended initially—IV preferred—; predictable.

INTEGUMENT

- IM absorption is prolonged and variable:
  - □ Depends on site selection
  - □ Exercise improves absorption
- Oral route after desired plasma level is achieved
- Antimicrobial choice
  - □ Superficial wounds—penicillin alone or in combination with trimethoprim—sulfa is usually effective
  - □ Deeper wounds including synovial structures—penicillin and an aminoglycoside (gentamicin or amikacin). The combination is synergistic. Ceftiofur or enrofloxacin are reserved for infections caused by bacteria that are resistant to penicillin and aminoglycosides
  - □ Deep fascial cellulitis/septic myositis due to Clostridia—high doses of penicillin and metronidazole, rifampin or ceftiofur.
  - □ Pyonecrotic processes—metronidazole and penicillin
- Duration of antimicrobial treatment:
  - □ Minimum course of 3-5 days
  - □ Established infections in:
    - □ Soft tissue, 7-10 days
    - □ Synovial tissue, 10-21 days
    - □ Bone, 3-4 months

TOPICAL ANTIBIOTICS

- Can retard wound healing, especially some ointments or creams (e.g., nitrofurazone [Furacin] and gentamicin cream).
- Solutions are most useful when applied to wounds before closure or as lavage solutions.
- Creams and ointments that remain in contact with the wound longer prevent desiccation of the wound surface and are best used under bandages and on exposed wounds.
- Topical antimicrobials are most effective when applied within 3 hours of the injury. However, if the wound is thoroughly debrided, thus creating a new wound, they can be applied within 3 hours of debridement and are considered effective.
- *Triple antibiotic ointment (TAO) (bacitracin, polymyxin B, and neomycin)*
  - □ Has a wide antimicrobial spectrum but is ineffective against *Pseudomonas aeruginosa.*
  - □ The zinc component of bacitracin stimulates epithelialization (a 25% increase) but can retard wound contraction.
  - □ These antimicrobials are poorly absorbed. Therefore toxicity is rare.
- *Silver sulfadiazine (SS)*
  - □ Has a wide antimicrobial spectrum, including *Pseudomonas* organisms and fungi.
  - □ Increases epithelialization 28% in some studies and in others it slows epithelialization.
  - □ Can cause wound fragility.
- *Nitrofurazone ointment (NO)*
  - □ Has a good antimicrobial spectrum against Gram-positive and Gram-negative organisms, but has little effect against *Pseudomonas* organisms.
  - □ Decreases epithelialization 24% and decreases wound contraction in horses.
  - □ The antibiotic nitrofurazone, not the vehicle, is responsible for the delay in wound healing.

- *Gentamicin sulfate (GS)*
  - □ Has a narrow antimicrobial spectrum but it may be applied to wounds infected with Gram-negative bacteria, particularly *P. aeruginosa*.
  - □ Treatment with 0.1% oil-in-water cream base slows wound contraction and epithelialization.
- *Cefazolin*
  - □ Effective against Gram-positive and some Gram-negative organisms.
  - □ When it is applied at 20 mg/kg, cefazolin yields a high-concentration wound fluid above minimal inhibitory concentration (MIC) for longer periods than does systemically administered cefazolin at the same dose.
  - □ The powder form provides a more sustained tissue concentration than does the solution. Because of this property, cefazolin may be effective in the management of established infections.

NOTE: Wounds with 10^9 microorganisms/g of tissue develop infection despite antibiotic treatment.

- Synovial lavage and drainage
  - □ Lavage with sterile salt solution (1-3 L) + 10% DMSO (1 L)
  - □ Arthroscopy/tenoscopy ± synovectomy
  - □ Arthrotomy
  - □ Closed suction drainage
  - □ Ingress/egress
- Intrasynovial injection of antimicrobials
  - □ Less than one systemic dose every 24 hours
  - □ The bactericidal effect of aminoglycosides is concentration dependent, as bacterial kill is proportional to the peak drug concentrations in the tissue. High peak concentrations are also associated with longer post antibiotic effect (PAE).
  - □ Amikacin, 250 mg every 24 hours; amikacin has good activity against equine orthopedic pathogens and resistance to amikacin is less likely compared to gentamicin.
  - □ Gentamicin, 150-250 mg every 24 hours; intraarticular administration of 150 mg of gentamicin results in peak concentrations of gentamicin of 4745 µg/ml compared to 5.1 µg/ml when administered systemically at 2.2 mg/kg. The concentration remains significantly higher than the MIC for *E. coli* for more than 24 hours. Gentamicin is effective against 85% of the bacterial isolates obtained from musculoskeletal infections in the horse.
  - □ Penicillin, 5 x 10^6 IU every 24 hours
  - □ Ceftiofur, 150 mg; intrasynovial (IA) treatment with 150 mg of ceftiofur results in synovial fluid concentrations that are significantly higher than those found after IV administration of 2.2 mg/kg. Synovial fluid concentration following IA administration remains above MIC for 24 hours; following IV administration MIC is maintained for only 8 hours.
- Regional limb perfusion (see Chapter 5, p. 16)
  - □ Allows delivery of an antimicrobial into ischemic tissue and exudates at very high concentrations; greater than that achieved by the parenteral route. Antimicrobial doses reported include:
    - □ Amikacin, 125-500 mg
    - □ Gentamicin, 500 mg-1g

NOTE: Doses in excess of 1 g may result in soft tissue sloughing and therefore 250 mg of amikacin or gentamicin is generally used clinically.

- The technique is primarily used for treatment of septic osteitis/osteomyelitis and for septic synovial structures of the distal extremities (below the carpus and tarsus). An Esmarch bandage is used to remove the blood and to prevent blood flow from the distal limb after which a tourniquet is placed proximal to the site of the infection. After the Esmarch bandage is removed, 60 ml of a sterile balanced electrolyte solution containing the antibiotic is delivered under pressure over a 1-10 minute period, either by the intraosseous or the intravenous route. The tourniquet is removed after 30 minutes.
- Intraosseous (IO) (see intraosseous infusion procedures, p. 15): A 4-mm diameter hole is drilled into the medullary cavity of the distal one third of the MC/MT-III. Then a centrally cannulated 5.5-mm ASIF cortical screw, with an IV adaptor welded to the top, or the male adaptor end of an IV delivery set is placed into the marrow cavity. If the screw is not self-tapping, a tap is used to create threads in the cortex before screw placement. If the male adaptor end of an IV set is used it can be wedged into the hole with needle holders using a to-and-fro rotating motion.
- Advantages to IO delivery:
  - Eliminates localization to a particular site and repeated venipuncture
  - Permits frequent local perfusion even in the standing horse
- Disadvantages of IO delivery:
  - Some leakage of the perfusate around the cortical hole particularly when the IV extension set method is used
  - A hole must be drilled in the medullary cavity
- Intravenous delivery involves placement of a 3.2-cm over-the-needle catheter in the lateral palmar/plantar digital vein at the level of the proximal sesamoid bone.
- Disadvantages of this technique are:
  - Vein identification can be difficult in cases of considerable swelling associated with the area.
  - Repeat IV injections or maintaining an IV catheter because there is the tendency to develop venous thrombosis
  - If there is excess swelling, a "cut-down" procedure is often needed to achieve access to the vein
- Antimicrobial impregnated beads
  - Increase the local concentration of an antimicrobial 200 times that achieved by systemic administration
  - Minimal inhibitory concentrations (MICs) exist for up to 80 days after implantation
  - Plasma concentrations do not reach toxic levels
- Biodegradable drug delivery systems are becoming available
- Poly (DL) lactide* ± co-glycolide flat discs + 500 mg of gentamicin (Boehringer Ingelheim).
  - An in vitro study of synovial explants infected with *S. aureus*
  - The discs released >500 µg/ml for 10 days
  - Infection was eliminated within 24 hours
  - Synovial morphology, viability, and function did not return to normal

---

*Poly (DL) lactide. Boehringer Ingelheim, Inc., Animal Health, 2621 North Belt Highway, St. Joseph, MI 64506.

□ May be useful in vivo in the future
- Gentamicin-impregnated collagen sponge + 130 mg of gentamicin* (Collatemp G/Schering Plough)
  □ Used commonly in humans for soft tissue surgery and injury with good results
  □ Higher concentrations of the antibiotic are achieved for 3 days (first day, 15 times; third day, 2 times) in wound exudates than with PMMA beads
  □ Collagen sponge is absorbed within 12-49 days depending on the vascular supply to the area.
  □ 7 of 8 horses with moderate to severe traumatic septic synovial structures (arthritis and tenosynovitis) responded to the treatment. The collagen sponges are implanted in the synovial space via the arthroscope cannula.
- Continuous intrasynovial infusion
  □ Catheter + balloon infuser placed in the tarsocrural joint.
  □ 17 of 24 remained functional.
  □ Gentamicin dosage 0.02-0.17 mg/kg/h results in concentrations 100 times the MIC for the common equine pathogens.

Antiseptics for Skin Preparation

- The two most commonly used surgical scrubs for skin preparation are povidone-iodine (Betadine) and chlorhexidine (Hibiclens).
- Rinsing with saline solution or 70% isopropanol does not make a difference in short-term antimicrobial effect.
- *Rinsing with 70% alcohol reduces the residual effect and antiseptic value of chlorhexidine.*
- A disadvantage of the use of povidone-iodine is skin reactions, particularly in small animals. An occasionally acute skin reaction occurs in horses treated with povidone-iodine but this is unusual.
  □ More common in the horse after clipping, scrubbing, and rinsing with 70% alcohol, spraying with povidone-iodine solution, and bandaging.
  □ Skin reactions include subcutaneous edema and skin wheal formation.
- A disadvantage to Hibiclens is that short exposure to the eye even in small concentrations results in corneal opacification and ocular toxicity.
- The mechanical effect of scrubbing the wound with antiseptic soaps can be helpful in removing debris and reducing bacterial concentration on the surface of the wound; smooth soft sponges are recommended. However, if the soap is not thoroughly rinsed from the wound, there is a marked delay in wound healing.

| **NOTE:** This is particularly true with Hibiclens.

Surgeon's Hand and Arm Preparation

- Hand cultures immediately following standard surgical hand preparation, and 4 hours in surgical gloves using alcohol (70% ethyl) and chlorhexidine (4%), serves as an effective surgical scrub with good residual properties. Povidone iodine has little residual benefit.
- Chlorhexidine preparations are superior.
  □ Povidone-iodine has poor prolonged effect.
  □ Triclosan is not effective in most experimental trials.

---

*Collatemp, Schering Plough. Animal Health Corp., 1095 Morris Avenue, Union, NJ 07083; (908) 629-3346.

□ 70% ethanol (V/V) shows low antibacterial function; 70% ethyl alcohol is preferred.

Antiseptics and Antibiotics for Wound Lavage

- *Bacteria adhere to the wound surface by an electrostatic charge. Lavage cleans the wound of debris and reduces the bacterial numbers and IPFs.*
- Lavage solutions are most effective when delivered by a fluid jet at an oblique angle on the wound using a minimum of 7 psi.
- This pulsatile pressure can be achieved by:
  □ Forcefully expressing lavage solutions from a 35-cc or 60-cc syringe through an 18-gauge needle
  □ Using a spray bottle
  □ A "Water Pik"
  □ Stryker InterPulse irrigation system*
  □ Pressure = to 7 psi *cannot* be achieved with gravity flow or lavage with a bulb syringe.
- Pressures of 10-15 psi have been shown to be approximately 80% effective in removing soil infection potentiating factors and adherent bacteria from a wound.
- The "Water Pik" delivers 40-50 ml/min at 10-15 psi at the low-intermediate setting and is most effective for heavily contaminated wounds. Pressures of 10-15 psi can also be achieved with a spray bottle.

CAUTION: Care must be taken so contaminants are not driven deeper within the wound and loose fascial planes are not inadvertently separated.

Antiseptics

POVIDONE-IODINE SOLUTION
- Commonly used to lavage wounds because of its broad antimicrobial spectrum against.
  □ Gram-positive and Gram-negative bacteria, fungi, and *Candida* organisms
  □ Bacterial resistance has not been identified
- Disadvantages:
  □ Inactivated by organic material and blood
  □ <0.1% concentration inactivated by a large number of neutrophils
  □ Concentrations >1% needed to kill *Staphylococcus aureus.*
- The free iodine gives the solution its antimicrobial activity, forms a complex with polyvinyl pyrrolidone to increase its stability, and reduce irritation and staining.
- The complexing tightly binds the iodine and reduces the free iodine for antimicrobial activity.
- Diluting the solution uncouples the bond, making more free iodine available for antimicrobial activity.

NOTE: Povidone-iodine solutions diluted to 0.1% and 0.2% (1-2 ml/1000 ml) concentrations are best for wound lavage.

CHLORHEXIDINE DIACETATE SOLUTION
- Chlorhexidine diacetate (CHD) solution has a broad antimicrobial spectrum.

---

*Stryker InterPulse irrigation system. Med-Vet Innovations, Inc., 1099 7th Street, Penrose, CO 81240; (719) 372-0490; email: medvet01@aol.com.

NOTE: CHD is not effective against fungi and *Candida* organisms, and *Proteus* and *Pseudomonas* organisms have developed or have an inherent resistance to CHD.

- Still commonly used as lavage solution.
- When CHD is applied to the intact skin, its antimicrobial effect is immediate and has a lasting residual effect caused by binding to protein in the stratum corneum.

NOTE: Currently, 0.05% CHD (1:40 dilution of 2% concentrate) solution is recommended for wound lavage. Greater concentrations can be harmful to wound healing.

- Disadvantages:
  - Avoid contact with eyes. Ocular toxicity is a concern
  - Full-strength CHD delays wound healing to a greater extent than does alcohol
  - >0.5% solutions inhibit epithelialization and granulation tissue formation
  - <0.05 % solutions result in significant survival of *S. aureus*

HYDROGEN PEROXIDE
- Common wound irrigant
  - Narrow antimicrobial spectrum
  - Has little value as an antiseptic
  - An effective sporicide
- 3% hydrogen peroxide is damaging to tissues and cytotoxic to fibroblasts
- It can cause thrombosis in the microvasculature adjacent to wound margins

NOTE: Hydrogen peroxide is not recommended for wound lavage

SODIUM HYPOCHLORITE 0.5% (DAKIN SOLUTION)
- Release of chlorine and oxygen kills bacteria
- More effective in killing *S. aureus* than are povidone-iodine and CHD
- Cytotoxic to fibroblasts
- Recommendation: Use at 0.25 strength (0.125%) for wound lavage

Antibiotics
- The addition of antibiotics to the lavage solution has been shown to markedly reduce the number of bacteria in a wound.
- Experimentally 1% neomycin is very effective in preventing infection in wounds contaminated with feces.
- *In a double-blind study of 260 sutured lacerations, penicillin sprayed on the wound before closure decreased the infection rate by 75%.*

NOTE: A biologically oriented surgeon never selects a solution to irrigate a wound that he is not willing to put in his conjunctival sac.

Amount of Fluid for Lavage
- Depends on the size of the wound and degree of contamination
- At minimum, the gross contaminants are removed
- Discontinue the lavage before the tissue becomes "water-logged"

Wound Debridement
- Debridement reduces the number of bacteria and removes the contaminants (e.g., dead tissue, foreign bodies) that alter the local defense mechanisms.

INTEGUMENT

- The standard approach is sharp debridement, which converts a contaminated wound to a clean wound. Types of debridement include:
  - Excisional
  - Simple or piecemeal
  - En bloc
- Laser
- Chemical debriding agents are available, however their effect on wound healing and reduction in the incidence of infection is unclear
- Debridement dressing includes:
  - Adherent open mesh gauze (e.g., 4 × 4 gauze sponges)
  - Wet-to-dry, using 4 × 4 mesh gauze or sheet cotton

NOTE: If exposed cortical bone is debrided to bleeding bone, granulation tissue proliferates from the surface.

Suturing Techniques and Suture Material
- Suturing and the material chosen influence wound healing
- Compared with simple continuous sutured skin wounds, simple interrupted sutured skin wounds have:
  - Less edema
  - Increased microcirculation
  - 30% to 50% greater tensile strength after 10 days

NOTE: Use interrupted sutures when impaired healing is anticipated and excessive tension is present.

- Simple interrupted sutures cause less inflammation than do vertical mattress and far-near/near-far patterns
- Loosely approximated wounds are stronger 7, 10, and 21 days postoperatively than are wounds tightly secured with sutures
- Recommendation:
  - Ensure that the wound edges are just apposed. Avoid overreduction of tissues

NOTE: Use a low number of sutures. Increasing the number of sutures increases risk of infection.

  - Deep suture only fascial planes, tendons, and ligaments.
  - Use tension suturing techniques when excessive tension is present (Fig. 36–4).
- Synthetic absorbable and nonabsorbable sutures cause less reaction than do surgical catgut, cotton, or natural silk sutures.
- Monofilament sutures are less reactive than are twisted and braided materials.

Hematoma and Seroma
- Collection of blood or serum in tissues delays healing by mechanically separating the wound.
- High expanding fluid pressure can alter the blood supply.
- Blood and serum are excellent media for bacterial growth.
- Hemoglobin inhibits local tissue defenses, and iron is necessary for bacterial replication. Ferric ion plays a role in increasing the virulence of bacteria.

Bandaging and Dressing
Bandaging is considered beneficial for the following reasons:

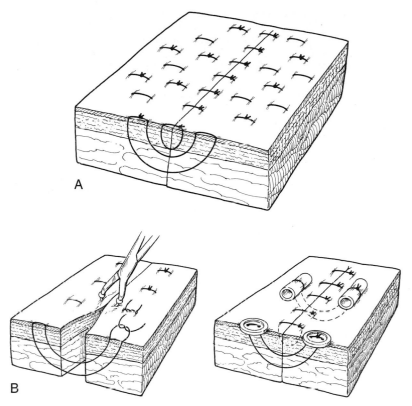

FIGURE 36-4. Tension suture patterns. **A,** Plain tension suturing technique with vertical mattress sutures. **B,** Quill tension suturing technique with vertical mattress sutures and supports. (From Stashak TS: *Equine wound management,* Philadelphia, 1991, Lea & Febiger.)

- The wound is protected from further contamination
- The pressure reduces edema
- Exudate is absorbed
- Bandages increase temperature and reduce CO_2 loss from the wound surface, thus reducing pH
- Bandages immobilize a part and reduce additional trauma (e.g., a wound on the dorsal surface of the hock)

Wound Dressings
Wound dressings are classified as adherent or nonadherent. Nonadherent dressings are further subdivided into semiocclusive and occlusive dressings.

ADHERENT DRESSINGS (WIDE MESH GAUZE)
- Beneficial when applied during the inflammatory and debridement phase
- Deleterious when used during the repair phase of wound healing
- Apply dry or wet

- □ Dry is used if wound fluids are of low viscosity
- □ Wet is applied if wound fluid has high viscosity or a scab has formed
- □ Sterile saline solution often is used as the wetting agent with or without antibiotics or antiseptics
- Aid the debridement of wounds by removing the absorbed exudate and necrotic tissue fragments
- Antimicrobial sponges and gauze dressing (Kendall Kerlix, AMD) containing polyhexamethylene biguanide (0.2%) are available commercially*

NONADHERENT DRESSINGS

CALCIUM ALGINATE DRESSINGS (CADS)

- Made of salts of alginic acid extracted from seaweed to form a flat nonwoven pad.
- Used during the transition from debridement to the repair phase.
- Form a gel when they absorb exudate and reportedly stimulate epithelialization and granulation tissue formation.
- CAD-dressed wounds heal at the same rate as Telfa-dressed wounds.
- CADs improve clotting and are useful in the management of deep wounds.

SEMIOCCLUSIVE DRESSINGS (SODS) (TELFA, MELOLITE, PETROLEUM JELLY–IMPREGNATED GAUZE, AND DERMAHEAL)

- Most beneficial when applied to the wound during the repair phase.
- Petroleum jelly–based SODs are inert, nontoxic, nonirritating, and water insoluble; the moisture that forms lubricates the wound and allows nonpainful removal.
- Petroleum jelly–impregnated (high melting point) SODs have been shown to delay epithelialization 17%.
- Wounds dressed with Telfa heal more rapidly than do wounds dressed with amnion, Mitraflex, and BioDres.

OCCLUSIVE DRESSINGS (ODS)

- Classified as synthetic or biologic.
  - □ Synthetic ODs include hydrogels, polyurethane film, hydrocolloid, and polyurethane foam.
  - □ Biologic ODs include amnion and collagen gels and sponges.
- Reported benefits include prevention of infection, reduced pain, increased concentration of growth factors, and improved rates of healing.
- Complete occlusion of wounds of the distal extremity with synthetic ODs for the entire healing period promotes formation of exuberant granulation tissue and mixed infections, which delay wound healing.
- Synthetic ODs are best used for healthy wounds within 6 hours of injury up to 48 hours and during the repair phase.
- Biologic dressings are developed from natural products.
  - □ Equine amnion has most of the qualities of an ideal bandage.
  - □ Despite its occlusive properties, equine amnion results in faster wound healing, less granulation tissue formation, and greater epithelialization.

---

*Tyco Healthcare Group LP, Mansfield, MA 02048; (800) 962-9888; www.kendallhq.com.

- □ Collagen gels, sponges, and membranes reportedly enhance wound healing in humans and experimental animals. Bovine collagen membrane bandages for use on horses show no benefit of this dressing over adherent bandages.
- Silver chloride–coated nylon dressings are effective in killing five equine pathogens in vitro.
  - □ Silver ions time-released from the dressing kill the bacteria.
  - □ Shows promise for future prevention of equine wound infection.

NOTE: No single dressing can produce the optimum microenvironment for all wounds or for the total healing stages in one wound.

Other Topical Agents

- *Hydrophilic preparations (HPs)*, such as copolymer flakes, powder, and dextranomer beads, cause effusion of fluids through the wound, which cleanses the wound and results in lower exudate viscosity. By this process, tenacious coagulum and debris on the wound surface are diluted and drawn into the dressing.
  - □ Dextranomer beads are chemotactic for neutrophils and mononuclear cells; this property reduces inflammation.
  - □ No studies have evaluated the efficacy of these HPs in horses.
- *Maltodextrin* is a polysaccharide powder that inhibits the growth of and is bactericidal to *P. aeruginosa, S. aureus,* and *Bacteroides fragilis* in vitro and provides energy for cell metabolism and wound healing.
  - □ Maltodextrin reduces pain and swelling, stimulates early growth of granulation tissue and epithelium, and improves overall healing in horses.
- *Live yeast-cell derivative (LYCD)* is a water-soluble extract of yeast reported to stimulate angiogenesis, epithelialization, and collagen formation.
  - □ Associated with improved wound healing in dogs.
  - □ In horses, use of LYCD has prolonged wound healing and resulted in excessive granulation tissue formation.
- *Aloe vera (AV)* is reported to have both antithromboxane and antiprostaglandin properties that maintain vascular patency and prevent dermal ischemia. AV is also effective against *P. aeruginosa.*
  - □ AV extract gel with allantoin stimulates epithelialization and improves wound healing.
  - □ AV extract gel with acemannan increases epithelialization and wound healing in open pad wounds in dogs at 7 days.
  - □ AV's efficacy in horses has not been investigated.
  - □ A delay in second intention wound healing in patients treated with topical Aloe Vera gel is reported.
- *Honey* may be beneficial in the management of chronic infected wounds.
  - □ Proposed advantages include wound debridement, antibacterial effect, and promotion of wound healing.
  - □ Honey-treated wounds show little neutrophilic infiltration but show a marked proliferation of angioblasts and fibroblasts.
- *Activated macrophage supernatant (AMS)* may improve wound healing in horses and ponies because of its inhibition in vitro of equine fibroblast proliferation. No significant in vivo effects are known.
- *Sugardine (S)* is Betadine ointment and sugar mixed to make a thick paste.
  - □ May accelerate wound healing.
  - □ *Effective for management of hoof wounds.*

□ *Gentian violet is a carcinogenic agent when used on open wounds and mucous membranes.*

Dehydration and Edema
- Dehydration of the wound surface delays epithelialization by desiccation of the marginal epithelial cells and scab formation.
- Poor perfusion of the peripheral tissues in a dehydrated patient is believed to delay wound healing.
- The cause, extent, and location of the edema determine its effect on healing.
  □ Mild to moderate dependent edema not associated with chronic disease or infection has little harmful effect on wound healing.
  □ Severe edema alters the vascular dynamics within a wound and affects wound healing.
- *Treatments with NSAIDs, pressure bandages, sweats under a bandage, and hydrotherapy are most beneficial in the management of edema associated with the limbs. Hand-walking exercise may be beneficial in the reduction of edema in regions of the upper body that cannot be bandaged.*

Blood Supply and Oxygen Tension
- Healing wounds depend on adequate microcirculation to supply nutrients and oxygen for healing.
- Alteration in the microcirculation can occur from:
  □ Applying bandages or casts too tightly.
  □ Seroma formation.
  □ Tying sutures too tightly.
  □ Local trauma.
  □ The use of local anesthetics with vasoconstrictive agents.
- Oxygen is needed for cell migration, multiplication and synthesis of collagen, and protein in healing wounds.
- The migration and synthetic capabilities of the wound fibroblast depend on the rate at which revascularization occurs.
- Anything that impairs blood flow and subsequent delivery of oxygen retards wound healing.

Temperature and pH
- Wounds heal faster at higher temperatures and lower pH.
- Healing is accelerated at an ambient temperature of 30°C (86°F) rather than 18°C-20°C (64.4°F-68°F).
- Lower temperatures (12°C -20°C, 53.6°F-68°F) reduce tensile strength in wounds 20%. Alternating warm and cold temperatures delays wound healing.
  □ The inhibitory effect on wound healing of decreasing temperature is a result of reflexive vasoconstriction and reduction of local blood flow.
- The use of warm hydrotherapy accelerates healing of sutured wounds and is beneficial during the inflammatory and debridement phases of healing of open wounds. (It delays healing of open wounds if applied during the repair phase.)
  □ Moist heat above 60°C (140°F) causes thermal injury to cells.
  □ Moist heat at 49°C (120.2°F) is optimum for acceleration of hemostasis in a newly incised wound.
  □ Warm hydrotherapy accelerates wound healing by increasing blood flow.

- Acidification of a wound promotes healing by increasing the release of oxygen from hemoglobin.
- Alkalinity results from loss of CO_2 from the wound or from the presence of urease-producing bacteria in the wound.
- Bandaging is beneficial in increasing the wound surface temperature and decreasing the loss of CO_2.

PRINCIPLES OF WOUND MANAGEMENT

- A rapid assessment of the wound should be followed by a physical examination, including vital signs.
- A minor wound should not divert attention from more serious problems, such as
  - Hemorrhagic shock
  - Exhaustion
  - Cerebral contusion associated with head injuries
- The goal is to return the patient to a functional and cosmetic status as soon as possible.

History

- Historical features of the injury can be helpful in determining the approach to wound care.
- How long since the injury? Initially it was accepted that wounds managed within 6-8 hours after injury could be sutured with little risk of infection—the golden period. Although this can be used as a rough guideline, other factors must be considered.
- The following factors contribute to the likelihood of wound infection:
  - Mechanism of injury
  - How the wound was managed
  - Degree and type of contamination
  - Location and type of wound
  - Virulence of the organism
  - Patient's immune status

Mechanism of Injury

- The cause of the injury influences the patient's susceptibility to infection.
  - Lacerations caused by sharp objects (e.g., metal, glass, and knives) generally are resistant to infection.
  - Shear wounds from barbed wire, sticks, nails, and bites are more susceptible to infection because of the degree of soft-tissue damage.
  - Soft-tissue trauma from entanglement or entrapment or impact with a solid object or from being kicked, is more susceptible to infection because the degree of soft-tissue injury alters the vascular supply.
  - *Wounds caused by an impact injury are 100 times more susceptible to infection compared to wounds caused by a shearing force.*
- *The greater the magnitude of the energy on impact, the more severe is the soft-tissue damage and the greater is the change in blood supply.*

Degree and Type of Contamination

- Wounds contaminated with feces and dirt are at a high risk of infection despite treatment.

- □ Feces contain as many as 10^{11} microorganisms per gram.
- □ Infection-potentiating factors in soil have organic components and inorganic clay fractions. These highly charged particles react directly with WBCs and antibodies modifying normal function and reducing bactericidal effectiveness. As few as 100 microorganisms cause infection in wounds contaminated with these substances.

Location and Type of Wound

- Wounds involving the head region are more resistant to infection than those of the distal extremities. Reason: The blood supply is better.
- Degloving wounds that encircle the limb and damage the periosteum and paratenon are more susceptible to infection due to a lack of blood supply (Fig. 36–5). Osteomyelitis and septic tendinitis can be sequelae. Provide a soft-tissue covering within 4 days if possible.
- Synovial structures penetrated. Open wounds are less likely to become infected than are puncture wounds.
- Wounds with flaps that lack a good blood supply are more susceptible to infection. Blood supply is assessed by:
  - □ Physical examination: Tissues feel cool
  - □ Fluorescein dye examination: Inject 5 g /450 kg, IV

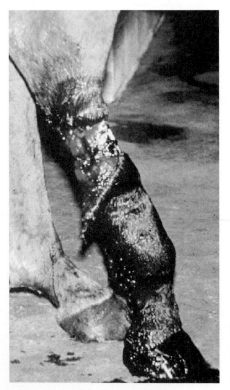

FIGURE 36–5. A degloving injury that occurred after the horse became entrapped in a wire fence. (From Stashak TS: *Equine wound management,* Philadelphia, 1991, Lea & Febiger.)

□ Nuclear medicine examination: assess the vascular phase

Virulence of the Microorganism
- In general, the more virulent the organism, the greater is the likelihood of infection.
- Fewer than 10^6 organisms can cause infection.

Immune Status of the Patient
- Poor health from chronic disease or inadequate nutrition can result in an altered immune status and make the patient more susceptible to infection.

Wound Preparation
- Preparation of the wound for additional examination is important.
- Some patients require sedation before wound evaluation.
- Avoid using phenothiazine tranquilizers in hypovolemic shock.
- Regional perineural anesthesia is useful for wounds of the distal extremity and regional infiltration of a local anesthetic is used elsewhere.
- Direct infiltration of the wound is acceptable after the wound is cleaned.
- Protect the wound with sterile moist gauze sponges, clip a wide area of hair around the wound and shave the wound edges with a recessed head razor to prevent damage to the infundibulum of the hair follicle. *Dampen the hair with water or coat lightly with K-Y water-soluble jelly to prevent hair from falling into the wound.*
- Sponges used to pack the wound are discarded and replaced by new ones.
- *Scrub the clipped area at least three times with antiseptic soap and rinse between scrubs with sterile 0.9% saline solution.*
- *The wound bed is gently cleaned with antiseptic soap and soft, smooth sterile gauze sponges, followed by lavage.*
- *The detergent base in antiseptics are neutralized with lavage.*

Initial Wound Examination
- *The most important criteria in the decision on management of a wound are based on the results of physical examination of the wound and of the patient.*
- Tissue adjacent to the wound edges is palpated for swelling and tissue temperature. Swollen, cool, discolored tissues indicate vascular compromise.
- The edges of the wound are separated to assess the extent of the wound and the degree of contamination.
- *Avoid direct digital palpation of the wound until the area is clipped, scrubbed, and lavaged.*
- Replace skin flap into its normal position to identify tissue deficits.
- Using this approach provides insight into choice of treatment and prognosis.
- Factors affecting selection of the treatment:
  □ Duration since injury
  □ Wound location and depth
  □ Whether a synovial structure has been penetrated
  □ Configuration of the wound
  □ Degree of contamination
  □ Severity and nature of the trauma
  □ Economics
  □ Patient temperament

□ Physical status
□ Intended use of the horse

Wound Lavage

- The mechanical effect of lavaging the wound with solutions under pressure is important for the removal of adherent contaminants and bacteria.
- Deliver lavage solutions by fluid jet and impact the wound with at least 7 psi (10-15 psi is most effective). These pressures can be achieved with a 35-ml syringe + 19-gauge needle, a spray bottle or Water Pik set at a low to intermediate setting, and/or a Stryker InterPulse irrigation system.
- Lavage solutions include sterile isotonic saline and Ringer's irrigation solution. Tap water from a hose can be used for a very large wound; this should be discontinued when a granulation bed is present. The continued use of tap water delays wound healing.
- The addition of antiseptics and antibiotics to the lavage solution is effective in preventing wound infection. Povidone-iodine (0.1%-0.2% 1-2 ml per 1000 ml of sterile solution) or CHD (0.05%) (1:40 dilution of the 2% concentrate) is effective and preferred.
- Lavage is discontinued before the tissues take on a water-logged appearance and become discolored, appearing as a gray hue.

Wound Exploration

- After cleaning the wound and freeing it of devitalized tissue and debris, explore the wound digitally while wearing sterile gloves.
- Consider use of a sterile probe to identify the depth of the wound, the presence of a foreign body, and whether bone has been contacted. The probe can be used in combination with plain radiography.
- Identify synovial fluid by stringing it between thumb and forefinger. If questions remain, submit a sample for cytologic examination and culture and sensitivity testing.
- If it appears that a synovial structure has been entered , place a needle in the synovial cavity at a site remote to the wound. If it is retrieved, synovial fluid is submitted for cytologic examination and culture and sensitivity testing. Inject sterile saline solution into the synovial structure. If the joint capsule has been breached, fluid is seen at the wound. If a synovial structure is involved, lavage with 3 to 5 L of sterile saline or crystalloid solution followed by lavage with 1 L of a 10% DMSO solution. Intrasynovial instillation of antibiotics is recommended.
- Radiographic examination
  □ Plain radiographs
  □ Contrast radiographs
- Ultrasound examination can:
  □ Identify tendon and ligament injury
  □ Assist in locating and identifying foreign bodies
  □ Recognize gas collection and muscle separation
- Arthroscopy/tenoscopy permits a more complete examination and debridement of a synovial structure

Wound Closure

- **Primary closure** is used for:
  □ Fresh, minimally contaminated wounds that have a good blood supply and do not involve vital structures

□ Wounds of the head region
□ Flap wounds with a good blood supply
□ Wounds of the upper body when a good cosmetic result is required
- **Delayed primary closure** is used for:
  □ Severely contaminated, contused, or swollen wounds (and for wounds that involve a synovial structure)
- **Secondary closure** is used for:
  □ Chronic wounds with a compromised blood supply. When a healthy bed of granulation tissue develops, the wound is closed.
- **Second intention healing** is used for:
  □ Large wounds over moveable areas such as the pectoral and gluteal regions
- **Skin grafting** is used when tissue deficits exceed the capability of wound contraction and epithelialization.
- **Reconstructive surgery** is used for a better cosmetic and functional result in a healed wound.

Primary Closure

WOUND PREPARATION

- Clean, lavage, explore, and debride the wound.
- Scrub the skin and wound with antiseptic soap, rinse the skin with sterile saline solution, and lavage the wound.
- Explore the wound digitally or with a probe.
- Perform excisional debridement, which is most effective in removing contaminants and bacteria in the superficial layers of the wound.
- After debridement is complete, lavage the wound and surrounding skin with 0.1% povidone-iodine–sterile saline solution.
- Change surgical gloves, redrape if appropriate, and use a new set of instruments for closure.
- Instill water-soluble, nonirritating antimicrobial agents in the wound if the blood supply is questionable.

SUTURING

- Ensure that sutures just appose the tissues with minimal tension.
- Use the lowest number of sutures to close the wound effectively.
- Use sutures in deeper tissue to appose fascial layers, retinacula, joint capsules, and transected flexor tendons or ligaments.
- *Avoid using a large number of sutures. An excessive number of sutures increase the risk of infection.*
- Use synthetic monofilament absorbable or nonabsorbable sutures, which cause minimal inflammatory response.

TENSION SUTURES

- Tension suturing patterns are used to reduce the pull on the primary suture line.
- Widely placed vertical mattress sutures with or without support by buttons, gauze, or rubber tubing are effective in reducing strain on the primary suture line (see Fig. 36–4).
  □ Tension sutures with supports are used in areas that cannot be effectively bandaged (e.g., upper body and neck regions).
  □ Tension sutures without supports are used in areas that are bandaged or to which a cast has been applied.

- Tension sutures are removed in 4 to 10 days, depending on the appearance of the wound. Staggered removal is preferred, whereby one half of the sutures are removed initially and the other half later.

DRAINS
- Drains are used when a large dead space remains after suture closure.
- Drains must be maintained in a sterile environment.
  □ Use a sterile bandage for the extremities.
  □ Use a sterile stent bandage for the upper body.
- *Drains should be sutured proximally. Traverse the wound adjacent to but not directly underlying the sutured skin edges and exit adjacent to the distal extremity of the wound. Drains also should be sutured at the point of exit.*
- The drain should exit from a separate incision adjacent to the wound edges. This placement of the drain reduces the risk of retrograde infection directly involving the suture line.
- Drains usually are left in place for 24-48 hours but may remain longer if drainage persists. Drains are a two-way street. Meticulous postoperative care of the drain exit site is most important to decrease the risk of infection.

Delayed Primary Closure
- Delayed primary closure is closure of a wound before granulation tissue forms, usually within 2-4 days after injury.
- Healing and a gain in tensile strength are not appreciably affected by delayed closure.
- Before suture closure, the wound is maintained in a sterile environment under a pressure bandage and assessed at bandage changes daily or every other day. Antibiotics and NSAIDs usually are administered during this period.
- *Clean wounds with reduced swelling and clear, serous, nonodiferous surface fluid are candidates for closure.*
- The wound is clipped, shaved, cleaned, and debrided as needed according to the principles described for primary closure.
- Degloving injuries require special consideration because they generally involve the cannon bone region, and the periosteum and paratenon often are compromised (see Fig. 36–5).
- Bone devoid of periosteum and tendon lacking paratenon lack sufficient blood supply to support the development of granulation tissue, and they are more prone to infection.
- There is increased risk of bone sequestrum or tendon degeneration with continued infection if the blood supply is not able to support healing.
- If delayed primary closure is used, the loose skin is held in place with a few sutures to provide soft-tissue covering of the exposed tendon and bone, which should provide sufficient blood supply to prevent bone infection and tendon degeneration until wound reconstruction.

Secondary Closure
- Secondary closure is used for chronic, severely contaminated, or infected wounds after formation of granulation tissue. Heel-bulb lacerations frequently are managed this way.
- The wound is cleaned, lavaged, cultured if necessary, debrided, and placed in a bandage.

- Appropriate antimicrobials and NSAIDs are administered. Bandages are changed daily until the exudative response is diminished and signs of infection are gone.
- It generally takes 4-6 days before a healthy bed of granulation tissue appears that is free of infection.
- Reconstruction involves removal of the exuberant granulation tissue and apposition of the wound edges.
- If a large dead space exists, a drain is used to prevent accumulation of serum within the wound.

Secondary Intention Healing

- Healing by secondary intention depends on wound contraction and epithelialization to close the wound. It is used in cases of large tissue loss and wounds of the upper limbs, torso, and neck.
- Wounds are prepared as for primary and delayed primary closure, except wounds above the extremities are left uncovered. Appropriate antimicrobial agents and NSAIDs are administered. Bandages are changed daily until the exudative response is diminished and signs of infection are gone.
- The uncovered wounds are cleaned daily to remove exudate and tissue debris.
- The exposed skin below the wound is cleaned and covered with petroleum jelly to prevent serum burns. The distal limb is supported with bandages.
- When a healthy bed of granulation tissue forms, the frequency of cleaning is reduced and antimicrobials discontinued unless skin grafting is planned.
- If a skin flap is present or the wound is gaping, use a few well-placed sutures to support the wound.

EXUBERANT GRANULATION TISSUE

- Wounds of the distal limb, below the carpus and tarsus, with large tissue deficits present a special problem with the development of exuberant granulation tissue.
- Factors believed to be involved in the formation of exuberant granulation tissue include:
  - □ Increased movement
  - □ Lack of soft-tissue covering
  - □ Excessive contamination
  - □ Reduced blood supply to the distal extremities
  - □ Body size: Individuals >140 cm in height and weighing more than 365 kg have a tendency to develop exuberant granulation tissue. Ponies have improved fibroblast organization and faster wound contraction.
  - □ Persistence of TGF-B (1) in the distal limb wounds compared to upper body wounds is believed to be important
- Treatment is directed at preventing the formation of exuberant granulation tissue with pressure bandages and casts.
- Excessive granulation tissue is managed in the following ways:
  - □ Application of steroid-antibiotic ointment and a pressure bandage.
  - □ *Steroids applied to newly formed granulation tissue have little effect on delaying wound healing when applied more than 5 days after the wound has occurred.*
  - □ Granulation tissue protruding above the skin surface to form a fibro-granuloma is excised, and a pressure bandage or cast is applied.
- Caustics and astringents effectively remove and prevent the formation of granulation tissue through chemical destruction. Chemicals are not selective

INTEGUMENT

and destroy migrating epithelial cells. The result is prolonged healing, increased inflammation, and excessive scarring.

SELECTION OF WOUND SUPPORTS

Bandages

- Bandages are applied over wounds of the extremities to protect the wound from additional contamination, prevent edema, absorb secretions, and prevent movement.
- Wounds generally are covered with an adherent or nonadherent dressing that is followed by application of conforming gauze.
- For pressure, elastic adhesive bandage is applied over the conforming gauze, which is followed by a cotton bandage.
- If further immobilization is important, additional layers of cotton are used, a polyvinyl chloride splint is incorporated into the bandage, or a cast is applied.

Casts

- A cast generally is recommended in the management of lacerations of the coronary band, heel bulbs, or dorsal surface of the fetlock, degloving injuries, and injuries to tendons and ligaments.
- Casts also are used after repair of deep lacerations perpendicular to the long axis of the wound to minimize movement of the fetlock, carpus, and hock and to place tension on the wound.
- If these wounds are not immobilized with a cast, dehiscence can occur.

NOTE: Wounds of the distal extremities that are sutured under tension generally are managed with a cast.

■ B. BURNS AND ACUTE SWELLING

Thomas J. Divers

THERMAL INJURY (BURNS)

Thermal injury to a horse is rare. Most cases involve barn fires, lightning, electricity, caustic chemicals, or friction. Most burns are superficial, easily managed, and inexpensive to treat, and heal in a short time. Serious burns, however, can result in rapid, severe burn shock or hypovolemia with associated cardiovascular changes (smoke inhalation and corneal ulceration also are of great concern). Management of these severe and extensive burns is difficult, expensive, and time consuming. Before treatment, it is recommended that the patient be carefully examined with respect to cardiovascular status, pulmonary function, ocular damage, and extent and severity of the burns, and that prognosis be discussed with the owner.

History and Physical Examination

- A well-taken history helps determine the cause and severity of burns. Skin typically takes a long time to absorb heat and a long time to dissipate the absorbed heat. Therefore, the longer the horse is exposed the worse is the situation and prognosis.

▶ ▪ It is **imperative** that the entire patient be examined, not just the burns. Horses frequently become severely hypovolemic and shocky and have respiratory difficulty. Thermal injuries may cause serious suppression of the immune system.

Clinical Signs and Findings
- Skin burns most common on the back and face
- Erythema, pain, vesicles, and singed hair
- Increase in heart and respiratory rates
- Abnormal discoloration of mucous membranes
- Blepharospasm, epiphora, or both, which signify corneal damage
- Coughing, which may indicate smoke inhalation
- Fever

Laboratory Findings
- Shock (decreased cardiac output, low total solids and blood volume, increased vascular permeability)
  □ Anemia may be severe and steadily progressive
- Hemoglobinuria
- Hyperkalemia early but hypokalemia later, often associated with fluid therapy

Classification of Burns
SUPERFICIAL
- Thickened, erythematous epidermis
- Typically painful
- Heal readily by epithelialization
- Prognosis excellent*

PARTIAL THICKNESS
- Severe subcutaneous edema
- Inflammation
- Typically very painful
- Heal by epithelialization from deeper skin appendages
- Prognosis good*

FULL THICKNESS
- No dermis remaining
- Damage to underlying tissue structures
- No cutaneous sensation
- Healing requires time and epithelialization from the wound edges. Skin grafting may be required.
- Prognosis can be poor, depending on extent.

Management
SUPERFICIAL BURNS
- Typically not life-threatening
- Immediately cool affected area with ice or cold water to draw heat out of tissues and decrease continued dermal necrosis.

---

*If there is minimal ocular and respiratory involvement.

INTEGUMENT

- Apply topical water-soluble antibacterial creams: aloe vera or silver sulfadiazine cream
  □ Prevents infection
  □ Decreases thromboxane activity
- Pain control: flunixin meglumine (Banamine), phenylbutazone (Butazolidin), ketoprofen (Ketofen)

PARTIAL-THICKNESS BURNS
- Typically not life-threatening.
- Management the same as that of superficial burns.
- Typically cause vesicle and blister formation. Leave intact for 36 hours, then open the lesion by removing the top and applying copious antibacterial cream.
- A bandage, if possible, is a good idea as long as it is not tight, allows drainage, and does not stick to the wound. Change the bandage daily.

FULL-THICKNESS BURNS
- Potentially life-threatening: *Manage shock first.*
- Treat as for superficial and partial thickness burns.
- Clip surrounding hair and debride all devitalized tissue.
- Perform copious lavage with sterile polyionic fluid with or without CHD (0.05% solution is beneficial.)
- Apply moist bandage with antibacterial cream. A shroud (sheet) soaked in antiseptic solution (e.g., povidone-iodine, CHD) and draped over the topline of the patient works well for dorsal burns.
  □ Change bandage frequently and debride devitalized tissue as it appears.
  □ Leave eschar intact.

BURN SHOCK: LIFE-THREATENING
- Large volumes of lactated Ringer's solution may be needed. An alternative is to use hypertonic saline solution, 4 ml/kg, with plasma, Hetastarch, or both followed by additional isotonic fluids. If there has been inhalation (smoke or heat) injury then crystalloids should be *limited* to the amount that normalizes circulatory volume and blood pressure.
- Use lactated Ringer's solution unless electrolyte values dictate otherwise.
- Flunixin meglumine 0.25-1.0 mg/kg IV q12-24h
- Pentoxifylline 7.5 mg/kg IV q12h
- Carefully monitor hydration status, lung sounds, and cardiovascular status.
- Administer plasma 2-10 L/adult.

NOTE: As a general rule, for a 450-kg adult, 1 L of plasma increases the total solids 0.2 g/L.

- Gradually increase grain availability; add 4-8 oz vegetable oil, and feed free-choice alfalfa hay.
  □ Patients with severe burns have a negative nitrogen balance and an increased metabolic rate with high energy demand. Gradually increasing the grain, adding fat, and offering free-choice alfalfa hay increases caloric intake and helps restore nitrogen balance.
  □ If smoke inhalation is a concern or there is evidence of burns around the face, hay should be water soaked and fed on the ground, paper should be used as bedding, and good ventilation should be provided.

- An anabolic steroid, boldenone undecylenate (Equipoise), may be used to help restore nitrogen balance.
- DMSO, 1 g/kg IV for the first 24 hours, may decrease inflammation and pulmonary edema.
  - If pulmonary edema is present and is unresponsive to DMSO and furosemide treatment, administer dexamethasone, 0.5 mg/kg IV once only.
- If there are respiratory signs or smoke inhalation is suspected, begin systemic antimicrobial therapy. Administer penicillin intramuscularly to protect against oral contaminants colonizing the airway. Broad-spectrum antimicrobial therapy may encourage fungal growth. If respiratory signs deteriorate, transtracheal aspiration should be performed, and additional broad-spectrum antimicrobial therapy administered according to the results of Gram stain, culture, and sensitivity.

Complications
WOUND INFECTION
- Severe burns become infected. Most infections are caused by normal skin flora.
- *P. aeruginosa, S. aureus, Escherichia coli*, β-hemolytic streptococci, other *Streptococcus* organisms, *Klebsiella pneumoniae*, and *Proteus, Clostridium*, and *Candida* organisms are commonly isolated.
- It is appropriate to change antibacterial creams as needed to control infection.
  - Silver sulfadiazine is effective against Gram-negative organisms such as *Pseudomonas*.
  - Aloe vera is reported to have antiprostaglandin and antithromboxane properties (e.g, to relieve pain, decrease inflammation, stimulate cell growth), in addition to antibacterial and antifungal activity.

SMOKE INHALATION
- See Chapter 43, Respiratory System, p. 513.
- For severe upper airway injury, a tracheotomy may be required. Perform only if there is obstruction. (see tracheotomy procedure, p. 69)
- Endoscopy of the trachea should be performed for prognostic purposes. If there is obvious sloughing of the mucosa, aspiration should be performed. This aspiration should last no longer than 15 seconds at a time because prolonged aspiration leads to hypoxemia.
- Supplemental oxygen should be provided through an intranasal catheter. (see nasal oxygen insufflation procedure, p. 66)
- Nebulization with albuterol, amikacin (1 ml) and acetylcysteine should be performed every 6 hours (see Chapter 52, p. 665).
- Systemic antioxidant therapy should include orally administered vitamin E and vitamin C.
- The mouth should be rinsed q4h with 0.05% CHD solution.
- Whether to use systemic antibiotics is controversial! One choice is penicillin alone as for burn shock. Another choice is ceftiofur (Naxcel), 2-4 mg/kg IV q12h), and metronidazole (15 mg/kg PO q6-8h).
- Flunixin meglumine, 0.25-1 mg/kg IV q12h, should be administered for both antiinflammatory effect and in the prospect of decreasing pulmonary hypertension.

CORNEAL ULCERATION AND EYELID BURNS
- If the lids are swollen, apply ophthalmic antibiotic ointment to the cornea q6h.

- Examine the cornea for ulceration initially and twice daily. If damaged, debride the necrotic cornea after tranquilization and application of a topical anesthetic.
- Apply antibiotics and cycloplegics (atropine) topically. Do **not** use corticosteroids.
- A third eyelid flap may be needed to protect the cornea from a necrotic eyelid. (see Chapter 41, p. 436)
- Silver sulfadiazine can be used around the eyes but CHD cannot.

LAMINITIS
- See Chapter 39 on the musculoskeletal system, p. 368.

KIDNEY DAMAGE
- See Acute Renal Failure in Chapter 44, p. 529.

PRURITUS
- Occurs frequently in healing burns and may necessitate sedation throughout most of the healing process
- Acepromazine (injectable or granules) works well.
- Antihistamines also may be effective.

ACUTE SWELLING: EDEMA

Acute edematous conditions in the horse most commonly result from increased hydrostatic pressure, septic inflammation, or a local or general immune response. Acutely occurring hypoproteinemia is a less common cause. Inflammatory conditions, both septic and immunologic, usually are painful to the touch. Edema resulting from increased hydrostatic pressure is less painful and in many cases nonpainful.

Purpura Hemorrhagica
- Consider purpura hemorrhagica with any unexplained vasculitis and edema.
- Edema is most common in the limbs and ventral abdomen and often moderately painful to the touch. It forms elsewhere in the body, causing *respiratory distress* (*laryngeal swelling* and *pulmonary edema*), *colic, heart failure* (*distress* and *trembling*), or *myositis* (*stiffness*).
- **Fever and petechiae of mucous membranes occur in approximately 50% of cases.**
- There is often a history of respiratory infection or exposure to *Streptococcus equi* (most frequent) or *Streptococcus zooepidemicus* in the preceding 2-4 weeks.

Diagnosis
- Based on a complete blood cell count, measurement of creatine kinase (CK) and aspartate aminotransferase (AST), platelet count, measurement of serum immunoglobulin A (IgA), and serologic testing for serum streptococcal M protein antibody and immune complexes (performed at Gluck Equine Research Center, University of Kentucky).
- A skin specimen from an edematous area obtained with a 6-mm Baker biopsy punch (Baker Cummins Pharmaceuticals Inc., Miami, FL 33178; [800] 347-4774) can be submitted in formalin to examine for vasculitis. Detection of

immunoglobulin deposition is rare, and submission in special medium (Michel's) or snap freezing is recommended. The biopsy specimen should not be harvested from an area over an important structure (e.g., tendon).

- There is often mature neutrophilia, and CK and AST levels frequently are elevated with or without signs of myositis.
- A normal platelet count >90,000 cells/ml is expected.
- An elevation in plasma protein measurement is usual, as are an elevated IgA level and a high antibody response to streptococcal M protein. However, a high antibody response to streptococcal M protein also occurs in some healthy individuals.
- Severe proteinuria and even *hematuria* occur in some patients!

Differential Diagnosis

Equine viral arteritis (EVA), equine herpesvirus, equine infectious anemia, *Anaplasma Phagocytophilia* infection, and Lyme disease. Be careful interpreting positive Lyme titers. Many normal horses in endemic areas have a titer to *Borrelia*. An indirect fluorescence antibody (IFA) titer greater than 1:1280 is considered suspect for Lyme disease, and additional testing with kinetic enzyme-linked immunosorbent assay (ELISA) (>300 units), immunoblots, and polymerase chain reaction (PCR) (performed at Cornell University Diagnostic Laboratory, [607] 253-3900) may be indicated. Most Standardbreds are serologically positive for EVA. (For more information see p. 331, Chapter 37.)

Treatment

- Corticosteroids: Dexamethasone, 0.04-0.16 mg/kg IV or IM q24h. Begin therapy at 0.08 mg/kg. If there is no response in 24-48 hours, the dosage should be increased or the diagnosis reconsidered. Continue at the clinical response dose for 2-3 days after signs abate and reduce the dosage over 7-14 days. Clinical signs may recur as the steroid dosage is decreased or withdrawn.
  - If corticosteroids are contraindicated, plasma exchange can be tried. Remove 8 ml/kg of the patient's blood and replace it with 8 ml/kg compatible plasma.
  - In mild cases, corticosteroids may not be needed.
- Antibiotic: Aqueous penicillin, 22,000 IU/kg q6h IV, or procaine penicillin, 22,000 IU/kg q12h IM during steroid therapy
- Furosemide, 0.5-1.0 mg/kg IV or IM q12-24h for 1-2 days for severe edema
- Leg wraps and hydrotherapy for limb edema
- Tracheotomy for life-threatening laryngeal edema (see p. 10).

> Purpura hemorrhagica is a serious disease with life-threatening complications in some cases. There is no single diagnostic test; purpura hemorrhagica is a clinical diagnosis. Owners should be informed of the risks of corticosteroid-associated laminitis, generally low, and that laminitis can result from purpura-induced vasculitis.

Acute Onset of Edema in All Four Limbs of More than One Horse

- This common occurrence can affect more than one individual on a farm, especially weanlings and yearlings.

- Fever often is present. Edema and fever affecting several horses often is caused by *equine herpesvirus I, influenza, unidentified viruses,* or, less commonly, *EVA.*
- EVA manifests as ventral edema and focal areas of painful edema elsewhere on the body. Vasculitis caused by EVA may result in sloughing of the skin. Other viral infections usually do not cause vasculitis this severe.

Diagnosis

- Made with history, clinical signs, virus isolation, and serologic findings

▶ *Hoary alyssum (see Chapter 53 on toxicology, p. 721)* poisoning is a toxic cause of limb edema, fever, and occasionally mild diarrhea affecting groups of horses in the northeastern and north central United States. A member of the mustard family, the plant is evidently palatable to horses. Clinical signs usually occur 18-36 hours after the horse consumes hay or pasture with large amounts of *hoary alyssum* and resolve within 2-4 days of removal of contaminated hay.

Treatment

- NSAIDs: Dipyrone, 22 mg/kg IV or IM, or phenylbutazone, 4.4 mg/kg PO q24h, as supportive therapy for viral infection
- Corticosteroids: Dexamethasone, 0.04 mg/kg PO, IV, or IM q24h, *if the edema is progressive or persists more than 7 days and there is no clinical or laboratory evidence of sepsis*
- Antibiotic: Ceftiofur, 1-5 mg/kg IV or IM q12h
- Cold hydrotherapy and leg wraps to decrease the swelling

Acute Edema Affecting Only One Horse

Acute edema of all four limbs or the ventral abdomen, generally accompanied by fever, may affect a single individual. The differential diagnosis includes

- Equine infectious anemia
- Ehrlichiosis
- Borreliosis (Lyme disease, which is probably rare)
- Onchocerca, especially after anthelmintic treatments
- Prefoaling or postfoaling ventral edema
- Purpura hemorrhagica (see p. 304)
- Autoimmune hemolytic anemia (see p. 310, Chapter 37)
- Autoimmune thrombocytopenia
- Right-sided heart failure (see p. 175, Chapter 34)
- Ventral abdominal hernia
- Acute septic cellulitis (see p. 311)
- Idiopathic or toxic conditions

Equine Infectious Anemia

The acute clinical syndrome caused by equine infectious anemia is rare but can cause *fever, edema, hemoglobinuria, jaundice, depression,* and *petechial* or *ecchymotic hemorrhage.* A Coggins test should be performed, although seroconversion may not be present at the onset of the disease, necessitating retesting 10-14 days later. The horse, if it survives and pending the diagnosis, should be kept in a screened stall at least 200 yards (180 m) from other horses.

Equine Granulocytic Ehrlichiosis

- *Anaplasma Phagocytophilia* infection is a common cause of edema and fever among horses in certain areas of the western United States (e.g., northern California), as well as eastern New York and other northeastern states.
- The organism is spread by ticks (incubation period may be 1-9 days), which can frequently be found on the horse.
- Signs: *Depression, anorexia, ataxia, limb edema, fever,* and *petechial hemorrhage*
- Laboratory findings: *Thrombocytopenia, leukopenia,* and *mild anemia.* The organism (morula) is sometimes seen in the neutrophils with a Giemsa stain (see Color Plate 11).
- Serologic testing (send sample to the University of California–Davis, Texas A & M University, or Louisiana State University) can be useful to confirm the diagnosis, if the disease has been present for several days. Some horses do not undergo seroconversion for several weeks.

Treatment
- Tetracycline, 6.6 mg/kg IV q12h for 5-7 days

Lyme Disease

Lyme disease frequently is cited as a cause of fever, lethargy, stiffness, edema, and malaise in horses in the northeastern United States. Lyme disease most commonly causes chronic lameness and rarely necessitates emergency treatment. Acute fever and edema in an endemic area would be much more compatible with *Anaplasma Phagocytophilia* infection.

A high IFA (>1:1200) or ELISA (>300) result and strong reaction on immunoblot support the diagnosis. PCR on a synovial membrane biopsy specimen (send to Cornell Diagnostic Laboratory) may be needed to confirm the diagnosis.

Treatment

If a patient exhibits the aforementioned clinical signs and has a high (>1:1200) or changing titer to *Borrelia* with a strongly positive immunoblot reaction and if other diseases have been ruled out, treat with tetracycline, 6.6 mg/kg IV q12-24h. A response should be seen in 3-5 days if the diagnosis is correct. Doxycycline, 10 mg/kg PO q12h, is used for longer-term management of Lyme arthritis.

Onchocerca

Reaction to *Onchocerca cervicalis* larvae after anthelmintic therapy does not necessitate treatment unless the ventral edema is very painful or the horse has a fever. In these cases, use dexamethasone, 0.05 mg/kg q24h, and an antibiotic such as ceftiofur, penicillin, or trimethoprim-sulfamethoxazole.

Prefoaling or Postfoaling Ventral Edema

Rule out hernia, ruptured prepubic tendon (see p. 494), mastitis (see p. 495, Chapter 42), and cellulitis. If the mare is in good health and the edema is progressive, administer two dexamethasone (5 mg)/trichlormethiazide (200 mg) boluses PO q24h (ground-up, mixed in molasses). *This dose of dexamethasone is unlikely to cause abortion in late-term pregnant mares. Nevertheless, it should be used only when infectious etiologies have been ruled out and the edema is progressive.*

Idiopathic Condition

Most individual cases are responsive to corticosteroids. Such cases occasionally occur as a herd outbreak in weanlings, yearlings, or adults, often with a respiratory or ocular component. If septic cellulitis or abnormal lung sounds are not present but there is progressive edema with severe pain, treat the patient with steroids.

Anaphylactoid Reactions Causing Edema

Previous sensitization to an antigen is not always required for an anaphylactoid reaction. The most common drugs causing a reaction are vaccines, vitamin E and selenium, anthelmintics, penicillin, trimethoprim-sulfamethoxazole, anesthetics, and NSAIDs. Many of the reactions to parenterally administered penicillin, trimethoprim-sulfamethoxazole, and anesthetics that cause collapse are not immunologic in origin and are covered under Adverse Drug Reactions (see Chapter 52, p. 650). *Anaphylactic reactions generally occur within minutes to 12 hours and may persist for several days.* The clinical signs are *urticaria, dyspnea, sweating, collapse,* and occasionally *laminitis.* The diagnosis is based on a history of exposure.

Treatment

- Urticaria only
  - □ Antihistamine: Doxylamine succinate, 0.5 mg/kg IV or IM slowly, if cardio-vascular status is stable. Urticaria persists in many cases and may have to be managed with oral prednisolone, 0.4-1.6 mg/kg q24h or every other day for several days. Dexamethasone, 0.25 mg/kg IV, may be used in addition to the therapies previously listed if the edema is rapidly progressive.
- Respiratory distress
  - □ Epinephrine 1:1000 (as packaged), 3-6 ml/450 kg given *slowly* IV or 3-10 ml/450 kg IM in less severe cases
  - □ Tracheotomy (see tracheotomy procedure, p. 10) if laryngeal edema is present
  - □ Furosemide, 1 mg/kg IV
- Cardiovascular collapse and hypotension (poor pulse, pale membranes)
  - □ Epinephrine or 2 L hypertonic saline solution or dobutamine, 50 mg/500 ml in dextrose solution administered over 10-20 minutes to a 450-kg adult (5-10 mg/kg per minute)

Idiopathic Urticaria

Idiopathic urticaria occurs in either a generalized or a local form. The generalized form often is a persistent problem, although the immediate response to corticosteroids or antihistamines is often good. Local edema (ocular, nasal, laryngeal) may occur without a known cause. Conjunctival edema of one or both eyes is the most common symptom.

Treatment

- Ocular
  - □ Ophthalmic corticosteroids after a *careful* and *complete* examination of the eye and fluorescein stain *reveal no corneal erosion*

- Skin urticaria
    - Antihistamine or corticosteroids: Hydroxyzine hydrochloride, 1.0-1.5 mg/kg q8-12h, or prednisolone, 0.5 mg/kg PO q24h. This form of urticaria may recur for weeks or months.

Cellulitis

Septic cellulitis, the most common cause of painful inflammatory edema in horses, is usually is associated with a wound or a local reaction to an injection. Pain and progressive swelling are the characteristic findings. Diagnosis is based on results of Gram stain and culture of a sample of the fluid. Anaerobic culture tubes* are recommended. Explore the wound to establish drainage and to search for a foreign body. Perform an ultrasound examination with a 7.5-MHz probe to localize and evaluate the fluid and to check for hyperechoic foreign bodies.

➤ **S. aureus or Clostridium organisms are common etiologic agents of severe and often rapidly spreading cellulitis in horses.**

Staphylococcal infection may result from blunt trauma, such as that caused by a starting gate or a bruise to the hock, without a noticeable break in the skin. *Staphylococcal and clostridial infections are considered the most pathogenic causes of cellulitis in horses.*

Treatment

- Antibiotics:
    - Penicillin, 40,000 IU/kg IV q6h, and gentamicin,[†] 6.6 mg/kg q24h IV, if cellulitis is severe and rapidly progressive and if there is the probability of a mixed bacterial infection.
    - *If an anaerobic infection is suspected because of the smell of the exudate or the presence of subcutaneous gas, add metronidazole, 15-25 mg/kg PO q6-8h, to the treatment.*
    - In less severe cases or when **only Gram-positive cocci (staphylococci) are seen on Gram stain, ceftiofur, trimethoprim-sulfamethoxazole, or both may be used.** Enrofloxacin, 7.5 mg/kg PO once a day or 5 mg/kg IV once or twice a day, is an excellent choice for staphylococcal and Gram-negative cellulitis but a poor choice for anaerobic or streptococcal infection.
    - Hydrotherapy: Septic and aseptic (injection site) cellulitis—cold water therapy for the first 24 hours followed by warm water therapy
    - Support: Wrap if an extremity is affected
    - NSAID: Phenylbutazone, 4.4 mg/kg q12h for 2-3 days

NOTE: Should tetanus toxoid or antitoxin or both be given to horses with a wound?
- Tetanus toxoid is administered to **all** patients. If on routine vaccination prophylaxis, antitoxin is not given.
- If the wound has occurred in an individual less than 2 years of age with questionable tetanus vaccination, use antitoxin (preferably a product with low incidence of serum hepatitis associated with administration of TAT).

---

*Port-a-Cul. Becton-Dickinson Microbiology Systems, Cockeysville, MD 21030.
†If using gentamicin, check serum creatinine every 2-3 days and be sure the patient is producing urine.

> Antitoxin should be administered to adults only if there is no history of previous tetanus toxoid vaccination.

- Surgical drainage—incision and drainage when and where appropriate

Malignant Edema: Clostridial Myositis

Malignant edema most commonly occurs on the chest from a wound, at the site of a nonantibiotic intramuscular injection, or from perivascular injections. *The most common intramuscularly administered drug associated with malignant edema is flunixin meglumine,* probably because it is the nonantibiotic drug with limited tissue irritation most frequently administered intramuscularly.

Clinical Signs
- Acute painful swelling, which is warm and soft and becomes cool and firm, subcutaneous crepitus, a stiff neck after a cervical injection, inability to lower the head, and, rarely, ataxia.
- **Subcutaneous crepitus is absent in many cases of clostridial myositis.**

Diagnosis
- Made with needle aspiration and Gram stain in search of large, Gram-positive bacilli. Place the fluid sample in anaerobic culture media (Port-a-Cul) and send a slide for fluorescent antibody examination.

Treatment
- Antibiotics: **Penicillin**, 40,000 IU/kg IV q4-6h, and metronidazole, 15-25 mg/kg PO q6h or 25-30 mg/kg per rectum q6h. Oxytetracycline is a second choice.
- **Surgical incision and drainage** or radical incision may be needed if the disease appears rapidly progressive or no improvement is seen after 24 hours of antimicrobial treatment. It is better to incise too early than to wait until it is too late! Hyperbaric oxygen may be useful but is not a substitute for *early* surgical drainage.
- Oral antiinflammatory therapy: Phenylbutazone, 4.4 mg/kg PO q12-24h
- Hydrotherapy
- Tetanus prophylaxis

Lymphangitis
- Lymphangitis is an emergency!
- The longer the leg remains swollen, the more severe is the anatomic disruption of the lymphatic vessels.
- The greatest chance of obtaining a positive bacterial culture is in the untreated acute case.

There is often an *acute progressive swelling of one hindlimb.* Acute bacterial lymphangitis may cause limb swelling, with serum oozing through the skin. Fungal infections usually are nodular and slower to develop. Acutely affected patients have a fever and frequently are very lame. Diagnosis is based on clinical signs and results of ultrasound examination with a 7.5-MHz probe that reveals numerous dilated vessels (lymphatics). The gross and ultrasound appearance of the limb is fairly uniform compared with that of cellulitis. A wound may or may not be present on the leg. Culture of the fluid should be attempted with a 22-gauge needle to minimize damage to the limb and avoid vessels. *An etiologic agent generally is not identified.*

Treatment

- Antibiotics: Trimethoprim-sulfamethoxazole, 20-25 mg/kg PO q12h, or tetracycline, 6.6 mg/kg IV q12h, or others, such as enrofloxacin, 5 mg/kg IV q12h, that are effective against *S. aureus*
- Antiinflammatory: Phenylbutazone, 4.4 mg/kg IV or PO q12h
- Aggressive hydrotherapy with cold water. Use a Jacuzzi or hydrotherapy tub or a cold boot* if available. If the patient can get its leg in the boot, the constant pressure of the water reduces the size. Prompt decrease in the swelling may prevent damage to the leg
- Pentoxifylline, 8.4 mg/kg PO q8-12h, to improve circulation in the severely swollen leg
- Support wrap of the opposite leg and close monitoring for laminitis
- Moderate walking
- Furosemide, 1 mg/kg IV or IM q12-24h for two treatments, or trichlormethiazide/dexamethasone (Naquasone) for *recurrent* cases *without* fever
- Support wrap with nitrofurazone (Furacin) sweat applied to affected leg

The owners should be advised that lymphangitis is a serious disease, the etiologic agent is rarely identified, the prognosis is guarded unless there is a rapid response to therapy, and recurrence is common.

Corynebacterium Pseudotuberculosis Infection

Corynebacterium pseudotuberculosis infection is acute and progressive swelling in the pectoral area, mammary gland, ventral abdomen, inguinal area (causing swelling of one limb), or sporadically elsewhere on the body. It can cause nodular lymphangitis and affects horses in the western United States. Ultrasound examination reveals deep abscesses proximal to the swelling.

Treatment

- Drainage and systemic procaine penicillin, 20,000-44,000 IU/kg q12h IM

Hematoma

Hematoma is acute swelling due to vessel rupture and blood collection. A common cause is a kick. If the swelling is not progressive, the hematoma is allowed to organize, and surgical drainage is considered later. If the skin is injured, administer an antimicrobial agent such as penicillin.

NOTE: Rule out thrombocytopenia as the cause of hematoma before administering intramuscular injections by examining the mucous membranes for petechial hemorrhage.

If a hematoma is rapidly progressive, an artery or, in rare instances, a large vein may have been ruptured. *Most rapidly progressive hematomas of the limbs are*

---

*P.I. Medical, Athens, TN; (800) 963-9632.

associated with a fracture, such as fracture of the pelvis with laceration of the iliac artery. Severe lameness also suggests a fracture. If no cause of hematoma is found and the hematoma is progressive despite medical treatment, consider surgery to identify and ligate the vessel.

Treatment

- Phenylbutazone, 4.4 mg/kg PO q12-24h, because it has little effect on platelet function
- Butorphanol, 0.01-0.02 mg/kg IV, 2-5 minutes after a low dose of xylazine, 0.2-0.4 mg/kg IV, for sedation
- Polyionic fluids: No hypertonic saline solution when first examined
- Pressure wrap if possible
- Whole-blood transfusion if bleeding is progressive, patient's condition is deteriorating, or PCV decreases to <18% within 12 hours after the start of bleeding

NOTE: Caution is advised in using PCV as a guide for transfusion because it can be quite variable between patients during the first 12-18 hours. If thrombocytopenia is present, the blood should be freshly collected in a plastic container for transfusion (see Chapter 37, p. 337).

- Aminocaproic acid, 20 mg/kg, mixed in 3 L of saline solution may be used to manage prolonged bleeding.

Nutritional Myopathy

Acute muscle swelling caused by selenium deficiency is rare but can occur. Swelling of the masseter and pterygoid muscles (masseter myopathy) results in a severe swelling of the facial muscles and protrusion of the conjunctiva. Affected individuals appear stiff and reluctant to chew but can eat. The urine is frequently dark and strongly positive for occult blood (myoglobin) on urine dipstick examination. This form of myopathy usually is a disease of poorly fed horses. Blood (whole blood, plasma, or serum) is collected for measurement of selenium (normal, 15-25 mg/dl) and serum level of creatine kinase. White muscle disease may occur in adults, newborn foals or weanlings.

Treatment

- Selenium, 0.05 mg/kg **IM**; repeat in 3 days if the diagnosis is confirmed
- DMSO, 1 g/kg diluted IV, once as ancillary therapy
- Warm compresses on the affected area
- Nursing care for any tissue compromised by the swelling, such as conjunctiva
- Phenylbutazone, 4.4 mg/kg PO q12h
- Intravenous fluids to correct hypotension, electrolyte abnormalities, and azotemia

Snake Bite, Spider Bite, and Bee Sting

These injuries occasionally result in severe swellings in horses. Snake bite is common on the noses of horses, causing airway obstruction and hemolysis (see nasal obstruction section, Chapter 43, p. 507). Bites of black widow spiders can cause hot, painful swelling. The diagnosis is supported by finding the spider in the stall. Bites of fire ants can cause acute swelling, particularly of the distal extremities. Fire ants are common in the southeastern United States, where they build large mounds (nests). Bee stings cause acute, painful swelling and can be fatal if they occur in large numbers. Bee stings are identified by circular areas of edema with a stinger in the center of the swelling.

Treatment
- Antihistamine: Doxylamine succinate, 0.5 mg/kg; hydroxyzine hydrochloride, 1.0-1.5 mg/kg
- Corticosteroids: Dexamethasone, 0.04 mg/kg IM, *if the injury is severe*
- Epinephrine, 3-7 ml (1:1000 solution)/450-kg adult slowly IV or SQ, only in cases of systemic (anaphylactic) involvement and respiratory distress
- Airway maintenance: Place a short endotracheal tube in the proximal nasal passages before the swelling becomes severe to prevent the need for tracheotomy. This is especially important in the treatment of individuals bitten on the nose by a snake.
- Broad-spectrum antibiotics for snake bite, such as penicillin, 44,000 IU/kg IV q6h, and gentamicin,* 6.6 mg/kg q24h, and metronidazole, 15 mg/kg PO q6-8h or 25-30 mg/kg per rectum q8h
- Tetanus toxoid
- NSAID therapy for snake bite: Flunixin meglumine, 0.8 mg/kg q12h IV for 3 days. *Because of the size of the patient, the frequent time delay between the bite and clinical recognition of the problem, and the possibility of an adverse reaction, antivenin is rarely indicated.*

Fly Bites

Fly bites rarely necessitate emergency treatment. Severe reactions to horse flies (core of necrotic tissue in the center of the swellings), stable flies, horn flies, or black flies (characteristic hemorrhagic center in the urticarial swelling) can occur. In rare instances, large numbers of black fly bites cause death.

Other Causes of Acute Dermatitis

Contact dermatitis, photosensitivity, and drug eruptions can necessitate emergency treatment. Photosensitivity is caused by liver disease, most commonly from toxic plants or less commonly from mycotoxins on the plants. Drug eruptions in the form of multifocal dermatitis bizarre in appearance or distribution can occur at any time during treatment or within a couple of days of discontinuation of treatment.

Treatment
- Corticosteroids, topical or systemic (in severe cases only), for contact dermatitis or photosensitivity
- Remove the causative agent

Acute and Severe Pruritus

Acute and severe pruritus is most common in the summer months owing to acute *Culicoides* hypersensitivity. Drug eruptions (see earlier), reaction to stinging nettle,

---

*Monitor serum creatine, hydration status, and urine production.

and bites by fire ants and other insects can cause intense pruritus. Also consider neurologic disorders such as rabies or self-mutilation syndrome in stallions.

Treatment

- Corticosteroids: Prednisolone, 2 mg/kg, to control itching in severe cases.

REFERENCES

Wound Healing and Management
Adams AP, Santschii EM, Mellencamp MA: Antibacterial properties of a silver-coated nylon wound dressing, *Vet Surg* 28:219-225, 1999.

Baxter GM, Doran RE, Moore JN: Management of lower leg wounds with delayed closure in horses. In *Proceedings of the 32nd annual convention of the American Association of Equine Practitioners*, 1986.

Bhandari M, Adili A, Schemitsch EH: The efficacy of low pressure lavage with different irrigating solutions to remove adherent bacteria from bone, *J Bone & Joint Surg* 83-A: 412-418, 2001.

Booth LC: Delayed wound closure and scar revision, *Vet Clin North Am Equine Pract* 5:615-632, 1989.

Butt TD, Bailey JV, Dowling PM, Fretz PB: Comparison of 2 techniques for regional antibiotic delivery to the equine forelimb: intraosseous perfusion vs. intravenous perfusion, *Can Vet J* 42:617-622, 2001.

Cook VL, Bertone AL, Kowalski JJ, Schwendeman et al: Biodegradable drug delivery systems for gentamicin release and treatment of synovial membrane infection, *Vet Surg* 28:233-241, 1999.

Ethell MT, Bennett RA, Brown MP et al: In vitro elution of gentamicin, amikacin, and ceftiofur from polymethylmethacrylate and hydroxyapatite cement, *Vet Surg* 29:375-382, 2000.

Farnsworth KD, White NA, Robertson J: The effect of implanting gentamicin-impregnated polymethylmethacrylate beads in the tarsocrural joint of the horse, *Vet Surg* 30:126-131, 2001.

Fogdestam I: A biomechanical study of healing rat skin incisions after delayed primary closure, *Surg Gynecol Obstet* 153:191-199, 1981.

Fretz PB, Martin GS, Jacobs KA: Treatment of exuberant granulation tissue in the horse: evaluation of four methods, *Vet Surg* 12:137-140, 1983.

Lindsay WA: Reconstructive surgery, *Probl Vet Med* 2:397-550, 1990.

Liptak JM: An overview of the topical management of wounds, *Aust Vet J* 75:408-413, 1997.

Murphey ED, Sanischi EM, Papich MG: Regional intravenous perfusion of the distal limb of horses with amikacin sulfate, *J Vet Pharmacol Ther* 22:68-71, 1999.

Peacock EE Jr: *Wound repair,* ed 3, Philadelphia, 1984, WB Saunders.

Rodeheaver GT et al: Wound cleaning by high pressure irrigation, *Surg Gynecol Obstet* 141:357, 1975.

Southwood LL, Baxter GM: Instrument sterilization, skin preparation, and wound management, *Vet Clin North Am Equine Pract* 12:173-194, 1996.

Stashak TS: Suture patterns used for wound closure in veterinary surgery. In *Proceedings of the 24th annual convention of the American Association of Equine Practitioners*, 1978.

Stashak TS: *Equine wound management,* Philadelphia, 1991, Lea & Febiger.

Swaim SF: Wound healing. In *Surgery of traumatized skin*, Philadelphia, 1980, WB Saunders.

Swaim SF, Lee AH: Topical wound medication: a review, *J Am Vet Med Assoc* 190:1588-1593, 1987.

Burns and Acute Swelling
NUTRITIONAL MYOPATHY
Perkins G et al: Electrolyte disturbances in foals with severe rhabdomyolysis, *J Vet Intern Med* 12:173-177, 1998.

SNAKE BITE
Dickenson CE et al: Rattlesnake venom poisoning in horses: 32 cases (1973-1993), *J Am Vet Med Assoc* 208:1866-1877, 1996.

PURPURA HEMORRHAGICA
Divers TJ, Timoney JF: Group C streptococcal antigen-antibody immune complex disease in horses. In *Proceedings of the 38th annual meeting of the American College of Veterinary Internal Medicine,* 1992.

EQUINE INFECTIOUS ANEMIA
Lucas MH, Davies THR: Equine infectious anemia, *Equine Vet Educ* 7:89-92, 1995.

IDIOPATHIC URTICARIA
Fadok VA: Overview of equine papular and nodular dermatoses, *Vet Clin North Am Equine Pract* 11:61-63, 1995.

MALIGNANT EDEMA
Rebhun WC et al: Malignant edema in horses, *J Am Vet Med Assoc* 187:732-736, 1985.

NUTRITIONAL MYOPATHY
Step DL et al: Severe masseter myonecrosis in a horse, *J Am Vet Med Assoc* 198: 117-119, 1991.

37 Liver Failure and Hemolytic Anemia

Thomas J. Divers

ICTERUS (JAUNDICE)

Icterus usually indicates *hemolytic disease, liver failure,* or a *physiologic disorder* (Fig. 37–1). These entities usually can be separated with a well-taken history, clinical examination, and a few laboratory tests. If a problem is found in another organ system that might cause anorexia, icterus is probably physiologic icterus. Physiologic icterus in adults is believed to result from anorexia, increased levels of plasma free fatty acids (FFA), and competition between FFA and bilirubin for hepatic uptake. *Icterus is common in young, septic foals and may be a result of several physiologic mechanisms.* The best way to detect clinical icterus is by examining the membranes of the sclera, mouth, and vagina.

History

- If icterus is caused by anorexia, the history indicates inappetence for more than 2 days.
- If neurologic signs or photosensitivity are present, suspect liver failure.
- If the icterus is severe, suspect liver failure or hemolytic disease.
- During late summer and fall in the eastern United States, the incidence of both liver failure and hemolysis increases because both red maple poisoning and Theiler's disease are more prevalent during this time.
- With either liver failure or hemolysis, urine is dark red, bright red, black, or orange.

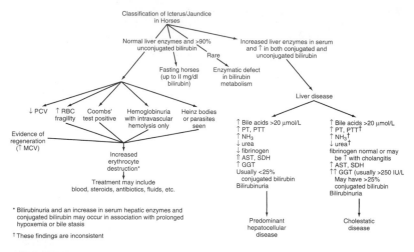

FIGURE 37-1. Classification of equine icterus/jaundice. *AST,* Aspartate aminotransferase; *GGT,* γ-glutamyl transaminopeptidase; *MCV,* mean corpuscular volume; NH_3, ammonia; *PT,* prothrombin time; *PTT,* partial thromboplastin time; *PCV,* packed cell volume; *RBC,* red blood cell; *SDH,* sorbitol dehydrogenase.

Diagnostic Tests

- If a urine sample is collected, a dipstick examination is helpful.
- *Physiologic icterus:* Usually no abnormalities on urinalysis.
- *Liver failure:* Usually bilirubinuria (shaking may produce a green foam).
- *Hemolysis:* Strong reaction to occult blood and occasional reaction to bilirubin if the hemolytic disease is of several days' duration.
- Best tests for determining the cause of icterus:
  - Packed cell volume (PCV) and total protein: Low PCV and normal to high total protein are most compatible with hemolysis. Pink plasma confirms intravascular hemolysis.
  - γ-Glutamyl transaminopeptidase (GGT): Elevations in the serum confirm liver disease.
  - Bilirubin: Increases in direct and indirect bilirubin with an elevation in GGT and a normal to high PCV indicate liver failure. An increase in only indirect bilirubin with a lower than expected PCV indicates hemolysis.
- Physiologic icterus: If suspected, manage the primary cause; should resolve in 24-36 hours. In rare instances, a healthy horse has persistent icterus and hyper-bilirubinemia (indirect) associated with a conjugation defect.
- Hemolysis: If suspected, see p. 328.

LIVER FAILURE

Patients with liver failure may be examined on an emergency basis because of bizarre, maniacal behavior, blindness, severe depression, acute dermatitis (photo-sensitivity), discolored urine (bilirubinuria), or jaundice. Theiler's disease is an example of a liver disorder necessitating emergency care. Affected horses may be either maniacal or obtunded and may have signs of colic.

► *Hyperlipemia in ponies and miniature equines is a common condition necessitating immediate medical care.* Affected horses are generally depressed rather than maniacal, and edema of the ventral abdomen is a frequent finding.

Chronic active hepatitis and diseases that cause progressive fibrosis, such as pyrrolizidine alkaloid toxicosis and cholangiohepatitis, can cause a sudden demise in which severe depression, yawning, or maniacal behavior necessitates emergency care.

► *Liver disease with elevations in serum hepatic enzyme activity is common with intestinal disorders and endotoxemia, but progression to liver failure is rare.*

HEPATIC DISORDERS CAUSING LIVER FAILURE
Theiler's Disease (Serum Hepatitis)
General Information

- Disease of adults
- Most commonly seen during summer or fall
- More than one horse on a farm may be affected over a period of several weeks
- *May* have a history of administration of tetanus antitoxin 4-10 weeks earlier
- ► In areas of the United States other than the western states, if you are called in late summer or fall to examine an adult horse with signs of acute encephalopathy without fever, Theiler's disease should be a differential diagnosis.

Clinical Signs

HEPATIC ENCEPHALOPATHY
- Depression or bizarre behavior
- Blindness
- Ataxia

HYPERBILIRUBINEMIA
- Icteric mucous membranes
- Neurologic signs may occur before the icterus in peracute cases.
- Discolored urine indicates bilirubinuria (with hemoglobinuria in some cases).

Laboratory Findings

- Marked elevations in serum hepatocellular enzymes
  - Aspartate aminotransferase (AST): Usually >1000 IU/L; more than 4000 IU/L is a poor prognosis.
  - Sorbitol dehydrogenase: marked elevation
- Moderate increase in biliary-derived enzymes: GGT usually between 100 and 300 IU/L
- Bilirubinemia: Direct (conjugated) bilirubin concentration is increased, but the most dramatic increase usually is in unconjugated bilirubin.
- Prolongation of prothrombin time (PT) and partial thromboplastin time (PTT) (submit in blue top/citrate tube with a control sample)
- Elevated levels of bile acids
- Increased blood ammonia (may be mild)
- Rarely hypoglycemia
- Variable acid/base profile

Diagnosis

- Ultrasound examination
  - Usually cannot see the liver on the right side of the abdomen, but it can be seen at the seventh-to-eighth intercostal space low on the left. The liver may look more anechoic than normal (see indications for biopsy of the liver, p. 324).

Treatment

- Supportive therapy for hepatic failure and hepatic encephalopathy (see p. 325)

Cholangiohepatitis and Cholelithiasis

Signalment and Clinical Findings

- Cholangiohepatitis: Clinical findings most commonly include fever, jaundice, and anorexia. Most common in adults.
- Cholelithiasis: Recurrent episodes of cholangiohepatitis, plus *colic, weight loss,* and, in rare instances, neurologic signs. Middle-aged or older horses with cholangiohepatitis are more likely to have stones than are younger horses.

Diagnosis

- History, signalment, and clinical signs

Laboratory Findings

- Marked elevation in GGT: 300-2500 IU/L
- Milder response in hepatocellular enzymes, AST usually <1000 IU/L
- Liver function tests: Increased bilirubin, often 50% or more is conjugated (direct) bilirubin; increased serum bile acids (normal <12 mmol/L in a horse that is eating or <20 μmol/L in an anorexic horse); PT and PTT often are normal.
- Increases often occur in white blood cell and neutrophil counts, fibrinogen, and total protein.
- Biopsy reveals periportal fibrosis, dilatation of bile ducts, and inflammation. Culture usually shows Gram-negative enteric aerobic and Gram-positive or negative anaerobic organisms, if anything, can be grown! *Positive culture results are obtained in only 50% of cases.*

Both aerobic and anaerobic cultures should be performed.
Rarely bile pigment and bacteria may be present in the peritoneal field.

Ultrasound Examination

- A subjectively enlarged liver
- Bile duct distention in some cases
- Possible acoustic shadows (stones)
- Evidence of fibrosis, which can be severe in chronic cases

Treatment

CHOLANGIOHEPATITIS

- Ceftiofur, 3.0 mg/kg IV or IM q12h, or trimethoprim-sulfamethoxazole, 20-30 mg/kg PO q12h, is a reasonable initial selection pending results of culture and sensitivity from the liver biopsy.
- Enrofloxacin, 5-7.5 mg/kg PO q24h, has been used successfully. Add metronidazole, 15 mg/kg PO q8-12h, to any of these regimens, especially if anaerobes are cultured.

- Administer vitamin K$_1$ IM or SQ for *chronic and severe* cholangitis. This agent may be ineffective if administered orally. *Do not administer intravenously.*
- DMSO 1 g/kg as a 10% solution administered IV q24h for 5-7 days can dissolve calcium bilirubinate stones.
- Ursodeoxycholic acid should be used only if other treatments are unsuccessful.
- Pentoxifylline 8.4 mg/kg IV q12h

GENERAL MANAGEMENT OF LIVER FAILURE
- Administer general therapy for liver failure when appropriate (see p. 325). *Hepatic encephalopathy is not as great a concern with cholangitis as it is in Theiler's disease. Some therapies for hepatic encephalopathy, such as oral neomycin, usually are not indicated in the management of cholangiohepatitis.*

Hyperlipemia

- Occurs mostly in ponies, miniature equines, adults with pituitary adenoma, and less commonly in late-term pregnant and azotemic mares. It can affect foals or adults.
- In ponies, most common in pregnant or early-lactation mares. Hyperlipemia usually is a disease of well-conditioned or fat ponies.
- Characterized by fatty liver and serum that is cloudy because of accumulation of lipids.
- Any disease that decreases appetite or results in catecholamine release and lipolysis can initiate hyperlipemia.

Clinical Signs
- Anorexia
- Depression
- Diarrhea
- Ventral edema

Diagnosis (Laboratory Tests)
- Increased triglycerides, >500 mg/dl
- Increased hepatocellular enzymes in the serum, but results of liver function tests may not be markedly abnormal.
- Whitish discoloration of the serum or plasma

Treatment
SPECIFIC MANAGEMENT OF HYPERLIPEMIA
- Provide both intravenous and oral calories along with intravenous polyionic fluids: 0.45 NaCl and 5% dextrose or Plasmalyte with 5% dextrose and additive KCl (20-40 mEq/L). Nasogastric intubation if the pony is not eating, with 0.5 g/kg glucose as a 15% solution and 10-20 g KCl. If appetite does not improve within 24 hours, start enteral feeding with Osmolyte HN (Ross Laboratories, Columbus, Ohio) or home-prepared gruel (see nutrition for the sick horse, Chapter 57) for foals. Administer the enteral feed in small volumes every 2 hours through an indwelling 18F nasogastric tube (Ross Laboratories).
- On the first day, give an adult patient 50 kcal/kg of Osmolyte or home-prepared gruel. If the feeds are well tolerated on day 1, increase to 75 kcal/kg on day 2 and 100 kcal/kg on day 3 and beyond. If the patient does not tolerate enteral feeding (diarrhea or reflux), use intravenous nutrition if possible. Do not use lipids.

LIVER

- For patients not tolerant of enteral feeding, use parenteral nutrition. This is one of the few indications for the emergency use of total parenteral nutrition (TPN) in the care of adults. Begin by placing a Mylar or Arrow catheter in the jugular vein. The TPN is a formulation of 50% dextrose and 4% branched-chain amino acid solution (BranchAmin, Clintec, Deerfield, IL). The final solution should be <20% dextrose and administered at a rate of 2 ml/kg per hour. In some cases, glucose will not be tolerated.
- Monitor plasma glucose level frequently; it should not be >180 mg/dl. Feed the pony anything it will eat.
- Heparin, 100 IU/kg IV q12h, is of questionable benefit.
- Flunixin meglumine, 0.25 mg/kg q8h, for endotoxemia or to improve overall attitude
- If there is persistent and marked hyperglycemia, insulin may be given.

NOTE: Aggressively treat the patient for the primary disease. Administer pergolide, 0.0017-0.01 mg/kg PO, to adults believed to have pituitary adenoma as an underlying cause. A low dose of 0.0017 mg/kg per day has been shown efficacious. If expense is a concern, the alternative is cyproheptadine, 0.25-0.5 mg/kg PO q12h. Pergolide may be more likely to suppress the appetite.

- Insulin is of questionable value but can be used if patients are being given 10% dextrose IV. Protamine zinc insulin, 0.4 IU/kg SQ q24h, or ultralente insulin, 0.4 IU/kg IV q24h, may be used.
- Ponies or miniature equines that have no appetite and cannot receive adequate nutritional support, have a primary disease that is difficult to manage, or have severe ventral edema have a very poor prognosis.
- Apply general principles for managing hepatic failure when appropriate, although fulminant hepatic encephalopathy is not common with hyperlipemia. It is important that affected horses eat something even if it is a higher-protein feed! Rehydration is especially important if triglycerides are to be lowered.

Pyrrolizidine Alkaloid Toxicosis
Geographic Incidence
- Predominately a disease of the western United States
- The most common plants containing pyrrolizidine alkaloid are *Senecio jacobea* (tansy ragwort), *Senecio vulgaris* (common groundsel), *Cynoglossum officinale* (hound's tongue), and *Amsinckia intermedia* (fiddleneck). *Crotalaria* (rattlebox), a common plant of the southeastern United States, contains pyrrolizidine alkaloid but is rarely ingested by horses.

Clinical Signs
- Although pyrrolizidine alkaloid toxicosis is a chronic disease, most affected horses have an acute onset of clinical signs.
- Central nervous system (CNS) signs are signs of acute hepatic encephalopathy: Depression, wandering, yawning, and so on. Rarely, acute laryngeal paralysis has been seen.
- Icterus is mild to moderate.
- Photosensitization

Diagnosis

LABORATORY FINDINGS

- The AST level usually is elevated. The GGT level is consistently elevated and remains elevated for as long as 6 months after removal of horses without symptoms from exposure to the toxin.
- Bile acids are elevated.

ULTRASOUND EXAMINATION

- Increased echogenicity (fibrosis)

Treatment

- Supportive therapy for fulminant liver failure and hepatic encephalopathy (see p. 325)
- Make sure horses with hepatic failure are housed out of direct sunlight.

NOTE: What about other horses that have been exposed to pyrrolizidine alkaloids?

- Monitor GGT and bile acids to determine whether the disease is progressing. If the horses appear clinically normal 6 months after exposure, and levels of GGT and bile acids are normal, the likelihood of development of hepatic failure from the exposure is minimal, and the horses can be put back to work.
- Find the contaminated feed and do not feed it to horses.

Tyzzer's Disease *(Clostridium piliformis)*

Signalment

- 8- to 42-day-old foal
- Usually only one foal on the farm is affected, although farm problems occur in certain areas, such as Oklahoma.

Clinical Signs

- Immediate death, depression, anorexia, hyperthermia or hypothermia, jaundice, convulsions, shock, diarrhea

Diagnosis

- Age and clinical signs

Laboratory Findings

- Elevated AST and sorbitol dehydrogenase levels
- Abnormal results of liver-function tests: Bilirubinemia (both direct and indirect fractions are increased)
- Hypoglycemia
- Severe metabolic acidosis
- Serologic testing for recovered and suspected cases
- Histopathologic examination of the liver or polymerase chain reaction on feces

Treatment

- Supportive therapy for fulminant hepatic failure and hepatic encephalopathy (see p. 325)

LIVER

- Antibiotics: Penicillin, 44,000 U/kg IV q6h, gentamicin, 6.6 mg/kg IV q24h (if the foal is urinating and is being treated aggressively with intravenous fluids), and metronidazole, 15 mg/kg PO q6-12h
- Aggressive management of septic shock
- Normalize blood pressure with a nonlactated polyionic crystalloid solution and colloid (hetastarch or Oxyglobin) administered intravenously. If systemic arterial blood pressure cannot be normalized with fluid therapy and central venous pressure becomes elevated (>11 cm H_2O), attempt dobutamine (5-10 µg/kg/min. Lastly, α-adrenergic drug therapy with dopamine, administered 5-10 µg/kg/min, or norepinephrine, 0.1-1.0 µg/kg per minute may be used in an attempt to normalize arterial blood pressure.
- Administer hyperimmune plasma incubated with 100 U heparin per liter.
- Pentoxifylline, 8.4 mg/kg PO q8-12h
- Intranasal oxygen, 5 L/min

Prognosis
- Grave.

Other Causes of Hepatic Disease that Lead to Liver Failure
Aflatoxicosis
- Rarely reported among horses

Leukoencephalomalacia (Moldy Corn)
- Uncommon cause of liver failure in horses, although it frequently causes liver disease

Obstruction of the Bile Duct
- Unusual
- *Colon displacement:* If an adult has mild, persistent colic, no fever, normal serum globulin and plasma fibrinogen levels, abnormal results of a rectal examination, and a high bilirubin level (usually >12 mg/dl and GGT level usually >100 IU/L), suspect approximately 180 degrees of displacement or volvulus of the large colon. On ultrasound examination of the caudal or midlateral abdomen, the displaced colon and enlarged colonic vessels can sometimes be visualized. A displaced colon in the horse occasionally obstructs the bile duct. Treatment is surgical correction. Bilirubin and GGT levels should decrease within 24-36 hours.
- Obstruction of the bile duct also occurs among foals in association with healing duodenal ulcer and stricture. Serum GGT concentration is increased, and the foal may be icteric, but there is no retrograde movement of barium into the biliary ducts 2 hours after the oral barium study (1 L/foal) as occurs with duodenal stricture posterior to the opening of the bile duct. The prognosis is very grave, although transposition of the bile duct and gastrojejunostomy or duodenojejunostomy can be attempted.

Portacaval Shunts
- Consider portacaval shunts if a foal 2 months or older has an acute onset of blindness, seizures, coma, or other signs of bizarre behavior. Relapsing episodes are almost enough to confirm the diagnosis. Foals rarely have clinical signs unless they are eating large amounts of grain, hay, or spring grass. Routine lab-

oratory findings often are unremarkable. Liver enzyme levels are typically normal, AST and creatine kinase levels may be increased because of seizure activity, and hypoglycemia may be present. Measurement of ammonia and bile acids in a blood sample is used to help confirm the diagnosis. Hepatic scintigraphy will further confirm the diagnosis, but a portogram will be needed too if surgery is contemplated.

NOTE: Proper handling of the sample to measure blood ammonia level is critical. The blood should be carefully (hemolysis interferes with the measurement) collected in a heparin tube, kept on ice, and taken to a laboratory within 1 hour. If this is not possible, harvest the plasma within 30 minutes and freeze it at $-4°F$ $(-20°C)$ for measurement within 48 hours. It is ideal to submit a control sample collected from a horse of similar age and diet.

LIVER

TREATMENT
- Medical stabilization for hepatic encephalopathy, including polyionic crystalloid fluid therapy with 5-10 g dextrose added per liter. Neomycin mixed with Karo syrup and administered three times 12 hours apart may be effective in decreasing intestinal production of ammonia. Sedation with low-dose xylazine, 0.2 mg/kg, followed by pentobarbital or phenobarbital administration, 3.0-11.0 mg/kg or *to effect*, may be needed to sedate a foal having seizures. *No diazepam!* Surgical correction can be performed after diagnostic venography is performed to find the shunt location.

Hyperammonemia and Liver Disease
- Can occur in weanling Morgan foals. This syndrome appears to be familial and may be associated with a metabolic defect in urea synthesis.

DIAGNOSIS
- Morgan breed, clinical signs occur after weaning, diminished growth rate, and depression. Moderately elevated liver enzymes. Normal or only mildly elevated bilirubin level. Blood ammonia levels are very high (>200 μmol/L). Terminal hemolytic anemia may occur in a few cases.

PROGNOSIS
- Some horses have temporary improvement in clinical signs but die days or weeks later.

Primary Hyperammonemia of Adult Horses
This may be seen in horses presented for abdominal pain. The horses exhibit cortical signs including blindness, and have severe metabolic acidosis, hyperglycemia, and blood ammonia >200 μmol/L. Supportive treatment with fluids and neomycin PO is often successful with recovery in 2-4 days.

Hyperammonemia in Dysmature, Premature Foals
Some dysmature, premature foals with persistent meconium impaction and/or constipation may develop high blood ammonia and worsening neurologic signs.

TREATMENT
Enema

Klein Grass and Fall Panicum

- Consider Klein grass as a cause of liver failure in areas (southwestern United States) where the grass is grown. In the eastern United States, fall panicum may produce a similar syndrome.

Alsike Clover

- Alsike clover poisoning is a cause of *photosensitization and jaundice* in horses in the northern United States and Canada. Outbreaks occur sporadically, likely associated with environmental conditions and increased growth of mycotoxin on the grass or a toxin (saponin) in the plant.

DIAGNOSIS

- Based on history and exposure, clinical findings of liver disease or failure, and ruling out other causes of hepatic failure. With fall panicum, Klein grass, or alsike poisoning, more than one horse on the farm may have increases in GGT, although they may not have liver failure. Laboratory findings are similar to those of pyrrolizidine alkaloid poisoning (moderate increases in GGT and a mild to moderate increase in AST).

TREATMENT

- Supportive therapy and removal from the hay or pasture

PROGNOSIS

- Usually good for panicum and alsike toxicity

Iron Intoxication

- May cause liver disease and rarely failure. It may result from parenteral administration of iron sulfate. It also may occur in a few horses because of abnormal liver uptake or storage (hemochromatosis) rather than excessive administration.

► Finding elevated iron concentration in the liver does not prove it is the cause of liver disease!

Ultrasound Examination of the Equine Liver: to Perform Biopsy or Not to Perform Biopsy?

- Ultrasound examination of the liver is performed with a 5.0-MHz probe of the right abdomen beginning at the 10th intercostal space just above the point of the shoulder and continuing caudally and ventrally. Also scan the left cranial quadrant of the abdomen at the 7th-9th intercostal space in a line drawn from the point of the elbow and moving caudally.
- Liver biopsy or aspiration can be performed for diagnostic purposes, such as detection of pyrrolizidine alkaloid toxicosis or suppurative cholangitis and culture or for prognostic purposes, such as assessment of fibrosis. These procedures rarely are needed as emergency procedures and are not necessary for proper management in most cases. The biopsy can be performed with a Tru-Cut biopsy needle introduced into a section of liver viewed at ultrasound examination as relatively *avascular*. Only local anesthesia is needed.

General Management of Fulminant Liver Failure and Hepatic Encephalopathy

- Tranquilize only if needed to control the horse. Use low doses of xylazine (0.2 mg/kg IV as needed). Do not use xylazine doses that will cause the head to be lower, below the point of the shoulder.
- Persistent lowering of the head may increase cerebral edema.

> **NOTE:** *Do not use diazepam.* If additional sedation is required, use pentobarbital or phenobarbital to effect, generally 5.0-11.0 mg/kg IV.

- Minimize stress and *feed small amounts of grain* (preferably grain with higher amounts of *branched-chain** amino acids, such as sorghum and corn) *frequently.* Remove alfalfa hay and feed grass hay or "soaked" beet pulp. Grazing on late summer or fall nonlegume grasses is acceptable if it is done in the evening to prevent photosensitization.
- Begin *IV fluid therapy:* 0.45% or 0.9% NaCl or plasmalyte if the horse is acidotic with 2.5% dextrose and additive, 40 mEq/L KCl. After volume deficits have been replaced, maintenance rates should be 80 ml/kg per day or greater. In many cases, the PCV remains elevated despite apparent rehydration. Fluids containing acetate are preferred over lactate-containing fluids in the management of hepatic failure.
- Administer 4-8 mg/kg neomycin sulfate orally q8h mixed in molasses when hepatic encephalopathy is present or a concern. This treatment may be continued at a lower daily rate for 3 days. Diarrhea may result with overzealous administration of neomycin. Metronidazole also may be used, 15 mg/kg PO q12-24h.
- For severe neurologic signs (ataxia or encephalopathy): Mannitol, 0.5-1.0 g/kg IV, DMSO, 0.1-1.0 g/kg, or both should be given.
- Flunixin 0.25 mg/kg q8h is routinely given because many horses with hepatic failure experience endotoxemia.

Special Considerations

- *No diazepam!*
- When hepatic encephalopathy is of major concern, do not pass a nasogastric tube unless it is needed to administer oral medication. Bleeding and swallowing of blood can worsen hepatic encephalopathy.

> **NOTE:** Do not administer 5% dextrose as the sole source of fluid replacement because it does not sufficiently expand the intravascular space.

- Do not administer bicarbonate unless plasma bicarbonate level is <14 mEq/L. Rapid correction of acidosis can increase the level of ionized ammonia and exacerbate CNS signs.
- *Maintain adequate serum potassium (K^+) concentration because this is important in reducing hyperammonemia.*
- Do not leave affected horses outside in the sun.
- For primary hyperammonemia or fulminant hepatic failure with confirmed or suspected high blood ammonia concentration, metronidazole, 15 mg/kg q12-24h PO, mixed with molasses, or lactulose, 0.1-0.2 ml/kg PO q8h can be given *in*

---

*A branched-chain amino acid paste also is available.

addition to the neomycin. Metronidazole is effective in decreasing enteric ammonia production, is a good antimicrobial against anaerobic infections of the liver, and has antiinflammatory and antiendotoxin properties.

- For patients with severe or uncontrolled (with the preceding treatment) hepatic encephalopathy: Flumazenil therapy (5-10 mg slowly IV to a 500-kg adult) can be attempted.
- Administer B vitamins IV slowly and vitamin E either PO or IM.
- Consider parenteral nutrition for foals and adults with fulminant hepatic failure caused by acute disease. Use only formulations prepared for patients with hepatic failure (Heptamine), and use a rate less than for routine TPN therapy. Experience with this form of therapy in the management of acute hepatic failure is limited to a few cases.
- S-adenosylmethionine (Denosyl-SDR) 20 mg/kg/day may provide antioxidant properties to the diseased liver.

HEMOLYTIC ANEMIA
General Diagnostic Considerations

Collect blood in EDTA tubes for a direct Coombs test if an immunologic reaction is suspected, as with isoerythrolysis or recent penicillin administration. Ask for a new methylene blue stain if exposure to a plant toxin, such as red maple, is a possibility. Collect serum for a Coggins test and streptococcus M protein antibody if edema and fever are present. Measure serum calcium if lymphoma is suspected. Examine thoroughly for other diseases (e.g., clostridial myositis) that may cause hemolytic anemia. For classification of anemia in horses, see Fig. 37–2.

Toxic or Heinz Body Anemia

Acute hemolytic anemia can be caused by plant toxins or occasionally can be a direct effect of intravenous administration of drugs (DMSO, tetracycline, propylene glycol). It also can occur in association with exposure to clostridial bacterial toxins or leptospirosis. Plants reported to cause intravascular hemolysis are wild onion and red maple. Red maple toxicity is most common during late summer and fall and results from ingestion of wilted leaves. It often occurs 3-4 days after a storm. This disorder occurs only in the middle or eastern United States.

Red Maple Toxicity
Clinical Signs
- Depression
- Jaundice
- Discolored urine

Diagnosis
- History
- Clinical signs

Diagnostic Tests
- PCV
- Total protein

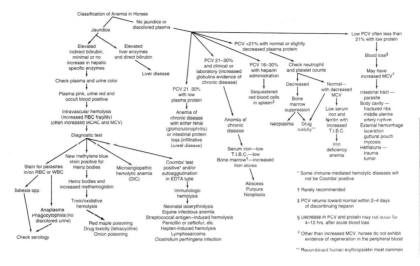

FIGURE 37-2. Classification of equine anemia. *DIC,* Disseminated intravascular coagulation; *MCHC,* mean corpuscular hemoglobin concentration; *MCV,* mean corpuscular volume; *PCV,* packed cell volume; *RBC,* red blood cells; *TIBC,* total iron-binding capacity; *WBC,* white blood cells.

- Bilirubin
- Urinalysis
- Methemoglobin*
- Red blood cell morphology
- Heinz bodies may be found with meticulous searching if the horse has red maple poisoning. These structures are more commonly found with onion poisoning. The PCV often decreases to a life-threatening value (<14%) with red maple toxicity; this is rarely the case with onion toxicity. Mean corpuscular volume (MCV) and mean corpuscular hemoglobin concentration (MCHC) may be increased, and the plasma protein level is usually normal or increased. The increase in serum bilirubin level is mostly indirect.

Treatment
- Blood transfusion (see p. 336)

When to Administer Transfusions to Horses or Foals with Hemolytic Anemia

There is no magical PCV that serves as a transfusion trigger.

All of the following *may* be used to make that determination:

- Clinical signs: Weakness, depression, pallor

---

*In some cases, the methemoglobin level may be very high (>50%), and death occurs rapidly. The membranes are dark but not icteric, and the PCV may be normal with severe methemoglobinemia. Methemoglobin usually can be measured at most hospitals for humans. A new methylene blue stain and examination for Heinz bodies should be performed.

- Clinical findings: Tachycardia, tachypnea
- Hematocrit and hemoglobin level: Generally hemoglobin values <5 g are unable to support tissue oxygen requirements
- Duration of the decline in hematocrit and hemoglobin level: The more acute the drop, the higher the probability a transfusion will be needed
- Pvo_2, Svo_2: Unless there is primary pulmonary disease, arterial samples provide little or no information about need for transfusion. A venous O_2 pressure <30 mm Hg in an anaerobic sample (heparinized syringe) collected from a vein that is only briefly held off and measured immediately (e.g., i-STAT), is a good laboratory determinant to suggest tissue oxygen deficit and time for transfusion. The same is true for Svo_2 <50%.
- Blood lactate concentration >4 mmol/L
- Perform transfusion if PCV decreases to <18% within 24 hours
- In cases with a slower decline in PCV, transfusion can be postponed until the PCV is <12%.
- Oxyglobin, 5-20 ml/kg can be used in either peracute cases or in severe cases while whole-blood transfusion is being organized.
- Administer isotonic fluids if there is clinical evidence of hypovolemia. Although fluids decrease the PCV, they do *not* decrease oxygen-carrying capacity. They increase oxygen supply through an increase in perfusion.
- Oral vitamin C, 250 g q12h for 2 days

Immune-Mediated Hemolytic Anemia

- May result from either an autoimmune reaction or more commonly another disease (lymphoma, equine infectious anemia [EIA], *Clostridium perfringens* or *Streptococcus* infection) or drug-induced hemolytic anemia (most commonly due to intravenous administration of penicillin or ceftiofur)

Clinical Signs and Findings

- Lethargy
- Depression
- Edema, usually in the limbs and ventral body, may be the result of sludging of red blood cell complexes in the microcirculation.
- Pale mucous membranes
- In a few cases, red urine and fever

Diagnosis

- History of penicillin, ceftiofur, or other drug administration within past 1-2 weeks
- Recent infection with *Streptococcus* organisms or less commonly *C. perfringens*
- Suspicion of lymphoma

Laboratory Findings

- PCV decreased
- MCV and MCHC may be increased.
- Look for severe autoagglutination in the EDTA sample; the plasma may be either yellow or pink, depending on the duration of hemolysis and whether it is intravascular or extravascular.

- Internal hemorrhage can be ruled out with the history and the presence of a normal or high plasma protein level.
- Autoagglutination can be differentiated from normal rouleaux formation by means of dilution of the sample 1:4 with 0.9% saline solution.

Additional Tests

- EIA: Coggins test (serology)
- Coombs test (EDTA sample): If autoagglutination is obvious, there is no need to perform a Coombs test.
- Antibody-coated red blood cells (RBCs) may be detected with flow cytometry (Kansas State).
- Heinz bodies may be seen with oxidant-induced hemolytic anemia but not with autoimmune hemolytic anemia.

Treatment

- Blood transfusion only if needed (see guidelines on p. 336) from donor compatible on the basis of cross-matching
- Dexamethasone, 0.04-0.08 mg/kg IV q24h

Neonatal Isoerythrolysis

- Suspect neonatal isoerythrolysis (NI) in young foals, especially mule foals, younger than 7 days of age that have icterus, tachycardia, and weakness.
- The foal is usually a product of a multiparous mare.
- Urine is usually discolored in peracute cases: Usually light red (hemoglobin), although it can be brown (bilirubin) in chronic cases.
- *There are many causes of jaundice in young foals,* such as sepsis. NI usually can be differentiated from other causes by means of measurement of the PCV, which usually is <20% in clinically ill foals with NI. NI is unrelated to the A or Q antigen in *mules.*

Additional Tests

- Use Coombs test with whole blood (EDTA) to confirm an immune reaction. Close examination of the sample may reveal autoagglutination (presence of clumps), in which case a Coombs test is not needed for confirmation.

Treatment

- If the foal is less than 48 hours old, do not allow it to nurse unless the mare's colostrum has a colostrometer value of <1.03 and the colostrum added to the sire's red blood cells does not result in agglutination. Accomplish this with as little stress as possible to the foal; use a muzzle.
- Peracute severe cases with PCV <20% within 24 hours:
  - Transfusion for horse foals from Aa- and Qa-negative donors. A cross-match (major and minor) is ideal. If a cross-match is not feasible, use of an Aa/Qa negative donor usually is safe and effective. The mare's blood may be used if it is washed three times and suspended in saline solution before each transfusion, which is time consuming.

The ideal time to use oxyglobin is in peracute cases while whole-blood transfusion is being organized.

LIVER

- *Mule foals:* Female donors should not have been previously bred with a donkey.

> All equine practices should have Aa/Qa-negative donors identified for emergency purposes. Blood typing can be performed by sending samples of acid-citrate-dextrose (ACD) anticoagulated blood to the Veterinary Genetics Laboratory, School of Veterinary Medicine, University of California, Davis, CA 95616; (916) 752-2211, or to the Equine Blood Typing Research Laboratory, University of Kentucky, Department of Veterinary Science, Lexington, KY 40546; (606) 257-3022. Donors should be free of Aa and/or Qa antigens and hemolytic or agglutinating Aa, Qa antibodies.

- Administer intravenous fluids at maintenance level (approximately 60 ml/kg per day).
- ➤ *Administration of needed intravenous fluids decreases PCV but does not reduce the total numbers of RBCs and does not exacerbate hypoxemia.*
- Administer dexamethasone, 0.04 mg/lb (0.08 mg/kg), only in peracute cases (foals 2 days of age or younger with PCV <12%), if donor cells cannot be administered immediately, or if compatibility is uncertain.
- Administer intranasal oxygen (5 L/min) bubbled through a nasopharyngeal tube if the foal is severely anemic.
- Administer antimicrobials or antibiotics to all foals with NI to minimize sepsis. Despite evidence of passive transfer of colostral antibodies, NI foals can become septic. Valuable foals should be administered a combination of intravenous penicillin and amikacin or ceftiofur; less valuable foals can be given a combination of trimethoprim-sulfamethoxazole (20 mg/kg PO q12h) and penicillin (22,000 IU/kg q12h IM).
- ➤ Antiulcer medication: Sucralfate, 1 g PO q6h with or without a histamine H_2-receptor blocker or proton pump blocker.
- Provide nutritional support (Land-O-Lakes) foal milk replacement, such as mare's milk or goat's milk, at 20%-25% of body weight per day during the time* the foal is not allowed to nurse.
- Provide supportive care, such as keeping the foal warm.
- Expect a second decline in PCV 4-11 days after the transfusion.

Other Causes of Hemolysis in Adults
Babesia Infection (Piroplasmosis)
- *Babesia caballi* and *Babesia equi*
- *B. equi* is more pathogenic.
- Found in North and South America, including the Caribbean region, Europe, Russia, Asia, Africa, and the Middle East

CLINICAL SIGNS
- All horses are susceptible; older horses are more severely affected. Once infected, survivors are carriers.
- Incubation period is 5-28 days.
- Fever 38.9°C-41.7°C (102°F-107°F)
- Hemolytic anemia
- Jaundice

---

*The foal should be 36-48 hours old before it is allowed to nurse.

- Hemoglobinuria
- Death

GENERALIZED SIGNS
- Depression, anorexia, incoordination, lacrimation, mucous nasal discharge, eyelid swelling, increased recumbency

DIFFERENTIAL DIAGNOSIS
- Equine granulocytic ehrlichiosis *(Anaplasma Phagocytophilia)*
- EIA
- Liver failure

DIAGNOSIS
- Serologic tests: Complement fixation, indirect fluorescence antibody assay, cytologic identification of the organism on a Giemsa-stained blood smear, although the result may be negative in infected horses even when the sample is drawn from a small-diameter vessel.

TREATMENT
- *B. equi* is more refractory to treatment than is *B. caballi*.
- Imidocarb: For *B. caballi*: 2.2 mg/kg two times q24h; for *B. equi*: 4.0 mg/kg 4 times q72h.

> **CAUTION:** Do not treat donkeys at the higher dosage; death results. Imidocarb may cause signs of colic.

- Tetracycline, 6.6 mg/kg q12h slowly IV diluted

PREVENTION AND CONTROL
- Tick control is key.
- No effective vaccine is available.

Granulocytic Ehrlichiosis (a Differential Diagnosis for Babesiosis and Equine Infectious Anemia)
GENERAL INFORMATION
- Rickettsial disease *Anaplasma Phagocytophilia*
- Recovery (without treatment) is usually within 2-3 weeks.
- The vector is a tick, *Ixodes* sp.
- Not contagious, but multiple cases may occur on the same premises.
- Abortion is not an expected complication of granulocytic ehrlichiosis.
- Common in northern California and in parts of the eastern coast and the surrounding states but has been reported in many other states

SIGNS
- Fever (38.9°C-41.7°C [102°F-107°F]), icterus, depression, anorexia, limb edema, mucosal petechiae, ataxia, reluctance to move (typically worse if horse is older than 3 years). Clinical disease is most common in the fall and winter in California.

DIAGNOSIS
- Cytoplasmic inclusions in neutrophils and eosinophils (see Color Plate 11)

LIVER

- Serologic test (Texas A & M Diagnostic Laboratory or University of California, Davis). Some horses may require several weeks for seroconversion.
- Leukopenia (mild to moderate)
- Thrombocytopenia, anemia

TREATMENT
- Supportive therapy
- Oxytetracycline, 6.6 mg/kg IV q12-24h, will shorten the disease course considerably.

Equine Infectious Anemia
GENERAL INFORMATION
- Necrotizing vasculitis of the horse, donkey, and mule
- Affected horses are carriers of the EIA retrovirus for life and may have periodic episodes of clinical signs
- Transmitted by the horsefly
- Infected mares may abort at any stage of gestation
- Clinical EIA can be recognized in different stages: Can be acute or chronic
- *Acute EIA is characterized by fever, depression, petechiae. An acutely affected horse may die in a few days.*
- *EIA is a reportable disease*

SIGNS
- Fever, anemia, icterus, ventral edema, weight loss, depression, petechiae (if disease is acute)

DIAGNOSIS
- Agar-gel immunodiffusion (Coggins test): Serum antibodies to EIA retrovirus. Result may be falsely negative in first 2 weeks after infection. Result may be falsely positive in foals born to infected mares. Use red-top tube (clot tube) sample for Coggins test.
- Anemia can be marked and progressive; Coombs test result may be positive.
- Mild lymphocytosis, monocytosis
- Thrombocytopenia is common during febrile episodes.

TREATMENT
- Isolate as soon as possible (200 yards [180 m] from other horses in a screened stall).
- No treatment other than supportive care is successful if the horse is in the carrier state. No treatment or vaccination exists specifically for EIA.
- EIA is a reportable disease. Contact the state veterinary medical office.

Other Less Common Causes of Hemolysis and Icterus (see discolored urine, Table 44–1)
- Hepatic failure (p. 316)
- Clostridial infection (pp. 309-311)
- Snake bite (p. 312)
- Disseminated intravascular coagulation (DIC): Microangiopathic hemolytic anemia may occasionally occur with DIC. Therapy is for the primary disease.
- Renal failure (p. 531)
- Leptospirosis: Rarely causes hemolysis or hematuria

NOTE: A common cause of acute anemia in the horse is *heparin* therapy. The PCV may decrease as low as 14%. The anemia is a result of both spurious lowering of the PCV and increased sequestration of the red blood cells by reticuloendothelial cells. Hemolysis does not occur, and PCV returns to the previous level within 2-4 days after discontinuation of heparin treatment.

HEMORRHAGE INTO BODY CAVITY

In adults, hemorrhage occurs most often into the abdomen. It can result from trauma (ruptured spleen or liver), foaling (ruptured middle uterine artery), surgery (e.g., ovariectomy), or idiopathic causes. *Idiopathic causes are common, especially among older horses.* In the newborn foal, rib fractures and umbilical cord hemorrhage are most common.

Clinical Signs
- Abdominal pain, increased respiratory rate, increased heart rate, pale mucous membranes, trembling, sweating, distress

Diagnosis
ABDOMINOCENTESIS
- Uniform stream of red fluid that does not clot with a PCV often ranging from 8% to 20%, confirms the diagnosis of bleeding. Platelets usually are not seen, and erythrophagocytosis may be present.

ULTRASONOGRAPHY
- Perform ultrasound examination of the abdomen for detection of cellular fluid in the abdominal cavity. Carefully inspect the liver and spleen if trauma is suspected. Tears in the liver and spleen may be seen with ultrasound and usually require corrective surgery.

Treatment
IDIOPATHIC
- Keep the patient quiet.
- Administer intravenous fluids (polyionic fluids), 20-80 ml/kg over several hours, depending on the degree of hypovolemia. *Low to normal blood pressure should be maintained (permissive hypotension).* Do not use hetastarch.
- ε-Aminocaproic acid (Amicar): 10-20 mg/kg IV *mixed* in the intravenous fluids
- Analgesics as needed to control pain and anxiety: Flunixin and phenylbutazone have little effect on platelet function.
- Intranasal oxygen in severe cases
- Do not perform surgery unless the patient continues to deteriorate, because the bleeding is likely to stop in older horses with no history of trauma. If there were a history of trauma, surgery would be indicated.
- Transfusion if PCV declines to <15% in subacute cases or chronic cases. In peracute cases, transfusion may be needed before a decrease in PCV occurs.

General Considerations for Blood Transfusion: When to Perform Transfusion for a Hemorrhaging Patient

> There is no magical cutoff for PCV and plasma protein that would definitely indicate transfusion.

LIVER

- Horses can generally lose 20%-30% of their blood volume (8%-10% of body weight) without a change in blood pressure, due to increased cardiac output, pressor responses, and renal and endocrine responses.
- If the hemorrhage is definitely stopped, crystalloids are probably all that is needed! Approximately 4 times the estimated blood loss.
  □ As fluid therapy is administered, blood pressure and the laboratory parameters listed for timing of transfusion for hemolytic patients (see p. 328) should be evaluated for markers of tissue hypoxia.
  □ Unneeded transfusion may result in immunosuppression.
- Fresh, frozen plasma can and probably should be used in the management of ongoing hemorrhage in the hope of replacing clotting factors.
- Hetastarch should not be used in the presence of uncontrolled bleeding or DIC.
- Autotransfusion is used if it is reasonably clear that the bleeding is not associated with sepsis (traumatized bowel, liver abscess or tumor).
- If bleeding into the abdomen or chest is so severe that it mechanically restricts ventilation, the blood should be removed. Otherwise, nonseptic blood should be left in the body cavity; the increased pressure helps promote clotting. The blood can be removed if immediate transfusion is required.

⮞ HEMORRHAGE WITH TRAUMA
- Keep the patient quiet.
- Administer intravenous fluids (polyionic fluids), 20-80 ml/kg over several hours or more, depending on the degree of hypovolemia and blood pressure.
- ε-Aminocaproic acid (Amicar): 10-20 mg/kg IV *mixed* in the IV fluids
- Analgesics as needed to control pain and anxiety
- Intranasal oxygen in severe cases
- Consider exploratory surgery. If a tear in the liver or spleen is found, splenectomy is possible. Gelfoam (gelatin foam sponge) may be used to manage liver lacerations. The prognosis is guarded with liver lacerations.

MIDDLE UTERINE ARTERY RUPTURE
If the affected horse is very agitated, use acepromazine, 0.02 mg/kg, along with balanced crystalloids and blood transfusion. If the heart rate is >100 beats/min and the membranes are white, *do not* use acepromazine. Use hypertonic saline solution *only* if rapid deterioration appears imminent and temporary improvement in the blood pressure is needed to pursue blood transfusion or surgery. Treatments that maintain systolic pressure between 70-90 are ideal (permissive hypotension).

RIB FRACTURES
- General considerations
  □ Hemorrhage into the thorax is common among foals but often is not recognized before death in adults.
  □ Look for evidence of pneumothorax. Provide intranasal oxygen and perform thoracocentesis; apply a Heimlich chest drain if dyspnea is severe. Keep the horse quiet and start antimicrobial therapy with a broad-spectrum antibiotic.
  □ Any physical examination of a foal, especially a neonate, includes a careful examination of the thoracic wall. Rib fractures can cause severe pneumothorax and hemothorax and rapid death.
- Fractures are generally just caudal to the elbow.
- Signs of hemothorax

- □ Hemorrhagic anemia
- □ Dyspnea
- □ Painful chest, reluctance to move
- □ Decreased or absent ventral lung sounds, frequently recognized bilaterally
- □ Possible jugular distention or jugular pulses
- □ Jaundice present or absent
- Diagnosis
  - □ Physical examination and ultrasound examination
  - □ Ultrasound examination of the thorax reveals cellular pleural fluid.
  - □ Diaphragmatic hernia may occur simultaneously.
  - □ Pleurocentesis reveals blood with no bacteria.
- Treatment
  - □ *Keep the foal quiet.* This is very important! Ideally, the foal is best lying on the fractured side to reduce fracture movement and laceration of a coronary artery.
  - □ Surgery should be strongly considered if there is any displacement of the fracture and/or flail chest or hemothorax are present.
  - □ Administer oxygen if dyspnea is severe.
  - □ Antibiotics: Broad-spectrum, especially if there is an open wound or evidence of pneumothorax.
  - □ Consider blood transfusion (see p. 336).
  - □ Pleurocentesis offers temporary improvement, but the foal should be monitored carefully because the pleural cavity frequently fills rapidly.
  - □ Administer antiulcer medication (see p. 210).

Ruptured Aorta

- Most common among older stallions during breeding
- Often results in immediate death

Diaphragmatic Hernia

- Thoracic bleeding can occur with chest trauma or diaphragmatic hernia.
- Suspect diaphragmatic hernia if a colicky horse has "negative" (or empty-feeling) rectal palpation and any evidence of respiratory compromise, especially if the lung sounds are quiet or absent, or gastrointestinal motility sounds are heard during auscultation of the thorax.
- Diagnosis is made by means of ultrasound examination of the thorax. Be careful performing thoracocentesis because compromised bowel can be penetrated even with a teat cannula.
- Treatment is corrective surgery.

Other Body Cavity Hemorrhage

- Bleeding from thoracic lymphosarcoma is common but rarely causes life-threatening anemia.
- Hemothorax develops in rare instances after exercise and pulmonary hemorrhage. Conservative management that includes therapy for pneumothorax often is successful.

EXTERNAL HEMORRHAGE

Bleeding of a major vessel can be life threatening. This is most commonly a result of trauma, although cellulitis occasionally erodes through a major vessel and causes life-threatening hemorrhage. Whenever possible, application of *pressure bandages* or *suturing the vessel* is performed to prevent additional blood loss. If the heart rate is elevated and the patient appears to be in hypovolemic shock, blood transfusion and administration of polyionic fluids are required. There may not be time for a cross-match; a horse known to be free of A and Q antigen and antibodies is a suitable donor.

➤ *With acute hemorrhage, the horse can die without a decrease in PCV.*

Hemorrhage from the Guttural Pouch

Hemorrhage from the guttural pouch is most often a result of fungal infection and erosion of the external or internal carotid or maxillary arteries within the pouch. The presence of this condition should be confirmed by means of endoscopic examination. Surgery is performed as soon as possible. Plans for a transfusion should be made as soon as the diagnosis is confirmed because acute, severe bleeding can occur.

➤ **Other causes of epistaxis** should be ruled out. Many require no specific treatment. Some can be managed medically (e.g., thrombocytopenia with immunosuppression therapy: dexamethasone, 0.1 mg/kg, and fresh blood transfusion collected in plastic), whereas others, such as ethmoid hematoma, are corrected with laser surgery or formalin injections if the cribriform plate is intact.

GENERAL CONSIDERATIONS IN BLOOD TRANSFUSION

Perform when:

- PCV decreases to <20% in the first 12 hours and hemorrhage or hemolysis is ongoing.
- PCV decreases to <12% over 1-2 days; hemoglobin values <5 g/dl have a marked effect on tissue oxygenation.
- *In peracute cases, death from hemorrhage can occur without a decrease in PCV. In these cases, the need for transfusion is based on the presence of severe tachycardia, white to gray mucous membranes, signs of hypotension (weak pulses, "cold sweat," general weakness, and evidence of severe bleeding).*

➤ ### Choice of Donor

- There are more than 400,000 blood types in the horse, and there is no universal donor.
- If time permits, use a cross-matched donor. The primary interest is in the major testing (donor RBC, plasma recipient). If the donor has not been previously tested for isoantibodies, also perform a minor match. Most of the testing detects agglutination, although a few laboratories (e.g., U.C. Davis or Stormont Labs) can test for lysis (rabbit serum is needed).
- If time does not permit, choose a gelding of the same breed and mix donor serum with patient RBCs and vice versa to look for evidence of agglutination.
- Consider *autotransfusion* for body cavity bleeding *without sepsis*. Blood can be collected from the abdomen or chest by means of insertion of a teat cannula and collection of the blood, with sterile technique, into a container with small amounts of ACD (approximately 1 part ACD per 15 parts blood).

- Store autologous blood for rare elective procedures (e.g., nasal surgery) in which severe hemorrhage is anticipated. Collect in citrate-phosphate-dextrose (CPD) rather than ACD. Can be stored at 4°C (39.2°F) for several days.

Collection and Administration

- Collect blood using aseptic technique in 2.5%-4% ACD: 9 parts blood to 1 part citrate.
- Use a blood collection set: 15%-20% of the blood volume (body weight in kg × 10% = liters of blood in the donor) of a healthy donor can be collected.
- Autotransfusion (see earlier): Use approximately ⅔ normal anticoagulant (ACD or CPD or sodium citrate) or 1 unit heparin per milliliter of blood. Filters should be changed every 2 L during autotransfusion.
- Blood bags, bottles, and anticoagulant can be purchased from Animal Blood Bank, Box 1118, Dixon, CA; (916) 678-7350. In the United Kingdom, telephone 441977-681523.
- Bottles are faster but are not ideal if platelet replacement is important.
  - The following anticoagulants can be used and are listed in order of ability to preserve red cells (least to greatest). This is generally not important unless storage of the red blood cells is planned.

  Sodium citrate
  ACD
  CPD: Red cells can be stored at refrigeration temperature for 2-3 weeks. Platelets are viable for approximately 3 days. (Plastic only)
  DPDA: Cells may be stored at refrigeration temperature for 2-3 weeks. Platelets are viable for approximately 3 days. (Plastic only)

- Administer whole blood with a blood administration set at a rate of 10-20 ml/kg per hour with close monitoring of vital signs. Filters should be replaced after 3-4 L.
- Blood for transfusion should be warmed to body temperature.
- Packed RBCs (80%) can be used to manage euvolemic hemolytic anemia. Example: washed RBCs given to a foal with NI.

Side Effects

If tachypnea, dyspnea, restlessness, pilocrection, and fasciculation occur, stop or slow the transfusion and administer epinephrine, 0.005-0.02 ml/kg of 1:1000 (if severe anaphylaxis), or doxylamine succinate, 0.5 mg/kg IV very slowly. Doxylamine succinate may be administered SQ as prophylaxis before transfusion.

How Much Blood to Administer?

- *At least* 6-8 L to an adult is an estimate or one-half the estimated blood loss.
- In addition, use polyionic fluids, plasma, and in some cases, hetastarch in the management of hypovolemic shock.
- With hemolysis, use the following formula to estimate blood volume needed:

$$\frac{\text{Desired PCV} - \text{PCV recipient } (0.08 \times \text{Body weight in kilograms})}{\text{PCV of donor}} = \text{Liters required}$$

- There is no universal recommendation for a desired PCV. A measurement of venous oxygen (PVO_2) may provide an estimate. An abnormally low PVO_2 or SVO_2 may be an indication of hypoxia.
  - ▫ Administer one third to one half of the calculated volume at 10-20 ml/kg per hour if there is no evidence of adverse reaction. The transfusion rate can be changed depending on the clinical conditions.
  - ▫ Expected life span of transfused "compatible" RBCs is:
    Autologous: At least 12-14 days
    Allogenic: As little as 2-5 days (foals, 3-4 days longer)
  - ▫ Blood collected in CPD maintains viable red blood cells for at least 2 weeks if refrigerated, but transfusion of stored whole blood increases the risk of a reaction.

Other Therapy for Hemorrhage/Hemolysis

- Dexamethasone, 40 mg q24h, for adults with immune-mediated hemolytic anemia. As the PCV stabilizes, dexamethasone dosage can be decreased.
- Isotonic fluids (up to 4 times the blood loss in shock) if the horse is hypo-volemic. Although the PCV decreases, it actually improves oxygen-carrying capacity. Nonisotonic fluids are not recommended except in severe shock.
- Intranasal oxygen is indicated if the horse is severely hypoxic.
- An alternative to whole-blood transfusion if a compatible donor cannot be found is bovine hemoglobin (Biopure Corp., Boston) administered at 1-20 ml/kg. The half-life is approximately 2 days. Oxyglobin is a potent colloid (35 mm Hg versus 21 mm Hg for plasma) and should be used with caution in the management of uncontrolled hemorrhage.

REFERENCES

George LW et al: Heinz body anemia and methemoglobinemia in ponies given red maple leaves, *Vet Pathol* 19:521-533, 1982.

Moore BR, Abood S, Hinchcliff KS: Hyperlipemia in nine miniature horses and miniature donkeys, *J Vet Intern Med* 8:376-381, 1994.

Oryan A et al: *Babesia caballi* and associated pathologic lesions in a horse, *Vet Clin North Am Equine Pract* 16:33-36, 1994.

Robbins RL et al: Immune mediated hemolytic disease after penicillin therapy in a horse, *Equine Vet J* 25:462-465, 1993.

Traub-Dargatz JL et al: Neonatal isoerythrolysis in mule foals, *J Am Vet Med Assoc* 206:67-70, 1995.

Liver Failure

Peek SF, Divers TJ: Medical treatment of cholangiohepatitis and cholelithiasis in mature horses: 9 cases (1991-1998), *Equine Vet J* 32:301-306, 2000.

Peek SF, Divers TJ, Jackson CJ: Hyperammonaemia associated with encephalopathy and abdominal pain without evidence of liver disease in four mature horses, *Equine Vet J* 29:70-74, 1997.

Hemolytic Anemia

Perkins GA, Divers TJ: Polymerized hemoglobin therapy in a foal with neonatal isoerythrolysis, *J Vet Emerg Crit Care* 11:141-147, 2001.

Piercy RJ, Swardson CJ, Hinchcliff KW: Erythroid hypoplasia and anemia following administration of recombinant human erythropoietin to two horses, *J Am Vet Med Assoc* 212:244-247, 1998.

Thomas HL, Livesay MA: Immune-mediated hemolytic anemia associated with trimethoprim-sulfamethoxazole administration in a horse, *Can Vet J* 39:171-173, 1998.

38 Blood Coagulation Disorders

T. Douglas Byars

Coagulation disorders are represented by hypercoagulation (thrombosis) and hypocoagulation (bleeding diathesis). A normal coagulation system can be present in the presence of a hemorrhagic crisis due to physical disruption of vascular integrity, as in external trauma or spontaneous internal vascular rupture (e.g., aortic root rupture, uterine artery hemorrhage, guttural pouch mycosis).

HYPERCOAGULATION: THROMBOPHILIA AND THROMBOSIS

Hypercoagulation is common in horses. It is associated with abnormally elevated platelet counts (thrombocytosis), arteritis (cranial mesenteric arteritis), vasculitis (purpura hemorrhagica), idiopathic iliac thrombosis, spontaneous or sepsis-associated limb arterial thrombosis as in foals, laminitis, pulmonary infarction, deficiencies of antithrombin III and protein C or S cofactors, inhibition of fibrinolysis, and related consumptive coagulopathies (disseminated intravascular coagulation [DIC]). DIC can exhibit laboratory evidence of hypocoagulation (prolonged clotting times and thrombocytopenia) while the individual has clinical evidence of hypercoagulation, such as vascular thrombosis without overt signs of bleeding.

HYPOCOAGULATION: BLEEDING DISORDERS AND DIATHESIS

Hypocoagulation in the horse can be associated with thrombocytopenia (immune mediated or acquired), toxicosis (warfarin toxicity, moxalactam and related antibiotics), inherited disorders (hemophilia A, von Willebrand disease), primary fibrinolysis (hyperplasminemia), and DIC as a consumptive coagulopathy with secondary fibrinolysis.

Clinical Signs of Thrombosis or Hemorrhage

- Obvious clinical signs of thrombosis or hemorrhage can be inapparent because of pigment and hair in the horse.
- Examination of the mucous membranes often supports the clinical recognition of disorders of either thrombotic lesions or a bleeding diathesis.
- Thrombotic lesions are consistent with partial or complete ischemia. Apparent clinical signs of thrombosis may not be present until identified at surgery or post-mortem. Antemortem diagnosis can be established with ultrasound identification of intravascular clot formation or with Doppler detection of decreased blood flow. Clinical thrombosis can be evident, as in jugular thrombosis, asymmetric cold limbs, hypothermic lameness related to increased exercise, or the presence of regional edema in conjunction with petechial or ecchymotic hemorrhage (purpura, vasculitis).
- Hemorrhagic disorders can be acute or chronic. An acute bleed is commonly accompanied by changes in vital signs (tachycardia, tachypnea, and hypothermia) and pale mucous membranes. Peracute aortic root rupture with collapse and death usually occurs in stallions after breeding. Uterine-ovarian artery rupture usually is acute and can occur before or after parturition. A

subcutaneous hematoma may follow trauma or spontaneous hemorrhage. Ultrasound evaluation of body cavities may show the presence of extraneous "ground glass" swirling fluid indicative of the presence of free blood within a space. Epistaxis, genitourinary hemorrhage, melena, and petechial or ecchymotic lesions may be present. Overt epistaxis can be caused by exercise-induced pulmonary hemorrhage (EIPH), guttural pouch mycosis, ethmoidal hematoma, sinusitis, trauma, and coagulation deficiencies, including thrombocytopenia.

Laboratory Assessment of Coagulation

The following laboratory tests are available in most equine testing laboratories. Clotting time assays also are available with point-of-care instrumentation. Specialized tests (coagulation factors, von Willebrand disease, antibody-coated platelet, protein assays) necessitate referral of samples to a research laboratory or for consultation.

NOTE: If known laboratory values are not available, a normal control sample is recommended for interpretation of results.

- Platelet counts: False platelet aggregation can occur in EDTA and therefore may necessitate sample collection in sodium citrate for quantitative counts. A scan of a hematology slide for adequate platelet numbers by a laboratory technician is accurate in detecting inadequate numbers. Qualitative function testing can be performed in vivo by means of the bleeding time assay with a sphygmomanometer cuff and a Simplate incision device or in the laboratory by means of instrumentation aggregometry.
- Activated coagulation time (ACT): Activated whole-blood clotting time. This test replaces the Lee-White whole-blood clotting test because it is easier to perform and more accurate.
- Prothrombin time (PT): Evaluation of the extrinsic coagulation system.
- Activated partial thromboplastin time (aPTT): Evaluation of the intrinsic coagulation system. Point-of-care automated coagulation systems are available for "bedside" coagulation testing. The SCA2000 system (Synbiotics, San Diego) is accurate and is used to measure ACT, PT, and aPTT.
- Fibrinogen: Quantification of fibrinogen can be performed by means of either heat precipitation or the use of a fibrometer.
- Fibrinogen and fibrin degradation products (FDPs): Evaluation of primary (activated plasminogen without clot formation, fibrinogenolysis) or secondary (clot dissolution) fibrinolysis. Commercial test kits may not differentiate the FDP fragments, XYDE, whereas measurement of D-dimer reflects recognition of secondary fibrinolysis and is the preferred test.

BLOOD CLOTTING DISORDERS

Thrombocytopenia

Thrombocytopenia is not an uncommon clinical finding in equine practice and is usually associated with a severe systemic inflammatory response or secondary to immune-mediated platelet removal by the spleen. The autoimmune phenomena can be secondary to a viral infection, abscessation, neoplasia, colostral antibodies or drug-associated causes (the platelet is the "innocent bystander") or is idiopathic. If thrombocytopenia occurs in conjunction with autoimmune hemolytic anemia (Coombs positive) the disorder is known as Evans's syndrome and is more commonly associated with a primary neoplasia or abscess.

➤ An unusual thrombocytopenia (often severe) with oral vesicles and skin lesions has recently been reported in foals and appears to be an immune reaction to colostral antibodies. Most foals have recovered with or without steroid therapy.

A low platelet count can be evident on a blood smear or by absolute count. Petechiation typically is observable with platelet counts in the 40,000-60,000/μl range. A more serious bleed (epistaxis) can occur in the 10,000-40,000/μl range, and *life-threatening hemorrhage can develop at less than 10,000/μl.* Blood samples can be tested at Kansas State for antibody-coated platelets and/or a regenerative platelet response. The platelet count can be normal even when platelet function is compromised, as in drug-induced (aspirin-induced bleeding has not been reported among horses) or an associated bleeding disorder (e.g., von Willebrand disease).

➤ **Management of platelet autoimmune deficiencies** consists primarily with the administration of corticosteroids.

Dexamethasone is considered the most effective drug as long as caution is practiced regarding laminitis. Doses may vary from a low of 10 mg to a high of 80 mg per adult, preferably administered IV with a 20-g needle. Platelet counts should be determined every other day until numbers reach levels consistent with near-normal values and then steroid administration can be tapered. In some cases the use of vincristine, 1 mg IV, can be combined with the steroid, once a day for 3-5 days, twice a week for 1-2 weeks and finally once a week until the platelet count remains stable. A plasma transfusion has been beneficial in some horses, allegedly as a source of blocking antibody. Plasma, freshly collected in plastic bags, or whole blood, provides a source of platelets that may inhibit bleeding. If the thrombocytopenia is a result of increased consumption, there is little benefit from the transfusion. Fresh frozen plasma may have hemostatically functional platelet microparticles.

Clotting Factor Deficiencies

Clotting factor deficiencies are relatively uncommon among horses. Hemophilia is the most common inherited disorder. Foals usually have hemarthrosis of many joints or bleed excessively from minor wounds. The aPTT (intrinsic system) is prolonged, and factor VIII is deficient. Factor VIII–associated deficiency occurs with von Willebrand disease and is linked with qualitative deficiencies in platelet function that cause an increase in the in vivo bleeding time test results.

Acquired factor deficiencies occur with toxicities such as to warfarin, which primarily affects the extrinsic coagulation system (factor VII) and prolongs the PT. Some lactam and β-lactam antibiotics (most notably moxalactam and carbenicillin) are capable of causing hypoprothrombinemia. Advanced liver disease may result in both intrinsic and extrinsic factor deficiencies.

Disseminated Intravascular Coagulation

DIC is an acquired thrombotic and bleeding disorder secondary to a primary disease process such as sepsis, systemic inflammatory response syndrome (SIRS), endotoxemia, trauma, immune reaction, or organ failure. It is a true consumptive coagulopathy and is associated with a poor prognosis. DIC can be acute or chronic and be either local or systemic. The diagnosis of DIC can be made by means of assessment of the results of the principal diagnostic tests of coagulation: ACT, PT, aPTT, platelet count, and measurement of fibrinogen and evaluation for the presence of FDPs. An additional test for antithrombin III is useful in the diagnosis of DIC. The level of this heparin cofactor often is less than 60% to 70% of normal. Other associated diagnostic signs include deficiency of anticoagulant proteins C and S, levels of which decrease in association with sepsis and SIRS and can contribute to thrombophilia before the consumptive coagulopathy of DIC occurs.

Management of DIC always should include treatment for the primary disorder if known and treatments that slow the consumptive process. Heparin in conjunction with normalizing plasma antithrombin III levels is traditionally recommended at dosages of 40-80 IU/kg three or four times a day SQ or IV in fluids. Subcutaneous dosing can result in local swelling, and heparin use has been associated with secondary anemia. Blood and plasma transfusions are controversial in regard to adding "fuel to the fire" by providing additional components for the continuation of the consumptive process. However, absolute contraindications also are controversial. If supported on the basis of clinical or laboratory results, plasma transfusion is indicated with low antithrombin III levels.

▶ Management of DIC often is difficult and must be individualized.

REFERENCES

General

Kopp KJ et al: Bleeding time effects of three nonsteroidal inflammatory drugs in the horse, *Equine Vet J* 17:322-324, 1985.

Rathegeber R et al: Von Willebrand disease in a Thoroughbred mare and foal, *J Vet Intern Med* 15:63-65, 2001.

Hemorrhage

Perkins G, Ainsworth DM, Yeager A: Hemothorax in 2 horses, *J Vet Intern Med* 13:375-378, 1999.

Waguespack R, Belknap J, Williams A: Laparoscopic management of postcastration hemorrhage in a horse, *Equine Vet J* 33:510-513, 2001.

Thrombocytopenia

Sellon DC, Levine J, Millikin E: Thrombocytopenia in horses: 35 cases (1989-1994), *J Vet Intern Med* 10:127-132, 1996.

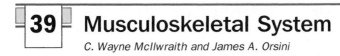

39 Musculoskeletal System

C. Wayne McIlwraith and James A. Orsini

Equine orthopedic emergencies include:

- Fracture
- Luxation
- Laceration of supporting structures
- Laceration of major peripheral blood vessels
- Puncture of synovial structures, including joints, bursae, and tendon sheaths and infection of these structures

Most of these injuries cannot be managed easily in the field and necessitate transport of the patient to another environment or referral to a surgical facility. The horse is frequently anxious as it attempts to use the injured limb, causing additional secondary soft-tissue injury that *complicates later repair efforts.*

Emergency Steps

- Calm the patient using tranquilization, sedation, and pain relief.
- Perform a cursory examination to determine whether repair is feasible.
- Apply protective splints, bandages, or a cast if appropriate.
- Continue the diagnostic examination.
- Transport the patient to an equine hospital.

TRANQUILIZATION, SEDATION, AND PAIN RELIEF

- There is a choice of sedative drugs and at least one tranquilizer (acetylpromazine) to calm the patient.
- Several opioid agonists (morphine, meperidine [Demerol]) and agonist-antagonist preparations (butorphanol, pentazocine) can be used to manage pain.

The goal is relaxation without ataxia. Table 39–1 lists suggested regimens to reduce anxiety with readily available drugs. The most commonly used are xylazine plus butorphanol and detomidine plus butorphanol; additional combinations are available. Use of these agents allows sufficient time to stabilize the limb, assess the degree of bony involvement, and obtain radiographs before transporting the patient.

COMMON ORTHOPEDIC EMERGENCIES

- Sedate or restrain the patient enough to examine the injury.
- Perform a cursory examination to determine the general category of injury.
- For *non–weight-bearing* lameness, rule out
  - Displaced fracture
  - Luxation
  - Infection
- Orthopedic emergencies that allow some degree of *weight bearing* include:
  - Laceration

MUSCULOSKELETAL

TABLE 39–1. Drug Combinations and Dosages Useful in Equine
Orthopedic Emergencies

Combination	IV Dosage	Effects
Xylazine (Rompun)* *plus*	0.3-1.1 mg/kg (average, 2 ml/ 500 kg)	Produces sedation and analgesia for up to 30 minutes Useful for limb stabilization and early transportation
Butorphanol (Torbugesic)†	0.02-0.05 mg/kg (average, 1.5 ml/ 500 kg)	
Xylazine (Rompun)* *plus*	0.3-0.6 mg/kg (average, 2 ml/ 500 kg)	May cause profound hypotension in the face of excitement or high blood loss
Acetylpromazine (Acepromazine)†	0.02-0.03 mg/kg (average, 1.5 ml/ 500 kg)	Horse may fall because of a dramatic decrease in arterial blood pressure
Detomidine (Dormosedan)§ *plus*	0.01-0.02 mg/kg (average, 0.5 ml/ 500 kg)	Ataxia is present at higher dosages, making control more difficult Sedation is profound, allowing more painful manipulation
Butorphanol (Torbugesic)†	0.02-0.05 mg/kg (average, 1 ml/ 500 kg)	May have to delay trailering for more than 1 h
Epidural morphine/xylazine	50 mg/500 kg morphine 80 mg/500 kg xylazine	Epidural catheter needed for frequent dosing. Morphine-preservative free
Fentanyl Transdermal System (Duragesic)#	2-100 ug/h/ 500 kg	Replace every 2-3 days. The withers works well for good skin contact

Concentrations:
*Rompun, 100 mg/ml (Miles, Inc., Shawnee Mission, KS)
†Torbugesic, 10 mg/ml (Fort Dodge Animal Health, Fort Dodge, IA)
†Acepromazine, 10 mg/ml (Fort Dodge Animal Health, Fort Dodge, IA)
§Dormosedan, 10 mg/ml (Pfizer Animal Health, Exton, PA)
#Duragesic, 100 μg/h Transdermal System (Janssen Pharmaceutica Products L.P., Titusville, NJ)

□ Puncture wound
□ Nondisplaced fracture
▪ *Determining whether the patient can bear weight allows an initial decision about how to proceed.*

FRACTURES
Long-Bone Fractures
▪ Emergency treatment focuses on calming or restraining the horse.
▪ Assess the severity of the fracture.
▪ Protect the injured limb to prevent further damage.
▪ Horses attempt to bear weight on even a grossly unstable leg. Protect the limb with splints or casts before radiographic examination or transportation to a surgical facility.
▪ Fractures can occur in many different situations. Suspect fracture when
  □ The horse is acutely non–weight-bearing.
  □ A loud crack is heard before the onset of lameness.

□ The limb is grossly unstable.
- Physical examination determines the level of the suspected fracture.
  □ Forelimb fracture divisions:

  Level 1: Phalanges and distal metacarpus
  Level 2: Midforearm to distal metacarpus
  Level 3: Middle and proximal radius
  Level 4: Proximal to the cubital (elbow) joint in the forelimb

  □ Hindlimb fracture divisions:

  Level 1: Phalanges and distal metatarsus
  Level 2: Middle and proximal metatarsus
  Level 3: Tarsus (hock) and tibia
  Level 4: Femur and above

Immobilization

- Closed fractures at *levels 1 and 2,* such as nondisplaced condylar fracture, have the best prognosis for repair and are managed initially with a cast, splint, or well-applied bandage immediately to *protect the soft tissues* from further damage.
- *Level 3* fractures, that is, of the middle and proximal radius and the tibia, carry a grave prognosis. They often are open fractures and difficult to immobilize for transport.
- In the treatment of foals, apply a splint and transport the patient to a hospital for repair if feasible.
- In the treatment of adults, because of the poor prognosis, euthanasia often is recommended.
- *Level 4* fractures are surrounded by a large muscle mass that provides protection against open fracture.
- Little is done to splint or support these fractures.
- Front limb splintage of the carpus allows the patient to balance on the limb for transport. Extension of lower limb with a large bandage improves the support.

Level 1 Fractures

▶ *A splint-cast is recommended before transporting the patient with a fracture of the digit or the distal metacarpal or metatarsal bones (level 1).*

Materials for a Splint-Cast
■ Leg bandage materials
■ Polyvinyl chloride (PVC) splint, 40-45 cm (~16-18 in) long
■ 4-6 rolls of 4- to 5-inch (10-12.5 cm) fiberglass casting material

PROCEDURE
- After application of a light cotton bandage to the limb from carpus or tarsus to the coronary band, elevate the limb and have an assistant hold it proximal to the carpus or tarsus.
- Maintain the leg in this position until application of the splint or cast is complete and the cast material cures.

- Place a PVC or wood splint on the dorsal surface of the forelimbs or the plantar surface of the hindlimbs (Figs. 39–1 and 39–2).
- PVC splints are constructed by cutting the appropriate length of 4-inch (10-cm) PVC pipe (available at any hardware store) into thirds longitudinally and rounding the edges.
- Incorporate PVC pipe into a fiberglass cast and allow it to set.
- Apply minimal padding to prevent cast slippage during transport.
- With the limb in a cast, the patient is able to support weight on the toe without additional damage.
- Incorporation of the foot with the heel elevated requires more cast material and helps the horse maintain better balance during transport. Radiographs taken through the cast provide a more accurate prognosis regarding the injury and treatment options.

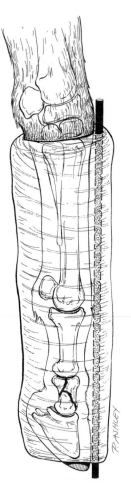

FIGURE 39–1. Splint-cast placement for a **level 1** fracture of the foreleg. The splint is placed on the dorsal surface of the limb, over minimal padding, and secured with cast material.

- An alternative limb immobilization is use of a preformed splint that holds the leg in a slight degree of flexion and allows weight bearing on the toe. The Leg-Saver* brace is an aluminum splint secured to the limb with Velcro straps.

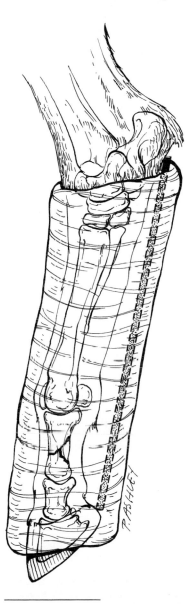

FIGURE 39–2. Splint-cast placement for a **level 1** fracture of the rear limb. The splint is placed on the plantar aspect of the limb.

---

*Leg-Saver splint. Kimzey Inc., 164 Kentucky Avenue, Woodland, CA 95695; (530) 662-9331; Fax: (530) 662-9178); www.kimzeymetalproducts.com.

Level 2 Fractures

- Fractures at level 2, proximal metacarpus to distal radius and proximal metatarsus, are supported with a Robert Jones bandage with caudal and lateral splints.

Materials for a Robert Jones Bandage

- 6-8 rolls of 1-pound-roll cotton
- 4-6 gauze bandages or elastic tape, 6-inch (15-cm)
- 1-2 Ace bandages, 6-inch (15-cm)
- 2-4 broom handles or wooden splints
- Duct tape, 2-inch (5-cm)

PROCEDURE
- Restrain the patient.
- Apply heavy cotton bandage to stabilize the limb and prevent fracture fragment shifting.
- Bandaging also reduces edema and hematoma formation at the fracture site.
- With this support, the patient can use the limb for balance, even though not fully weight bearing, which helps reduce anxiety.
- Apply multiple layers of cotton directly to the limb if the fracture is closed and over a sterile dressing if there is a skin wound.
- After application of two rolls of cotton, place a 6-inch (15-cm) gauze or elastic bandage with enough pressure to hold the cotton securely in place.
- The internal pressure of the bandage protects the overlying soft tissues. In the forelimb, the resultant bandage extends from elbow to ground and is three times the diameter of the limb when completed.
- In the rear limb, the bandage extends from tuber calcaneus to the ground and is two times the diameter of the limb.
- If splints are used, they are incorporated into the last layer of cotton and gauze.
- The outermost layer of tape is inelastic material, such as duct tape (available at any hardware store), for rigidity.

Level 3 Fractures

- Fractures at level 3, middle and proximal radius, tarsus, and tibia, are difficult to splint because of abduction of the lower portion of the limb.
- The lateral muscles of the upper forearm pull the lower portion of the limb outward and displace the fracture fragments medially.
- A long extension of the lateral splint to the shoulder or hip after placement of a Robert Jones wrap is used to neutralize lower limb abduction (Figs. 39–3 and 39–4).
- Apply the splints with nonelastic tape to minimize slippage during transportation.

Transportation of the Patient

- Loading should be as atraumatic as possible and is facilitated by bringing the trailer as close to the patient as feasible.
- Adults do best when trailered in a confined space; they can use the sides for support.
- The patient is tied loosely, or not at all, to allow use of the head and neck for balance.

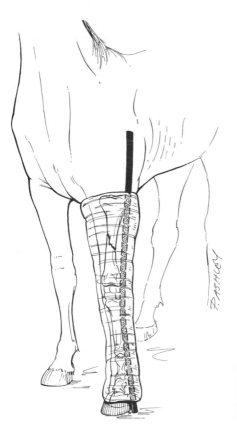

FIGURE 39-3. Robert Jones bandage plus splint for a **level 3** fracture of the forelimb. The extended splint helps reduce lower limb abduction.

- For a forelimb fracture it is helpful that the patient face backward in the trailer so it can support itself and use its rear limbs when the trailer stops.
- If the patient has never been trailered, the added anxiety may not warrant this approach.
- A patient with a hindlimb fracture is transported facing forward; extreme care is needed during unloading to protect the injured limb.
- A large stock trailer with a partition is best for a mare and injured foal. The mare is restrained on one side so she can see the foal. The bedding is deep on the foal's side for comfort.
- An assistant cradling the foal's head to prevent struggling is helpful.

Prognosis for Long-Bone Fractures

- *The prognosis for successful repair decreases as age and weight increase.*
- Owners frequently base their decisions about transporting a horse for surgery on the veterinarian's advice.
- The prognosis for return to athletic function or, at a minimum, reproductive function is often the basis for the decision.

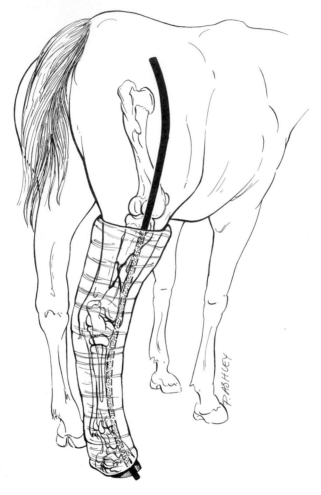

FIGURE 39-4. Robert Jones bandage plus splint for a **level 3** fracture of the rear limb.

- After general evaluation and limb stabilization, obtain radiographs of the affected area to determine treatment options.
- Consult the nearest surgical facility treating long-bone fractures for experiences and costs.
- Some owners pursue all possibilities and therefore should be referred as soon as a splint is in place; radiographs can be obtained at the referral center.
- Open fractures have a poorer prognosis than do closed fractures.
- Fractures more proximal on the limb have a poorer prognosis than do those more distal.

NOTE: A rule of thumb is that repair of proximal fractures in horses that weigh less than 600 lbs (272 kg) may be feasible.

- Each fracture must be considered with regard to the following additional information:
- The owner's intended use of the horse
- Temperament of the horse
- Surgical expertise available
- Economics
- Specific prognoses for fractures and their treatments are summarized in Table 39–2.

Incisive Bone, Mandibular, and Premaxillary Fractures

These fractures are common. The mandible is the most frequently fractured bone in the head.

Etiology

- Unilateral or bilateral
- Fractures occur when teeth are caught on a fixed object
- Iatrogenic during tooth extraction or repulsion or pathologic as a result of chronic alveolar periostitis
- Interdental space most common site

Diagnosis

- Malocclusion of the incisor teeth
- Pain on palpation
- Crepitation
- Food packed into open fracture
- Fetid odor if fracture is several days old
- Salivation, dysphagia, tongue protrusion
- Radiographs: Lateral, dorsoventral, and oblique projections

Treatment

- Horizontal and vertical fractures generally do not require surgical intervention because soft tissues support rami (pterygoid and masseter muscles).
- Stable, nondisplaced unilateral fractures generally require a conservative approach.
- Fractures involving deciduous teeth necessitate removal of involved teeth.
- Unstable fractures necessitate surgical management:
  - Intraoral wire fixation
  - Orthopedic pin and wire fixation
  - Lag screw fixation
  - External thermoplastic brace
  - Intraoral U-bar technique
  - Intraoral acrylic splint
  - Intramedullary pinning
  - External skeletal fixation device
  - Dynamic compression plating

Prognosis

- Generally good.

| **NOTE:** Adequate immobilization is necessary.

TABLE 39–2. Treatment and Prognosis for Return to Former Use for Various Equine Fractures

Fracture Location	Fracture Type	Treatment	Prognosis
Distal phalanx	Articular	Medical or surgical	Guarded
	Nonarticular	Medical	Good
Middle phalanx	Comminuted	Medical or surgical	Guarded
Proximal phalanx	Comminuted	Surgical	Guarded to poor
	Noncomminuted	Medical or surgical	Good
Proximal sesamoids			
Apical	Small/large fragments	Surgical	Good
Midbody	Displaced	Surgical	Guarded
Abaxial	Small fragments	Surgical	Fair to good
Basilar	Small fragments	Medical/surgical	Guarded to poor
Comminuted/ biaxial	Several fragments	Medical/surgical	Poor
Sagittal	Complete	Medical/surgical	Poor
Metacarpal/tarsal III			
Condyle (lateral)	Nondisplaced	Surgical	Good
	Displaced	Surgical	Guarded
Condyle (medial)	Articular	Surgical	Good
Dorsal cortical	Nonarticular	Surgical	Good
Transverse	Displaced	Surgical	Poor
	Nondisplaced	Surgical	Good
Small metacarpals	Distal	Surgical	Good to excellent
Tarsals	Proximal	Surgical	Good
Carpal bones	Chip	Surgical	Guarded to excellent
	Slab	Surgical	Poor to guarded
Tarsal bones			
Talus	Trochlear ridges	Surgical	Good
	Sagittal	Surgical	Good
	Comminuted	Surgical	Poor
Calcaneus	Small/large fragments	Medical or surgical	Guarded
	Calcaneal tuberosity	Surgical	Guarded
	Comminuted	Medical or surgical	Fair
Central and third tarsal fractures	Slab	Surgical	Favorable
Ulna	Open	Surgical	Fair
	Closed	Surgical	Good
Radius	Open	Surgical	Poor
	Closed (<400 lb)	Surgical	Good to fair
	Closed (>400 lb)	Surgical	Poor
Humerus	Stress	Medical	Excellent
	Complete	Medical	Poor
Scapula			
Supraglenoid tubercle	Displaced	Surgical	Fair
Neck/body	Complete	Surgical	Grave
Tibia	Physeal	Surgical	Good
	Diaphyseal	Surgical	Guarded to poor
Patella			
Sagittal	Displaced	Surgical	Fair to good
Comminuted	Displaced	Surgical	Fair to good
Femur	Physeal	Medical or surgical	Guarded to poor
	Diaphyseal	Surgical	Guarded to poor

MUSCULOSKELETAL

Temporomandibular Fractures

- Unusual occurrence
- Surgical intervention when
  - Fractures enter joint
  - Septic arthritis occurs as the result of lacerations or puncture wounds
  - Osteoarthritis occurs as the result of fracture healing

Clinical Signs

- Soft-tissue swelling overlying the joint
- Crepitation
- Inability to open mouth
- Masseter muscle atrophy

Diagnosis

- Physical examination
- Radiographs, including oblique projections

Treatment

- Conservative approach if fracture is nondisplaced
- Mandibular condylectomy, unilateral or bilateral

Prognosis

- Guarded outcome because secondary arthritis may affect mastication.

Cranial Fractures

Etiology: Trauma

- Halter breaking
- Trailering
- Kick
- Impacting a fixed structure

Clinical Signs

- Increase in intracranial pressure because of edema and hemorrhage
  - Ataxia
  - Anisocoria
  - Nystagmus
  - Head tilt
  - Bradycardia
  - Depressed respiration
  - Hyperthermia
  - Altered state of consciousness
- Hemorrhage from nose and ears

Diagnosis

- Two most common types:
  - Dorsal and dorsolateral fractures
  - Basilar skull fractures
- Radiographic examination of all suspected fractures of the skull

Treatment
NONSURGICAL MANAGEMENT
- Corticosteroids: 0.25 mg/kg aqueous dexamethasone IV
- Dimethyl sulfoxide (DMSO), 1 g/kg in a 10%-20% solution with 0.9% saline solution
- Furosemide to decrease circulating blood volume and pressure
- Broad-spectrum antimicrobial agents

SURGICAL MANAGEMENT
- Closed, nondisplaced fracture associated with hemorrhage and edema
- Open fracture with brain trauma:
  - *Class I:* Does not penetrate dura mater
  - *Class II:* Inner portion of fracture penetrates dura, resulting in hemorrhage
  - *Class III:* Injury to dura mater and brain parenchyma

Prognosis
- Guarded to poor if surgery is needed

Orbital and Periorbital Fractures
Clinical Signs
- Pressure on globe may result in permanent eye damage
- Periorbital soft-tissue structures may be distorted

Diagnosis
- Physical examination and palpation
- Swelling, heat, and pain around eyelids
- Chemosis and subconjunctival hemorrhage
- Strabismus
- Radiographs, including oblique projections

Treatment: Surgical Reduction
- Open technique
- Closed technique

Prognosis
- Cosmetic appearance and functional status generally good
- Older and more severe fractures, poorer prognosis
- Injuries resulting in neuropathies to eye, edema, and severe trauma to globe, and fractures with injury to nasolacrimal system, guarded to poor prognosis

Nasofacial Fractures
Clinical Signs
- Common injury to the horse, involving maxilla, nasal, and frontal bones
- Marked respiratory compromise if severe bony displacement with significant soft-tissue swelling obstructing the airway
- Facial deformity

Diagnosis
- Physical examination
- Facial bone asymmetry
- Local pain on palpation
- Subcutaneous emphysema
- Bone crepitation
- Epistaxis
- Soft-tissue disruption overlying the fracture
- Radiographs not always conclusive

Treatment
- Surgical treatment preferred to minimize potential sequelae:
  □ Permanent facial deformity
  □ Bone sequestration
  □ Chronic sinusitis
  □ Upper respiratory tract compromise

Prognosis
- Generally good
- Monitor for sinus infection and bone sequestrum formation

LUXATION
- Luxation occurs after disruption of one or more support structures of the joint.
- Clinical manifestations range from complete instability of the joint to full weight bearing with minimal malalignment of the joint.
- Luxation confirmed by gross instability or severe pain when attempting weight bearing
- The interrupted soft-tissue structures may include
  □ Collateral ligaments
  □ Intraarticular ligaments
  □ Fibrous joint capsule
  □ Synovium
- The luxation may be open if the skin is torn over the joint.
- The luxation can spontaneously reduce and recurs with weight bearing.
- In the most extreme cases, the joint remains dislocated.
- The prognosis depends on:
  □ The degree of instability
  □ Whether the luxation is open or closed

Diagnosis
- *After the patient is tranquilized, the severity of damage to the collateral support structures is evaluated by means of palpation, plain radiography, stress radiography, and ultrasound examination of the supporting soft tissues.*
- Palpation of the limb helps determine the level of the luxation if it has spontaneously reduced.
- Stress radiographs with the limb manipulated to open the affected joint space aid in determining which soft-tissue structures are involved.

- If ultrasound examination is needed the results confirm complete disruption of a supporting structure.

Types of Luxation
Lower Limb Luxation
- Necessitates reduction and external coaptation.
- If the luxation is open, debridement of tissue if necessary and copious lavage of the joint are needed before cast application.
- If the patient is to be transported to another facility for treatment, protect the limb as described for fractures.

Luxation of the Scapulohumeral and Shoulder Joint
- These fractures are rare and involve rupture of some or all of the soft tissues that stabilize this joint, including the following:
  - Biceps brachii
  - Supraspinatus muscles
  - Tendon of insertion of the infraspinatus muscle
  - Joint capsule

Stifle Luxation
- Involves damage to at least one collateral ligament in addition to one or more cruciate ligaments.
- Damage to the menisci often occurs.
- The prognosis for use is very poor; degenerative joint disease (osteoarthritis) is a common sequela.
- The exception is *patellar luxation* (lateral luxation) that is surgically managed in foals and usually is not a traumatic event necessitating emergency treatment. Dorsal patella luxation occurs in adults and is usually a result of trauma. It can also have a good prognosis.

Luxation of the Hip and Coxofemoral Luxation
- Usually result in disruption of the surrounding joint capsule and the round and accessory ligaments of the femur.
- Anesthesia is needed to reduce the luxation, and maintaining reduction is difficult in all but the smallest patients.
- Arthritis is generally the sequela.

Carpometacarpal Luxation and Subluxation
- Injury to the periarticular soft-tissue structure and proximal metacarpals II and IV as a result of trauma, usually a kick.
- Subluxation is reduced under sedation, and a PVC splint is placed on the limb dorsally and laterally. The splint should extend from the foot to the proximal radius and be incorporated in a cotton bandage.
- A radiograph of carpal region is obtained for assessment of severity of injury.
- Treatment options include:
  - Full-leg external coaptation.

CAUTION: Plaster-based materials (plaster of Paris) and casting tape (synthetic materials) can cause soft-tissue problems, especially over the accessory carpal bone.

- □ Internal fixation to stabilize lateral or medial aspects of the carpus.
- ▪ Degenerative joint disease of the carpometacarpal joint is a sequela.

Prognosis

- ▪ Closed luxation of the distal tarsal, metacarpophalangeal or metatarsophalangeal, and proximal interphalangeal joints is successfully managed with long-term (12 weeks) external coaptation (cast application). Arthrodesis of the proximal interphalangeal (pastern) joint is commonly performed.
- ▪ The limb is cast in normal alignment, the foot included in the cast. General anesthesia is required for correct limb orientation. *Arthritis is a potential sequela,* so advise the owner of this.
- ▪ Horses treated with external coaptation often are functional.
- ▪ Luxation of the distal interphalangeal joint is rare and is associated with advanced degenerative joint disease and biaxial neurectomy used to manage chronic pain. The prognosis is poor. Arthrodesis is difficult.
- ▪ Affected horses with luxation of the shoulder or hip that spontaneously reduces usually recover function of the joint.
- ▪ Patients that need manual reduction of the luxation under general anesthesia have a guarded prognosis for a pain-free joint.
- ▪ If reduction of the luxation is not maintained the joint becomes nonfunctional and arthritis results; euthanasia is recommended.
- ▪ Luxation of the stifle generally is associated with severe damage to supporting structures; limb instability makes treatment impossible.

INFECTION

- ▪ Non–weight-bearing lameness often indicates infection in the following:
  - □ A joint
  - □ Bursa
  - □ Tendon sheath
  - □ Other soft-tissue structure
- ▪ Sepsis often is secondary to a laceration or puncture wound that occurred before and was not diagnosed or treated early and aggressively to prevent contamination progressing to infection.
- ▪ Lacerations, punctures, and management of secondary infections are covered in the following section.

Summary

A patient unable or unwilling to bear weight on a limb needs rapid intervention to reduce anxiety and prevent further damage to the limb. Figure 39–5 summarizes the steps required to minimize damage, establish a preliminary diagnosis, and prepare for referral to a medical facility.

LACERATIONS

- ▪ *One of the most common reasons for emergency assistance.*
- ▪ The initial and most important first step: Determine which structures are involved.
- ▪ *Adequate treatment is impossible until all affected structures are identified.*

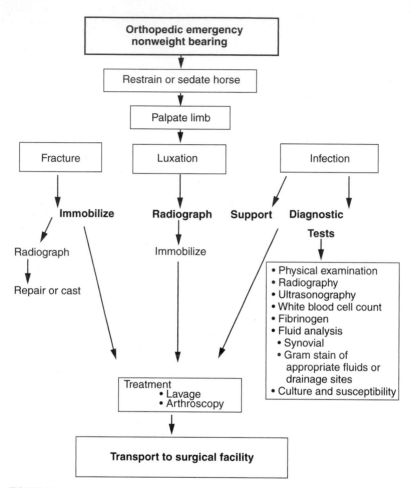

FIGURE 39–5. Algorithm for emergency management of non–weight-bearing problems.

- The patient is restrained for evaluation, then treated or referred to a surgical facility if needed.
- Referral is based on whether the injury requires facilities or expertise not available locally and is made after the initial examination.
- Lacerations necessitating special treatment include
  - Tendons and tendon sheaths
  - Extensive degloving injuries
  - Periosteum
  - Veins and arteries
  - Coronary band and hoof wall
  - Joints

- Lacerations involving less critical structures are cleaned, debrided, and sutured primarily or bandaged for several days and then sutured (delayed primary closure).
- With any laceration, adequate *tetanus prophylaxis* and appropriate antibiotic therapy are mandatory.

Lacerations Requiring Special Care
Lacerations to Flexor Tendons and Their Sheaths

- Tranquilize the patient and assess the damaged structures.
- The depth and cause of the laceration determine which structures are injured or severed.
- Superficial lacerations cause damage to the flexor tendon sheath only.
- Deeper lacerations affect first the superficial digital flexor tendon, next the deep digital flexor tendon, and then the suspensory ligament.
- Degree of damage, contamination, duration of injury, temperament, and extended use contribute to the prognosis. *The prognosis is best if*:
  □ *Blood and nerve supply are intact*
  □ *Contamination is minimal*
  □ *Injury is located outside the tendon sheath*
- If a flexor tendon or the suspensory ligament is completely severed, changes in the axial and flexure alignment of the limb are useful in determining the degree of damage.
- Complete laceration of the superficial flexor tendon causes the fetlock to drop slightly. When both the superficial and deep flexor tendons are severed, the fetlock drops slightly and the toe dorsiflexes and *elevates with weight bearing*.
- *Severe* loss of fetlock support results from severance of the superficial and deep flexor tendons *and* the suspensory ligaments, accompanied by toe elevation.
- "Breakdown injuries" (traumatic disruption of the suspensory apparatus) demonstrate the same bony malalignment and are caused by rupture of the suspensory ligament, distal sesamoid ligaments, or biaxial fracture of the sesamoid bones. Radiographs depict the involved structures.

TO TRANSPORT

- Apply a splint to minimize hyperextension of the limb. This limits tendon end distraction and preserves blood and nerve supply. Several commercially produced splints can be used:
- Leg-Saver Splint (preferred), Klimzey, Inc., Woodland, CA
- A board splint made from readily available materials can be used if necessary.

Materials Needed for a Board Splint

- Leg bandages
- 1 roll of cotton padding
- Elastic tape
- 1 hardwood board, 40 cm long × 12 cm wide × 2 cm thick
- Hand drill
- Steel drill bit
- Heavy wire

APPLICATION OF THE BOARD SPLINT

- After cleaning the laceration, place a nonadherent dressing on the wound and cover the limb from the coronary band to the carpus or tarsus with a cotton wrap. Place a 2-cm-thick hardwood board, 12 by 40 cm, flat on the ground. Drill holes through the hoof at the toe and matching holes in the board at one end (Fig. 39–6A). If a shoe is in place, leave the shoe intact and drill holes through the shoe. Secure the board to the toe with heavy wire (16- to 18-gauge). Pad the board, flex the limb at the fetlock, bring the board parallel to the caudal aspect of the cannon bone, and incorporate it in the bandage (Fig. 39–6B).
- The patient bears weight on the toe, sparing the flexor tendons, and can be safely transported to a hospital facility.
- The splint can be used as a conservative treatment; the wraps are changed as needed by means of lowering the splint and replacing it after wound dressing.
- If both flexor tendons, or a tendon sheath, is involved, *the prognosis is guarded* for return to athletic soundness.
- Induce general anesthesia and perform surgical debridement, reapproximate the tendon ends, and flush the tendon sheath (lavage of the tendon sheath with a balanced crystalloid solution with or without antibiotics added).
- If the laceration is surgically repaired, clean the site meticulously, debride the tendon ends to healthy tissue, and use heavy monofilament absorbable suture to reappose the tendon ends.

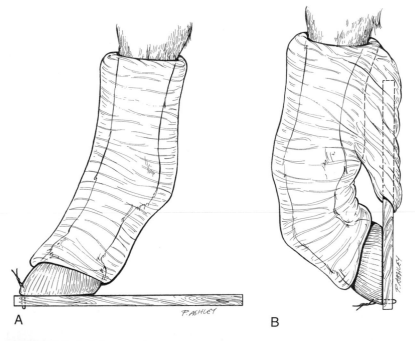

FIGURE 39–6. **A,** A flexor tendon laceration splint can be fashioned by wiring a hardwood board to the toe and flexing the limb to reduce tension on the severed tendon. **B,** The board is then incorporated into the bandage.

- The risk of tendon sheath infection is high, and adhesions usually occur as the tendon heals.
- Even minor tendon lacerations of the tendon sheath are expensive to manage properly, so prepare the owner for this before undertaking treatment.
- Perform cultures of the lacerated area at surgery. Start broad-spectrum antibiotic therapy immediately and make adjustments when results of the culture and sensitivity are final. Intrathecal antibiotics can be injected into the tendon sheath to increase tissue levels of the drugs. Broad-spectrum antibiotic regimens recommended for orthopedic emergencies are listed in Table 39–3.

Lacerations to Extensor Tendons

- These injuries rarely involve a tendon sheath and have a better prognosis than do flexor tendon injuries.
- Frequently they can be cleaned, bandaged, and maintained in an extensor splint and heal well without primary reapposition of the severed tendon ends.
- Fashion an extensor splint by drilling two holes in the toe of the hoof with the shoe in place; an alternative is a bandage and PVC splint alone.
- Make a splint of heavy PVC the length of the limb from toe to just below the carpus or tarsus.
- Drill holes matching those on the hoof in one end of the splint.
- Clean and debride the wound, then apply a dressing and bandage.
- Wire the splint to the cranial aspect of the limb, bring it up over the bandage, and secure it in place with elastic tape (Fig. 39–7).
- Lower the splint periodically for wrap changes during healing.
- This splint prevents knuckling of the foot during walking and helps ensure that the extensor tendon heals in the normal position.

TABLE 39–3. Broad-Spectrum Antibiotic Regimens for Orthopedic Emergencies

Combination	Dosage	Route and Frequency
Penicillin G	22,000–44,000 IU/kg	IM, IV q6h
plus		
Gentamicin	2.2 mg/kg	IM, IV q6-8h
or	6.6 mg/kg	IM, IV q24h
Amikacin	6.6 mg/kg	IM, IV q8h
	15-25 mg/kg	IM, IV q24h
Ampicillin sodium	25-100 mg/kg	IV q6h
plus		
Gentamicin	2.2 mg/kg	IM, IV q6-8h
or	6.6 mg/kg	IM, IV q24h
Amikacin	6.6 mg/kg	IM, IV q8h
	15-25 mg/kg	IM, IV q24h
Ceftiofur (Naxcel)	1-4 mg/kg	IM, IV q12-24h
Trimethoprim/ sulfamethoxazole	20-30 mg/kg	PO q12h
Ticarcillin/clavulanic acid	100 mg/kg loading dose then 50 mg/kg	IV q6h
Enrofloxacin	5 mg/kg	IV q12-24h
	7.5 mg/kg	PO q24h

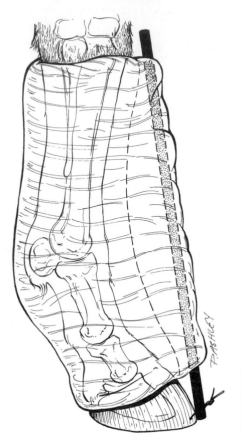

FIGURE 39-7. An extensor tendon laceration can be protected by means of wiring a polyvinyl chloride splint to the toe, extending the digit, and incorporating the splint into the bandage.

Degloving Injuries

- Lacerations that remove large amounts of tissue from the lower limb are referred to as **degloving injuries** because the superficial tissues pull away as a glove does from the hand.
- Assessing tissue viability when the wound is first examined is difficult.
- Clean, dress, and bandage the wound.
- Start broad-spectrum antibiotic therapy (see Table 39–3) immediately. If the degloving injury is extensive, use general anesthesia to debride and reapproximate the tissues.
- Meticulously remove dirt, and use large mattress sutures to reappose the injured tissues.
- A cast is advisable for 7-10 days to immobilize the injured tissues, reduce edema, and promote revascularization.
- *Large areas of skin can be salvaged by means of rapid cleaning and cast immobilization.*
- After the cast is removed, which tissues are viable and which need to be debrided is apparent.

- Debride dark brown or black, leathery tissue back to healthy, pink, and bleeding tissue.
- Skin grafting may be needed later to cover unepithelialized areas.
- When a degloving injury has exposed bone, osteitis, osteomyelitis, and bone sequestration are frequent sequelae.
- Suspect these conditions if healing of the original injury is slow, or if the wound reopens after closing.
- Obtain radiographs of the limb if healing does not progress as expected to determine whether a sequestrum or other bony problem exists.
- If the bone shows areas of lysis, periostitis, or sequestration, additional debridement or antibiotic therapy is needed for the overlying tissues to heal.

Large-Vessel and Nerve Lacerations

- If a large vessel of the distal limb is lacerated, it is possible, but uncommon, for exsanguination to occur.
- The bleeding is reduced or stopped by means of compression, with pressure wraps over the bleeding area, heavy padding of the area, and reinforcing the bandage with elastic tape.
- If the severed vessel is the major blood supply to the area, perform suture repair with the patient under general anesthesia.
- Leave the pressure bandage in place until the patient is under anesthesia, to minimize additional blood loss.
- Lacerations of major arteries such as the brachial and femoral arteries **can** be rapidly fatal and usually accompany fractures of the humerus or radius (brachial artery) or femur and pelvis (femoral artery). Repair usually is not feasible.
- Lacerations of nerves in the lower limb are more common than is clinically recognized (unless neuromas form during healing) and generally cause few problems.
- Severance of major nerves high in the limb is caused by fractures of the humerus or femur and is not repaired.
- Complete severance of nerves is difficult to differentiate from nerve trauma (neuropraxia) that resolves with time.
- When in doubt, use nonsteroidal antiinflammatory drugs (NSAIDs) to decrease edema and inflammation around the nerve. An improvement in the limb is seen within several days with neuropraxia; no change is evident if the nerve is severed.
- In most cases, damage to large nerves is recognized clinically by a change in limb carriage.
  - Damage to the main trunk of the radial nerve interrupts innervation of the triceps muscle, causing the elbow to drop, and is most common with a fracture of the humerus.
  - Damage to lower branches of the radial nerve cause stumbling or poor placement of the foot and is caused by injury to the antebrachium.
  - Damage to the femoral nerve supplying the quadriceps muscles causes the affected horse to be unable to fix the stifle or bear full weight on the limb.
  - Damage to the tibial and peroneal nerves results in stumbling and the inability to extend the digit.

Coronary Band and Hoof Wall Lacerations

- The coronary band supplies blood to the germinal tissue of the hoof wall; any interruption in its integrity results in a permanent hoof wall defect.

- Clean lacerations of the coronary band carefully and place a large, horizontal mattress suture of #1 or #2 nonabsorbable suture material to bridge the defect.
- Minimizing the gap in the coronary band defect minimizes the hoof wall defect.
- If a portion of the coronary band is displaced, repair it at the time of injury.
- If such a wound heals by secondary intention, the abnormal hoof wall growth requires lifelong hoof wall management because of the defect.
- Lacerations of the hoof wall are examined for the following:
  □ Depth of the defect
  □ Instability of the hoof capsule
  □ Involvement of the distal interphalangeal joint and soft tissues
- To evaluate deep lacerations properly, use local or general anesthesia.
- To transport, place a clean, well-padded bandage around the foot, including the sole, and extend the bandage to the fetlock joint.
- If bleeding is excessive, use several layers of cotton applied over the initial bandaging material.
- Placing a plastic bag between cotton layers helps confine the hemorrhage, keeps the outer layers from becoming blood-soaked, and minimizes contamination during transport.
- When the wrap is complete, place impervious tape (duct tape) over the outside to waterproof and provide wear resistance until repair.
- Broad-spectrum antibiotic therapy (see Table 39–3) and tetanus prophylaxis are recommended.
- After cleaning and debriding a hoof wall laceration, achieve stability by using a slipper cast (Fig. 39–8) or by using a bar shoe and bandages.
- Hoof wall lacerations require 4-8 months to heal by new hoof formation rather than healing from side to side.

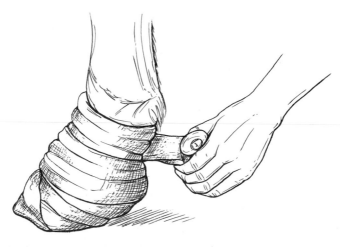

FIGURE 39–8. A short, slipper cast can be used to stabilize lacerations of the hoof wall or coronary band. The cast can be applied with the horse standing and should extend to just beneath the fetlock joint.

Joint Lacerations

- A joint laceration is an emergency and is confirmed if bone and cartilage are seen.
- Even if the joint surface is not seen, the proximity of the laceration to the joint may suggest involvement.
- If joint involvement is even suspected, broad-spectrum antibiotics (see Table 39–3) are started immediately, followed by additional diagnostic procedures to rule out joint involvement.

NOTE: Prognosis is markedly improved if antibiotics are started within 24 hours of injury.

- Techniques to determine joint involvement include:
  - Sedate the patient.
  - Surgically prepare the opposite side of the joint, inject sterile saline solution intraarticularly, and check to see whether it communicates with the laceration.
  - Sterile methylene blue dye can be used.
  - An alternative is to inject sterile contrast medium and obtain a radiograph focused on the lacerated area to determine whether the joint capsule is open.

NOTE: Plain radiographs with gas density in the joint indicate communication with the skin.

- *If the joint is involved, place the patient under general anesthesia and lavage the affected joint copiously.*
  - After sterile preparation, place a 14-gauge needle intraarticularly opposite the laceration.
  - Infuse a continuous ingress flow of lactated Ringer's solution plus 10% DMSO through the joint during debridement of the wound.
  - Infusion of an antibiotic solution after lavage is advocated in addition to broad-spectrum systemic antibiotics.
  - Avoid antibiotics with a low pH; they are irritating to the synovium.
  - Crystalline penicillin (1×10^6 IU) or a solution of gentamicin (50 mg/ml) or amikacin (250 mg/ml) buffered with sodium bicarbonate (1 mEq/ml) is safely infused after thorough lavage.
  - Gentamicin is supplied at a pH of 2.0, and a near-normal pH is achieved by means of adding 2 ml of sodium bicarbonate to 1 ml of gentamicin
  - If the laceration is clean and can be closed primarily, maintain an intra-articular closed suction drain for 2-4 days.
  - Apply antibiotic ointment at the drain exit site and cover the area with a sterile bandage.
  - When fluid is removed from the suction system, be careful not to contaminate the drain and the exit portal.
  - Superficial contamination can lead to ascending infection and therefore necessitates careful monitoring.
  - After drain removal (<10 ml q6-8h), leave sterile wraps in place until joint fluid is no longer evident on the bandage.
- *If the patient becomes progressively more lame as the laceration heals, suspect infection.*
- Aspiration of joint fluid for cytologic examination and culture and susceptibility testing is essential in determining the cause.

- A white blood cell count >30,000 cells/dl in synovial fluid is presumptive evidence of infection.
- Repeat culture and sensitivity testing of the fluid until sepsis is ruled out.
- If antibiotic therapy has been discontinued, reinstitute it.
- Sequential joint lavage, with continuous suction drainage between, reduces the bacterial count and joint destruction caused by the septic inflammation.
- Joint lacerations carry a guarded prognosis: **Early, aggressive** diagnosis and treatment maximize the chance for recovery.

PUNCTURE WOUNDS

- Punctures into synovial structures, including joints, tendon sheaths, and bursae, are emergencies:
  - Introduction of bacteria into these closed spaces can result in life-threatening infection.
  - Joint and tendon sheath punctures are managed as small lacerations to these structures.
  - Aspiration of synovial fluid for culture and sensitivity, meticulous cleaning of the area, copious lavage, broad-spectrum antibiotic therapy (see Table 39–3), and bandaging are recommended.
- *Puncture wounds of the sole* with injury to the frog or the bars are likely to involve deeper structures, such as the digital cushion, navicular bursa, deep digital flexor tendon and sheath, and distal interphalangeal joint.
- If these structures are involved, *conservative treatment with soaking and systemic treatment alone is **not** sufficient to prevent infection.*
- If a puncture wound is found in this area, aggressive diagnosis and treatment are required.
- Obtain radiographs of the foot with the penetrating object in place, if possible, to give an indication of the depth of penetration.
- If the object or foreign body has been removed, locate, open, and clean the tract and introduce a sterile probe before obtaining the radiograph. *Do not force* the probe into the deeper tissues.
- Extension of a tract can be delineated with contrast medium.
- If radiographs indicate that the navicular bursa, deep digital flexor tendon sheath, or distal interphalangeal joint has been entered, synovial samples of these structures are confirmatory for involvement:
  - Distal interphalangeal joint fluid is obtained by means of aspiration 1 cm above the coronary band, 1 cm medial or lateral to the extensor tendon (Fig. 39–9b).
  - Flexor tendon sheath fluid is obtained by means of aspiration of the most fluctuant area of the sheath (Fig. 39–9a).
  - The navicular bursa fluid is difficult to aspirate. Aseptically prepare the area on the lateral aspect of the pastern proximal to the collateral cartilage; insert a 20-gauge, 1.5-inch (3.8 cm) needle palmar to the second phalanx and dorsal to the deep digital flexor tendon. Advance the needle toward the sole of the medial hoof (Fig. 39–9c).
- If the white blood cell count is increased with degenerate neutrophils, suspect infection and lavage the joint or tendon sheath, ideally with the patient under general anesthesia.

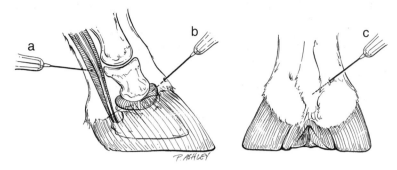

FIGURE 39-9. Placement of needles for centesis of the deep digital flexor tendon sheath *(a)*, distal interphalangeal joint *(b)*, and navicular bursa *(c)*.

- If the navicular bursa is involved, make a surgical window into the bursa from the frog and establish ventral drainage (Fig. 39–10). This is called a *street nail procedure.*
- Endoscopy of the navicular bursa is *now* the preferred technique for management of contaminated and septic bursa (see p. 00).
- Punctures are misleading because they appear benign when first encountered; thus aggressive therapy is frequently delayed until clinical signs of infection occur.
- *At this point the prognosis is guarded for return to athletic function.*
- When penetration is suspected, aggressive treatment is recommended.
- Perform lavage while the patient is standing. Use xylazine and butorphanol sedation (see Table 39–1). Most horses need general anesthesia.
- Bandaging after lavage includes sterile dressings over the puncture site. If a portion of the sole or frog is removed, bandaging is needed until horn tissue covers the area. Fabricate a treatment or medicine plate shoe that allows easy bandage changes to minimize the work and cost of daily treatment.
- Keep the foot dry and clean and limit exercise until the wound is covered with granulation tissue and a cornified layer forms.

Summary

- Many equine orthopedic emergencies manifest themselves when the patient bears all or some weight on the affected limb.
- This is true in cases of minor, or incomplete, fractures, lacerations, and puncture wounds.
- Because the patient appears to be in less distress, the injury is not viewed as serious or necessitating emergency care.
- *If treatment is not initiated soon after injury, the sequela can be life threatening.*
- Fig. 39–11 provides guidelines for managing injuries in which the patient has an injury that allows weight bearing and is managed as an emergency.

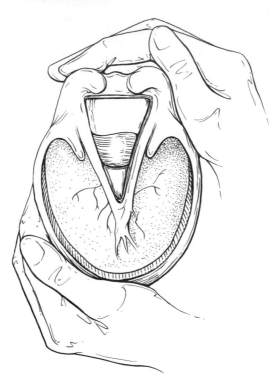

FIGURE 39–10. With punctures in the middle third of the frog, damage to the navicular bone or its bursa should be suspected. A street nail operation or the preferred technique of "Endoscopy of the Navicular Bursa" (see pp. 000) may be needed to drain the bursa and see the navicular bone.

LAMINITIS (FOUNDER)

David M. Hood

Types

- Developmental laminitis
- Acute laminitis
- Subacute laminitis
- Chronic laminitis

Developmental Laminitis
Definition

- High risk of development of laminitis because of exposure to an identifiable cause or predisposing factor

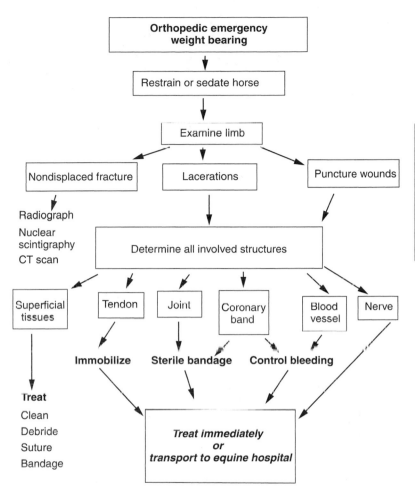

FIGURE 39-11. Algorithm for emergency management of weight-bearing problems.

Causes: Events and Factors Correlating with the Onset of Acute Laminitis

- Carbohydrate overload
- Retained placenta
- Gastrointestinal disease
- Trauma
  - Overexercise on hard surfaces
  - Continuous forced weight bearing on a single foot
- Exposure to black walnut (*Juglans nigra*) wood shavings
- Any systemic problem resulting in hypovolemia or a hypotensive state

MUSCULOSKELETAL

Predisposing Factors
- Corticosteroids
- Obesity
- Equine Cushing's disease

Signs
- Asymptomatic relative to digital pain
- Feet may be cold and insensitive

Principal Pathologic Changes
- Submural blood flow reduced
- Laminar epidermal cells show mild nuclear pyknosis and cytoplasmic vacuolization (edema)

➤ Preventive Measures
- Remove or limit exposure to the cause or predisposing factors
- Mineral oil through a nasogastric tube in cases of carbohydrate- or protein-rich feed overload
- Manage primary systemic disease, such as colic, diarrhea, sepsis, retained placenta
- Provide sole support for foot exposed to continued loading
- NSAIDs
  - Phenylbutazone (2.2 mg/kg IV or PO q12h)
  - Flunixin meglumine (1.1 mg/kg IV q24h)
- Improve digital blood flow
  - Maintain adequate circulatory volume
  - Vasodilator therapy (acepromazine 0.02-0.06 mg/kg IV q6h)
  - Rheologic therapy (pentoxifylline, 8.4 mg/kg PO q12h)

Acute Laminitis
Definition
- Signs of pain with or without evidence of an associated cause or predisposing factor

Causes
- See earlier.

Digital Signs: Digital Pain and Lameness
- Pain, if recognized early, usually is subtle but can rapidly progress to severe lameness in 6-12 hours.
- Lameness generally involves more than one foot. One foot may be more severely affected and lameness referable to one foot.
- Increased digital pulse due to systemic hypertension and inflammation.

| **NOTE:** Not a consistent finding; depends on severity and duration of disease.

- Heat felt over hoof wall owing to hyperemia and inflammation.

| **NOTE:** Not a consistent finding; depends on severity and duration of disease.

- Altered stance: Patient typically stands with the forefeet and hindfeet forward of the normal position. The classic stance for laminitis may not be present if the disease is mild or if all four feet are affected.
- Altered gait: Varies markedly depending on the severity of disease. In early, mild disease the patient may only have a shortened or stilted gait and an unwillingness to turn.

Systemic Signs
- Hypertension, tachycardia, pyrexia, mild metabolic acidosis and inappetence

Principal Pathologic Changes
- Submural blood flow is increased.
- Digital changes demonstrate a cascade that includes reperfusion hyperemia, reperfusion injury, and a secondary vascular compartment injury.
- Lesions seen: Dermal endothelial cell activation, microthrombosis, occasional perivascular hemorrhage, epithelial cell pyknosis, vacuolization, and necrosis affecting the peripheral regions of the submural laminar interface in the early acute stages. If the disease progresses in severity, lesions may extend to the axial areas of the laminar interface, and separation of the epithelial basement membrane may occur.

Diagnosis
- Based on presence of acute digital pain and lameness with or without elevated digital pulses and warm feet
- Radiographs and physical examination of the feet are needed to rule out preexisting laminar disease and chronic laminitis:
  - Rotation
  - Sinking
  - Flat feet
  - Widened white line
  - Depressed coronary band
- Judicious use of diagnostic nerve blocks is useful to rule out other causes of lameness.

Treatment Goals
- Limit the pathologic cascade occurring in the submural laminar interface.
- Reduce pain.
- Protect the damaged interface from mechanical overload that predisposes to mechanical failure.
- Administer NSAIDs:

  NOTE: Administer NSAIDs as early as possible to limit the progression of the disease and improve comfort.

  - Phenylbutazone (2.2 mg/kg IV followed by 2.2 mg/kg q12h PO for 3 days)
  - Flunixin meglumine (1.1 mg/kg IV q24h)
- Minimize injury to foot.
  - Sole support with deep sand bedding if the horse is standing, or wood shavings if recumbent.

□ Sole support for the posterior part of the foot. Pads should provide support and be nonrigid. Examples include Styrofoam, Equilox, and Lily pads.

| **NOTE:** Pads should not extend in front of the point of the frog.

□ Do not walk or trailer the horse. Increased loads damage the laminar and sole interface and can result in mechanical failure of the foot.

Although controversial, continual application of ice to the foot may decrease reperfusion injury. This can be easily achieved by placing crushed ice in an empty 5 L fluid bag and using it as a boot.

Subacute Laminitis
Definition
- The patient recovers from an acute episode without mechanical failure of the foot.

Cause
- An episode of acute laminitis

Signs
- Affected horses are mildly lame but frequently have no symptoms of digital disease.

Principal Pathologic Changes
- Submural laminar interface changes with mild epithelial hyperplasia and bleeding in the hoof wall and sole

Diagnosis
- History of acute laminitis within the last 3-6 months combined with radiographic and physical examination findings revealing no abnormalities of the foot

Treatment Goals
- Protect the healing laminar interface during healing; analgesics as needed.
  □ Analgesics: NSAIDs use in subacute laminitis should be limited to the lowest dose for pain management.
- Protection of the foot:
  □ After an acute episode, exercise is limited for 3-6 months depending on the severity of the initial disease: No riding, hand trotting, or walking on hard roads.
- *No* long distance trailering is recommended; if trailering is necessary, provide good sole support.
- Treatment support shoes can be used to reduce laminar interface loading.

➤ Chronic Laminitis
Definition
- The radiographic or physical findings show mechanical collapse of the foot.

Cause
- A previous episode of acute laminitis
- Acute mechanical collapse in a horse with subacute laminitis caused by excessive loading of the healing foot
- Serial episodes of laminitis associated with mechanical injury, vascular insults, or sepsis

Signs
- Pain, lameness
  - Asymptomatic: Compensated chronic laminitis
  - Symptomatic: Uncompensated chronic laminitis with severe pain and lameness
  - Many horses with chronic laminitis have no symptoms
- Evidence of digital collapse or altered growth of the hoof includes:
  - Sunken coronary band
  - Coronary shear lesions
  - Founder rings
  - Long curved toes or an acute change in the dorsal wall contour
  - Evidence of repeated sole or wall hemorrhage
  - Overgrown heels
  - Flattened or dropped soles
  - Widened white line
  - Sole or coronary abscesses
  - Sole penetration

Systemic signs
- Endocrine disease
  - Equine Cushing's disease
  - Stress-induced hypothyroidism (euthyroid sick syndrome)
- Systemic hypertension
- Hyperreactive immune system
- Renal disease

Principal Pathologic Changes
MECHANICAL COLLAPSE OF THE FOOT
- Displacement of the distal phalanx relative to the hoof capsule
  - Phalangeal rotation
  - Capsular rotation
  - Vertical displacement of P3
- Digital instability: An increased mobility of the distal phalanx and hoof capsule associated with the type of healing occurring in the submural tissue.
- Reduced strength of the laminar interface: Weakening of the laminar interface due to changes in the architecture and the healing response.

METABOLIC DISEASE OF THE LAMINAR INTERFACE
- The healing of the laminae exists as a noncornifying, basal cell hyperplasia predisposed to digital instability and reduced strength of the laminar interface. More appropriate healing leads to a cornifying or partially cornifying laminar hyperplasia predisposed to a clinically compensated, less painful patient.

VASCULAR PATHOLOGIC CHANGES

- Regional vascular insufficiencies and avascularities are commonly present and associated with mechanical failure of the foot.
- Vascular hyperplasia and a vascular hyperreactivity may be present in the dorsal submural region.

SEPSIS

- Infection can be present with chronic laminitis, and its clinical significance varies with the site and the bacteria present.
- Infection may be located in the following areas:
  □ Fully cornified areas of the wall: Contamination
  □ Viable submural soft tissues
  □ The distal phalanx

Diagnosis

COMPLETE PHYSICAL AND RADIOGRAPHIC EXAMINATION

- Document the presence of chronic laminitis changes.

NOTE: For the clinically compensated patient, a complete diagnostic evaluation is necessary to prevent inappropriate shoeing or overexercise that may lead to clinical decompensation.

- If the patient is clinically uncompensated, diagnostic evaluation is essential to plan the appropriate rehabilitation.

PAIN

- Identify the cause of foot pain and determine whether other causes of pain are present. Minimal examination includes palpation, hoof testers, limb flexion, and nerve blocks.

NOTE: Gait evaluation should be restricted after nerve blocks.

RADIOGRAPHIC EVALUATION

- Radiographs *always* should be obtained in cases of chronic laminitis.
- Radiodense markers attached to the dorsal hoof wall at the coronary band are important for the diagnosis of displacement of the distal phalanx and are helpful in orienting the farrier for therapeutic shoeing.
- Serial radiographs are useful for assessing disease progression and the effectiveness of treatment.
- Specific radiographic changes include air lines, severity of rotation, and sinking of the distal phalanx.

NOTE: Stress remodeling of the distal phalanx should not be used solely for prognosis and clinical status.

BLOOD SUPPLY

- The severity of damage to the digital circulation is assessed with:
  □ Contrast angiography
  □ Nuclear scintigraphy
  □ Submural laminar biopsy
- The presence of large areas of loss of blood supply under the sole or wall suggest a poor prognosis and poor shoeing.

METABOLIC STATUS
- Submural laminar biopsy is currently the only technique for assessing laminar healing.

INFECTION
- It is difficult to identify specific bacteria in chronic laminitis because of severe contamination. Radiographs and nuclear scintigraphy are helpful diagnostic aids.

REHABILITATION GOAL
- Rehabilitation versus short-term treatment: The primary focus is to return the patient to a *clinically compensated state* that allows return to function.

Treatment
THERAPEUTIC SHOEING GOALS
- Stabilize and protect the mechanically failed foot so that healing of the submural and subsolar tissues occurs.
- Decrease the pain resulting from biomechanical changes in foot axis.
- Return the foot to a *normal* conformation if possible.

SHOEING OPTIONS
- Several types of shoes are used to reach the goals, and which shoe to use for each patient is poorly defined.

  NOTE: Clinical experience indicates that *no* single shoe benefits all horses with laminitis. The therapeutic approach should be changed as needed for each patient.

ANALGESIC THERAPY
- Rational use of systemic analgesics is appropriate in chronic laminitis. NSAIDs should be administered at the lowest effective dosage and for a minimum of 3 days. Chronic pain and non–weight-bearing lameness can result in contracture of the foot and flexor tendons. High levels of analgesics can lead to further mechanical damage of the foot and to toxic renal and gastrointestinal side effects.

CONTROL OF INFECTION
- Infection in chronic laminitis is difficult to manage.
- Superficial infections, between layers of cornified tissue, rarely necessitate treatment.
- Infections involving viable submural areas should be managed with antibiotics and bactericidal-bacteriostatic foot soaks. Local debridement can be beneficial.
- Bone infections (P3) frequently necessitate surgical curettage through a dorsal wall resection.

SURGICAL CONSIDERATIONS
- Deep digital flexor tenotomy and inferior check ligament desmotomy may result in improved comfort, especially if clinical contraction is present.
- Hoof wall resection and grooving are used in the care of some patients to access focal infections or stimulate dorsal hoof wall growth.

| **NOTE:** Hoof wall resection or grooving is contraindicated without foot support through therapeutic shoeing.

NUTRITIONAL SUPPORT

- Nutritional support is directed at providing the laminar tissues with substrates needed for optimal healing. Because of vascular insufficiencies in chronic laminitis, the use of oral supplements containing biotin, essential amino acids, trace minerals, and vitamins increases plasma concentrations of these nutrients and the delivery of substrates.
- The diet for a patient with chronic laminitis is changed to maximize body condition. This is challenging because of the presence of concurrent disease: endocrine, gastrointestinal, and renal problems associated with chronic laminitis.

➤ Contraindicated Therapies for Laminitis

- Highly reactive vaccines
- Corticosteroids
- Neurectomy
- Unproven treatments in place of conventional proven treatments

Prognosis

- See Table 39–4.

PEDIATRIC ORTHOPEDIC EMERGENCIES

- The principles for emergency treatment of foals parallel those for adults:
  - □ Sedate or tranquilize the patient.
  - □ Examine the injury.
  - □ Apply protective splints or bandages.
  - □ Consider the advisability of and options for further treatment.
- Compared with those in adults, fractures in foals respond to treatment well and heal more rapidly.
- Internal fixation is more successful in foals than it is in adults because of lower body weight.
- With open fractures or puncture wounds, the foal may be more prone to complications of septicemia or focal infection owing to
  - □ Greater blood flow to the growing bone
  - □ The immaturity of the immune system

➤ Splints and Casts

- A splint can be constructed from half-shell PVC pipe applied over sufficient cotton wrapping.
- Remove and reset twice a day to prevent pressure sores from developing.
- If used, a cast should leave the foot free (sleeve/cylinder cast).
- Full-leg casts can produce osteopenia and severe flexor laxity.
- Two products that can be adapted for treating orthopedic injuries in foals:
  - □ A semirigid support wrap*

---

*Scotchrap, 3M Animal Care Products, 3M Center 270-2N-03, St. Paul, MN 55144; (800) 848-0829); Fax: (651) 733-9151.

TABLE 39–4. Prognosis for the Chronic Laminitis Patient

	Prognosis		
Characteristic	Good	Fair	Poor
Pain severity	Variable	Variable	Variable
Response to pain medication	Good	Good	Poor to none
Hoof appearance			
Sunken coronary band	–	Dorsal only	Dorsal and
Founder rings	Rare	±	quarters
Flattened sole	±	±	+
Redirection of wall tubules	–	±	+
Coronary shear lesions	–	–	+
Radiographic findings			
Capsular rotation	±	±	+
Phalangeal rotation	–	–	+
Vertical displacement	±	±	+
Remodeling of P3	±	±	±
Thickened dorsal wall	+	+	±
Air densities			
Acute separation	–	–	+
Submural airlines	±	±	±
Irregular spaces	–	–	±
Hoof Instability	Normal	Normal	Increased
Blood supply			
Decreased perfusion	–	–	+
Avascular regions	–	–	+
Laminar morphology			
Dysplastic	Mild	Mild	Severe
Basal cell hyperplastic	–	Mild	Severe
Laminar cornification	+	±	–
Infection			
Epidermal	±	±	+
Laminar interface	–	–	+
Bone involvement	–	–	+

- A one-step splint (Scothcast/Primacast, 3M Immobilization Products)
- When rigid immobilization is not needed, use a semirigid support.
- The one-step splint consists of
  - Several layers of knitted fiberglass fabric impregnated with polyurethane resin
  - One side has an air- and moisture-permeable nonwoven fabric, and the other is padded with a permeable open-cell foam.
  - After it sets on exposure to water, the splint is lightweight, strong, and radiolucent and conforms to the limb.

Tendon Rupture

- Bilateral extensor tendon rupture can occur in a foal with flexural contracture that is straining to keep up with the mare at pasture.
- Most often seen in large foals with mildly bucked knees (often a primary condition) and marked by soft, fluid-filled swelling on the carpus
- Heavy wraps reduce the swelling but can cause tendon laxity.

- Larger foals need more rigid support, and for them, splints or fiberglass-reinforced wraps are added to the support wraps.
- Surgery usually is not needed to reappose the tendon ends, which reunite over the course of several months.

Rupture of the Gastrocnemius Tendon

Anatomy Review

The gastrocnemius is the largest muscle of the caudal hindlimb. Its theoretical action is to flex the stifle and extend the hock. However, because of the anatomy of the peroneus tertius (fibularis tertius), the hock and stifle always flex or extend in unison, leaving the gastrocnemius with a primarily supportive role. The gastrocnemius is the most superficial muscle of its group. It originates as two heads from the supracondylar tuberosities of the femur. The semitendinosus and semimembranosus muscles cover the gastrocnemius proximally. The two-headed unit forms a single strong tendon at the level of the mid tibia composing the major portion of the calcanean tendon and inserts on the point of the hock with the superficial flexor tendon winding around its medial surface.

General Information

- Rare. Affected horses usually are <1 week old. Gastrocnemius rupture is believed more common among premature or dysmature foals struggling to rise, particularly on slippery floors.
- An incomplete rupture is more common than a complete rupture.
- Frequently occurs in association with rupture of the superficial digital flexor tendon.
- Generally a result of hyperflexion of the hock when the horse falls with the hock flexed under the body.
- Also occurs during recovery from anesthesia or as the result of improper cast or bandage application, which leads to pressure necrosis of the tendon and to rupture.
- Occurs at the muscle-tendon junction of the gastrocnemius rather than at the insertion and therefore heals rapidly.

Clinical Signs

- Hock flexed without stifle flexed indicates complete rupture.
- Lack of weight bearing
- Hock lower than opposite leg
- If injury is not acute, atrophy of gluteal muscles may be present on the side of the injured leg.
- If injury is not severe enough to produce non–weight-bearing stance, calcaneus may rotate laterally and toe medially (on side of affected limb) during weight bearing.
- A large hematoma on caudal aspect of the affected hindlimb is commonly recognized on physical examination.

Ancillary Testing to Confirm Diagnosis

- Ultrasonography
- Radiography to rule out avulsion fractures

Treatment

▶ | **NOTE:** Treat as an emergency.

- Apply Schroeder-Thomas splint as soon as possible or apply another type of external coaptation bandage.
- Assist foal in standing on three legs to
  - Nurse
  - Prevent decubital sores
- After 5-7 days, apply an external coaptation bandage, such as a Robert Jones bandage with splint; reset every 2-3 days.
- Remove Schroeder-Thomas splint after a maximum of 10-12 days to prevent severe contraction and problems with soft tissues.

Prognosis
- Good for use as a pleasure horse. Poor for use as a performance athlete.

Prevention
- Avoid slippery surfaces, especially if foal is weak. Assist and support the weak horse and improve footing.

Luxation of the Superficial Digital Flexor (SDF) Tendon
- Occurs among adults as the result of trauma; rare among foals and presumed to be traumatic in origin or caused by overexercise in rapidly growing foals
- Caused by disruption of the supporting structure of the tendon; may be bilateral

Diagnosis
- Large unilateral or bilateral swelling in area of tuber calcaneus
- Acute lameness that improves with symptomatic treatment
- Ultrasonography diagnostic procedure of choice:
  - Disruption of medial attachment with tendon displaced laterally most common
  - Disruption of lateral attachment with tendon displaced medially
  - SDF splits longitudinally with a portion of the tendon on each side of the tuber calcaneus

Treatment
- Conservative
  - Stall confinement
  - External coaptation
  - NSAIDs
- Surgical correction
- Mesh onlay graft to repair disrupted tissue

Prognosis
- Varies with expectations for athletic use.

Rupture of the Common Digital Extensor Tendon in Foals

General Information

- Frequently misdiagnosed, occurrence unknown
- Congenital to within days of birth
- May have a heritable component
- Increased incidence among Arabians and Quarter Horses
- Large foals with bucked knees predisposed
- Site of rupture at level of carpus at the musculotendinous junction
- Occurs with or without flexor tendon contraction or deformity
- A tight bandage, trauma, stenosis, and constriction of the annular ligaments can lead to reduced blood flow to the peritendineum and to rupture

Diagnosis

COMMON CLINICAL SIGNS

- Characteristic swelling over the dorsolateral surface of the carpus at the level of the intercarpal and carpometacarpal joints
- Fluid distention of tendon sheath nonpainful to palpation; ruptured ends frequently can be palpated.
- Normal carpal or fetlock flexion on ambulating foals with flexural deformities. Differentiate radial nerve injury and brachial plexus damage secondary to the flexural deformity problem.

ANCILLARY TESTING

- Radiographs to rule out fracture
- Ultrasonography to evaluate the tendon
- Aseptic aspiration of tendon sheath for improved palpation of tendon

Treatment

- If flexural deformity does not exist and the foal walks without flexion of the fetlock, no treatment is indicated; tendon heals more quickly without immobilization.
- If flexural deformity is present, external coaptation (supportive wrap) and stall confinement are needed.
- External coaptation and a splint or sleeve cast may be necessary if fetlock flexion is a consistent finding.

Prognosis

- Good if independent of flexor tendon contraction or deformity
- Guarded if moderate to severe flexural contraction or deformity is present

Prevention

- Manage flexor tendon deformities early (inferior check ligament desmotomy).
- Minimize overexercise and stressful conditions.

Fractures

Management

- Fractures of any bone of the hindlimb or forelimb are relatively common among foals because of their playful disposition and the vulnerability of the growing bone to the effects of a kick or a fall. In most cases treatment is surgical.

- Compared with adults, foals respond well to methods of internal fixation because:
  - Bone remodeling and periosteal growth are more rapid.
  - The body weight of foals approximates that of adult humans, for whom the orthopedic implants were originally designed.
  - Foals are more easily restrained after reduction and fixation, making refracture less likely during recovery from anesthesia.
- Fractures to the third metacarpal/metatarsal necessitate immediate stabilization because of the sparse soft-tissue covering; prognosis depends on the success and stability of fixation.
- Suspensory disruption occasionally occurs as a result of biaxial fracture of the proximal sesamoid bones in youngsters that are overexercised (Fig. 39–12).
- Management with splints has generally been more successful than has surgical treatment.

Physeal Fractures

LONG-BONE PHYSEAL FUSION TIMES (see Appendix IX on physeal times and growth plate closures.)
Physeal fusion times are important for radiographic interpretation and are not always indicative of true growth plate closure. The fusion times listed are for the long bones of the thoracic and pelvic limbs. Breed variations occur. (The growth

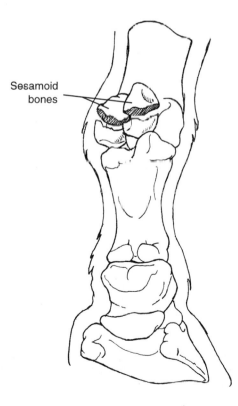

Sesamoid bones

FIGURE 39–12. Biaxial fractures of proximal sesamoid bones; palmar dorsal view.

MUSCULOSKELETAL

plates of lighter breeds close earlier than do those of heavier breeds.) The bones also differ in terms of fusion age, and the proximal and distal growth plates close at different times.

KEY POINTS

- The most rapid growth period in foals is birth to 10 weeks.
- The distal radius has continuous growth up to 60 weeks.
- Angular limb deformities should be recognized and managed early in life (before 70 days of age for fetlock deformities).
- The radiographic appearance of the growth plate does not directly reflect the ability of chondrocytes to proliferate.
- Growth plates determine bone length and to some extent, bone shape.
- Endochondral ossification abnormalities affect bone length, axial alignment of bone ends, and joint contour.
- The physis is the vulnerable point in the immature skeleton.
- The physis is weaker than mature bone, joint capsule, ligaments, or tendons; sufficient shearing or avulsion force often results in a fracture through the cartilaginous cells in the growth plate.
- Physeal fractures are the *most common* fractures among foals; suspect them when any foal has signs of joint fracture or dislocation.
- Physeal fractures are considered more serious than diaphyseal fractures because of the risk of disturbed growth patterns and of involvement of adjoining articular surfaces.
- Early recognition and treatment are essential to prevent development of angular limb deformity or arthritis.
- The Salter-Harris classification (Fig. 39–13) is a useful guide to determine prognosis and treatment options.
- In general, the prognosis worsens as the classification number increases, but other relevant prognostic factors include:
  - Severity of the trauma to the growth plate
  - Integrity of the vasculature
  - Location of the physis
  - Foal's age
  - Time elapsed after injury before treatment is initiated
- Types I and II are the most common physeal fractures and involve the third metacarpal/metatarsal bones. The prognosis is relatively good for healing without lameness.
- Femoral capital physeal fractures or proximal femoral physis fractures are among the most common of types I and II and are generally managed more successfully with internal fixation than with stall confinement.
- Proximal femoral fractures have a better prognosis than do fractures of the distal femoral physis because the contour of the distal femur makes repair difficult and the strength of the available implants is often inadequate.
- Younger foals appear to have better prospects for achieving a sound, straight limb than do older foals.
- Physeal fractures heal rapidly, in approximately half the time needed for metaphyseal fractures.
- Commonly occurring complications include:
  - Infection
  - Flexor muscle atrophy

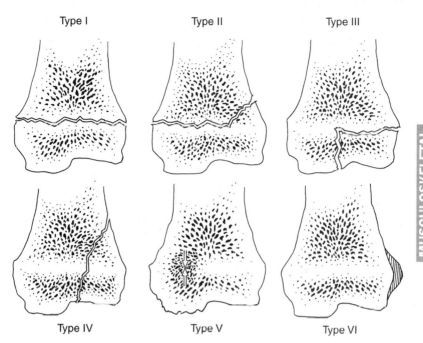

FIGURE 39-13. Salter-Harris fracture classification. (Adapted from Salter RB, Harris WR: Injuries involving the epiphyseal plate. In Stashak TS: *Adams' lameness in horses,* Philadelphia, 1987, Lea & Febiger.)

- Tendon contracture
- Cast sores
- Gluteal muscle atrophy in the affected limb
- Stretched flexor tendons
- Angular limb deformity in the contralateral limb
- Premature closure of the growth plate may occur regardless of the method of treatment.

Infection

- Infection can cause serious physeal damage and leads to instability and failure in repaired fractures.
- The extensive vasculature of equine long bones promotes bacterial spread, septic arthritis, osteomyelitis, and physitis, which often are present concurrently.
- For this reason, assume that a foal with septic arthritis and osteomyelitis in one or more joints has septicemia, although there may be few clinical signs of systemic infection.
- Because of increased blood flow to the developing bone, septicemia quickly spreads to involve the joints. Bacteria are carried across the growth plates by the transphyseal vessels that supply the area.

- Bacterial penetration of the physis is followed by an acute inflammatory reaction and subsequent ischemia and bone necrosis.
- Once marked necrosis has occurred, antimicrobial therapy alone is not adequate. Debridement and drainage of the inflammatory by-products from the joint by through-and-through lavage are needed.
- Most common sites of focal infection (osteomyelitis or septic arthritis):
  - Medial and lateral femoral condyles
  - Tibial tarsal condyles
  - Lateral styloid process of the radius
  - Distal tibia
  - Patella
  - Distal metacarpal/metatarsal III
- Foals with septic arthritis or osteomyelitis have
  - Lameness
  - Pain
  - ± Increased rectal temperature
  - Warmth and swelling in the affected joints
  - Involvement of more than one joint also supports a diagnosis of septic arthritis or osteomyelitis.
- Radiographic findings:
  - Osteomyelitis is recognized by the presence of bone lysis with or without associated soft-tissue swelling.
  - Septic arthritis appears as soft-tissue swelling and widening of the joint space and is differentiated from incomplete ossification primarily on the basis of the physical signs of swelling and warmth in the affected joints.
- Infection in epiphyseal bone is marked early on by:
  - Swelling at the level of the physis and sensitivity to point pressure at this site
  - Radiographic signs may not be present for 3-7 days, at which time the prognosis has worsened considerably.
  - Suspect septic epiphysitis (and septic arthritis) in any foal with lameness, synovial fluid white blood cell count > 40,000 cells/μl, total protein > 2.5 g/dl, and bacteria isolated from the joint
- Musculoskeletal infections in newborns and foals are most frequently caused by:
  - Gram-negative organisms; Gram-positive pathogens are sometimes isolated in foals with septic arthritis.
  - Broad-spectrum antibiotic treatment is indicated, pending results of culture and sensitivity studies.
  - A combination of an aminoglycoside (gentamicin or amikacin) with a penicillin or cephalosporin provides broad, relatively safe coverage pending culture results.
  - Foals are believed to be more sensitive to the nephrotoxic effects of aminoglycosides because of their slower rate of elimination.
  - If use of an aminoglycoside is contraindicated because of the presence of renal disease, a third-generation cephalosporin provides the needed Gram-negative coverage.
  - Dosage guidelines are presented in Table 39–5.
  - Polymethylmethacrylate (PMMA) antibiotic-impregnated beads placed at the site of infection increase the tissue concentration of drugs such as gentamicin and amikacin.

TABLE 39–5. Antibiotic Therapy for Infection in Newborns and Foals

Agent	Dose	Route and Frequency
Procaine penicillin G	22,000-44,000 IU/kg	IM q12h
Sodium/potassium penicillin G	22,000-44,000 IU/kg	IV q6h
Gentamicin	2.2 mg/kg/6.6 8.8 mg/kg	IM, IV q6-8h/q24h
Amikacin	6.6 mg/kg/15-25 mg/kg	IM, IV q8h/q24h
Ceftiofur	1-4 mg/kg	IM, IV q12h
Ticarcillin/clavulanic acid	50-100 mg/kg	IV q6h
Imipenem	15 mg/kg	IV q6-8h diluted
Azithromycin	10 mg/kg	PO q24h

Angular Limb Deformity

Not considered an orthopedic emergency but important to recognize early in any foal with "crooked" legs. Three major types:

Laxity of the Periarticular Supporting Structures

- Usually knock-kneed (valgus deformity)
- *Must* be differentiated from incomplete ossification of the cuboidal bones by means of radiographic evaluation
- Responds with moderate exercise over 7-10 days

Incomplete Ossification of Cuboidal Bones of the Carpus and Tarsus

- *Most commonly* recognized in the premature, dysmature, or twin foal
- Radiographic evaluation *essential* to confirm the presence of incomplete ossification (Fig. 39–14)
- Affects cuboidal bones of carpus and tarsus primarily
- Results in permanent deformity and early degenerative joint disease if not recognized *early* in life
- Treatment includes external coaptation with well-padded splints or tube casts in addition to assisted standing and restricted walking.

Disproportionate Growth of Epiphysis/Metaphysis

- A growth imbalance above the affected joint
- Generally occurs among foals several weeks of age or older
- Differentiated by means of radiographic evaluation of epiphysis
- Treatment is designed to promote growth on affected side.
- Many times this is normal for the foal's age.

SUMMARY

- Orthopedic emergencies are not uncommon among foals, whose immature bones are vulnerable to kicks, falls, infection, and the ill effects of overfeeding and inappropriate exercise.
- Foals respond to treatment more readily and rapidly than do adults.
- Internal fixation is most often the preferred treatment option.
- Infection should always be a concern with any trauma to the bone or joint.

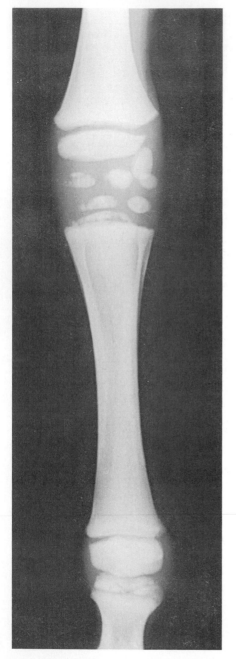

FIGURE 39-14. Dorsopalmar radiograph of the carpus shows incomplete ossification of cuboidal bones. Wide joint spaces are evident around small, rounded bones.

REFERENCES

Bramlage LR. Emergency first aid treatment and transportation of equine fracture patients. In Auer JA, editor: *Equine surgery,* Philadelphia, 1992, WB Saunders.

Cohen ND et al: Results of physical inspection before races and race-related characteristics and their association with musculoskeletal injuries in Thoroughbreds during races, *J Am Vet Med Assoc* 215:654-661, 1999.

Cohen ND et al: Frequency of musculoskeletal injuries and risk factors associated with injuries incurred in Quarter horses during races, *J Am Vet Med Assoc* 215:662-669, 1999.

Dyson S: Musculoskeletal injuries in the horse: the uses and limits of diagnostic ultrasonography, *Pferdeheilkunde* 12:681-683, 1996.

Embertson RM, Bramlage LR, Gabel AA: Physeal fractures in the horse: management and outcome, *Vet Surg* 15:230, 1986.

Hogan PM, Mc Ilwraith CW, Honnas CM et al: Surgical treatment of subchondrial cystic lesions of the third metacarpal bone: results in 15 horses (1986-1994) *Equine Vet J* 29(6):477-82, 1997.

Holland M: Preanesthetic medication and chemical restraint. In White NA, Moore JN, editors: *Current practice of equine surgery,* Philadelphia, 1990, JB Lippincott.

Honnas CM: Surgical treatment of selected musculoskeletal disorders of the forelimb. In Auer JA, editor: *Equine surgery,* Philadelphia, 1992, WB Saunders.

Mc Ilwraith CW, Bramlage LR: Surgical treatment of joint injury in joint disease in the horse. In Mc Ilwraith CW, Trotter GW, editors: *Joint Disease in the Horse,* Philadelphia, 1996, WB Saunders.

Nixon AJ: Tendon lacerations. In White NA, Moore JN, editors: *Current practice of equine surgery,* Philadelphia, 1990, JB Lippincott.

Orsini JA: Pharmacotherapy of the critically ill neonate. In Higgins AJ, Wright IM, editors: *The equine manual,* London, 1995, WB Saunders.

Orsini JA, Kreuder C: Musculoskeletal disorders of the neonate, *Vet Clin North Am Equine Pract* 10:137-166, 1994.

Richardson DW: Fractures. In White NA, Moore JN, editors: *Current practice of equine surgery,* Philadelphia, 1990, JB Lippincott.

Stashak TS: *Adams' lameness in horses,* Philadelphia, 1987, Lea & Febiger.

Stashak TS: Wounds. In Stashak TS, editor: *Adams' lameness in horses,* Philadelphia, 1987 Lea & Febiger.

Todhunter RJ: Therapeutic principles for joint disease and repair of articular tissues. In Stashak TS, editor: *Adams' lameness in horses,* Philadelphia, 1987, Lea & Febiger.

Turner TA: Abscesses and punctures of the foot. In White NA, Moore JN, editors: *Current practice of equine surgery,* Philadelphia, 1990, JB Lippincott.

Watkins JP: Treatment principles of tendon disorders. In Auer JA, editor: *Equine surgery,* Philadelphia, 1992, WB Saunders.

Wright IM, Phillips TJ, Walmsley JP: Endoscopy of the navicular bursa: a new technique for the treatment of contaminated and septic bursa, *Equine Vet J* 31:5-11, 1999.

40 Nervous System

Thomas J. Divers with contributions from Alexander deLahunta

Neurologic disorders frequently have an acute onset, may rapidly worsen, and often necessitate emergency diagnostics and therapeutics.

- The *first goal* of the examination is to determine that the nervous system is the origin of the clinical signs.
- The *second goal* is to determine the anatomic location of the abnormality within the nervous system; doing so shortens the list of differential diagnoses. Incoordination or ataxia suggests involvement of the long tracts in the spinal cord. Change in mentation indicates a cerebral or brainstem disorder. If the brainstem is involved, cranial nerve deficits and ataxia may be observed. Always consider metabolic disorders as a potential cause of change in mentation, such as hepatic or uremic encephalopathy. In the evaluation of horses with acute neurologic disorders, it is important to consider rabies. Weakness without ataxia causes a support problem and is characteristic of neuromuscular or ventral motor neuron disease.
- The *third goal* is to be able to complete the examination and provide reasonable diagnostics and therapeutics without further bodily injury to the patient, personnel, or facilities.

GAIT EVALUATION
Unwilling or Unable?

That is the first question to be answered in the examination of a horse with a gait abnormality. This is especially true when the horse is short-strided or does not support its weight on a limb. A loss of support from a femoral or radial nerve injury mimics a severe, painful disorder causing a reluctance to bear weight.

Patterns

With experience, clinicians recognize specific "patterns" in abnormal gaits that suggest the anatomic diagnosis. There are five components to these patterns: two qualities of paresis (weakness) and three qualities of ataxia (incoordination).

PARESIS

In neurologic terms, *paresis* means deficiency in generation of gait or the ability to support weight. This definition covers the two qualities of paresis: upper motor neuron and lower motor neuron, respectively.

Lower motor neuron (LMN) paresis reflects degrees of difficulty in supporting weight and varies from a slightly shortened stride (easily mistaken for musculoskeletal lameness) to complete inability to support weight, which leads to collapse of the limb whenever weight is placed on it.

Upper motor neuron (UMN) paresis causes a delay in the onset of protraction, the swing phase of the gait. Usually the stride is longer than normal. Stiffness (spasticity) may be apparent in the stride. The UMN comprises numerous neuronal systems that initiate the gait through LMN recruitment and modulate muscle tone for normal posture and smooth locomotor function. In domestic animals most of these neuronal cell bodies are located in the pons and medulla, and their processes descend the spinal cord in the lateral and ventral funiculi. Most lesions affecting these components of the UMN also affect the general proprioceptive sensory system and cause ataxia because the involved tracts are adjacent to each other.

ATAXIA

Ataxia has three qualities that reflect the functional system involved: general proprioception, the vestibular system, and the cerebellum.

General Proprioceptive Ataxia

The general proprioceptive (GP) sensory system has its dendritic zones in specialized receptors in muscles, tendons, and joints. The GP system is responsible for "informing" the central nervous system (CNS) of the degree of muscle contraction (tone) at any time. It tells the CNS where the animal's "parts" are in space at any instant. Loss of this system affects the gait by contributing to the delay in the onset of protraction. The result is excessive adduction (swing in) or abduction (swing out) of the limb and occasionally overflexion in the swing phase and scuffing-dragging of the hoof and standing on the dorsal aspect of the hoof.

The GP system and the UMN are affected by the same lesions because of their proximity.

It is difficult *but not necessary* to differentiate the UMN and GP signs.

Horses with UMN-GP deficits from a lesion anywhere between C1 and C6 have a tendency to overreach at the end of protraction; the result is a floating motion to the stride. This is referred to as a "UMN-GP deficit" because one does not know which system is responsible for preventing this action and because that differentiation is unnecessary to make the segmental anatomic diagnosis.

Neurologists do not try to differentiate conscious (cerebral) and unconscious (cerebellar) GP pathways. If an individual stands on the dorsal aspect of its digits, is this an LMN, UMN, conscious GP, or unconscious GP deficit? One cannot differentiate the latter three and must use other features of the examination to determine whether the deficit is LMN.

Vestibular (Special Proprioceptive) Ataxia

This quality of ataxia reflects the loss of orientation of the head with the eyes, trunk and limbs: a loss of balance. Lesions in this system cause the patient to lean, drift, or fall to one side, usually the side of the lesion. It generally is accompanied by a head tilt to that side and sometimes abnormal nystagmus.

These same signs result from a lesion in any part of the vestibular system: peripheral or central. The difference is in the other clinical signs exhibited by the patient. A horse with only vestibular ataxia and facial paralysis most likely has otitis. These same signs with UMN-GP deficits indicate the presence of a pontomedullary lesion.

Cerebellar Ataxia

Individuals with cerebellar disorders classically have dysmetria characterized by sudden bursts of motor activity with marked overflexion on protraction—hypermetria. This is accompanied by a stiff-spastic quality to the movement. The horse is unusual in that spasticity is much more pronounced than the hypermetria. This is most obvious in the thoracic limbs, which are thrown forward on protraction with marked extension of the limbs. This spastic overreaching movement differs in its degree and abruptness from the overreaching-floating that occurs with UMN-GP disorders. There are vestibular components in the cerebellum, so there usually is some loss of balance. When the individual runs, it often swings its head and neck side to side with a stiff appearance. The presence of an obvious intentional head tremor also helps with the anatomic diagnosis.

ACUTE ATAXIA

Evaluation and Management of Neurologic Conditions in Weanlings and Adult Horses

Ataxia (incoordination) results from loss of the ability to sense the position of the limbs in space. It is the hallmark of spinal cord disease in the horse but can also be a feature of vestibular disease.

Physical Examination

- Proceed with caution to avoid injury to the patient and personnel. An open grassy area with a slight incline is ideal.
- Observe the patient for inappropriate circumduction, adduction, or abduction of the limbs; basewide stance; delay in protraction of the limbs; scuffing or abnormal wear of the hooves; and striking one limb with another. Tight circles, backing, and serpentines often exaggerate these deficits.
- Careful examination of the cranial nerves is helpful in formulating a differential diagnosis.

Equine Protozoal Myelitis

- Equine protozoal myelitis (EPM) may manifest as acute onset of ataxia with or without cranial nerve deficits (vestibular disturbance, facial paresis, and dysphagia are the most recognizable cranial nerve deficits).

Diagnosis

- Signalment is useful in arriving at a diagnosis, because the disease is most common among horses between 15 months and 4 years of age, although it can affect adults of *any* age. It is rarely diagnosed among individuals younger than 1 year.
- EPM appears to affect performance horses more frequently, seems more prevalent in the eastern United States, and less common in the winter.

Clinical Signs (Acute Onset)

- *Depression, if present, often serves to separate EPM from many other spinal cord diseases.*
- Ataxia (often asymmetric) may progress to recumbency. In some cases the ataxia is symmetric, and then it is almost impossible at clinical examination to differ-

entiate EPM from equine degenerative myelopathy (EDM) or cervical stenotic myelopathy (CSM).

- Trembling (one or two limbs) can be mild to severe (rare) and indicates LMN involvement. Trembling may be seen with acute disease, whereas noticeable atrophy requires 10 days or more.
- Head tilt: Rule out stylohyoid osteoarthropathy with an endoscopic examination.
- Facial paralysis: Same as above.
- Difficulty swallowing: See Dysphagia, p. 430 of this chapter.
- Dragging one or more limbs.
- Blindness is rare but can occur.
- Seizures may occur as the only clinical sign.
- Urinary incontinence: Rare.

Laboratory Testing: Serology

A serum or cerebrospinal fluid (CSF) sample or both can be sent to:

1. EBI, A153 Astecc Building, University of Kentucky, Lexington, KY 40502-0286; (606) 257-2300 ext. 226; (Fax) (606) 257-2489;
2. Neogen Corp., 628 East 3rd Street, Lexington, KY 40505; (800) 477-8201; or
3. Michigan State University Diagnostic Laboratory for measurement of antibodies against *Sarcocystis neurona* or for polymerase chain reaction (PCR) to determine the presence of *S. neurona* DNA.

A negative result of a serum or CSF antibody test has a good negative predictive value, but a positive result of a serum or even of a CSF antibody test *does not* have a strong predictive value for disease. Blood contamination of CSF or the presence of blood-brain barrier abnormalities as occur with herpes myelitis further lower the positive predictive value of the CSF test for EPM.

If the CSF test result is reported as weak positive, this further reduces the positive predictive value. Although there is approximately a 15% disagreement between laboratories on weak positive versus negative, there is no consistent pattern among the three laboratories in the "disagreement" cases. All three laboratories are reliable in their test results.

Treatment

- Antiprotozoal therapy
- Ponazuril, 5 or 10 mg/kg PO q24h for at least 30 days, is one treatment that is available and approved for use in horses.
- Sulfadiazine, 30 mg/kg PO q24h
  with
- Pyrimethamine, 1.0 mg/kg orally q24h (do not mix with feed or administer at time of feeding). A 2.0 mg/kg dosage may be used for the first 2 weeks in nonpregnant mares.
- Treat patients that show improvement for a minimum of 12 weeks. Test all pregnant and treated mares for plasma folic acid concentration and supplement with folinic acid if needed.
- Combination of ponazuril and pyrimethamine/sulfa.

Supportive Therapy

- Feed patients that cannot eat or drink with gruel at least twice a day by stomach tube (see Chapter 57, p. 769).

- Administer penicillin, metronidazole, or both if aspiration pneumonia is evident.
- Apply ophthalmic ointment four times a day to the eyes of patients with facial paralysis.
- Perform partial tarsorrhaphy if a corneal ulcer is already present (see treatment, Chapter 41, p. 442).
- ☛ *Corneal ulcers that develop as a result of facial nerve paralysis can be refractory to treatment.*
- Long-term use of corticosteroids is contraindicated. Short-term (1 or 2 days) dexamethasone at an antiinflammatory dose (0.1-0.2 mg/kg) in severe cases may improve clinical signs but is recommended only in cases that are rapidly progressing to recumbency.
- Flunixin meglumine, 0.5-1.0 mg/kg IM q12-24h if signs are more severe after treatment is started.
- Dimethyl sulfoxide (DMSO), 1 g/kg IV in saline solution or other polyionic fluid as a 10% solution, administered over 30-60 minutes once per day for 5 days.
- Levamisol, 2.2 mg/kg PO q24h for 5 days followed by once weekly therapy, as an immune modulator.
- Vitamin E, 2000 to 5000 units/day in feed, for nonspecific antioxidant properties.

Prognosis
- Fair for return to function for horses receiving *early* and appropriate treatment.
- There should be a noticeable response within 3 weeks of treatment.

Cervical Stenotic or Compressive Myelopathy ("Wobblers")

Horses with CSM or cervical compressive myelopathy may be brought for emergency treatment because of a traumatic accident that acutely worsens the underlying compressive disease.

Signalment
- Often a young, rapidly growing horse; may have a history of clumsiness, which suggests a preexisting condition.
- Trauma can exacerbate clinical signs to the point of extreme ataxia or recumbency.
- Males are more commonly affected.

Clinical Signs
- Symmetric ataxia (in most cases) involving all four limbs. Deficits in the thoracic limbs may be subtle.
- No cranial nerve deficits unless secondary to trauma.
- Neck pain inconsistent; abnormal resistance to neck flexion may be seen.
- Most patients are bright and alert with no depression.
- Stiffness of the neck and more pronounced forelimb signs are present with C6-7 to T1 lesions. Caudal cervical osteoarthritis is more common among older horses.

Diagnosis
Survey radiographs may *suggest* CSM characteristics: vertebral canal stenosis (minimal sagittal diameter ratio <0.52 at C2-6 and <0.56 at C6-7, determined by comparing the narrowest dorsal-ventral measurement of the cranial vertebral

canal with the widest dorsal-ventral measurement of the corresponding cranial vertebral body) (Fig. 40–1A), osteoarthritis of the articular processes, malalignment, or a ski jump appearance of the dorsocaudal vertebral body (Fig. 40–1B).

- Obtain definitive diagnosis through myelographic demonstration of impingement on the spinal cord (>50% impingement of the dorsal column). The 50% rule does not have a high specificity unless it is on nonflexed views.
- CSF usually is normal unless a previous centesis was performed within 7 days, in which case xanthochromia, an elevated protein level, and pleocytosis may be present.

Treatment

- Dexamethasone, 0.1-0.2 mg/kg IV once per day for 1-2 days, and DMSO, 1 g/kg IV as a 10% solution in saline or lactated Ringer's solution, once per day for 5 days, may provide transient improvement in cases made abruptly worse by trauma.
- Long-term dietary and exercise restrictions may help stop the progression of the disease in some youngsters.
- Surgical arthrodesis may benefit some patients, determined by neurologic status, number of vertebrae involved, myelographic findings, and duration of clinical signs.

Prognosis

- Fair to poor, depending on the site of compression, number of compressed sites, age of the patient, and severity of signs.

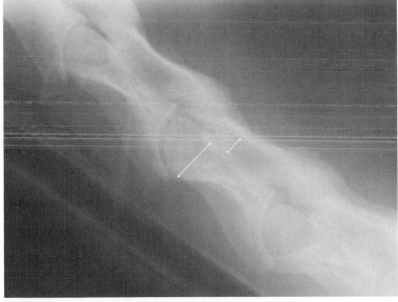

FIGURE 40-1A. Cervical radiograph demonstrating areas of measurement for intravertebral sagittal diameter ratios.

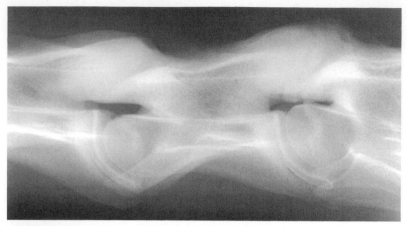

FIGURE 40-1B. Cervical radiographs of caudal C4, C5 and rostral C6. At C5-6 there is evidence of severe osteoarthropathy of the dorsal facet and malalignment of the vertebral body.

Equine Herpesvirus 1 Myeloencephalitis

Equine herpesvirus 1 (EHV-1), or rhinopneumonitis, causes respiratory disease and abortion as well as neurologic disease. The neurologic form occurs sporadically, often as a sequela to either of the other two forms.

Signalment
- Most commonly adults (rarely occurs in foals).
- Race track, breeding farm, boarding stable, or training facility.
- Often multiple cases on the same farm within a short time period. Isolated cases have been reported.
- No seasonality.
- May be a risk factor among horses housed with donkeys or mules.

Clinical Signs
- *Abrupt* onset of (usually) symmetric ataxia and paresis that may progress rapidly to recumbency.
- Neurologic deficit of pelvic limbs is worse than thoracic limbs in *most cases*.
- *Urinary bladder paralysis with urine dribbling is a* common *clinical sign.*
- Hypotonic tail and fecal retention in a few cases.
- May rarely have vestibular signs and other cranial nerve deficits.
- Fever may be detectable early in the disease course. Individuals without signs on the same farm may have fevers. Initial fever generally occurs 2-8 days before onset of clinical signs.

Diagnosis
- Several horses from the same farm with an acute onset of hindlimb ataxia and bladder paralysis and an episode of previous respiratory disease on the farm is the classic presentation.
- Hematology and serum biochemistry profile usually are unremarkable.

- CSF generally has an elevated protein level with few nucleated cells. The CSF may be yellow (xanthochromia).
- Fourfold increase in serum neutralization titer in samples drawn 10 days apart is highly suggestive of EHV-1 infection but is not always present in neurologically affected horses.
- Virus isolation from the buffy coat, nasal swab, CSF, or CNS from a neurologically affected horse is only occasionally successful. Immunocytochemistry findings demonstrating herpes antigen in the CNS vascular endothelium is the preferred postmortem test.
- Examination of nasal and pharyngeal swabs and buffy coat for virus isolation in individuals with respiratory or neurologic disease should be attempted and is helpful if the results are positive. Adjacent horses that have normal neurologic findings but a fever are more likely to have positive culture results.
- Many, but not all, affected horses have relatively high serum neutralization titers (1:640 or more) at the onset of clinical signs.
- The authors find little value in performing CSF titers.

Treatment

- DMSO, 1 g/kg IV as a 10% solution mixed in saline solution or any isotonic polyionic fluid once per day for 5 days.
- Mannitol, 0.25-1.0 g/kg IV.
- *Urinary bladder catheterization and drainage three to four times per day in cases with dysuria and bladder distention.*
- Bethanechol, 0.04 mg/kg SQ q8h, to manage bladder distention. Injectable bethanechol is expensive and difficult to obtain and therefore is not an option in some cases. Bethanechol tablets for oral administration, 0.2-0.4 mg/kg PO q8-12h, are not as expensive and are not as effective as the parenteral product. *The oral product can be easily dissolved and filtered through a 0.5-μm filter for intravenous or subcutaneous injection.*
- Antibiotics for cystitis, which is unavoidable with frequent catheterization.
  - Trimethoprim-sulfamethoxazole, 20 mg/kg PO q12h, or ceftiofur, 2.2-4.4 mg/kg IV q12h.
  - Urine culture is recommended because resistant infections can develop despite antibiotic therapy and enrofloxacin, 7.5 mg/kg PO or 5 mg/kg IV q24h, may be needed.
- *Administer corticosteroids in progressive or severe cases;* use caution because this therapy can potentiate secondary bacterial infections. Clinical signs may worsen 2-4 days after a single corticosteroid treatment.
- The potent antiinflammatory effects of short-term (1-2 days) dexamethasone, 0.1-0.2 mg/kg IV, may prove lifesaving to a recumbent or nearly recumbent patient. Corticosteroids should be used only in the care of patients whose condition is rapidly progressing toward recumbency or is acutely recumbent.
- Acyclovir, 20 mg/kg PO q8h. It is not clear that acyclovir therapy improves the prognosis or shortens the recovery time. It may be of greater benefit in the early management of EHV-1 infection before neurologic signs develop. Bioavailability and efficacy against EHV-1 are unproven. Newer drugs in the same family may be more effective in treating horses and foals with EHV-1 infection.
- Supportive care: Protective leg wraps, laxative diet, intravenous or oral fluids to maintain hydration, topical care of decubitus ulcers, and avoidance of urine scalding.

| **NOTE:** *Do not overhydrate!*

- Fecal evacuation, laxative treatment, and feeding low residue diets (pellets) are recommended for patients with fecal incontinence (approximately 10% of cases).
- Use of a sling (Anderson) is recommended for recumbent horses. Horses that sustain pressure sores in the sling can be slung in a pool or, if the horse is very calm, in a bovine float tank (see p. 736).

Prognosis

- Highly variable. Many individuals make a full recovery; others are left with residual deficits; some are euthanized because of paralysis and secondary complications. Nursing care can be very intensive and full recovery can take months. Determining the prognosis at the beginning of the clinical course often is difficult, although those that rapidly become recumbent rarely return to normal function. Bladder dysfunction may be the last clinical problem to resolve in many cases.

Management of an Outbreak

- Quarantine the facility for at least 30 days after confirming the *last* case.
- Minimize movement of horses within the facility to avoid spread of the virus.
- Assign specific personnel to care for affected horses; these employees should not handle healthy horses.
- Monitor temperature (twice per day) of all at-risk horses to detect a fever that generally precedes clinical disease by 2-8 days.
- Steam cleaning and phenol- or iodophor-based disinfectants kill the virus.
- *Vaccination in the face of an outbreak is not known to be useful and may exacerbate the problem. Vaccination after clinical signs have resolved is recommended.*
- There is no reported recurrence of the neurologic syndrome in a patient that has recovered from this disease.
- Individuals that have to be moved into a stable that has had EHV-1 should be vaccinated, but the vaccines may not protect against the neurologic form of EHV.
- Horses with suspected EHV-1 infection sent to referral hospitals should be isolated!

Vestibular Disease

Clinical Signs

The vestibular system controls balance and maintains orientation of the head, eyes, and trunk. Ataxia often is a manifestation of an acute vestibular disturbance.

- Low-grade fever in a few cases
- Head tilt
- Staggering, leaning, drifting sideways
- Abnormal nystagmus (quick phase away from the affected side) observed only in the acute stages of vestibular disease in the horse
- Strabismus, especially ventral strabismus on the affected side when the head is elevated
- Loss of balance exacerbated by blindfolding
- Other cranial nerve deficits, especially of cranial nerve VII (facial nerve), may occur with peripheral or central vestibular disease

- History of ear rubbing or head shaking or difficulty chewing
- If severe, recumbency and inability to maintain sternal recumbency
- If recumbent, patient may refuse to be positioned on side opposite the lesion

Differential Diagnosis

- *Cranial trauma* (see Cranial Trauma, p. 420): *Common,* generally central vestibular disease but may be peripheral
- *Otitis media* and *interna* with or without temporohyoid osteoarthropathy: *Common* peripheral vestibular disease, but affected horses may be depressed because of inflammatory extension to dura mater
- EPM (see Equine Protozoal Myelitis, p. 390): *Common* central vestibular disease
- Polyneuritis equi (cauda equina): Central vestibular disease
- Space-occupying mass: Central vestibular disease
- Encephalitis or encephalopathy: Hepatic failure, viral or parasitic encephalitis; central vestibular disease
- Guttural pouch mycosis with extension to the middle ear: Peripheral vestibular disease
- Idiopathic vestibular disease: Peripheral vestibular disease
- Cranial cervical lesion: May have vestibular signs

The distinction between a peripheral (outside the brainstem) and central (within the brainstem) lesion is as follows:

Peripheral	Central
Normal mentation (except for some cases of temporohyoid osteoarthropathy)	Depression
No proprioceptive deficits	Proprioceptive deficits
Normal strength	Weak
Possible involvement of the seventh cranial nerve	Possibly multiple cranial nerve involvement (other than VII and VIII)

Occasionally seen is a horse with an acute onset of *body leaning* (with no head tilt) and *drifting to that side.* This is most commonly a prosencephalon lesion on the *ipsilateral* side and frequently is EPM.

Diagnosis of Vestibular Disease

- Palpate the base of the ear for any signs of pain.
- Skull radiographs: Lateral, oblique, and ventrodorsal (most useful) views. Evaluate stylohyoid bone, tympanic bullae, petrous temporal bone, and guttural pouch. Lateral and oblique views may not be very sensitive.
- Computed tomography (CT): Excellent for evaluating lesions in this area.
- Endoscopic evaluation of upper airway and guttural pouch. In the guttural pouch, look for proliferative changes (bulging) of the proximal stylohyoid bone or the temporohyoid joint and lack of movement when external pressure is applied to the hyoid bone (see Color Plate 1).
- Careful aural examination and culture of any exudate. Usually unrewarding!
- CSF analysis, including *S. neurona* antibody titer to rule out EPM (see p. 391).
- The few patients with drainage from the ear most often have *Staphylococcus aureus* infection. *Streptococcus* and *Actinobacillus* organisms also have been isolated from infected ears.

Treatment

- DMSO, 1 g/kg IV as a 10% solution in saline or any isotonic fluid intended for IV administration, once per day for 5 days.
- Trimethoprim-sulfamethoxazole, 20 mg/kg PO q12h for 30 days. *This is an effective therapy for many staphylococcal infections in the horse!*
- Phenylbutazone, 2.2 mg/kg PO once or twice daily for 7-10 days.
- Corticosteroids: dexamethasone 0.05-0.1 mg/kg IV q24h. Judicious use is advised and not recommended unless the vestibular dysfunction is *traumatic* or *rapidly progressive.*
- Supportive care: *Ophthalmic ointment and tarsorrhaphy for patients with facial nerve paralysis;* protective leg wraps; good footing; and easy access to food and water.
- Surgical resection of a portion of the ceratohyoid bone is recommended for cases of osteoarthropathy to improve chewing ability and to decrease risk of future fracture.

Prognosis

- Fair to good for otitis media or interna.
- Fair with stylohyoid osteoarthropathy, which can be caused by otitis media or interna and fracture of the fused bone.
- Uncontrolled otitis interna or fracture can progress to meningitis.
- Fair to poor for central vestibular disorders except EPM.
- Rare cases of idiopathic vestibular disease resolve without treatment over several days.

Plant-Induced Ataxia

In certain areas of the United States (especially the south), during certain summers (probably associated with environmental conditions and proliferation of mycotoxins), ataxia may occur in one or more horses at pasture when grazing rye grass, Bermuda grass, or fescue grass.

Clinical Signs

- Affected horses usually are adults.
- Ataxia may be severe.
- Head tremors and hypermetria may occur.
- Occurs more commonly among individuals at pasture than those fed hay.
- Sorghum and Sudan grass and black locust bark also can cause ataxia.
- Distinctive clinical signs are as follows:

Sorghum or Sudan Grass	Black Locust Bark
Dribbling urine	Anorexia, depression
Abortion	Mild colic
Arthrogryposis in utero	Irregular heart beat
Stringhalt-like gait	

Treatment

- No specific therapy for mycotoxin, Sorghum and Sudan grass and black locust bark poisoning other than removal from the source of the poison.
- Treat with DMSO, 1 g/kg IV, as a 10% solution in saline solution or any isotonic fluid q24h for 3 to 5 days, or dexamethasone, 0.04-0.08 mg/kg IV q24h for 1-2 days with a tapering dose, or use both treatments.

- Horses affected by mycotoxins often return to normal within 5 days.

Other Causes of Acute-Onset Ataxia

- **Spinal cord trauma:** See p. 423 in this chapter.
- **Fibrocartilaginous emboli:** Rare but can cause acute hemiparesis and ataxia without evidence of vertebral pain.
- **Equine ehrlichiosis:** Affected horses are occasionally ataxic, depressed, jaundiced, febrile, and have petechiations. The organism can be seen in neutrophils. Treatment is tetracycline, 6.6 mg/kg IV q12h.
- **Grove poisoning:** A syndrome causing ataxic and convulsion-like signs with oral mucous membrane congestion. Reported to occur among adults in proximity to large crop farms or orchards. Toxicity is suspected. Signs may wax and wane, and affected horses may recover. There is no known treatment.
- *Neospora*-associated EPM: Looks like *S. neurona* EPM except the patient may have nerve root signs (pain, hyperesthesia). *Neospora hughesi* does not cross react serologically with the organism that causes EPM, so affected horses may have negative results on the current EPM test.
  - *Diagnosis:* Clinical signs, serologic testing for *Neospora caninum* (*N. hughesi* cross reacts with *N. caninum*).
  - *Treatment:* Same as for EPM.
- **Postanesthetic myelopathy** is a *rare* but fatal complication to horses positioned in dorsal recumbency for surgical procedures (mostly elective procedures such as bilateral hock arthroscopy). It appears to be most common among weanlings and young adults. There is generally complete paralysis of the rear limbs with areflexia of the hindlimbs, tail, and anus. Antiedema, antiinflammatory treatment (methylprednisolone sodium succinate, 30 mg/kg IV) can be tried, but the prognosis is grave.

Acute Ataxia in Foals
Causes

- Most commonly a result of **trauma** (see spinal cord trauma, p. 423).
- Congenital anomalies, such as spina bifida, should be considered when an ataxic newborn foal does not improve with standard antiinflammatory and antiedema therapy.
- Young foals, especially Arabian foals, with ataxia, extended neck posture, or a clicking noise caused by head movement should undergo radiography, CT, and/or fluoroscopy to rule out occipitoatlantoaxial malformation or subluxation or fractures of this area.

Vertebral Body Abscess

- Vertebral body abscess can cause acute pain and ataxia and paresis in foals.
- Affected foals are generally 2-8 months of age and appear healthy just before the onset of pain and neurologic signs.
- The clinical signs vary depending on the site of the infection.
- Sacrococcygeal abscess causes decreased tail tone and ataxia and weakness in the rear legs (often asymmetric).
- Thoracolumbar lesions cause stiffness and UMN signs in the rear limbs.

- Cervical lesions cause neck pain, tetraparesis, and ataxia (worse in the front limbs if the lesion is low cervical).
- The most common organisms are
  - *Rhodococcus equi*
  - *Salmonella* organisms
  - *Streptococcus equi*
  - *Streptococcus zooepidemicus*

Diagnosis
- Clinical examination and localization of site of pain
- Radiography
- Ultrasonography
- CT
- Serologic testing for *R. equi*—sensitivity not proved
- Fecal cultures for *Salmonella* organisms, *R. equi*
- Tracheal wash
- Nasal swab for *S. equi*

Treatment
- Surgical drainage.
- Antibiotics: Begin with either K penicillin and amikacin or azithromycin if *R. equi* is the more likely organism.
- Nursing care (e.g., splints, physical therapy).

TREMBLING IN HORSES

Etiologies include weakness, pain, shock, adverse drug reactions, hypothermia, and toxicity. Diseases presented are neurologic and neuromuscular problems that cause trembling. Trembling from pain and shock is discussed in Chapter 48.

Physical Examination
A careful physical examination shows whether the trembling is a result of weakness, pain, shock, or other causes. In conditions with generalized weakness (e.g., botulism), the eyelids, tongue, tail, and anus all are dull. Botulism, equine motor neuron disease, and severe cachexia cause affected horses to stand with all four feet closer together than is normal. If the weakness is a result of electrolyte abnormalities, hypocalcemia, or periodic paralysis, a tetanic appearance may be seen. Trembling associated with abdominal pain or endotoxemia is common and can be detected with a complete clinical examination. Sweating may occur with either weakness or pain. Trembling due to a primary muscle disorder may be difficult to separate from other causes of trembling. Trembling in one limb also is common with EPM, *vertebral osteomyelitis*, myopathy, and any peripheral neuropathy.

Botulism
Signalment
FOALS
- Often 2-8 weeks of age; most are 21-28 days of age
- Generally occurs because of toxic-infectious botulism

- Most common among foals in Kentucky, Maryland, Pennsylvania, and New Jersey

ADULTS

- Most often a result of ingestion of a preformed toxin (although it is rarely found)
- Associated with a closed wound in rare instances
- Endemic in the middle Atlantic states (*Clostridium botulinum* type B is common in the soil)
- Outbreaks of *C. botulinum* types C and D have been reported in other parts of the United States in association with contamination of the feed with dead animals.

Clinical Signs

- Generalized (and therefore symmetric) weakness in most, but not all, cases
- Decreased tail, eyelid, and tongue tone (the tongue can easily be pulled from the mouth and held with two fingers)
- Trembling
- Lying down
- Dysphagia in most but not all cases; if the horse can swallow, it takes >2 minutes to consume 1 cup (approximately 140 g) of grain
- Standing with all four limbs close together
- The disease often progresses to severe paresis with inability to stand and subsequent respiratory failure
- The onset usually is acute, with rapid progression within 18-48 hours, although some cases may progress more slowly or even stabilize without treatment
- Mydriasis and ptosis

Diagnostic Tests

- The diagnosis of botulism is made by consideration of the signalment, clinical signs, and geographic location.
- Anaerobic culture of soil, feed, or wound tissue for identification of *C. botulinum* and its toxin may be submitted to Dr. R. H. Whitlock* to support the diagnosis in adult horses. In foals, the presence of organisms in the feces is considered to confirm the diagnosis if appropriate signs are present. Anaerobic conditions can be maintained by packing an airtight container full with the sample.
- Muscle enzymes are normal or only slightly elevated (unless the patient has been recumbent).
- Endoscopy often reveals a displaced soft palate, even in mild cases.
- Arterial or venous PCO_2 >70 mm Hg suggests hypoventilation and a poor prognosis.

Treatment

- *Do not stress!*
- Remove hay and water; muzzle if patient attempts to eat the bedding.

---

*University of Pennsylvania, New Bolton Center, Kennett Square, PA 19348-1692; (610) 444-5800.

- Administer polyvalent botulism antiserum IV (approximate cost is $1500/foal and $2500/adult). Contact Dr. Whitlock. Signs may progress for 12-24 hours after administration of the antitoxin.
- Broad-spectrum antibiotics: Ceftiofur, 4.4 mg/kg IV q12h, or potassium penicillin, 22,000 IU/kg IV q6h. Metronidazole is not effective against *C. botulinum*.
- Procaine penicillin, aminoglycosides, and tetracycline should not be administered because of their effect on the neuromuscular system.
- *Debride wound (in the unusual case of wound botulism).*
- Supply feed and water or milk by means of *nasogastric* intubation (see Nutritional Guidelines, Chapter 57, p. 769). *In the care of acutely affected adults, passage of a nasogastric tube should be postponed until the antitoxin has been administered (at least 24 hours) to reduce stress.*
- If laxatives are needed, mineral oil is preferred.
- In foals, the standard approximately 22% of milk per kilogram of body weight per day usually is not required because the activity level of these foals is markedly decreased, and abdominal distention should be prevented. Antiulcer medication is recommended.
- Supportive care: Urinary catheterization if needed in the treatment of recumbent horses. Good bedding and ventilation. Turning of recumbent horses every 2-4 hours but only after placing in sternal recumbency for 5 minutes.

Prognosis

FOALS
- *Foals that can stand* have a fair to good prognosis with antitoxin therapy.
- *Recumbent foals* without respiratory distress have a guarded to fair prognosis.
- *Foals with respiratory distress and PCO$_2$ >70 mm Hg* have a poor prognosis without ventilatory support, which is expensive and requires 2-3 weeks of hospitalization. These foals can be maintained with intranasal intubation and an Ambu Bag until they can be admitted to an intensive care facility for ventilatory support.

ADULTS
- *Adults that have a 3-5-day history of weakness and are still standing* have a fair to good prognosis, sometimes even without antitoxin treatment.
- *Adults that cannot stand or that have a peracute course of disease* have a poor prognosis even with antitoxin.

Equine Motor Neuron Disease

Equine motor neuron disease (EMND) affects adults, usually in a management situation in which there is little or no pasture and poor hay quality, most commonly in the northeastern United States. The disease is closely linked to prolonged (>14 months) deficiency of vitamin E.

Diagnosis

- Clinical signs provide a tentative diagnosis:
  - Weight loss of more than 150 lb (70 kg)
  - Trembling
  - Weakness of the limbs and neck
  - Generalized muscle atrophy

- Standing with all four limbs close together
- Increased periods of recumbency
- Good appetite
- *No dysphagia, ataxia, or weak tail*
- Raised tailhead in many cases
- Fundoscopic changes (see Color Plate 2)

Definitive Diagnosis
- Laboratory test (result is suggestive, not diagnostic). Serum (creatine kinase [CK]) level is mildly or moderately elevated (500-2000 μ/L) in approximately 90% of horses with EMND that are trembling.
- Measurement of plasma vitamin E; all horses with EMND have had <1 μg/ml.
- Muscle biopsy of the sacrocaudalis dorsalis medialis (tailhead) muscle. This is the most superficial muscle on either side of midline at the base of the tail. To perform the biopsy, sedate with xylazine and administer local anesthesia subcutaneously and into the muscle. Make a 3-inch (7.5-cm) skin incision and dissect through any subcutaneous fat to the muscle. Undermine the muscle before cutting to obtain a 1-inch-long by 0.25-inch-wide (2.5- by 0.6-cm) specimen. Place the specimen in formalin after sticking on a tongue depressor and ship it to a pathologist experienced in the evaluation of equine muscle.
- Perform biopsy on the ventral branch of the spinal accessory nerve (submitted in formalin). The results are approximately 94% accurate in predicting the presence of the disease, if the biopsy is performed by an experienced pathologist.

Treatment
- None known. Possibly vitamin E, 6000 IU *without added selenium* PO q24h.
- Buckeye Feeds and other companies produce a supplement, sold only to veterinarians, that contains vitamin E, folic acid, and thiamine.
- Prednisolone, 0.5-1 mg/kg PO q24h, appears to improve the signs in acute, severely affected horses.

Prognosis
- Poor for return to previous function.
- The condition in more than half of affected horses begins to stabilize after 2-4 weeks.

Tetanic Hypocalcemia in Horses
Causes
- Lactation: More common in draft horses and miniature horses.
- Blister beetle toxicity (see p. 258 in Chapter 35).
- *Idiopathic: Most common.*
- Transport and stress.
- Hypoparathyroidism: More common among foals (frequently 2-5 months of age); grave prognosis.
- Farm problems may occur among foals, in which case low dietary magnesium as a cause of diminished parathyroid hormone (PTH) activity or vitamin D deficiency should be investigated.
- Colitis and colic in *adults* or *exhaustion syndrome* in endurance horses (see p. 622).
- Excessive bicarbonate administration!

Clinical Signs
- Generalized stiffness
- Trismus
- Trembling
- Dysmetric flared nostrils
- *Synchronous diaphragmatic flutter*
- Prolapsing third eyelids (some of the signs of hypocalcemic tetany are similar to those of hyperkalemic periodic paralysis [HYPP])
- Respiratory distress
- Stringhalt or goose-stepping gait
- Recumbency
- Dilated pupils
- Sweating
- Elevated heart rate
- Hyperesthesia
- Choke
- Elevated temperature
- Seizures in foals
- *Colic (often severe) due to ileus*

Laboratory Findings
- Ca* usually <5.0 mg/dl (<1.25 mmol/L)
- Ionized Ca <0.6 mmol/L (<2.4 mg/dl)
- Mg <1.0 mg/dl
- May be alkalotic and hypochloremic due to sweating, which further aggravates hypocalcemia

Treatment
- 11 g (500 ml) 23% calcium borogluconate *slowly IV* over at least 15 minutes for a 450-kg adult. The calcium borogluconate can be mixed in 4-5 L of 0.9% NaCl and administered over 30-45 minutes. Adults in severe distress may be given 200 ml calcium borogluconate slowly IV without fluid dilution.
- Monitor heart rate and rhythm.
  - The expected cardiovascular response is an increase in the intensity of heart sounds.
  - An infrequent extrasystole may be expected, but pronounced change in rate or rhythm is an indication to discontinue the treatment immediately.
- Complete recovery from hypocalcemia may require several hours to days. Treatment may have to be repeated. Foals often are refractory to treatment.

Prognosis
Good except for horses with hypoparathyroidism, which is more common among foals. Laboratory samples for PTH (to diagnose hypoparathyroidism) can be sent to the Endocrine Diagnostic Section, Animal Health Diagnostic Laboratory, Michigan State University; (517) 353-0621. Blood samples must be clotted, centrifuged, and sent overnight on ice. Normal values are reported to be 0.25-2.0 pmol/L. The prognosis is poor for foals with hypoparathyroidism.

---

*Conversion factor: mg/dl to mmol/L divide by 4; mmol/L to mg/dl multiply by 4.

Hyperkalemic Periodic Paralysis

HYPP is a defect in muscle membrane transport that is inherited through an autosomal-dominant gene. Homozygous HYPP horses usually have more severe clinical signs.

Signalment

- Quarter Horses, Appaloosas, and Paints that are descendants of the Quarter Horse sire "Impressive."

ADULTS
- Typically 2-4 years of age at initial episode.
- Some are older when they first exhibit clinical signs.
- High-potassium diet, stress, or fasting can cause the onset of clinical signs.

FOALS
- May be neonates to weanling in age.
- Dam may have no history of clinical disease.

Clinical Signs
ADULTS
- Anxious attitude; remains alert
- Episodic muscle tremors, often seen first in the muscles of the face and neck, then progress to diffuse body tremors
- Swaying, staggering
- Dog-sitting posture (hindquarter paresis), which may progress to involuntary recumbency
- Prolapse or "flash" of the third eyelid
- Usually completely normal after recovery from an incident
- Signs may develop after a stressful event (e.g., colic), cold weather, anesthesia, or after feeding
- Increased respiratory rate and upper airway noise

FOALS
- Loud inspiratory noise
- Respiratory distress
- Collapse
- Most often exhibit respiratory signs when exercised, restrained, or nursing
- These foals usually are homozygous for the gene

Diagnosis

Signalment, clinical signs, endoscopy in foals, laboratory data, and response to treatment provide a tentative diagnosis. HYPP genetics testing leads to identification of homozygous and heterozygous individuals.

Laboratory Data

- Hyperkalemia (5-12.3 mEq/L) *during an incident.* Affected adults and foals rarely are reported to be *normokalemic* during clinical episodes.
- Muscle enzyme (CK and aspartate transaminase) levels are normal or only mildly elevated. Muscle biopsy does not provide enough information for a diagnosis.

- HYPP testing by the Veterinary Genetics Laboratory at the University of California, Davis, CA; (916) 752-2211. In Canada: Dr. Doug Nickel, Health Science Center, 3330 Hospital Drive, Calgary, Alberta, Canada TZN 4N1. Submit 5-10 ml of blood in an EDTA (purple top) tube. Results available in 3-5 working days.

Treatment
FOALS
- *Do not stress!*
- Tracheotomy may be needed for foals with excessive pharyngeal collapse.

ADULTS AND FOALS
- 23% calcium gluconate (0.2-0.4 ml/kg) in 1-2 L of 10% dextrose or 250 ml 50% dextrose or sodium bicarbonate (0.5 mEq/kg), administered IV over 30 minutes.
- Milder cases respond to dextrose or Karo syrup with or without sodium bicarbonate (baking soda) administered orally or through a nasogastric tube.
- Acetazolamide, 2.2 mg/kg PO q12h. This is a potassium-wasting diuretic used to lessen the incidence of clinical signs.
- Decrease potassium content of diet. Change from alfalfa to a *tested* grass hay but not brome grass. (Potassium in hay can vary widely!) Feed more oats and less of sweet feed or pellets. Avoid supplements (e.g., molasses, Litesalt, kelp) that contain potassium. Make certain there is enough calcium in the diet.

Prognosis
- Acetazolamide therapy and dietary changes control clinical signs in most affected horses.
- Recurrent episodes are reported in some individuals that initially respond to treatment.
- Sudden death is occasionally reported.
- Discourage breeding of horses with positive genetic test results for the disease, even those horses with no clinical signs.

Tetanus

Tetanus is caused by an exotoxin produced by *Clostridium tetani* that blocks the release of inhibitory neurotransmitters and results in spasticity of skeletal muscles.

Signalment
- Any unvaccinated horse is susceptible.
- Clostridial organisms usually are introduced through a soft-tissue or hoof wound.

Clinical Signs
- Initial signs are colic and vague stiffness.
- Trembling, spasm, and paralysis of voluntary muscles. Masseter muscle is commonly affected.
- Protrusion of the third eyelid, especially when menaced.
- Eyelid retraction, flared nostrils, and erect ear carriage.
- Sawhorse stance, stiff spastic gait, may progress to recumbency.
- Inability to open jaw, difficulty swallowing, aspiration pneumonia.

- Raised tailhead.
- All of these signs are exacerbated by activity or excitement. Stimulation of a horse that has tetanus may precipitate panic, recumbency, and a long-bone fracture or other secondary trauma.

Diagnosis
- Clinical signs in an unvaccinated horse.
- There are no diagnostic blood tests.
- Anaerobic culture of *C. tetani* from the primary wound may be attempted.

Treatment
- Provide a quiet environment with good footing and without barriers.
- Pad stall walls to reduce risk of injury.
- Minimize stimulation: Darken stall and stuff cotton in the ears.
- Provide deep bedding with straw, especially if the patient is recumbent.
- Provide muscle relaxation and tranquilization.
  - Acepromazine, 0.05 mg/kg IM or IV q6h. Increasing doses or shorter intervals may be required with time. Or use phenobarbital, 6-12 mg/kg slowly IV, followed by oral phenobarbital, 6-12 mg/kg q12h. Or use haloperidol, 0.01 mg/kg once every 7 days IM, as a long-acting tranquilizer.
  - Remove the source of infection.
  - Debride the wound, do not suture.
  - Infiltrate wound with procaine penicillin.
  - Administer potassium penicillin, 22,000 IU/kg IV q6h for a minimum of 7 days.
- Neutralize unbound toxin.
  - 100-200 U/kg tetanus antitoxin, IV or IM, should bind any residual circulating toxin but poorly crosses the blood-brain barrier to neutralize toxin in the CNS.
  - Intrathecal administration of antitoxin: Remove 50 ml of CSF by means of atlanto-occipital aspiration (30 ml in a foal), replace with an equal volume of tetanus antitoxin. Anesthetize with xylazine and ketamine for the CSF collection.
- Maintain hydration and nutritional status.
  - Place food and water off the ground in an easily accessible place.
  - Intravenous administration of fluids may be necessary to maintain hydration.
  - Oral fluids and gruel may be administered through a small bore nasogastric tube in some cases. Intubation may be difficult because of muscle spasms and pharyngeal paralysis. *Feed or intubate at peak tranquilization periods to reduce stress.* Leave tube in place.
- Establish active antitoxin immunity.
- Amount of toxin necessary to produce disease often is insufficient to stimulate an immune response. Vaccinate with tetanus toxoid in a separate site from the antitoxin administration.

Prognosis
- Fair to poor
- Contingent on the severity of clinical signs and the attitude of the affected horse
- Clinical signs may persist for weeks
- Secondary complications include aspiration pneumonia, myopathy, and long-bone or pelvic fracture

NEURO

- If the affected horse cannot stand, the prognosis is grave; if the horse is ambulatory after 5 days of clinical signs, the prognosis is fair to good

Myopathy, Myositis

Trembling can occur with myositis or myopathy. These conditions include the following:

NON–SELENIUM-DEFICIENT TYING-UP SYNDROMES

- Rule out glycogen storage disease if the patient is a draft horse, Warmblood or Quarter Horse (see Polysaccharide Storage Myopathy on the next page), and rule out other specific causes of myopathy.

EXERTIONAL MYOPATHY

- If the myopathy is believed to be caused by exertion and is unrelated to the specific causes listed, treatment includes:
  - Fluids to correct dehydration and electrolyte abnormalities. Remember, most horses with mild to moderate myopathy and exhausted horses are likely to be hypochloremic and alkalotic. Therefore, 0.9% NaCl with 20-40 mEq KCl/L often is the preferred fluid. Fluid diuresis may prevent myoglobinuric nephropathy. Hypertonic saline solution also can be used. In severe cases (myopathy, exhaustion, or both) acidosis may be present.
- Analgesic: phenylbutazone 2.2 mg/kg IV q12h for 1-2 days.
- Acepromazine, 0.02 mg/kg IV or IM q6h after correction of fluid deficits.
- Hot packs for affected muscles.
- Methocarbamol 10-30 mg/kg PO or IV q 24h.

COMPARTMENTALIZATION SYNDROME

- Associated with ischemia (localized myositis from trauma). Treatment is similar to the preceding, but if the disease is progressive and severe swelling occurs in areas of important nerves such as the radial nerve, perform fasciotomy to relieve the pressure.

SELENIUM-DEFICIENT TYING-UP

- Consider this syndrome in certain areas of the United States (e.g., northeast and north central) and Canada, especially (but not always) if the individual is poorly fed. May affect limb muscles or *masseter muscles.*
- Diagnosis and treatment (see below).

WHITE MUSCLE DISEASE

- White muscle disease (selenium-deficient myopathy) most commonly occurs in foals from birth to 60 days of age. It is most common in the northeast and northwest United States. If the cardiac muscle is affected, death may occur without clinical signs. With skeletal muscle involvement, dyspnea, dysphagia, recumbency, and stiff gait are typical. Hyponatremia, hypochloremia, hyperkalemia, and marked elevations in muscle enzyme levels are standard biochemical abnormalities.
- Diagnosis: Clinical signs, increased serum muscle enzyme activity, serum selenium <10 mg/dl.

NOTE: If selenium has already been administered and confirmation of the diagnosis is needed, blood can be collected in an anticoagulant tube and submitted to Michigan State Diagnostic Laboratory for measurement for glutathione peroxidase activity. After selenium administration, several days are required before the selenium molecule is incorporated into the red blood cell glutathione peroxidase. Repeated intramuscular injections of selenium, 0.06 mg/kg IM, may be needed for treatment, along with supportive treatments employed for exertional myopathy.

PURPURA HEMORRHAGICA MYOSITIS
- Clinical findings and diagnosis
- History of exposure to *S. equi*
- High streptococcus M protein antibody
- Acute trembling, stiffness, or recumbency
- Elevated levels of muscle enzymes (often marked)
- May have other signs of purpura
- Edema and severe colic may occur!
- Treatment: See treatment of purpura hemorrhagica (see p. 513)

PARASITIC MYOSITIS (*SARCOCYSTIS FAYERI*)
- Rare
- Trembling and stiffness
- Elevated muscle enzymes. Confirm with muscle biopsy

Treatment
- Phenylbutazone, 2.2 mg/kg PO q12-24h
- Trimethoprim-sulfamethoxazole, 20 mg/kg PO q12h
- Pyrimethamine, 2.0 mg/kg PO as a loading dose, then 1.0 mg/kg PO q24h

POLYSACCHARIDE STORAGE MYOPATHY
- May progress to recumbency and death.
- A glycogen storage disease.
- Common in draft horses and Quarter Horses. Less common in Warmbloods.
- Trembling and stiffness that can progress to recumbency.
- Serum selenium concentration may be normal or abnormal (often abnormal in draft horses).
- No response to treatment with selenium.
- Recurrent episodes and persistent elevation in muscle enzymes may be reported.

Diagnosis
Muscle biopsy sample of semimembranous or semitendinosus muscle just below the tuber ischii is placed on a tongue depressor and then immersed in formalin or placed in a *slightly* damp 4 × 4 sponge for overnight (chilled) shipment to Cornell University or the University of Minnesota, respectively. The muscle enzyme activity in the serum is high in severely affected cases but *may* not be dramatically elevated because this is not a myositis.

Treatment
MILD TO MODERATE CASES
- 2 cups (480 ml) vegetable oil PO q24h (in feed or through a nasogastric tube)

SEVERELY RECUMBENT CASES
- 2 cups (480 ml) vegetable oil PO.
- Intralipid, 0.2 g/kg IV administered slowly over 1-2 hours.
- Rice bran, 1-5 pounds (0.45-2.25 kg) per day is an excellent source of fat. Most companies have a high-fat feed.
- Withhold carbohydrates!
- Maintain daily routine with respect to exercise!
- Supportive care including slinging.

Other Causes of Trembling

There are many other causes of acute trembling besides those listed, including trauma, hypothermia, cachexia, and drug reactions.

WHITE SNAKE ROOT POISONING
- Signs of weakness leading to recumbency in horses eating white snake root. Increased frequency of urination is commonly seen (see Chapter 53, p. 709).

ACUTE LEAD POISONING
- Trembling, depression, ataxia (see Chapter 53, p. 706). *Laryngeal paralysis may or may not be present with acute lead poisoning!*
- Diagnosis: Exposure, clinical signs, and blood lead concentration >0.3 ppm.
- Treatment: Calcium disodium EDTA, 110 mg/kg in 5% dextrose, administered IV q24h for 2 days. Further interval treatment may be needed.

EAR TICK (*OTOBIUS MEGNINI*) INFESTATION
- Muscle spasms, sweating, prolapse of the third eyelid, and coliclike signs have been associated with ear tick infestation. On percussion, some muscles have prolonged and severe contracture. Muscle enzyme levels are generally mildly to moderately increased. The spinose ear tick can be found in the ear of affected horses. Signs resolve within 24-96 hours after treatment of the ticks with the pyrethrin piperonyl butoxide.

AORTOILIAC THROMBOSIS (SADDLE THROMBUS)
- Although most cases are chronic and intermittent, a few individuals may have acute onset of trembling of the rear limbs, violent shaking of the limbs, and weakness in the hindlimbs. The diagnosis is established with transrectal ultrasonography (7.5-linear-MHz probe). Palpation of limbs for decreased pulse yields inconsistent findings.
- Treatment: Pentoxifylline, 8.4 mg/kg PO q12h, can be attempted but is not proved; aspirin 15 mg/kg PO every other day. In the treatment of severely affected patients, surgical removal of the thrombus should be attempted by way of the femoral artery using a Fogarty Venous Thrombectomy Catheter.*

---

*6F Fogarty Venous Thrombectomy Catheter. Edwards Lifesciences, 1 Edward Way Irvine, CA 92614; (800) 424-3278. Catalog #320806F.

PERIPHERAL NEUROPATHY OR GRAY-MATTER LESIONS

- Any peripheral neuropathy caused by trauma or inflammation can cause trembling in a leg. Focal gray matter lesions, such as EPM, also can cause shaking in one leg or more.

CHANGE IN MENTATION

A change in the demeanor or behavior of a horse may be the first neurologic clinical sign recognized by an owner and suggests cerebral dysfunction. Erratic behavior or depression combined with ataxia or apparent blindness can be a sign of a bacterial, viral, or metabolic disease that affects the CNS.

Hepatic Encephalopathy

Hepatic encephalopathy is perhaps the most common cause of acute cerebral signs in adults (see Chapter 37, p. 317).

Primary Hyperammonemia

A sporadic cause of acute behavior change, blindness, circling, and seizure activity in an adult horse. Colic usually precedes the CNS signs by 12-24 hours, and diarrhea often occurs during recovery of CNS signs.

Diagnosis

- History of gastrointestinal signs immediately before CNS signs.
- Hyperglycemia
- Metabolic acidosis
- Hyperammonemia >150 µmol/L
- Normal liver enzyme values
- Normal hepatic function

Treatment

- Sedation with phenobarbital, 3-12 mg/kg IV
- Neomycin 0.02 g/kg PO q6h
- Normosol-R or Plasmalyte-A intravenously
- No sodium bicarbonate!
- Magnesium sulfate 1 g/kg PO

Prognosis

- Approximately 50% of patients recover in 2-3 days with supportive therapy.

Mycotoxic Encephalopathy

Known by many pseudonyms (moldy corn poisoning, blind staggers, leukoencephalitis, foraging disease), mycotoxic encephalopathy is caused by a toxin elaborated by the mold *Fusarium*, a common contaminant of corn. The clinical syndrome is highly variable and depends on the dose of toxin ingested, species of *Fusarium*, duration of the exposure, and individual susceptibility.

NEURO

History

- Highest occurrence in late fall to early spring; incidence varies from year to year.
- Contaminated corn is part of the diet for at least 2 weeks.
- Multiple horses on the farm are often affected.
- Death occurs within 1-3 days of onset of clinical signs.

Clinical Signs

NEUROLOGIC SYNDROME

- Afebrile
- Behavioral changes (depression to mania)
- Ataxia and weakness, may proceed to recumbency
- Blindness
- Asymmetric cranial nerve deficits
- Seizures
- Coma and death

No consistent pattern of neurologic signs is typical because of the variability of the CNS lesion produced.

HEPATOTOXIC SYNDROME (see Chapter 37, p. 315)

- Severe icterus
- Swelling of the muzzle and nose
- Difficulty in breathing
- Coma and death
- Associated with high dose of the toxin

Diagnosis

- History of feeding corn contaminated with *Fusarium* and multiple individuals with sudden onset of bizarre neurologic signs.
- Laboratory data usually are nonspecific: Stress leukogram and normal to elevated liver enzyme values.
- Results of CSF analysis may be normal or show neutrophilic pleocytosis with increased protein and xanthochromia.
- Postmortem finding of focal areas of liquefaction necrosis of cerebral white matter confirms the diagnosis.
- Feed can be quantitatively analyzed for *Fusarium*.
- Feed may look grossly normal.

Differential Diagnosis

- Hepatic encephalopathy
- Viral encephalopathy
- Trauma
- Equine protozoal myeloencephalopathy
- Cerebral abscess
- Rabies
- Space-occupying mass
- Botulism
- Herpes myelitis

Treatment

- Remove the source of the corn.

- DMSO, 1 g/kg IV as a 10% solution in saline solution, or any isotonic fluid once a day for 5 days.
- Maintain hydration with intravenous fluids.
- Corticosteroids, dexamethasone 0.1-0.2 mg/kg IV once per day for 1-2 days.
- Broad-spectrum antibiotic therapy.
- Thiamine, 10 mg/kg in IV fluids q12h.
- Good nursing care.

Prognosis
- Poor because of extensive CNS damage; few survive

Viral Encephalitis
When any horse has an acute onset of behavior change and fever, viral encephalitis should be on the differential diagnosis list.

➤ The absence of fever does not exclude viral encephalitis.

ALPHAVIRUSES
The alphavirus subcategory of the family Togaviridae is the classification of Eastern (EEE), Western (WEE), and Venezuelan (VEE) equine encephalitis. These diseases, clinically indistinguishable, manifest as an acute onset of fever and depression followed by diffuse CNS signs. Sporadic outbreaks may occur in the eastern, Gulf Coast, and north central United States after excessive seasonal rainfall.

Signalment
- Any age or breed and either sex. Not common among foals younger than 3 months of age.
- Disease occurs most commonly at the height of the vector (mosquito and tick) season. In the southeastern United States, this can be year round.
- EEE and WEE: Usually one horse in a herd.
- VEE: Morbidity as high as 50%. The last U.S. outbreak of VEE occurred in 1971.

Clinical Signs
- High fever
- Malaise
- Colic
- Anorexia

Neurologic Signs
- Depression: May progress to somnolence
- Dementia: Compulsive walking, excitability, aggressiveness
- Head pressing
- Hyperesthesia
- Ataxia
- Blindness
- Circling
- Seizures
- Head tilt
- Recumbency
- Paralysis of pharynx, larynx, and tongue

NEURO

- Irregular breathing
- Cardiac arrhythmias

Diagnosis
- Fourfold increase in serum titer over 2-3 weeks.
- PCR analysis of brain tissue.
- CSF analysis: Leukocytosis, elevated total protein value, xanthochromia. Most dramatic CSF changes with EEE, less dramatic with WEE and VEE. May be able to isolate virus from the CSF. Early and mild cases have mononuclear pleocytosis; more severe cases have an equal number of neutrophils.
- Histopathologic examination of the brain and spinal cord: No gross lesions characteristic of the disease. Best microscopic lesions in the cerebral cortex, thalamus, and hypothalamus. Submit fresh or frozen brain specimen for virus isolation.

CAUTION: Sufficient viral particles for human infection may be present in the CNS, especially with VEE. Use caution at postmortem examination. Do not use power tools.

Treatment
- No specific treatment is effective.
- DMSO, 1 g/kg IV, as a 10% solution in saline or lactated Ringer's solution once per day for 5 days.
- Dexamethasone, 0.1-0.2 mg/kg IV, once or twice per day for 1-2 days.
- Nonsteroidal antiinflammatory drug (NSAID): Phenylbutazone, 2.2 mg/kg IV or PO q12h or flunixin meglumine, 0.25-0.5 mg/kg IV or PO q12h.
- Anticonvulsant: Diazepam, 0.1-0.4 mg/kg IV for a 450-kg adult, phenobarbital, 3-12 mg/kg IV or to effect.
- Monitor hydration.
- Provide a laxative diet.
- Supply nutrients.
- Protect from self-induced trauma.

Prognosis
- EEE: 75%-100% mortality; complete recovery is unusual. Many may be recumbent for 3-4 days before dying.
- WEE: 20%-50% mortality; persistent neurologic deficits common.
- VEE: 40%-80% mortality; viremia may be present for 3 weeks after recovery. Keep the patient isolated.

Report cases of EEE, WEE, or VEE to public health officials. The affected horse is not a source of WEE and EEE for human infection, whereas VEE can be readily transmitted to humans directly or by mosquitoes.

Rabies

Because rabies becomes endemic throughout certain areas of the United States, serious consideration of this disease in cases with change in mentation, acute ataxia, and recumbency is imperative.

The antemortem diagnosis of rabies is difficult because of the wide spectrum of clinical signs and the lack of an accurate antemortem diagnostic test. Horses usually are infected by the bite of a rabid wild animal, but physical evidence of such a wound often is not found. The incubation period can vary from 2 weeks to several months, but once clinical signs develop, a short course (average, 3-5 days) of progressive neurologic deterioration usually ends in death.

Signalment
- No sex, breed, or age predilection.
- Young horses, being more curious, may be at increased risk.
- Although vaccination is thought to be highly protective, consideration of rabies in any horse with an acute onset of neurologic signs is advised regardless of vaccination status!

Clinical Signs
- Highly variable (Box 40–1).
- Individuals with rabies do not intentionally eat or drink.

Rapid progression of clinical signs is a feature of equine rabies. Most patients are terminally recumbent within 3-5 days after the onset of clinical signs, although one patient is reported to have remained ambulatory for 9 days after the onset of clinical signs.

Diagnosis
- Complete blood count and serum biochemical testing provides little useful information. Severe hyperglycemia may occur as the result of stress.
- CSF: May be normal or of low cellularity, the predominant cell type being lymphocytes. Total protein level in the CSF may be normal or elevated.
- No accurate antemortem test is available.

CAUTION: Handle with care any body fluid from a patient with suspected rabies. *Label specimens properly and inform laboratory personnel.*

Precautions in Dealing with a Horse with Suspected Rabies
- Minimize human exposure, especially individuals with open wounds.
- Wear gloves.

BOX 40-1. Clinical Signs of Rabies

COMMON	LESS COMMON
Recumbency	Head tilt
Ataxia and paresis	Circling
Hyperesthesia	Teeth grinding
Muscle tremor	Blindness
Lameness	Pharyngeal paralysis
Anorexia	Tenesmus
Loss of tail and anal tone	Drooling
Loss of hindlimb sensation	Roaring
Fever	Sweating
Colic	Paddling while recumbent
Depression	Abnormal vocalizations
Convulsions	
Paraphimosis	
Aggressiveness	

NEURO

- Wash hands thoroughly; the virus is relatively fragile and is killed by most detergents.
- Keep a list of all persons who come in contact with the horse believed to have rabies.

Treatment

Treatment may not be advisable if the findings are highly suggestive of rabies. Postmortem diagnosis is imperative because of zoonotic implications. Vaccination of horses after a bite has occurred may not be effective. Horses that have been vaccinated and later bitten by a rabid animal should be vaccinated again two to three times, 4 to 7 days apart, and quarantined for 6 months. Unvaccinated horses bitten by an animal that is confirmed to be rabid should be euthanized or quarantined for at least 6 months.

Submission of Rabies Material to State Diagnostic Laboratory

- Brainstem and cerebellum are the brain samples of choice. Do not submit the entire head.
- Appropriate samples can be obtained with minimal contact through the foramen magnum. Wear latex gloves, surgical mask, and glasses during sample collection.
- Remove the head, and using a hacksaw, remove the back of the calvaria. *Do not* use power saws (including Stryker saws), which can aerosolize the virus.
- Refrigerate specimens before shipment. Do *not* fix tissues with chemical preservatives.
- Place specimens in at least two separately sealed plastic bags with gel-type cold packs in a Styrofoam-insulated cardboard box.
- Test results are generally reported within 24-48 hours of laboratory receipt.
- Disinfect all instruments and surfaces with a 10% solution of household bleach in water.
- Veterinarians are encouraged to undergo rabies prophylaxis. Human serum for assessing current titer status may be submitted to Kansas State University, (913) 532-5660. Titer assessment is recommended before booster vaccination. *With proper precautions*, the risk that a human acquires rabies from a large animal is low. In the United States there have been no reported cases of human rabies transmitted from large animals.

West Nile Virus

Epidemiology

- A mosquito-borne flavivirus that affects horses in many areas of the United States (so far) from late summer into fall. Horses in the eastern parts of all states from Massachusetts to Florida have been affected. In Florida, the Panhandle area has had a large number of occurrences. Sporadic cases have been reported in central Pennsylvania, Kentucky, and Louisiana. West Nile infections are reported in the West!

Clinical Signs

- Ataxia: More severe in the rear legs and may progress to recumbency within 2-5 days

- Paresis
- Fever: Present in some but not all patients at examination
- Blindness (only occasionally)
- Fasciculation of facial and neck muscles!
- Stupor: Not always pronounced
- Hyperesthesia
- Hyperexcitability
- After acute signs, a late recrudescence may occur 2-3 days later

Diagnosis
- Geographic location, season of the year, clinical signs.
- Serology: Immunoglobulin M (IgM) capture enzyme-linked immunosorbent assay; many horses in endemic areas may be seropositive without clinical signs.
- CSF: Lymphocytic pleocytosis.
- Virus isolation or PCR analysis of brain tissue from euthanized horse.

Treatment
- Supportive: NSAIDS, maintain on good footing and safe environment.
- For recumbent horses, treatment may include dexamethasone (0.1 mg/kg IV q24) and/or mannitol (0.5-2.0 mg/kg IV).

Prognosis
- Variable, but apparent complete recovery in approximately 60% of cases in the United States.
- Affected horses either become rapidly recumbent or stabilize in 72-96 hours.

Prevention
- *A vaccine* is available;* mosquito control.

Other Viruses

In Canada and the western United States, Bunyavirus encephalitis has been described. Recovery is possible. Other unidentified or identified (Cache Valley, snowshoe hare, St. Louis) viruses may also sporadically produce encephalitis with recovery. Horses with fever, lymphocytic pleocytosis in the CSF and encephalitic signs can be tested (serologically) for these viruses if serum is sent to the Centers for Disease Control and Prevention.

Verminous Encephalitis

Verminous encephalitis can cause acute ataxia and change in mentation. *Halicephalobus (Micronema) deletrix* (gingivalis) is the most common nonsarcocystis parasite causing verminous encephalitis.

Clinical Signs
- *Halicephalobus* encephalitis most often results in signs resembling cerebellar or vestibular ataxia (hypermetria, head tremors). Seizures may occur.
- Hematuria and signs of renal disease may be present along with the ataxia.

---

*Although not approved for pregnant mares, adverse effects in pregnant mares have not been reported.

- Optic neuritis, retinitis, or osteomyelitis (head) may be found.

Diagnosis
- It is unlikely that a confirmatory diagnosis can be made ante mortem unless there is a lesion elsewhere in the body where a biopsy can be performed, such as kidney or bone.
- Urine should be examined for the presence of the parasite.
- CSF has pleocytosis, which suggests the presence of mixed (lymphocytes, polymorphonuclear leukocytes) inflammatory disease, but this could also be seen with EPM.

Treatment
- May be attempted with fenbendazole, 10 mg/kg PO q24h for 5 days, and diethylcarbamazine 50 mg/kg after meals daily along with corticosteroids: dexamethasone, 0.04-0.16 mg/kg IV q24h on days 1 and 2, with tapering dosage thereafter.
- There are no known reports of successful treatment of horses with CNS infection.
- Use of ivermectin, 0.22 mg/kg PO in a single dose, is controversial and may exacerbate neurologic signs.

Verminous encephalitis caused by *Strongylus vulgaris* is rare. Profound neurologic disease results from the migration of larvae within the brain or thrombosis of multiple small arteries to the brain. The thrombosis is caused by embolism of pieces of the verminous plaque, which may originate at the bifurcation of the brachycephalic trunk. The lesion is *asymmetric*, and in the case of thromboembolism, results in clinical signs that most closely resemble an intracarotid injection (see p. 429) or acute, severe EPM (see p. 390). In one report, more than one horse on a farm was affected. Rare episodes of CNS migration by the cattle bot fly *Hypoderma bovis* or *Hypoderma lineatum* and by *Setaria* organisms, filarial nematodes common in the peritoneal cavity, have been reported in horses. *Parelaphostrongyles tenius* may migrate along the dorsal grey column in young horses causing acute loss of sensation to one side of the neck and concavity on the same side. Corticosteroids and fenbendazole can be used as treatment, but efficacy is unproved. The CSF in affected horses may be normal.

Cerebral Abscess
Signalment
- Usually a young foal, 3 months of age or older
- Often a history of strangles, pneumonia, or head trauma a few weeks before the onset of signs

Clinical Signs
- Acute onset, may be febrile
- Depression progressing to stupor
- Often episodes of violent behavior, head pressing, or circling
- Hindlimb ataxia, falling, acute recumbency
- Unilateral or bilateral blindness
- Often multiple cranial nerves affected
- Head tilt and signs of neck pain common

- Seizures and coma
- Signs frequently wax and wane; affected horses may improve with treatment and then suddenly worsen despite treatment

Etiology

- *S. equi* is the organism most frequently reported; *S. zooepidemicus* or *R. equi* rarely
- Access to CNS through hematogenous spread from suppurative lesion (bastard strangles), *or* extension of suppuration from sinus, nasal cavity, guttural pouch, middle ear, *or* direct seeding of a variety of organisms from penetrating wound or fracture!

Diagnosis

- History
- Clinical signs
- CSF sample (elevated protein value and nucleated cells, culture of spinal fluid)
- Brain scan (CT) ideal

Differential Diagnosis

- Neoplasia, rare even in adults
- Intracranial hematoma
- Cholesterol granuloma: Middle-aged overweight adult
- EPM
- Rabies
- Hepatic encephalopathy
- Vestibular disease
- Encephalitis
- Idiopathic seizure syndrome in Arabian foals

Treatment

- Potassium penicillin, 22,000 IU/kg IV q6h
- Trimethoprim-sulfamethoxazole, 20 mg/kg PO q12h
- DMSO, 1 g/kg IV as a 10% solution in saline solution or any isotonic fluid
- Flunixin meglumine, 0.5 mg/kg IV q12h
- Dexamethasone, 0.1-0.2 mg/kg IV, single dose, if necessary to reduce cerebral edema
- Phenobarbital to effect, 3-12 mg/kg IV as needed to control seizures
- Surgical drainage

Prognosis

- Poor to grave.

Fungal Meningitis

Cryptococcus is the most common fungal infection of the CNS. Affected horses may have predominantly cerebral or spinal cord signs. Fever usually is present. The CSF has marked neutrophilic pleocytosis (generally greater than the clinical signs would indicate). The organism can be identified on *close* inspection of the CSF.

Treatment
- Itraconazole, 2.6 mg/kg PO q12h

Equine Self-Mutilation Syndrome

Equine self-mutilation syndrome is a self-mutilating behavior, described as biting at the flank area, tail, or lateral thoracic wall. It often is precipitated by stress (anticipation of eating or interaction with others) and is equated with Tourette's syndrome in humans. Males are seven times more likely than females to develop the condition, which most often starts during the first 2 years of life. Heritable factors, inactivity or confinement, and stimulation of endogenous opioids may be involved in the development of the behavior. Castration, change in diet, stabling changes, and the use of opioid antagonists (nalmefene) are used to manage the behavior with partial success. Imipramine, a tricyclic antidepressant drug, 1 mg/kg PO q12h, has been used successfully.

SUDDEN COLLAPSE

Examining a horse that has suddenly collapsed is an intimidating diagnostic and therapeutic challenge. Metabolic, respiratory, cardiovascular, and orthopedic causes of sudden collapse must be considered, as should the neurologic differential diagnosis list. The prognosis for future use often is the determining factor in the owner's decision to treat. An accurate anatomic diagnosis is the first, and occasionally the most difficult, step. *Always consider the likelihood of rabies* (see p. 414 in this chapter).

Cranial Trauma

Cerebral edema with hemorrhage is the most harmful pathology of cranial trauma and is the primary lesion to treat. Clinical signs are most severe within 12 hours, but uncontrolled cerebral edema can result in progression of intracranial signs.

Causes
- Collisions
- Penetrating wounds
- Falls: Over a jump; rearing and falling over backward
- Injury
  - Direct injury to neural parenchyma radiating from the point of impact
  - Indirect injury by displacement of basioccipital and basisphenoid bones into the overlying brainstem

Clinical Examination
- Obtain an accurate history
- Perform as complete a physical examination as possible. Look for hemorrhage or leakage of CSF from wounds, ears, and nose; respiratory distress (abnormal respiratory patterns); evidence of laryngeal injury.
- *Perform an ophthalmic examination (fixed, dilated pupils are a poor prognostic finding).* Retinal detachments may occur after head trauma, although optic nerve injury is more common.
- Stabilize the medical condition.

□ Maintain a patent airway. It is very important that the *PaCO$_2$ be maintained at a low-normal value* because elevations in PaCO$_2$ increase cerebral blood flow and edema. Hyperventilate if necessary to decrease PaCO$_2$ to low-normal range.

□ Intubate if necessary; supply oxygen.

□ Control blood loss.

Neurologic Examination

- Assess mentation (alert, depression, stupor, coma).
- Assess visual response (menace); cortical injury often results in contralateral blindness.
- Cranial nerve examination, especially pupil size, symmetry, pupillary light response, menace response (a severely depressed horse may not menace, even though it is visual), presence of nystagmus, strabismus, or dysphagia.
- Assess caudal brainstem function: Respiratory pattern, swallowing, tongue tone, and vestibular signs.
- Voluntary limb movement and quality of the gait. Evaluate for concurrent spinal cord or orthopedic injury.
- Pain perception
- Noxious perception by placing finger in the patient's nose; contralateral cortical response
- Abnormal body position or head tilt
- Keep an accurate written record of all observations; serial reassessment is crucial to evaluate progress and modify therapy.
- The presence of changes in pupil size from normal to miotic to dilated and fixed is a grave prognostic finding!

Ancillary Procedures

- If feasible, the following may prove valuable:
  □ Skull radiography
  □ CT, MRI
  □ CSF aspiration and analysis. If the fluid is grossly contaminated with blood, think fracture and a grave prognosis. Cisternocentesis (aspirate) and removal of a small volume of fluid should be done with *caution* because removal of excessive fluid from a patient with cerebral edema may result in tentorial herniation. If there is an opportunity (gas anesthesia) to provide brief hyperventilation (PaCO$_2$ <35 mm Hg) before CSF collection, this may decrease the risk of herniation. CSF may be normal even with severe hemorrhage in the forebrain.
  □ Upper airway and guttural pouch endoscopy: Bleeding may occur with fracture of basioccipital bones and ruptured capitis muscle.

Treatment

- Methylprednisolone, 5-30 mg/kg, may be of benefit if administered within the first hour of the injury. It is expensive and should not be administered if the injury occurred more than 1 hr before.
- Dexamethasone, 0.1-0.2 mg/kg IV q6-8h for the first 24 hours after injury, then q24h for 2-3 days (of questionable value for cerebral injury).
- DMSO, 1 g/kg IV, as a 10%-20% solution in saline or other polyionic fluid q12-24h for 5 days

NEURO

- Mannitol,* 0.5-2 g/kg IV as a 20% mixture, repeated once or twice at 4-8-hour intervals.
- Hypertonic saline solution: Can increase cerebral perfusion and decrease brain water but a rebound phenomenon can occur. Isotonic fluids should be administered at a maintenance rate to support normal cerebral perfusion.
- Furosemide, 1 mg/kg IV q12h for 1-2 days: Potent diuretic; monitor for electrolyte imbalances and *maintain hydration*, especially when combined with mannitol.
  - □ *Keep the head elevated at 30 degrees* if possible and *do not occlude the jugular veins.*
- Assess for signs of shock and begin treatment.
- Monitor systemic blood pressure.
- Broad-spectrum antibiotics, especially if palpable fracture or evidence of hemorrhage is present!
- Thyrotropin-releasing hormone: 1 mg IV q12h.
- Vitamin E, 20,000 units PO q24h for an adult.
- Calcium channel blockers.
- Magnesium sulfate, 4 ml of 50% $MgSO_4$ added to each liter of fluids.
- Fracture repair.
- Oxygen therapy if there is hypoventilation or pulmonary disease.
- Pentoxifylline, 8.4 mg/kg PO or IV q2h.
- *Do not administer the following:*
  - □ Glucose unless the patient is confirmed hypoglycemic.
  - □ Calcium unless the patient is confirmed hypocalcemic (low ionized calcium).
- Do not try to warm the patient too fast if hypothermia present!
- If sedation is necessary (try to assess neurologic status first):
  - □ Xylazine 0.1-0.2 mg/kg IV, may *transiently exacerbate* intracranial hemorrhage because of brief hypertensive effects. If the individual is standing, may cause *lowering of the head and worsening of the cerebral edema.*
  - □ Diazepam, 0.1-0.2 mg/kg (5-15 mg) IV for foals.
  - □ Phenobarbital to effect, 3-12 mg/kg IV. May have a protective effect on the brain.
- Protect the patient from further injury by using a helmet. and keeping the horse quiet and confined to a safe stall.
- CT and exploratory craniotomy are available at some centers.

Poor Prognostic Indicators

- Deterioration in vital signs
- Altered respiratory patterns (brainstem injury)
- Slow heart rate, decreasing blood pressure (medullary lesion)
- Unresponsive dilated pupils (midbrain lesion)
- Miotic pupils that become mydriatic (progressive midbrain edema or compression)
- Deterioration of mental status
- Tetraparesis or paraparesis to recumbency
- Progressive loss of cranial nerve function (compression, hypoxia)

---

*Use of mannitol if bleeding in the cranial cavity has not been controlled (i.e., if there is bleeding from the nose or ears or a palpable skull fracture or a grossly bloody CSF sample). This treatment is controversial.

- Opisthotonos (cerebellum, midbrain)
- Fracture of the skull with severe CNS signs
- Intensifying seizures
- Gross hemorrhage into CSF

Basisphenoid and Basioccipital Fractures

Fractures of one or both of these bones are particularly common among horses that flip over backward. Hemorrhage often is seen in both the nose and the ear.

If the displacement is minimal, clinical signs may improve, and the individual recovers or is left with a mild residual head tilt. Minor displacement can be difficult to recognize on standard radiographs. If the displacement is severe, cerebral hemorrhage occurs, and the patient does not recover.

A bloody CSF sample may or may not be obtained with cerebral hemorrhage, depending on the location of the bleed in the brain.

Some horses that flip over backward may rupture the muscles within the guttural pouch and sustain a fracture. Hemorrhage and a mild head tilt occur as a result of the muscle rupture.

Treatment

- As for cerebral injury if localizing signs are present. Head tilt may be the only clinical sign.

Spinal Cord Trauma

Causes

- Falls, including over a jump and rearing over backward
- Collision with a fixed object
- Pathologic fracture secondary to osteomyelitis (diskospondylitis), especially *R. equi* or *S. equi* in 2- to 10-month-old foals

Clinical Signs

- Acute ataxia after an injury or in the case of diskospondylitis, often unassociated with a traumatic event. The ataxia may be posterior ataxia, tetra-ataxia, or hemi ataxia depending on the location of the lesion.
- Progression to recumbency may be rapid.
- Perform a complete physical examination. The horse may be unmanageable because of pain.
- *Remember that spinal cord trauma may or may not be associated with a fracture.*
- Acute concussion from flipping over can cause severe edema or hemorrhage in the cord, which may progress for 24 hours.

Stabilize Medical Condition

- Support ventilation.
- Control hemorrhage.
- Manage shock with intravenous fluids (e.g., hypertonic saline solution and corticosteroids).
- Assess and manage other injuries, such as orthopedic injuries.

Neurologic Assessment of Spinal Cord Trauma

- *If the horse is standing,* evaluate attitude, posture, and gait. Look for ataxia: Are forelimbs involved or only hindlimbs? Examine for palpable cervical abnormalities and neck pain.
- *If the horse is recumbent,* carefully assess whether the horse can become sternal, rise with assistance, or support weight.

Localizing the Lesion

- C1-3 lesion: Horse may only lift head if recumbent
  - Hyperactive reflexes of all four limbs
  - May prefer to lie on one side
- C4-6 lesion: Horse can elevate head and neck if recumbent and is tetraparetic if standing
  - Hyperactive reflexes of all four limbs
- C6-T2 lesion: Tetraparesis or tetraparalysis
  - Most severe signs in front legs
  - Decreased spinal reflexes and tone in forelimbs
  - Normal or hyperactive reflexes and tone in the pelvic limbs
- T3-L3 lesion: Horse may be able to dog sit
  - Thoracic limbs are normal
  - Pelvic limb paresis to paralysis
  - With severe lesion, bladder paralysis and loss of anal and tail tone
  - May have patchy sweating along the trunk from damage to sympathetic nerves
- L4-6 lesion: Horse may dog sit
  - Pelvic limb paresis or paralysis
  - Loss of patellar reflex
- Sacral fracture: Bladder paralysis with severe lesion
  - Possible pelvic limb gait deficit
  - Pain on rectal palpation and manipulation of the tail
  - Fecal retention and decreased anal and tail tone may be evident
  - Hyperesthesia of perineum, anus, and tail may be present
- Schiff-Sherrington syndrome
  - Rarely occurs in horses
- Horner syndrome
  - May result from a severe cervical spinal cord lesion or a T1-3 lesion involving sympathetic nerves. Signs are ipsilateral facial, neck, or truncal sweating; miosis; ptosis; and third eyelid prominence to the side of the lesion

Diagnosis

- Radiographs
- Obvious blood in CSF indicates a poor prognosis.
- Myelogram
- CT: Most CT machines allow placement of only the proximal half of the neck of an adult horse in the cylinder.

Treatment

- Stall rest for ambulatory patients.
- Dexamethasone, 0.2-0.4 mg/kg IV q12h for the first 1-2 days.

- Methylprednisolone sodium succinate, 10-30 mg/kg IV within 1 hour of trauma (expensive).
- DMSO, 1 g/kg IV, as a 10% mixture in saline or lactated Ringer's solution.
- Broad-spectrum antibiotics if patient is recumbent or wounds are present.
- Maintain hydration and nutrition.
- Catheterize and drain bladder if necessary.
- Provide good nursing care.
- Surgery: Decompression or stabilization.
- General anesthesia should be undertaken with caution. Death can result from respiratory failure if the horse has severe cervical spinal cord lesions. Relaxation of muscle tone can cause displacement of fractures and exacerbate neurologic injury.
- A sling may be useful in the care of some recumbent patients that have nondisplaced vertebral fractures impinging on the cord.

Prognosis

Many weanlings or foals that fall over backward recover completely within a few days. Adults seem to be more predisposed to fractures and therefore have a poorer prognosis. *Fracture of the sacrum may result in cauda equina syndrome!* Blindness is a common sequela among horses of all ages that flip over and have acute concussion injury to the head (see Chapter 41, p. 438).

Occipital or Atlantoaxial Injury or Malformations and Fracture of the Cranial Cervical Spine

Fracture of one or more of these bones and subluxation are common problems in *foals.*

Clinical signs

- Tetra-ataxia
- Tetraparesis
- Stiff neck
- Head or neck tilt
- May progress to recumbency

Diagnosis

- Palpation: Crepitus
- Radiographs: Sometimes can be difficult to image the lesion even when a fracture is present
- CT
- Fluoroscopy for those that have only dynamic compression

Treatment

- Fracture without ataxic and cord compression: Stall rest, adapt feeding methods if needed, and antiulcer medication.
- Fracture with ataxia: DMSO 1 g/kg IV q12-24h, flunixin meglumine if pain is so severe the foal does not move, antiulcer medication. If compression seems likely, myelography should be performed and the fracture surgically stabilized or decompressed.

- Fracture or subluxation with head tilt, neck tilt: Neck brace. The brace should be developed to help support the neck and maintain some extension.

Seizures

Seizures may be either generalized or localized (partial seizure). *Generalized seizures* are characterized by tonic-clonic muscle activity, involuntary recumbency, and loss of consciousness. Postictal blindness and depression are common.

Partial seizures have postictal localized clinical signs, such as facial or limb twitching, compulsive circling, self-mutilation of a particular area, and excessive chewing.

The diagnostic goal is to uncover a treatable underlying cause of the seizure, if one exists.

Etiology

- Seizures can be classified as a manifestation of structural brain disease, metabolic disease, or an idiopathic condition.

STRUCTURAL BRAIN DISEASE
- Neoplasia
- Abscess
- Parasitic (EPM; fairly common)
- Embolism due to *Strongylus*
- Encephalitis (viral, bacterial, fungal)
- Meningitis
- Effect of trauma (hemorrhage, edema)
- Intracarotid injection
- Arterial air embolism
- Other masses: Cholesterol granuloma
- Ischemic, hypoxic damage: Mostly newborn foals (see p. 549)
- Do not misinterpret normal, vigorous rapid-eye-movement sleep in foals as seizure activity
- Developmental, such as hydrocephalus, microencephaly
- If the lesion is in a quiet area of the brain, the affected individual is normal in an interictal period. If the lesion is in an active area of the brain, the individual shows signs of depression or a cranial nerve or proprioceptive deficit in the interictal period.

METABOLIC DISEASE
- Hypoglycemia in foals and adults causes depression
- Neonatal maladjustment syndrome (ischemic, hypoxic damage): Foals have seizures, depression, or ataxia (see Chapter 45, p. 561)
- Hepatic encephalopathy: Portosystemic shunt
- Hyperammonemia without liver disease: 4- to 8-month-old Morgans and, infrequently, adults of any breed with colic
- Renal encephalopathy
- Hyperlipemia, hyperlipidemia
- Hyperkalemia (HYPP)
- Hyperthermia

- Kernicterus: Generally foals with neonatal isoerythrolysis with a bilirubin value in excess of 20 mg/dl. When bilirubin approaches this significance, prevention of kernicterus includes plasma exchange or transfusion and small doses of pentobarbital 0.5-1 mg/kg IV q8h
- Intoxication
  - Organophosphates
  - Propylene glycol
  - Mushroom toxicosis
  - Lead
  - Arsenic
  - Strychnine
- Hypocalcemia and hypomagnesemia (see p. 403)
- *Hyponatremia!* Common among foals with severe diarrhea or newborn foals with bilateral hydroureter or inappropriate secretion of antidiuretic hormone

MANAGEMENT OF SEVERE (<120 mEq/L) HYPONATREMIA

- If severe hypotension is present, hypertonic saline solution can be administered until the serum Na^+ concentration is 125 mg/L and further correction is made over several hours with isotonic crystalloids.
- Mannitol can be administered while the serum sodium level is *slowly corrected*. Rapid correction can result in a permanent neurologic disorder.
- Hypernatremia generally causes depression rather than seizure. Sodium concentration should be returned to a normal value slowly. Do not use 5% dextrose alone for hypernatremia.

IDIOPATHIC EPILEPSY OF FOALS

- Onset usually at 3-9 months of age
- Generalized seizures with or without involuntary recumbency
- May be hereditary in Egyptian Arabians
- Responds well to anticonvulsants
- Usually outgrown after 3 months of anticonvulsant therapy

LAVENDER FOAL SYNDROME

- Egyptian Arabians with abnormal hair color (not always lavender) that are born with opisthotonus. Foals continue to nurse, but their condition does not improve, and they are euthanized.

SEIZURES DURING ESTRUS IN MARES (RARE)

- Related to elevated estrogen level
- Occur during estrus only
- Underlying etiologic factor is unknown
- Control with progesterone or ovariectomy

OTHER IDIOPATHIC CAUSES OF SEIZURES

- Primary cerebral vascular disease (stroke) that is not related to an infectious or traumatic cause has been reported.
- On a rare occasion, acute and extensive (rostral) thrombosis of the jugular vein may cause seizures and circling.

Differential Diagnoses of Seizures

- Colic

- Exertional myopathy
- Syncope: Cardiac problems such as severe bradycardia, prolonged Q-T syndrome, obstruction of cerebral blood flow, and so forth. Two types of non-cardiac syncope appear to exist.
  - □ The presence of a mass in the lower thoracic region, such as *Corynebacterium pseudotuberculosis*. Can cause fainting when the horse lowers its head.
  - □ Some individuals faint when the head is rapidly elevated.
  - □ With both conditions recovery is rapid when the head and neck are returned to a normal position.
- Upper airway problems, such as laryngeal obstruction or acute pulmonary edema
- *Narcolepsy, cataplexy:* Primarily in Miniature Horses and Shetland ponies! Some horses respond to imipramine, 1 mg/kg PO q12h.
- Tetanus
- A normal sleeping foal may exhibit eyelid, lip, and limb movements that owners misinterpret as seizure activity.
- HYPP, hypocalcemia, and other tetanic disorders have seizurelike signs.

Diagnosis
- Laboratory tests (immediately after a seizure if possible), glucose, electrolytes, and so forth.
- Establish an accurate description of the seizure.
- Interictal examination: Closely examine cranial nerves.
- CSF sample and analysis.
- Skull radiographs.
- Fundic examination.
- Brain scan (CT or radioisotope imaging).

Treatment
TO STOP A SEIZURE
- Diazepam, 5-20 mg IV for a foal.
- Pentobarbital (administer IV to effect): Approximately 3-10 mg/kg IV for immediate effect.
- Phenobarbital (administer IV to effect): Approximately 6-15 mg/kg. May require 15 minutes for full effect.
- Xylazine, 0.5-1.0 mg/kg IV: Not recommended as the first choice because it reduces cerebral blood flow after transiently increasing intracranial pressure potentially exacerbating seizures. It can be used as a last resort if only a small-volume injection is feasible due to uncontrollable seizure activity.

ANCILLARY TREATMENTS
- DMSO, 1 g/kg IV as a 10% solution in saline or any other isotonic fluid once a day for 3-5 days.
- Flunixin meglumine, 0.5 mg/kg IV q12-24h. Potentially ulcerogenic in foals.
- Antibiotics if a bacterial cause is suspected.
- 10% dextrose IV for hypoglycemia, HYPP, and hepatic encephalopathy.

MAINTENANCE THERAPY
- Phenobarbital, 5-15 mg/kg PO q12h (wide individual variation in dosage). May take 2-3 weeks to adapt to dosage. Reduce the dosage if patient is too sedated. Therapeutic range is considered 10-40 μg/ml but some individuals seemingly respond to lower concentrations.

Prognosis
- Depends on the cause, that is, whether there is a treatable intracranial or extracranial condition. Poor prognostic signs include increasing frequency of seizures, escalating intensity of seizures, and poor response to maintenance therapy.

Drug-Induced Hyperexcitability, Seizure, or Collapse

Caused by inadvertent intracarotid injection, procaine penicillin reaction, or drug-induced hypotension.

Inadvertent Intracarotid Injection
- Onset during injection or a few seconds after injection.
- Acute seizure with recumbency and paddling.
- May be preceded by facial twitching and a wide-eyed appearance.
- Severity of signs depends on volume injected, properties of the drug, and individual sensitivity.

CAUTION: It is very difficult to differentiate arterial and venous (blood) puncture when a 20-gauge needle is used to administer intravenous medication.

- If drug is *water soluble* (xylazine, acepromazine):
  - The affected individual can usually stand in 5-60 minutes.
  - The horse's condition usually is clinically normal in 1 7 days if no secondary injuries occur.
  - The following clinical signs may occur in addition to collapse: Contralateral blindness, contralateral nasal septum hypalgesia, contralateral subtle hemiparesis.
- Treatment may be unnecessary because most recover on their own.

TREATMENT
- DMSO, 1 g/kg IV as a 10% solution in saline
- Dexamethasone, 0.1-0.2 mg/kg IV q12h for the first 24 hours
- Phenobarbital to effect, 3-12 mg/kg IV q12h or q24h
- If drug administered into the carotid is insoluble or oil based (e.g., phenylbutazone, procaine penicillin, trimethoprim-sulfamethoxazole):
  - Acute death often occurs.
  - Recovery is usually unsatisfactory.
  - Seizure is more severe.
  - Persistent stupor or coma may occur.
  - Euthanasia is commonly justified.

Reaction to Intramuscular Procaine Penicillin Injection
- Result of rapid intravenous absorption of procaine penicillin after intramuscular administration.
- Reaction may occur even with correct injection technique.
- Response is most common after several intramuscular injections have been given causing the injection site to be more vascular.
- The "reaction" usually begins after the injection or when it is nearly completed.
- Affected individuals act as if spooked, circle wildly, snort and/or bang around in their stall, and collapse associated with a seizure.

▶ ▪ Keep the patient confined! Often the most serious consequence is self-inflicted injury, which can worsen if the patient is loose.
  ▪ *Acute death can occur if a large volume is absorbed intravenously.*
  ▪ Treatment usually is not possible. If the patient has collapsed and appears in a stupor, administer dexamethasone, 0.1-0.2 mg/kg IV.
  ▪ If treatment can be administered during the seizure, diazepam, 0.2-0.5 mg/kg IV, is the drug of choice. Do not administer phenytoin.

Drug-Induced Hypotension
  ▪ Usually occurs with intravenous administration of acepromazine.
  ▪ May also occur with xylazine or detomidine, especially in draft horses and Warmblood horses.
  ▪ Do not have seizures.
  ▪ Treatment with intravenous fluids containing calcium or administer a hypertonic saline solution.

Drug-Induced Hyperexcitability
  ▪ Butorphanol produces bizarre head tremors in some horses, especially when xylazine is not given several minutes before. No treatment is needed, although naloxone may reverse signs.
  ▪ Abnormally high plasma and CSF concentrations of aminophylline result in bizarre behavior.
  ▪ Treatment: Discontinue aminophylline, give fluid therapy, and control any seizures with xylazine.
  ▪ Lidocaine may cause CNS signs when used in individuals *with cardiac dysfunction*. It seldom causes a problem when treating ileus.

Bizarre Behavior
  ▪ May occur after treatment with the long-acting tranquilizer fluphenazine decanoate (Prolixin)
  ▪ The reaction appears to be idiosyncratic.
  ▪ Treatment: Antihistamines such as diphenhydramine, 0.5-2.0 mg/kg slowly IV or IM, may be beneficial, but pentobarbital, 5-15 mg/kg IV, may be needed to calm the patient. Phenobarbital, 5-15 mg/kg PO, may be needed for several days to keep the patient from injuring itself.
  ▪ Gross overdosing of piperazine can cause recumbency and dementia.
  ▪ Treatment: Supportive.

DYSPHAGIA
Dysphagia (difficulty in swallowing) has many possible causes, such as oral irritation or injury, esophageal obstruction, a brainstem disease, and peripheral *damage to cranial nerves IX and X. Individuals with a cerebral disease and severe depression also may have decreased tongue function; the tongue may remain extended or be slow to return to the mouth.*

Differential Diagnosis
  ▪ Choke (see Chapter 35, p. 202)
  ▪ Presence of an oral foreign body and irritation (see Salivation, p. 201). Look carefully for sticks or injury to and infection of the mouth and pharynx. This

examination may necessitate sedation and use of a mouth speculum or general anesthesia and endoscopy through both the mouth and the nose and manual examination of the mouth and pharynx. Wooden tonguelike infections do occur in horses; if there is no foreign body, these infections respond satisfactorily to penicillin and trimethoprim-sulfamethoxazole

- EPM (see p. 390)
- Guttural pouch disease: Mycotic plaques in the dorsomedial compartment or melanoma of the pouch or flushing a pouch with an irritating substance. Severe empyema can cause mechanical problems
- Surgery on the guttural pouch, such as removal of chondroids, can cause mild dysphagia
- Botulism (see p. 400)
- Yellow star thistle intoxication (see p. 711)
- Viral encephalitis (see p. 413)
- Cerebral abscess (see p. 418) or any cerebral mass or injury
- Pharyngeal swelling or obstruction (see p. 202)
- Severe pharyngitis
- Rabies (see p. 414)
- Organophosphate or lead intoxication
- Grass sickness (exotic) (see p. 776)
- White muscle disease (see p. 408)
- Neonatal maladjustment syndrome or soft palate dysfunction in foals (see p. 561)
- Cleft palate
- Fractured mandible or stylohyoid bone (see p. 351)

Fractured Jaw

- Can cause deliberate head tilt, tongue protrusion, and salivation.
- Diagnosis can be made at physical examination, inability to properly align teeth, and radiographs. Common in horses with narcolepsy!
- Consider surgical treatment if signs are severe.

PERIPHERAL NERVE DISEASE
Suprascapular Nerve (Sweeny)

- Almost invariably caused by trauma:
  - Collision with a fixed object or a kick
  - Ill-fitting driving collar on draft horses
- Other possible causes:
  - Peripheral nerve neoplasm or abscess compressing C6 area or suprascapular nerve
  - EPM: A rule-out
- Atrophy of supraspinatus and infraspinatus muscles that results in an abnormal gait
  - Initial stumbling, dragging of the toe
  - Abduction (popping) of the shoulder on weight bearing
- If neurapraxia (nerve contusion), function returns in days to weeks.
- If the nerve has been severed, regrowth of the nerve along the fibrous framework occurs at a rate of 1 mm/month.

- Most horses return to near normal function with stall rest after 3-18 months
- Surgery can be performed to decompress the nerve if there is no return of function within 3 months
- The *suprascapular nerve* is motor only, so loss of sensation in any part of the limb indicates damage to other nerves
- Electromyelograms can be useful 2-4 weeks after injury to detect involvement of other nerves
- Anesthetic recovery can be physically difficult for any horse with nerve injury, muscle atrophy, or disuse of a limb!
- General treatment (see p. 435 in this chapter).

Musculocutaneous Nerve

- The musculocutaneous nerve originates from spinal cord segment C7-8.
- Musculocutaneous dysfunction causes:
  - Inability to flex the elbow, which results in an abnormally pronounced lifting of the shoulder to advance the limb and
  - Dragging the limb when backing
  - With severe lesions there may be loss of sensation on the dorsomedial aspect of the limb from the carpus to the fetlock

Radial Nerve

- May accompany humeral fractures:
  - Evaluation before surgery may be difficult because there is no reliable autonomous zone for skin sensation. Examine nerve at the time of surgery.
- May be caused by prolonged lateral recumbency:
  - Most likely a combination of ischemic myopathy and ischemic neurapraxia.
- Direct trauma is less likely because of protection by surrounding muscle.
  - If trauma is the known etiologic factor, it is more likely the lesion is contusion or avulsion of the brachial plexus (see below).
- Affected individual is unable to bear weight due to the radial nerve paralysis causing an inability to extend the elbow, carpus, and fetlock. The elbow drops during locomotion, toe drags; pectoral muscles may be able to advance the leg forward half a stride. When the patient is standing, the leg rests on the front of the toe and is able to paw with the limb.
- The limb must be supported with a splint or cast to avoid additional injury and muscle contracture.
- Recovery, in cases of neurapraxia, may take several weeks. If no improvement occurs in 6-8 weeks, the prognosis is poor. Radial nerve damage and separation combined with humeral fracture justify an extremely guarded prognosis.
- Rule outs include septic arthritis of the elbow, fracture, EPM, rupture of the medial collateral ligament of the elbow (with ultrasound), and focal myopathy.
- General treatment (see p. 435 in this chapter).

Brachial Plexus Avulsion

Many cases of shoulder injury with signs of radial paralysis are likely caused by damage to the roots of the brachial plexus.

- Limb carriage is almost identical to that described for radial nerve paralysis.
- Total avulsion results in flaccid paralysis of the entire limb and sensory loss distal to the elbow.
- Injury to the median and ulnar nerves, without radial nerve damage, results in a stiff, goose-stepping gait and hyperextension of the lower limb. *Analgesia may be present over the lateral aspect of the cannon bone and pastern.*
- The condition of patients that have sustained contusions progressively improves over 6-18 months. Physiotherapy (especially swimming) has been useful in returning the individual to function. Return to racing after brachial plexus injury has been reported.
- Neoplasia (nerve sheath) and EPM may have identical clinical signs.
- Prognosis in general is guarded to poor.
- The opposite limb should be bandaged for mechanical support!
- The affected limb should be bandaged or in a light cast in extension to protect the dorsal pastern area and serves to prevent tendon contracture.

Femoral Nerve

- The nerve is well protected from external trauma but may be damaged by:
  - Penetrating wound of the caudal flank.
  - Abscess, neoplasia.
  - Aneurysm in the region of the external iliac arteries.
  - Dystocia (hip or stifle lock) in a newborn foal.
  - Femoral or pelvic fracture (rare).
  - Compression during anesthesia or complicated by myopathy (may be bilateral).
  - EPM.
- The patient is unable to support its weight if femoral paralysis is present. The limb is advanced with difficulty. When the individual attempts to bear weight, the stifle collapses (flexes), and the hock and fetlock flex because of the reciprocal apparatus.
- At rest, all the joints are flexed.
- Atrophy of the quadriceps is evident in 2-4 weeks.
- Patellar reflex is depressed or absent.
- Hypalgesia may be evident over the medial thigh if the saphenous nerve or the femoral nerve dorsal to the iliopsoas muscle is involved.
- Prognosis is guarded regardless of etiologic factor.

Sciatic Nerve

- In foals, sciatic nerve damage is caused by *Salmonella*, *Rhodococcus*, or *Streptococcus* osteomyelitis of the sacrum and pelvis or, more commonly, an intramuscular injection into the caudal aspect of the thigh. Damage to the nerve occurs because of
  - Needle puncture of the nerve
  - Irritation due to drug injection
  - Pressure from a hematoma
  - Scarring around the nerve
- In adults, damage to the sciatic nerve is caused by
  - Pelvic fracture, especially the ischium

NEURO

- □ Coxofemoral luxation
- □ Other injuries (kick), especially the peroneal branch of the sciatic nerve
- □ Postfoaling, such as dystocia with delivery of a large foal
- □ EPM
- Gait and posture
  - □ Patient can support its weight if the limb is positioned under the body
  - □ At rest, the limb is held toward the rear, stifle and hock are extended, fetlock is flexed, and the front of the foot rolls forward
  - □ The toe drags because limb flexion is poor
  - □ Hypalgesia exists over most of the limb, except the medial thigh
  - □ Postfoaling mares with sciatic damage may be unable to stand entirely on the hindlegs

Peroneal Paralysis Versus Tibial Paralysis

Because the *peroneal nerve* is associated with sciatic nerve paralysis, the clinical findings are similar. In peroneal paralysis, hypalgesia may exist over the craniolateral gaskin, hock, and metatarsus. Paresis of the peroneal nerve is common after prolonged recumbency, and recovery generally occurs within 1-3 days; frequently the individual is found standing on the fetlock. Tibial paralysis is less common than is peroneal nerve paralysis. The gait in tibial nerve paralysis resembles stringhalt. Flexion of the hock and extension of the digit are unopposed, so the individual overflexes the limb and raises the foot higher than normal. The hock is flexed (dropped hock), and the fetlock knuckles forward at rest. Sensation may be reduced in the caudal and medial coronet region.

Cranial Gluteal Nerve

Damage to the gluteal nerve results in profound atrophy of the gluteal muscles of the rump. There is little alteration in gait. This condition may be seen with a pelvic fracture or EPM involving the L6 ventral gray column.

Lumbar, Sacral, and Caudal Roots

Most commonly injured as the result of a vertebral fracture. Improvement or recovery may occur with supportive therapy. Radiographs and CT (in foals) may aid in recognizing a fracture or soft-tissue swelling. Surgical decompression may be indicated. Ultrasonography in foals may identify an abscess.

- L6, L7, S1: Damage presents as sciatic nerve paralysis.
- S1, S2, S3: Inability to close the anal sphincter, analgesia of anus and perineum, distention of bladder and rectum.
- Caudal nerves: Analgesia of perineum and penis, but not prepuce, and inability to move tail.

Polyneuritis of the cauda equina may also affect the lumbar, sacral, and caudal roots; however, the onset of signs is insidious, and progression is slow.

Facial Nerve

Facial nerve paresis or paralysis can result from *vestibular syndrome* (see p. 396), *EPM* (see p. 390), trauma, or polyneuritis equi, or it can be idiopathic. If the facial nerve is affected at the nucleus (e.g., EPM) or as it courses through the middle and inner ear, all branches (auricular, palpebral, and buccal) are involved. With more distal injury, only one or two branches are usually affected (e.g., injury to the buccal branch caused by halter pressure during anesthesia).

Injury to Buccal Branch of Facial Nerve: Clinical Signs

- Lower lip droop and decreased nostril diameter on affected side and deviation of nose to the contralateral side

Idiopathic Facial Paralysis

- Idiopathic paralysis often involves both the buccal and the palpebral branches and usually is permanent.
- *With any cause of facial paresis affecting the palpebral branch, monitor closely to prevent corneal ulceration.*
- If no corneal ulcer is present at the first examination, apply ophthalmic ointment (Lacri-Lube) q6h for 1-2 weeks. Most affected individuals eventually compensate for the paresis and do not need further treatment.
- For corneal ulceration, see p. 451.

Management of Peripheral Nerve Disease

- Generally supportive, including bandaging of distal limbs to prevent abrasions of the front of the limb and support wraps on the opposite limb.
- Cold water hydrotherapy over the injured area.
- If an identifiable mass is compressing the nerve (e.g., hematoma, fracture), surgical decompression is indicated.
- NSAID therapy: Flunixin meglumine 1.0 mg/kg once or twice a day.
- Treat postfoaling mares with sciatic nerve damage aggressively with DMSO, 10% IV and mild sedation if anxiety is a problem. Physical support (e.g., tail tie) for short periods is important to enable the mare to stand. If the mare cannot stand with this regimen, administer a single dose of dexamethasone, 0.2-0.4 mg/kg IV.
- Postfoaling mares that cannot stand are difficult to treat and often have severe myopathy secondary to being down.
- Injection of neurotropic growth factor as close to the damaged nerve as possible has been done; however the effectiveness is unknown.

REFERENCES

General

Mayhew IG: The equine spinal cord in health and disease. In *Proceedings of the 45th annual convention of the American Association of Equine Practitioners,* Albuquerque, 1999.

Acute Ataxia

DeLahunta A: *Veterinary neuroanatomy and clinical neurology,* ed 2, Philadelphia, 1983, WB Saunders.

Mayhew IG: *Large animal neurology,* Philadelphia, 1989, Lea & Febiger.

Equine Protozoal Myeloencephalitis

MacKay RJ et al: Equine protozoal myeloencephalitis, *Vet Clin North Am Equine Pract* 16:405-425, 2000.

Equine Herpes Myeloencephalitis

Van Maanen C, Sloet van Oldruitenborgh-Oosterbaan MM, Damen EA: Neurologic disease associated with EHV-1 infection in a riding school: clinical and virological characteristics, *Equine Vet J* 33:191-196, 2001.

West Nile Virus Encephalitis
Ostlund EN, Andresen JE, Andresen M: West Nile encephalitis, *Vet Clin North Am Equine Pract* 16:427-441, 2000.

Ophthalmology

Nita L. Irby

EQUINE OCULAR EMERGENCIES

Many problems involving the equine eye are true emergencies, including:

- Blunt head trauma
- Acute orbital cellulitis
- Eyelid lacerations
- Corneal ulcers or corneal stromal abscessation
- Uveitis
- Glaucoma
- Acute blindness or visual disturbance
- Other traumatic injury to the eye

➤ These patients need to be examined immediately by a veterinarian or veterinary ophthalmologist because *long-term prognosis for vision or retention of the globe may depend on immediate, accurate diagnosis and treatment.*

Because many systemically administered drugs do not reach adequate intraocular levels, owners or caregivers should be prepared to administer topical ocular medications as frequently as every hour, or in acute conditions, even more often. In such cases, medication administration is greatly facilitated by the placement of a transpalpebral lavage apparatus (recommend reorder no. 6612 from Mila International; [888] MILA-INT). Referral to a facility providing 24-hour care 7 days a week may be necessary.

DIAGNOSTIC AND THERAPEUTIC AIDS TO TREATMENT

All of the equipment in Box 41-1 fits inside a small, three-tiered fishing tackle box and can travel with you wherever you go.

Auriculopalpebral Nerve Block

➤ - The equine orbiculus oculi muscle is very powerful. To safely examine a painful, squinted eye the orbiculus oculi muscle must be partially or completely paralyzed with a palpebral nerve block. This block should be performed any time a tightly closed eye is examined and the history is unknown.
- Branches of the auriculopalpebral nerve can be palpated in a number of sites as they cross the bony orbital rim dorsal or dorsolateral to the eye. Cleanse one or more sites and inject local anesthetic subcutaneously (1-3 ml per site) through a 25-gauge needle.

BOX 41-1. Contents of Equine Ophthalmology Kit (The Basics)

1. Welch-Allyn 3.5V rechargeable halogen direct ophthalmoscope with Finoff transilluminator
2. Cobalt blue filter for transilluminator to enhance fluorescein stain fluorescence
3. 20-Diopter or 2.2D indirect ophthalmoscopy lens
4. 4× magnifying loupe
5. Sterile cotton-tipped applicators and sterile gauze pads
6. Fluorescein stain strips, sterile
7. Mosquito hemostats
8. Allis or Bishop-Harmon tissue forceps
9. Small Metzenbaum or Stevens tenotomy scissors
10. Small needle holder (Derf or large Castroviejo)
11. 2-0 nylon on a straight needle
12. 4-0 to 6-0 polyglactin 910 (Vicryl) on small cutting needle
13. Schirmer tear test strips
14. Xylazine, detomidine, and butorphanol
15. Mepivacaine or lidocaine
16. Tropicamide 1% (short-acting mydriatic to dilate pupils)
17. Proparacaine 0.5% (topical anesthetic)
18. 10% phenylephrine
19. Sterile eye collyrium, eye-irrigating solution in a spray bottle or sterile saline solution
20. 5% povidone-iodine solution
21. Alcohol swabs
22. Cyanoacrylate tissue adhesive
23. #11, #12, and #15 Bard-Parker scalpel blades (#12 works well for suture removal)
24. Glass slides (cleaned and in carriers)
25. Matches: Nonessential but good to have with you!
26. 20-gauge intravenous catheters for normograde nasolacrimal cannulation, teat cannula, TomCat catheters, or 3.5F and 5F polypropylene canine urinary catheters for retrograde nasolacrimal lavage and cannulation
27. 30-, 25-, 20-, and 18-gauge disposable needles
28. Tuberculin, 3-cc, 5-cc, and two 12-cc syringes
29. Blood tubes, particularly red top (include one or two filled with formalin)
30. Culturettes, preferably minitip
31. Broth for bacterial culture
32. Mila subpalpebral lavage apparatus kits

- An alternative is to anesthetize most of the palpebral nerve branches by fanning 3-5 ml of local anesthetic subcutaneously immediately caudal to the most dorsal portion of the zygomatic arch. The nerve may not be palpable at this location.
- A properly performed block results in akinesia (temporary paralysis) of the upper eyelid within 5 minutes and greatly facilitates a complete and safe examination of the eye.

Never attempt to forcefully open a patient's closed eyelids without eyelid akinesia. This can result in rupture of a deep corneal ulcer or evisceration of a lacerated globe.

Frontal Nerve Block

- This block provides analgesia to most of the upper eyelid and good, albeit partial, upper lid akinesia.
- 2-3 ml of local anesthetic is instilled subcutaneously over the palpable supraorbital foramen (located in the zygomatic process of the frontal bone dorsal to the medial canthus of the eye).
- Preferred for routine eye examination because the patient does not feel the manipulation of the eyelids; a difficult patient is thus less resistant to the examination.

Topical Anesthesia

- Proparacaine (0.5%) and other topical anesthetics cause mild stinging on instillation and hyperemia of the conjunctiva. They also are mildly toxic to the corneal epithelium. There is faint, diffuse corneal epithelial thickening and *faint*, diffuse fluorescein uptake after administration of a topical anesthetic.
- A complete external examination of the eye that includes fluorescein staining always should be performed before instillation of an anesthetic.
- Apply by means of spray from a stock solution placed in a tuberculin or 3-cc syringe with a 25-gauge needle hub attached *but with the needle broken off.*
- Repeated administration of a topical anesthetic every 15-30 seconds for 3-5 minutes greatly enhances the depth of topical anesthesia.

ACUTE HEAD TRAUMA WITH EYE INJURIES

- Traumatic injuries to the head, orbit, or globe, self-inflicted or induced, are common among horses because of the large size of the eye, the prominent lateral placement of the eye in the head, the nervous temperament of many horses, and the powerful reflex throwing of the head.
- Head, ocular, or orbital trauma is always an emergency.
- After injury, immediately restrain the patient's head to avoid additional, self-induced injury that occurs from rubbing the eye and periocular area against the stall, wall, or forelimb.
- Avoid examination or manipulation of the ocular or periocular tissues until adequate restraint and tranquilization are completed.

Blunt Trauma to the Head with Secondary Optic Neuropathy

- A common sequela to occipital trauma, rearing and striking the head, and falling backward.
- May result in sudden unilateral or bilateral visual impairment or blindness secondary to partial or complete shearing or injury to the optic nerve fibers. Often associated with hemorrhage and fracture of the basisphenoid bone.
- Pupillary light reflexes, menace responses, obstacle course evaluation, and complete ophthalmic examination (including careful fundus and optic nerve examination) must be performed in all cases of blunt head trauma. Orbital ultrasound examination may be helpful diagnostically. Computed tomography (CT), magnetic resonance imaging (MRI), or both, with or without a contrast agent, often provide enough information to establish a diagnosis.

- Follow-up examination of a normal-appearing eye should be performed 6-8 or more weeks after trauma.

Immediate Findings
- Visual impairment! Most horses that have sustained head trauma are acutely, totally blind and remain so forever. Occasional patients may be affected unilaterally or have some vision in each eye (*oculus uterque* [OU]).
- Blind patients have widely dilated and unresponsive pupils (OU).
- Partially sighted horses have variable pupil positions and responses.
- The fundus may be normal, but optic nerve edema, hemorrhage, myelin loss, or alteration may be present. These are rare findings because the most common site of injury is proximal on the optic nerves, quite a distance from the globe.

Chronic Cases (6 or More Weeks after Injury)
- Optic nerve atrophy: Pallor, slight cupping, change in texture of the optic nerve head as scleral fibers become visible, and decreased diameter of the nerve head.
- Decreased or absent retinal vasculature.
- Peripapillary retinal or choroidal atrophy or pigment alteration may be present.

Treatment and Prognosis
- Partially sighted horses (with some intact optic nerve fibers) may improve with time and immediate, aggressive, appropriate management of central nervous system trauma (see p. 421).
- Most patients are permanently visually impaired.
- Prognosis is guarded to grave in all cases. Vision loss may progress for the first several days after the injury.

Blunt Trauma to the Eye without Laceration or Rupture
- Always perform careful physical, neurologic, and ophthalmic examinations, including fundus examination and evaluation of direct and consensual pupillary light reflexes (if possible). The eye may appear normal or have any combination of injuries.
  - Indirect ophthalmoscopy is recommended because it is more useful for fundus examination through cloudy media than is direct ophthalmoscopy.
- Some patients may be normal, others may have mild to severe optic nerve edema or hyperemia with or without peripapillary retinal and choroidal edema.
- Check the sclera carefully, especially in the equatorial region, for occult ruptures, which if not repaired can lead to phthisis bulbi (shrinkage and wasting of the eyeball).
- Perform repeat fundus examinations 1, 3, 6, and 12 months after injury because some patients sustain "butterfly lesions" (areas of peripapillary choroidal and retinal pigment, epithelial pigment disturbance, or atrophy), possibly as a result of compression of the posterior eye wall around the stalk of the optic nerve (see Color Plate 3). Visual disturbance has not been documented in these cases, and electroretinograms obtained in several cases were normal.
- Similar butterfly lesions have been associated with equine recurrent uveitis (ERU), an unsoundness in the horse; therefore document all trauma-induced butterfly lesions to prevent any question of a diagnosis of ERU-associated unsoundness during future prepurchase examinations.

- Acute **hyphema** often is present.
- If >50% of the anterior chamber is filled with blood or if spontaneous intraocular rebleeding occurs, the eye has a very poor prognosis, and phthisis bulbi often results.
- See Hyphema section in this chapter (p. 464).
- Monitor the cornea carefully for several days after any blunt traumatic injury. An initially normal cornea may slough its epithelium a few days later as a consequence of the contusion.

Orbital and Periorbital Fractures

The dorsal (frontal bone) and temporal (temporal and zygomatic bones) regions of the bony orbit are most commonly injured.

Clinical Signs

- Edema, swelling, pain, blepharospasm, chemosis, and subconjunctival hemorrhage may or may not be accompanied by lacerations, contusions, or other injuries of the face or lids.
- Subcutaneous or orbital emphysema may be present if the frontal or maxillary sinuses have been fractured (see Color Plate 4).
- Palpable disruption of the bony orbital rim if fracture fragments are displaced. Fractures generally are more extensive on radiographs than on palpation.
- Abnormal nasal or ocular discharge.
- Strabismus or displacement of the globe.
- Enophthalmic, exophthalmic, or normally positioned globe.
- Upper eyelid function may be impaired because of lid swelling or injury to the palpebral nerve.

Diagnosis

- Generally straightforward if a known traumatic event has occurred.
- Rule out orbital cellulitis.
- Complete physical, ocular, and neurologic examinations
- Be sure to check the cornea at presentation and again daily for several more days.
- Palpate the affected area and perform a digital examination through the palpebral fissure once the patient can be safely tranquilized and the eye topically anesthetized. Swelling and pain may prevent thorough palpation.
- Fully evaluate eye motility by moving the patient's head dorsally, ventrally, laterally, and in small circles while simultaneously observing for normal vestibular eye movements.
  - This may be difficult when there is significant periocular swelling.
  - Forced duction may be needed for complete evaluation (after moderate sedation and topical anesthesia or under general anesthesia). Grasp the limbal conjunctiva with a small tissue forceps and "force" the globe through all planes of motion.
- Any combination of skull radiographs, CT, ultrasonography, and MRI may be needed for a complete diagnosis.

Treatment
SYMPTOMATIC
- Cold compresses, analgesics, and antiinflammatory agents

- Systemic corticosteroids are not recommended because of concerns relative to a sinus infection.

NOTE: If optic nerve damage is present, administration of systemic corticosteroids is instituted.

- Hot compresses may be used after the first 24 hours: Apply for 5-10 minutes q2h.
- Systemic antibiotic therapy if open fractures, sinus fractures, or skin wounds are present.
- Frequent (6-8 or more a day) application of topical eye lubricants if there is any impairment of eyelid function or integrity. A membrane nictitans flap may be used to protect the globe.

> Symptomatic treatment alone is *not recommended* if there is sinus compromise, marked displacement of fracture fragments, or marked facial deformity or whenever there is **any** displacement of the globe or **any** impairment of normal eye movements. Fracture repair is urgently needed in cases of optic nerve injury.

FRACTURE REPAIR
- Most easily accomplished in the first 24-48 hours as a general anesthetic procedure if the patient's physical condition is stable.
- May be accomplished by digital manipulation and bony traction; however, most cases necessitate extensive orthopedic manipulation and instrumentation.

EYELID EMERGENCIES
Acute Blepharitis
Etiology
- Possible known causes include:
  - Allergic reaction
  - Bacterial hypersensitivity
  - Parasite infestation (e.g., *Demodex, Habronema*)
  - Noxious chemical irritation or chemical sensitivity
  - Exposure to noxious plants
  - Insect stings or sprays (e.g., from bombardier beetles)
- Cause unknown in most cases

Clinical Signs
- Lid swelling, edema, chemosis
- Blepharospasm
- Epiphora
- Exposure keratitis secondary to poor lid-to-globe contact and poor tear film distribution

Diagnosis
- Careful history: Has this occurred before? To what chemicals, fertilizers, feed additives, soaps, cleansers, and plants has the patient been exposed?
- Careful examination of the head and eye, including all conjunctival surfaces of the lids, globe, and membrane nictitans

- Requires sedation, eyelid akinesia, and topical anesthesia
- Remove any foreign material present.
- Perform copious lavage with saline solution or ocular collyrium.
- Perform fluorescein staining (see Chapter 28, p. 112).

Treatment
- Most cases only require symptomatic therapy.
  - Apply cold compresses.
  - Apply sterile ophthalmic lubrication with an agent such as Lacri-Lube (white petrolatum, mineral oil, and lanolin alcohol) until the lids have returned to normal.
  - Monitor the cornea carefully for any exposure keratitis that may develop as the result of poor lid-to-globe contact with resultant poor tear film distribution.

Facial Nerve Palsy or Paralysis
Facial nerve injury or inflammation (central or local) may result in the inability to close the eyelids with exposure keratitis and possible corneal ulceration a consequence.

Etiology
- Periocular trauma to palpebral nerve or nerve branches
- Temporohyoid osteoarthropathy
- Chronic, severe otitis media
- Equine protozoal myelitis
- Vestibular syndrome
- Polyneuritis
- Other

Diagnosis
- Signs usually obvious
  - Ptosis
  - Absent or reduced palpebral reflex
- Present or absent mucoid to mucopurulent ocular discharge due to impaired lacrimal pump system
- Corneal epithelial thickening, erosion, or ulceration
- Positive rose bengal or fluorescein stain uptake (rose bengal stains dead or devitalized corneal epithelium), usually in a horizontal elliptical pattern just above the lower lid margin

Treatment
- Treat the patient for the primary disease (see p. 435).
- Provide frequent (q4h) topical lubrication with artificial tear solution or ointment.
- Manage corneal ulceration (see p. 455).
- **Temporary tarsorrhaphy**
  - 2-3 horizontal mattress sutures placed split thickness in the eyelids may be adequate for 1-2 weeks. If the sutures are left in place longer, chronic lid thickening, depigmentation, and necrosis can result.
  - 4-0 silk is the recommended suture.

- □ Sutures should be tightened just apposing the lids, no tighter, or tissue necrosis can result.
- □ Use of sutures preplaced through rubber band stents and tied in a bow allows the lids to be easily opened for corneal examination.
- **Permanent "Split-Lid Tarsorrhaphy" That Preserves Lid Margins**
  - □ A simple procedure is used to close the temporal half of the palpebral fissure, and the tarsorrhaphy can be left in place for months to years. It allows the eyelids to be opened later, when lid function has returned. While the tarsorrhaphy is in place, vision is possible from the open medial palpebral fissure. The lid margins are left relatively intact and return to normal function if the tarsorrhaphy spots are opened later.
  - □ Heavy sedation and local anesthesia or, preferably, general anesthesia
  - □ Using a no. 15 scalpel blade, make two 6- to 7-mm incisions splitting to the upper eyelid margin, following the meibomian gland openings and incising to a depth of 4-6 mm. One incision should be placed centrally in the upper lid and the second in the temporal third of the upper lid. *The eyelid margins are not removed or excised; they are simply split into two layers.*
  - □ Make corresponding incisions (same position, length and depth) in the lower lid margin. *The lower lid margin is less defined than the upper. Pay careful attention to ensuring that the lid is split properly into an outer skin-muscle layer and inner tarsal plate–conjunctiva. The inner layer (upper or lower lid) must not contain ANY hairs or hair follicles; otherwise after closure it inverts towards the cornea.*
  - □ Using 5-0 absorbable suture, place one single, deep suture in the apex of each upper lid incision parallel to the lid margin and a corresponding suture in the lower lid incision. When these sutures are tied, they bring similar upper and lower eyelid wounds together, inverting the inner (tarsal plate–conjunctiva) layers toward the cornea. The skin-muscle layers evert outward.
  - □ Place 6-8 simple interrupted 5-0 absorbable sutures in the everted skin-muscle layers to ensure wound security.
  - □ The eyelid margins appear overcorrected (closed) initially because of lid swelling.
  - □ Medications can be applied through the open medial half of the palpebral fissure.
  - □ Suture removal is unnecessary if absorbable sutures are used in the skin.
- Depending on the cause of the paralysis, normal eyelid function may be delayed for weeks, months, and possibly forever. Ask the owner to monitor eyelid function on a regular basis for any changes. As the blink reflex returns, the medial spot tarsorrhaphy can be opened initially with a small scissors; the more temporal spot can be opened once normal function returns, or it can be left in place for life. Vision usually is good through the medial canthal opening.

Prognosis
- Guarded, but a number of patients have partial to complete return of nerve function over a 6- to 18-month period.

Eyelid Lacerations
- Usually the upper eyelid
- Perform a *complete* ocular examination including:

- Fluorescein staining
- Fundus and lens evaluation
- Make sure the eye is lubricated and protected from self-mutilation before, during, and after the examination
- If the cause is unknown, skull radiographs are indicated to rule out the presence of metallic foreign bodies. Explore the wound carefully before closing it

Etiology

- Lacerations usually occur because the patient has caught the upper or lower eyelid on a hook, nail, or other pointed object. The apparent laceration often is an avulsion.
- May be a result of blunt compression or trauma

Diagnosis

- Usually obvious!
- May be a simple laceration perpendicular to the lid margin, a flap of eyelid hanging from a pedicle, or a laceration that has removed the lid margin (uncommon)
- The wound usually is edematous and bloody.
- Blood, tears, and a mucoid to mucopurulent ocular discharge are seen on the lid and periocular area. The discharge is moist or dry depending on the time since the injury.
- The individual usually is in mild to moderate pain.
- A fluorescein dye test *must* be performed to assess the integrity of the cornea. Manage any corneal injury appropriately.

Treatment

- Tetanus prophylaxis.
- Systemic broad-spectrum antibiotics.
- *Any periocular laceration that breaches the eyelid margin must be surgically repaired as soon as possible!*
- *Never remove seemingly redundant eyelid tissue or eyelid flaps!*
  - □ Prepare the periocular tissues with 10% povidone-iodine solution, *never scrub* and *never* chlorhexidine.
  - □ Eyelids are well vascularized and very "forgiving" if properly repaired.
  - □ Tissue appearing hopelessly desiccated, inflamed, or infected can heal well if properly repaired.
  - □ No other tissue in the body can substitute for lost eyelid margin.
  - □ Removal or improper repair of an eyelid margin leads to chronic corneal disease from irritation by eyelid hairs (trichiasis), exposure keratitis due to improper spreading of the tear film over the cornea, and chronic keratoconjunctivitis due to an inability of the eye to properly cleanse itself.
  - □ *Preserve eyelid marginal tissue, even when viability is in doubt.* Debride conservatively!
  - □ *Preserve lid function* or otherwise ensure that the lids can protect the globe (e.g., tarsorrhaphy).
  - □ Prevent self-mutilation.

ANESTHESIA AND WOUND PREPARATION
- Local anesthesia and sedation if the patient is cooperative and the repair is a simple one. Use general anesthesia for all complicated repairs or if the patient is difficult to manage.
- In either case, application of topical anesthesia is a useful adjunct to repair.
- Avoid clipping the lid hair around the wound, because the small cut hairs are difficult to eliminate from the wound. Wounds that extend into the longer hair of the lid or face may need clipping.
- Cleanse the wound *thoroughly* with sterile saline solution or a 5% dilution of povidone-iodine solution (avoid most detergent or scrub cleansers because they are highly toxic to ocular tissues). Chlorhexidine *never* should be used in the periocular area.
- Debride the wound margins with sterile gauze until the cut surfaces bleed freely. Minimize sharp debridement to preserve the maximum amount of eyelid tissue.

ACUTE INJURIES (<12 HOURS OLD)
- 4-0 or 6-0 absorbable suture material on a small needle is preferred.
- Perform at a minimum a two-layer closure on all full-thickness lacerations. Some lacerations may require three layers.
- Examine the deeper layers of the eyelid until the thin connective tissue layer of the eyelid (the tarsal plate) is identified. This is the layer in which to place deep sutures.
- *The first suture placed is the most important.* It should appose the eyelid margins perfectly.
    - The first suture is a buried figure-of-eight, mattress, or cruciate suture that securely closes the tarsal plate and conjunctiva and leaves the knot deeply buried beneath the conjunctiva and well away from the eyelid margin.
    - If placement is not exact and a *"step"* develops in the eyelid margin, remove and replace the suture.
- This suture may be preplaced but not tied to facilitate placement of other sutures.
- Place additional deep sutures, as needed, depending on the length of the laceration.
- Confirm that these deep sutures *do not* penetrate the conjunctiva **at any point**.
- Perform routine skin closure.
- Place simple, interrupted sutures of 4-0 or 5-0 absorbable material in the sub-cuticular layers or skin.
- Make certain the cut ends of the skin sutures *do not* touch the cornea.
- Severe lacerations may benefit from a stent made with the opposing eyelid by means of tarsorrhaphy with split-thickness horizontal mattress sutures in the eyelid margins.
- If the eyelids must be closed, plan ahead and place a transpalpebral lavage apparatus for administration of topical medications (if needed) *before* closure of the lids (see Chapter 31, p. 117).

Postoperative Medical Management
- Apply warm compresses, if possible, for 10 minutes q2-3h for 2 days.
- Avoid topical corticosteroids.

- Administer topical broad-spectrum antibiotics q4h for 24 hours then q6h for 7-10 days if tissue injury is excessive or if corneal integrity is in doubt; otherwise antibiotics are unnecessary.
  - Avoid placing excessive tension or stress on the eyelid during application of topical medications.
  - If topical application is impossible, ophthalmic antibiotic solutions can be sprayed onto the cornea with a tuberculin syringe with the needle hub attached but *with the needle broken off* the hub. This makes a very effective, simple, medication "squirt gun."
- If the cornea is injured, administer topical medications more frequently and judiciously.
- Administer systemic antibiotics for 5-7 days.
- Use of a systemic antiinflammatory or antiprostaglandin is indicated depending on the degree of inflammation and discomfort. Minimally, administer phenylbutazone, 2.2-4.4 mg/kg PO q12h for 3-5 days.
- Assure tetanus prophylaxis.
- Prevent self-trauma.
- Gently clean the periocular area as often as exudate and discharge accumulate.
- After cleaning and drying, coat the drainage area of the face beneath the eye with a film of petrolatum jelly to prevent hair loss from irritation by the eye secretions.
- Check daily to ensure normal eyelid function and absence of suture irritation.

SUBACUTE TO CHRONIC LACERATIONS (>12 HOURS OLD)
- Postpone repair for a few days, if needed, to stabilize the patient's condition if other injuries are present or to allow any infection to be controlled by medications.
- Provide topical and medical management as described earlier.
- Restore the wound edges by means of sharp scarification with a #15 scalpel blade. Take care not to remove tissue but to restore a liberally bleeding surface.

CHEMICAL INJURIES TO THE EYE OR ADNEXA
- **Lavage, lavage, lavage.** Owners should immediately and thoroughly wash the affected tissues and maintain continuous lavage for at least 45-60 minutes or until a veterinarian arrives. If the patient is to be transported, attempts should be made to maintain the lavage during transporting if this can be done safely.
- Under no circumstances instill any product into the injured eye in an attempt to neutralize the offending agent. Further tissue damage results.
- In general, alkali burns carry a much poorer prognosis than do acid injuries because alkaline injuries progressively damage tissues for a considerable time after the insult. As a consequence of the tremendous tissue damage, severe, progressive keratomalacia occurs in most cases.
- Treat the patient as for complicated, melting ulcers (see p. 455 in this chapter).
- The prognosis is guarded to poor in all cases of alkaline corneal burn.

EMERGENCIES INVOLVING THE GLOBE
Acute Exophthalmos

> Acute Exophthalmos is *always* an emergency!

Clinical Signs
- The eye protrudes any abnormal amount from the orbit.
- The nictitating membrane protrudes or is recessed.
- Fever varies with cause.
- Pain, redness, swelling, and discharge of purulent material vary depending on the duration and cause.

Differential Considerations
ORBITAL INFLAMMATION, INFECTION, CELLULITIS
- Possible causes
  - Foreign body
  - Extension from an infected tooth root or sinus infection
  - Secondary to a penetrating injury
  - Myositis (rare among horses)
- Fever, pain, and leukocytosis are present in almost all cases

GLAUCOMA
- Rarely an acute problem among horses but may have gone unrecognized for long enough that exophthalmos is the first sign.
- The eye usually has obvious abnormalities (see Glaucoma, p. 469) and the patient has no systemic signs.

ORBITAL NEOPLASIA
- Numerous neoplasms can affect the equine orbit, primarily or as extensions from adjacent regions, particularly sinuses and the nasal cavity.
- Rarely an acute problem.
- Most patients have other clinical abnormalities (nasal discharge, sinus or facial swelling, neurologic abnormalities), depending on the location of the tumor.

PROPTOSIS
- RARE among horses. Most cases develop as the result of orbital neoplasia.
- If proptosis is secondary to trauma, the prognosis for the eye usually is grave. The eye should be enucleated if ruptured or if there is extensive extraocular muscle avulsion.

Diagnosis
- Complete physical and ophthalmic examination
- Complete blood cell count and chemistry profile
- Further diagnostic tests based on examination findings may include:
  - Radiography
  - Ultrasonography
  - Endoscopy of the caudal nasal passage and pharynx
  - CT, MRI

□ Anesthesia and exploration

Treatment
IMMEDIATE THERAPY
- Prevent self-mutilation.
- Careful cleansing of the eye and periocular tissues with sterile saline solution or sterile eyewash. Contact lens solutions in squeeze bottles are readily accessible and commonly used.
- Fluorescein staining to rule out exposure keratitis.
- Consider placing a transpalpebral lavage apparatus (see p. 117) because the eyelids may be temporarily closed as part of the therapy.
- After cleaning, heavily lubricate the eye and any exposed periocular tissues with a sterile ophthalmic lubricant such as Lacri-Lube.
- Perform temporary or split-lid tarsorrhaphy (see p. 443) to keep the eyelids closed.
- Use extreme care placing the tarsorrhaphy sutures so they do not rub the cornea and cause additional problems (see p. 442).
- Protect the cornea as the sutures are tightened.

FURTHER THERAPY
- Varies with the etiologic factor.

Lacerations and Ruptures of the Cornea and Sclera

> If there is any question that a laceration of the cornea or sclera has occurred, instruct the owner to prevent the patient from self-mutilating the eye. Any examination of the eye or periocular area by the owner or veterinarian should await heavy sedation and akinesia of the lids. Failure to follow these guidelines can cause a simple laceration to become a hopeless evisceration. Also instruct the owner that *nothing*, particularly ointments, should be instilled into the eye.

LACERATIONS OR RUPTURES WITH **POOR** PROGNOSIS
- Any laceration associated with:
  □ Proptosis
  □ 50% or greater hyphema
  □ Lacerations of >24 hours duration with flat anterior chamber
  □ Lens rupture or dislocation
  □ Rupture: The blunt force required to rupture an eye usually results in multiple, severe intraocular damage
- *Extensive laceration* with prolapse of intraocular contents *other than* aqueous or iris tissue
  □ *If you believe there is vitreous prolapse, be **sure** before you enucleate that it is not just clotted aqueous humor!*
  □ Repair of a globe (other than placement of an intraocular prosthesis) after partial evisceration usually ends as phthisis bulbi (a small, shrunken, and often painful or irritating eye). If the owner wants to preserve the appearance of an eye, an intraocular prosthesis can be placed through the wound after complete removal of the intraocular contents.

- *Lacerations that extend across the limbus* into the sclera have a poorer prognosis if uveal tissue has prolapsed through the wound.
  - □ Uveal tissue in these cases usually includes the ciliary body.
  - □ Damage to the ciliary body results in decreased production of aqueous humor, hypotony, and phthisis bulbi.
  - □ Enucleation or prosthesis implantation often is indicated in these cases.

LACERATIONS WITH A **FAIR** PROGNOSIS
- Formed anterior chamber
- Small amount of hemorrhage or fibrin; iris may protrude through and close the wound but there is minimal distortion of intraocular structures
- Simple lacerations with minimal contamination and minimal iris prolapse

---

At no time during the examination or surgery should ophthalmic ointments be placed on an open eye! *Use solutions only!*

Transpalpebral ultrasonography can be a useful prognostic tool to assess the posterior segment and lens but only if performed with extreme care on a heavily sedated patient. Gel *must not* enter the palpebral fissure.

Full-Thickness Lacerations

- **All full-thickness lacerations of the equine eye necessitate immediate surgical repair under general anesthesia.**
- **Referral to a veterinary ophthalmologist is recommended for all but the most simple cases. Do not attempt surgery unless standard ophthalmic surgical instruments and appropriately sized suture material are available. The surgery is usually more difficult than anticipated.**

Diagnosis
- Usually obvious
- Corneal or scleral defect, usually plugged with fibrin, iris, or other uveal tissue
- Decreased intraocular pressure
- Decreased depth or total collapse of the anterior chamber
- Fibrin, hypopyon, and hyphema present or absent in the anterior chamber
- Fluorescein stain
  - □ Usually stains corneal wound margins
  - □ May cause fluorescence of the aqueous humor if the wound has not sealed
  - □ Streaming of aqueous may be seen in the stained precorneal tear film
- Assess dazzle and indirect papillary light reflexes.

Treatment
- **Do not** use ketamine for general anesthesia. Consider muscle relaxants as part of the anesthesia protocol.
- **Protect the eye during induction.**
- **Culture the wound and any excised tissue.**
  - □ *Gently* lavage, cleanse, and carefully replace healthy-appearing prolapsed uveal tissue (usually iris) into the anterior chamber in acute injuries.

NOTE: Postoperative uveitis is proportional to the degree of uveal damage and handling.

- □ Carefully debride necrotic, desiccated, or otherwise devitalized uveal tissue if necessary.
- □ Uveal excision can result in severe hemorrhage. Be prepared!
- Irrigate and re-form the anterior chamber with balanced salt solution or lactated Ringer's solution.
  - □ Viscoelastic substances may be used to assist chamber formation and dissection of uveal tissue but should be removed before complete wound closure, or postoperative ocular hypertension may result.
- Wound apposition should be precise.
  - □ Binocular magnification should be used if possible.
  - □ 6-0 or 8-0 polyglactin 910 or nylon *ophthalmic* suture.
  - □ Sutures should be placed 1-2 mm apart, as deep as possible in the stroma, but **NOT** full thickness. Entry and exit points of the suture should be perpendicular to the corneal surface and wound edge, respectively. Tighten sutures just to appose.
- Re-form the chamber after wound closure as described earlier.
- Apply fluorescein stain and mild external pressure to assess wound integrity.
- Unstable, irregular wounds or repairs may be reinforced with a conjunctival flap.
  - □ This is not generally necessary unless the security of the wound closure is in doubt.
  - □ Flap placement almost always results in a more dense, opaque corneal scar postoperatively.
- **Consult ophthalmic textbooks for additional information!**
- Place a transpalpebral lavage device if desired.
- ▶ The eye should **not** be covered by a tarsorrhaphy or membrana nictitans flap. Such flaps frequently cause complications and potentially increase intraocular pressure, which results in wound leakage and prevents direct examination of the globe, which is important postoperatively.

Postoperative Care
- Examine the eyes daily or more often for 7-10 days.
  - □ Severe secondary uveitis is common.
  - □ Endophthalmitis may develop.
- Treatment is facilitated by placement of a transpalpebral lavage apparatus (p. 117) while the patient is under general anesthesia.
- Medications:
  - □ Topical 1% atropine solution, to effect or 4-6 times a day, to facilitate pupillary dilation, for cycloplegia, and to stabilize the blood-aqueous barrier.
  - □ Topical broad-spectrum antibiotic solutions, q1-2h for 24h then q2h for 3-7 days and finally q4-6h, depending on the condition of the eye.
  - □ Systemic broad-spectrum antibiotics with a good Gram-positive spectrum.
  - □ A systemic nonsteroidal antiinflammatory agent (NSAID) until the wound is healed and any associated uveitis controlled.
  - □ A topical NSAID may be used with caution (see following section on corneal abrasions and ulcers).

Partial-Thickness Lacerations

- Wound margins separated by more than 2-3 mm necessitate surgical repair under general anesthesia (see p. 449).
- Manage superficial nonpenetrating lacerations as corneal ulcers, but perform a careful examination every 1-2 days to identify secondary infection, especially if the laceration is caused by plant material.
- Medications:
  - Topical 1% atropine, q8h to q12h or to effect, to maintain pupil dilation
  - Topical broad-spectrum antibiotics, q1-2h for 24h then q2-6h, depending on the condition of the eye.
  - Systemic NSAIDs until the wound is healed and any associated uveitis controlled.
  - Monitor the wound for enzyme activity (collagenase) as described in the ulcer section. Topical acetylcysteine should be added q2h if there is doubt about enzyme activity.

Partial-Thickness Flaps

- Deep flap wounds of varying thickness that remain attached to the cornea are repaired in the same manner as any laceration.
- Flaps should be very thin with minimal edema.
  - Carefully replace the flap over the wound bed, and press it firmly in place by rolling the flap with a cotton swab and securing the wound margins with points of tissue adhesive.
  - If the flap detaches, excise it but preserve corneal tissue whenever possible.
  - Medications: As for uncomplicated ulcers (see p. 456)

CORNEAL ABRASIONS AND ULCERS

- Tables 41–1 and 41–2 cover ophthalmic antibiotic usage and dosages.
- The cornea fills almost the entire interpalpebral space in the horse, prominently protrudes from the side of the face, and is easily traumatized.
- Corneal ulcers are self-induced or have numerous external sources.
- **Any lesion that breaches the corneal epithelium is an emergency** because:

TABLE 41–1. Commercially Available Ophthalmic Antibiotic Preparations

Name of Drug	Concentration	Ophthalmic Preparations Available
Bacitracin	500 U/gram	O
Chloramphenicol	0.16-1.0%	O, S
Ciprofloxacin	0.35%	O, S
Erythromycin	0.5%	O
Gentamicin	0.35%	O, S
Norfloxacin	0.3%	S
Ofloxacin	0.3%	S
Tobramycin	0.3%	O, S

O, Ointment; *S,* solution.
All drugs are commercially available in the United States. Some drugs are approved for human use only.

OPHTHALMOLOGY

TABLE 41–2. Antibiotics That Can be Formulated for Ophthalmic Use

Name of Drug	Topical Dose (mg/ml)	Subconjunctival Dose (mg)
Amikacin	10	25-50
Ampicillin (Na)	50	50-100
Carbenicillin disodium	5	100
Cefazolin sodium	50-65	100
Ceftazidime	NA	200
Clindamycin	50	15-50
Erythromycin	50	100
Gentamicin sulfate	15-20	20-30
Methicillin sodium	50	50-100
Penicillin G	100,000 units/ml	0.5-1.0 million units
Ticarcillin disodium	6	100
Tobramycin sulfate	15	20-30

NA, Not applicable.
Final dilutions in artificial tear solutions may enhance contact time. Consult package inserts for shelf life, which varies by drug from 3 to 30 or more days.

- □ The cornea is an avascular tissue and corneal defense mechanisms are markedly reduced compared with those of well-vascularized parts of the eye or body.
- □ A normal cornea is continually exposed to environmental contaminants, bacteria, and fungi.
- □ The maximum thickness of the cornea is approximately 1 mm; therefore a superficial ulcer can perforate the cornea in a short time.

> All equine corneal ulcers, regardless of size or depth, should be considered emergencies, and the patient should receive prompt, aggressive treatment and follow-up care. All corneal ulcers should be considered infected until proved otherwise.

Clinical Signs

- Examine *immediately* any patient with a suspected ulcer.
  - □ Pain (mild pain indicated by a slightly dropped eyelash angle compared with the normal eye).
  - □ *The severity of the problem and degree of pain are* **not** *directly proportional.* A horse with a superficial corneal abrasion may exhibit more signs of pain than does a horse with a descemetocele or perforated ulcer!
- Blepharospasm, rubbing the eye, swelling of one or both eyelids.
- Epiphora
- Redness and swelling of the conjunctiva
- Corneal clouding from edema or inflammatory cell infiltrate may be present or absent.
- Change in corneal contour may be present or absent. Examine the corneal surface from all oblique angles.

NOTE: Downer foals should be examined carefully every day for corneal disease. The examination should include fluorescein staining. Young foals generally have decreased corneal and blink reflexes, particularly when they are neurologically or systemically compromised, and may have decreased tear production. Thick foam helmets can be used effectively in the care of recumbent foals to raise the down eye above the stall bedding. Artificial tear ointment q6h is recommended prophylactically for the eyes of downer foals.

Diagnostic Reminders

- The classic hallmark of corneal abrasions or ulcerations is the uptake of fluorescein stain by the corneal stroma. The examiner should be careful, however, because *dye uptake does not occur in all cases.*
- *Stromal* ulcerative processes can occur with active infection, stromal dissolution, and necrosis in the presence of an intact, overlying epithelium (see Color Plate 5). The cornea in these cases may not retain fluorescein dye. General guideline: If the eye looks like it has an ulcer, treat it for an ulcer even if it does not stain with fluorescein!
- Deep ulcers that extend to Descemet's membrane retain stain only in the circumferentially adjacent stroma, even when the stroma is covered with healing epithelium.

Diagnostic Steps

1. Assess *tear production,* preferably as early as possible in the examination.
   - Dry eye is rare among horses but it does occur. If the eye is painful and an ulcer is suspected, the patient should have epiphora. If not, suspect decreased tear production as a cause of the ulcer.
2. Assess *lid function.* Abnormal lid function (facial nerve dysfunction or decreased corneal sensation with resultant failure of reflex blinking) causes corneal disease.
   - *Assess the palpebral reflex!* Be *sure* to do this before the lids are blocked.
   - *Assess corneal sensation!* Carefully touch the cornea with a sterile cotton swab before applying topical anesthetic.
3. Tranquilize and restrain the patient as necessary and establish eyelid akinesia.
4. Culture the cornea with a sterile, moist swab.
   - This step may be unnecessary for simple ulcers of known cause or when wound contamination is not expected. However, a culture specimen obtained at the start of the examination can be discarded if not needed.
   - Avoid lid contamination when obtaining the culture specimen.
5. Examine carefully the cornea, conjunctiva, sclera, nictitating membrane, and eyelids, especially the conjunctival surface, in the dark with a bright, focal light.
   - Perform a thorough examination, *particularly* if the etiologic factor is unknown.
   - Examine with magnification if possible, concentrating on the areas of the conjunctiva, nictitans, and eyelid that *correspond to the position of the ulcer.* Evert the corresponding area of the eyelid over a finger and examine it carefully.
   - Careful examination of these areas in ulcer cases of unknown causation frequently discloses a foreign body, plant awn or spicule, or aberrant hair (rare) as the cause of the problem.
   - Document the size, position, and depth of the ulcer, corneal clarity, presence of edema and infiltrate, depth and contents of the anterior chamber, and size, shape, and response of the pupils.

OPHTHALMOLOGY

6. Apply **fluorescein stain** to the eye, making sure that it covers the entire cornea. Lavage excess fluorescein from the eye, if necessary, and look for dye retention in the cornea.
   - If dye retention is not obvious, use an ultraviolet or Wood's lamp or illumination through a cobalt blue filter (standard on many veterinary ophthalmoscopes) to enhance dye fluorescence.

Perform this examination meticulously because failure to detect even focal erosion has serious consequences, particularly if corticosteroids are prescribed to treat the eye.

- Record the size, shape, position, and depth of the corneal wound and document the amount of corneal edema present (the presence and extent of edema can help less experienced examiners assess the depth of a corneal lesion).
- *Corneal abrasions* (surface epithelium lost but underlying basement membrane intact).
  - Eye painful with marked blepharospasm.
  - Lesion may not be visible to the naked eye.
  - No change in contour of the cornea.
  - *Little to no corneal edema because the basement membrane or superficial stromal layers are intact and maintaining their barrier to fluid uptake by the corneal stroma.*
  - Fluorescein dye uptake is patchy to marked depending on the extent and depth of epithelial loss.
- *Corneal ulcers* (extending through epithelium into the underlying stroma).
  - Painful eye (some with deep ulcers are less painful, however, because the more abundant superficial nerve endings have been lost by necrosis).
  - Lesion is readily seen in most cases.
  - *Corneal edema is obvious within and adjacent to the ulcer bed.*
  - Intense fluorescein dye uptake.
- *Be sure to show the lesion to the owner and instruct the owner about signs that may indicate a worsening problem* (see Color Plate 6):
  - *Any increase in edema*
  - Change in contour
  - Change in color
  - Originally clear cornea turning white (edema), or yellowish-white (inflammatory cell infiltrate)
  - Originally cloudy cornea turning
    - More intense white (increasing edema)
    - Yellow to white (inflammatory cells increasing),
    - Clear (may indicate that a descemetocele is developing)
    - Developing a black spot (descemetocele or impending iris prolapse)
  - Pigment or blood may indicate focal perforation.
  - Decrease in the size of the pupil
  - Purulent ocular discharge

- Ulcer beginning to develop a mucoid appearance may indicate that keratomalacia is occurring. This can occur under intact epithelium!

MELTING ULCERS: *Pseudomonas* is the commonly blamed culprit in most melting ulcers, but keratomalacia can develop with a number of Gram-positive or Gram-negative bacterial infections, with fungal infections, or with corneal ulcers secondary to alkali injuries. Collagenases, proteases, and other tissue-toxic and tissue-digesting enzymes are released during normal corneal wound healing by rapidly dividing corneal epithelial cells, from fibroblasts, and from polymorphonuclear leukocytes. Some bacteria and fungal organisms induce collagenolysis, and some tissue destruction occurs during corneal vascular ingrowth. An imbalance of normal enzyme production or a corneal disease resulting in rapid, severe destruction or influx of neutrophils can cause keratolysis, keratomalacia, and perforation within hours.

- Other changes indicating complications, but that the owner may not be able to see, include *poor epithelial regrowth and corneal neovascularization.*
7. Apply a topical anesthetic and obtain a corneal cytologic sample (see corneal scraping, p. 111) for interpretation and culture.
   - Four to six applications of topical anesthesia over a 5-minute period maximize the depth of anesthesia.
   - The noncutting end of a sterile scalpel blade makes an excellent sampling instrument.
   - Remove surface debris before scraping.
   - Obtain three or four samples from stroma at the wound margins and smear them on four or five clean glass microscope slides.
     - Cover the slides at once to prevent environmental contamination.
     - Place a final scraping on a sterile swab that has been moistened with transport medium for bacterial and fungal culture or inoculate directly into broth.
8. Immediately stain cytologic samples with Gram and Giemsa stains for the presence of and Gram classification of bacteria and for fungi. *All initial treatments are based on this cytologic interpretation.*
   - Microorganisms invading the corneal stroma usually are resident conjunctival flora, most of which are Gram-positive bacteria, usually staphylococci and streptococci. After treatment with antibiotics or corticosteroids, isolated flora are predominantly Gram-negative.

Treatment Generalities

- *Regardless of size, all ulcers necessitate aggressive management and careful follow-up care!*
- Remove, treat, or correct the cause, if known.
- Control microbial growth.
- Control collagenase and protease activity.
- Maintain corneal hygiene.
- Maintain patient hygiene and comfort.
- *Never* use topical corticosteroids to manage an equine ulcer (except under daily supervision by an ophthalmologist and rarely even then) or within 6-8 months after healing. These agents *never* should be used to control posthealing vascularization or scarring in the horse.

- Topical NSAIDs should be avoided (see references at the end of this chapter).

Simple Ulcers

- Simple abrasions and erosions are managed conservatively.
- Topical broad-spectrum antibiotics, q4-6h for 24-48 hours then tapering of the intervals if the lesion is resolving
  □ Ointment or solution? Solutions are preferred. They are easily applied with a simple spray device (see p. 438) that is cleaner to use, and less likely to cause an injury to the eye from a medication tip.
  □ Triple antibiotic combinations (e.g., bacitracin-neomycin-polymyxin) are the drugs of choice for uncomplicated abrasions or erosions.
  □ If a wound is likely infected, use a topical aminoglycoside (topical tobramycin or fortified gentamicin).
- Mydriatics, cycloplegics
  □ Stabilize the blood-ocular barrier and decrease ciliary muscle spasm
  □ 1% atropine solution, q12-24h to effect on the first day, usually is sufficient to relieve the pain caused by the ciliary body spasm and counteracts reflex pupil constriction.

  The need for more frequent treatment may indicate that the ulcer is progressing. *Can be used safely q4-6h in the care of most horses, but the patient must be monitored carefully for prolonged gastrointestinal transit time, decreased bowel sounds, or bowel stasis, because atropine can cause idiosyncratic ileus and colic in certain horses. Instruct the owner to monitor gastrointestinal motility by observing bowel sounds and fecal output. If these diminish, discontinue atropine until motility is normal, and monitor the individual carefully for signs of colic.*

- Systemic NSAIDs as needed for 1-2 days in uncomplicated abrasion cases
  □ Phenylbutazone, 2.2-4.4 mg/kg IV or PO q12h
  □ Flunixin meglumine, 0.5-1.0 mg/kg IV q12h

Complicated Ulcers
Treatment

- **Recognize a melting ulcer!** The affected cornea **swells**, becomes blue-white and **edematous** and develops a **gelatinous, mucoid appearance** as the substances that "glue" corneal collagen fibrils together are dissolving.
- Horses with severe corneal disease usually have moderate to severe secondary uveitis. Most of these patients have some degree of hypopyon because the inflamed anterior uveal tissue exudes inflammatory cells. The hypopyon does *not* necessarily mean that the eye is infected intraocularly!
- Requires more aggressive treatment and most cases benefit by subpalpebral lavage (SPL) placement (see p. 117) Choose one drug from each of the following categories:
- Antibiotics q1-2h *or more often* until there are no signs that the ulcer is progressing then q1-2h for 48h then q4h or as indicated. Drug choices are based on cytologic and Gram stain results.
  □ Recommended empirical regimen for topical use in suspected bacterial ulcers until the offending organism and sensitivities are identified:

Cefazolin, 50 mg/ml q1h, in combination with
Tobramycin, 10-15 mg/ml q1h, *or*
Gentamicin, 10-15 mg/ml, may be used instead of tobramycin *or*
Amikacin 10 mg/ml

- □ Alter treatment, if necessary, on the basis of culture and sensitivity results. Recommended drugs for *Gram-positive organisms*: penicillin G, erythromycin, cefazolin, ciprofloxacin, ofloxacin; for *Gram-negative rods*: tobramycin, gentamicin (only at 10-15 mg/ml concentrations), carbenicillin, ciprofloxacin, piperacillin, or ticarcillin
- □ Subconjunctival medications may be indicated for difficult patients and are indicated in any deep or rapidly deteriorating infections.
- □ Medications may be administered through the SPL catheter 5 minutes apart. Each medication is followed with a gentle flush of 3 cc of air.
- Mydriatics, cycloplegics
  - □ 1% atropine topical ophthalmic solution, q4-6h, occasionally more often if the pupil does not dilate
  - □ *See atropine discussion (opposite page)*
- Acetylcysteine and other anticollagenase or antiprotease products are beneficial in some cases of melting ulcers (see p. 455)
  - □ Acetylcysteine (5%-10% Mucomyst), 1-2 drops q1-2h, more often in acute cases, tapering as the ulcer stabilizes and malacia decreases
  - □ Autologous serum
    - □ Contains macroglobulins that are excellent antiproteinases
    - □ Apply a few drops or small spray topically q1-2h or more often, tapering as the ulcer stabilizes.
    - □ Serum *must* be collected and administered aseptically, refrigerated, *and replenished q24-48h*
    - □ Can be used in combination with acetylcysteine
  - □ 0.05% disodium EDTA is particularly helpful in the management of ulcers caused by *Pseudomonas* organisms
  - □ Progressive keratomalacia is an indication that the ulcer must be reevaluated.
- Systemic NSAIDs
  - □ These drugs provide invaluable relief of the severe secondary uveitis that often develops in complicated ulcers.
  - □ Flunixin meglumine, 1 mg/kg, IV or PO, is subjectively more effective than is phenylbutazone, 1 g PO q12h, in these cases.
  - □ *Use judiciously* because NSAIDs can decrease angiogenesis (corneal neovascularization is desirable in many infectious corneal diseases that affect horses).
- Topical NSAIDs are successfully used in many cases to control inflammation, but recent reports (Guidera et al, 2001) and personal experience indicate that topical NSAIDs can worsen keratomalacia, delay wound healing, and suppress corneal neovascularization. It is no longer recommended to use these agents to manage ulcerative disease.
- Systemic antibiotics are recommended in cases of severe ulceration.
- Stall rest

Adjunctive and Supportive Therapy: Ulcer Debridement
- Daily debridement is beneficial in cases of melting ulcers (see Color Plate 7).

- □ Decreases necrotic material and thereby reduces numbers of bacteria and the quantity and activity of proteolytic enzymes
- □ May enhance drug penetration
- □ Helps maintain a more even corneal contour, which facilitates the spread of tear film
- Perform, under tranquilization, lid block, and repeated administration of a topical anesthetic. Use a small, toothed forceps to pick up the malacic cornea and small corneal or eyelid scissors to excise it. The malacic cornea cannot be simply rubbed off or pulled off! The collagen fibrils are still attached peripherally.
- Cleanse the ulcer bed with swabs of povidone-iodine *solution* (0.5%-1% dilution in sterile saline solution).
- Surgical debridement, debulking, and keratectomy of necrotic debris is very beneficial. Perform these procedures with general anesthesia.

Ocular and Periocular Hygiene
- Enhancing patient comfort and appearance and preventing periocular alopecia and dermatitis cannot be overemphasized.
- Clean ocular exudates as often as possible.
- Apply a thin coat of petrolatum to the tear drainage area.

Surgical Intervention for Severe Cases
- Conjunctival flap
  - □ A routine procedure that provides an immediate blood supply to the ulcer to aid healing and act as a source of fibrovascular tissue to reinforce the wound.
  - □ Use judiciously and only when necessary for ulcers located in the central cornea, because the resulting scar is much more dense and permanent. This is of particular importance in the care of performance horses.
- Corneoscleral transposition, lamellar keratectomy, and penetrating keratoplasty are recommended as possible surgical aids to healing. These procedures require specialized instrumentation and operating microscopes.
  - □ Useful in some severe cases
  - □ May result in more dense scar
  - □ May require referral to veterinary ophthalmologists trained in the procedure
- Use of a third-eyelid (membrana nictitans) flap or tarsorrhaphy is **never** recommended in cases of corneal ulceration. The resultant elevation in temperature can increase the rate of bacterial growth. The inability to continuously monitor the eye covered by a flap and the possibility that the flap may cause additional problems completely preclude use of these techniques.

Antibiotic Treatment
Commercially available antibiotic preparations may not have sufficient antibiotic concentration to be clinically effective in deep corneal infections. For example, commercially available gentamicin ophthalmic solution contains 3-mg/ml drug, and the clinically effective dose is considered 10-15 mg/ml. The commercial preparations can be "fortified" by adding to the ophthalmic solution an appropriate volume of the parenteral antibiotic to achieve the desired concentration.

Selected antibiotics *not* available in ophthalmic formulations can be used if the parenteral medication is diluted in artificial tears to the topical dose concentrations listed in Table 41–2. Cefazolin, for example, a favorite drug when Gram-positive cocci are found at cytologic examination, is made by diluting intravenous cefazolin to 500 mg/ml with sterile saline solution then adding 1.5 ml (750 mg) of the intravenous solution to 13.5 ml of artificial tears. This makes a 50 mg/ml concentration for topical use in the eye. The preparation is refrigerated and replenished every 3 days.

FUNGAL ULCERS

- Rarely manifest as emergencies, occurring instead as secondary infections of primary ulcers or as chronic stromal abscesses.

Diagnosis

- Corneal scraping (see p. 111) and cytologic examination. Special stains, such as calcofluor white, acridine orange, periodic acid–Schiff, or Grocott-Gomori methenamine-silver nitrate, are necessary in some cases.
- Culture and sensitivity are of minimal clinical use because results often are not complete for several weeks.

Treatment

- Daily debridement and cauterization with swabs of povidone-iodine *solution* (0.5% dilution in sterile saline solution)
- Daily removal of malacic tissue
- 1% atropine to effect mydriasis
- Natamycin is the most potent and the only approved ophthalmic antifungal medication and is the drug of choice
- Fluconazole, itraconazole, thiabendazole, ketoconazole, miconazole, and other antifungal medications can be used systemically or compounded for topical use

Author's recommendation: Minimize the frequency of topical antifungal medications for the first few days after diagnosis, or acute keratomalacia and severe uveitis may result (q6-12h, increasing slowly from that point as needed).

- Topical chloramphenicol 0.5% or neomycin-polymyxin-bacitracin, q4-6h.
- Flunixin meglumine, 1 mg/kg PO q12h.
- Most patients benefit from surgical removal or debulking of infected, necrotic tissue by means of lamellar keratectomy, full-thickness keratoplasty, or posterior lamellar keratoplasty
- For a complete discussion of fungal keratitis, consult standard ophthalmology references.

EOSINOPHILIC KERATITIS

- *Can manifest as an emergency in some cases because of the peracute onset and rapid progression.*
- A frustrating type of corneal ulcerative disease, usually seen in the summer and fall. Can take 1 to many months to resolve.
- Similar lesions have been attributed to ocular onchocerciasis, but this parasite has not been found in these cases. May affect both eyes simultaneously and recur in same patient several times in one season or in subsequent years.
- Mini outbreaks have occurred in some groups of horses.

Clinical Findings
- See Color Plate 8.
- One or multiple, acute, *superficial* corneal ulcers.
- Both eyes may be affected simultaneously, and there may be more than one ulcer in each eye.
- Usually found in the *peripheral or perilimbal cornea*, often beneath the nictitating membrane.
- May be covered partially to completely with a firmly *adherent, caseous white plaque* that may be *thin and translucent* or several millimeters *thick and opaque.*
- Ulcers enlarge, primarily *paralleling the limbus,* but may encroach on the central cornea as they increase in size.
- Ulcers may or may not have associated neovascularization, depending on the duration of the disease.
- There is minimal corneal edema peripheral to the ulcer bed, but the ulcer bed can appear quite white.
- The presence of pain, blepharospasm, epiphora, conjunctival hyperemia, and chemosis is variable. Some individuals are quite uncomfortable, whereas others barely squint.
- Some horses have acute, copious, caseous ocular discharge.

Diagnosis
- Fluorescein dye results may be difficult to interpret because of the large amount of (usually white) surface debris. Remove debris and repeat the stain.
- Exfoliative cytology. The **classic** finding is large numbers of eosinophils with some mast cells and neutrophils, a large amount of amorphous cellular debris with degenerated to normal epithelial cells. Bacteria and fungi rarely are present but may be present extracellularly, particularly within the amorphous debris.
- Cultures should be performed after all surface debris is removed. The results usually are negative.
- Perform histologic examination of excised lesion if keratectomy is performed.

Treatment
- Control flies!
- Worm with ivermectin.
- Administer prophylactic topical triple antibiotic q6-12h.
- Administration of a topical corticosteroid (0.1% dexamethasone or 1% prednisolone q4-6h, **not** hydrocortisone) may shorten the course of the disease in a few but **not** all cases. *Equine eosinophilic keratitis is the **only** disorder for which topical steroids should be used in the presence of a corneal ulcer.* Do *not* use corticosteroids unless
  - □ The diagnosis is **certain**.
  - □ Results of bacterial and fungal cultures are negative.
  - □ Daily reexaminations are possible for the first 7-10 days of corticosteroid treatment to make certain that the ulcers do not worsen with the therapy.
- Mast cell stabilizers such as lodoxamide tromethamine (Alomide) may be beneficial in some cases.
- Refractory cases necessitate excisional lamellar superficial keratectomy.
- Topical organophosphate drugs such as 0.125% echothiophate iodide may be used if available again.

- Horses with acute eosinophilic keratitis may benefit from keratectomy and are generally able to return to work more quickly than are medically treated patients.

Prognosis

- The ulcers may noticeably increase in diameter and number for the first several days after onset of the disease.
- Eosinophilic ulcers rarely increase in depth. Monitor the depth of the ulcer subjectively by noting the degree and extent of corneal edema adjacent to the ulcer.
- Neovascularization of the ulcer bed is variable. In some cases, it is very slow, whereas in others vascularization is very rapid and extensive (see Color Plate 9).
- Some cases heal in 3-6 weeks. Healing usually is accompanied by intense corneal neovascularization and granuloma formation; other cases remain unchanged for 6 weeks or longer, despite aggressive therapy. Lamellar superficial keratectomy is recommended in chronic cases or in selected acute cases to speed disease resolution (the cornea usually heals 10-14 days postoperatively).

CORNEAL FOREIGN BODIES

Etiology

- Plant material is most common. Metal, glass, gunshot, and many others have been reported. An eyelash can become a foreign body after traumatic injury.

Clinical Signs

- Similar to those of corneal ulcer (see p. 451, *but* signs vary with the size, location, nature, and extent of the injury and the type of foreign body.

Diagnosis

- Sedation, eyelid block, and topical anesthesia are necessary for diagnosis because most cases are quite painful with intense blepharospasm.
- Corneal foreign bodies may be readily seen *or* may be very small and difficult to see even with magnification.
- Examine the iris and anterior chamber very carefully for evidence of penetration.
- Flare, fibrin, hyphema, and similar lesions can be subtle to obvious.
- Foreign body penetration into the anterior chamber has a guarded prognosis.
- Keep patient sedated.
- Prevent self-trauma.
- Remove the object with magnification with the patient under general anesthesia.

> **BE AWARE!** Small black bodies in the cornea that appear to be foreign bodies may be a piece of iris or corpora nigra sealing a corneal perforation. Approach with caution because disturbing the lesion can cause the aqueous humor to leak. The results of careful examination of the anterior chamber and iris should confirm the diagnosis.

Treatment

- Regardless of the treatment used, it is critical to make sure that all foreign material is removed. This requires a very bright focal light source, magnification, time, and patience.

- Patients with large or deep foreign bodies should be referred to a specialist trained in microsurgical technique who is capable of managing a potential perforation.
- After removal, send *all* foreign particles for bacterial and fungal culture and sensitivity.
- Medical management is as for complicated ulcers (see p. 456).

SUPERFICIAL, NONPENETRATING FOREIGN BODIES
- Remove with the patient under topical anesthesia, sedation, and a lid block. Use a sharp stream of sterile saline solution directed tangentially at the foreign body.
- Removing the foreign body is facilitated with a 25-gauge needle or small, toothed forceps (e.g., Bishop-Harmon 1 × 2).

DEEP, NONPENETRATING FOREIGN BODIES
- General anesthesia usually needed for surgical removal and is much safer than local anesthesia in case the anterior chamber is entered during removal.

PENETRATING FOREIGN BODIES
- Refer to a specialist.
- Prognosis is guarded, particularly if perforation by plant material or hair has occurred, owing to the high incidence of secondary endophthalmitis.

ACUTE CORNEAL EDEMA SYNDROME
Acute corneal edema can have many *known* causes, such as trauma and uveitis, but edema with no apparent cause is a poorly understood syndrome among horses and may be a form of primary viral endotheliitis. In most cases the cause is never determined.

Clinical Signs
- Any age, breed, and sex
- Partial to complete corneal edema of mild to severe nature
- Minimal pain in most cases
- One or both eyes may be affected.
- Affected cornea has marked "bulge" because of the intense edema and hydrops.
- Uveitis usually is mild to absent.

NOTE: Corneal edema is *common* in cases of ERU. What differentiates this syndrome is the *intense* corneal edema with minimal intraocular pathologic changes.

Etiology
- Usually unknown
- Toxins or toxic reaction
- Venous stasis due to jugular thrombosis
- Herd "outbreaks" have occurred in two groups of yearlings and weanlings; 11% and 15%, respectively, of affected animals had some degree of retinal detachment acutely or over time. Detachment was bilaterally complete in several animals (see Color Plate 10). Affected horses need repeated fundus examinations for 12-18 months.

Diagnosis
- Results of complete ocular examination before and after complete mydriasis may necessitate referral to an ophthalmologist:
  - Careful slit biomicroscopic examination

    A fine fibrinous membrane often is apparent on the endothelial surface of the affected area

    Fine endothelial cellular precipitates and small keratic precipitates in affected area

    Acute demarcation between edematous and normal cornea (cellular precipitates and keratic precipitates stop abruptly and distinctly at the edema margins)

    Patients with chronic cases have fibrosis of the Descemet's membrane and endothelium.

  - Peripheral indirect fundus examination with scleral depression (if possible)
  - Ocular ultrasonography, especially if the cornea is opaque.
  - Bullous keratopathy (subepithelial "water blisters") may be present at the initial examination or may develop later. These lesions may stain positively with fluorescein.
- Complete physical examination
- Serum and aqueous samples for equine herpesvirus (EHV), leptospirosis, and equine viral arteritis (EVA) analysis
- If enucleation becomes necessary, the eyes should be submitted to a veterinary ophthalmic pathologist for evaluation.

Medical Treatment
- Can be extremely unrewarding if the edema is extensive and severe.
- Mild cases improve in 1-3 weeks.
- *Monitor for corneal ulcer formation* as bullae rupture.
  - Use topical broad-spectrum antibiotics q6-8h because of the likelihood of epithelial slough or bulla rupture.
- Topical corticosteroids are useful **only if** the corneal epithelium is intact and likely to remain so.
  - 1% prednisolone acetate or 0.1% dexamethasone q6h, *not* hydrocortisone
  - Affected horses *frequently* sustain corneal bullae or blisters as the edema accumulates under the tight junctions of the epithelium.
  - *Steroids should be used with extreme caution in this case because they may cause bullae to rupture and turn into ulcers.*
- Topical hyperosmotic agents such as 5% NaCl q4-6h may be used but are of no apparent benefit in some cases.
- Systemic NSAIDs: Standard dosages for 7-10 days
- Topical NSAIDs q8-12h may be beneficial (diclofenac, ketorolac, flurbiprofen) but should not be used if ulcers are present because they can induce melting corneal ulcers (Guidera et al, 2001).
- Systemic antihistamines may be beneficial in rare cases.

Surgical Treatment
- Temporary or split-lid tarsorrhaphy (see p. 443) may be indicated if sizable bullae develop in the cornea.

- Thermokeratoplasty: Meticulous multiple pinpoint thermal cauterization of the affected superficial stroma has been beneficial in some cases but should be performed *only* by a specialist because corneal perforation can occur. The procedure induces adhesions between corneal collagen lamella that may provide stability, reduce lesion thickness, and decrease bullae formation.

Prognosis
- Guarded. Affected horses rarely return to normal but may improve slightly during the first 4-6 weeks.
- Fibrovascular ingrowth from the limbus develops in some cases and reinforces and reorganizes the swollen cornea.

ACUTE HYPHEMA
Etiology
- Trauma, penetrating injuries, uveitis, glaucoma, intraocular neoplasia, retinal detachment, blood dyscrasia, congenital anomalies, and tumors.

Clinical Signs
- Variable: Small amount, or the entire globe may be filled with blood.
- Clotted red blood usually is the result of recent trauma.

Diagnosis
- Complete blood cell count (CBC), chemistry, clotting profile, if the etiologic factor is not apparent or known
- Complete ophthalmic examination of **both** eyes
- Complete physical examination
- Ocular ultrasonography

Treatment
- Controversial at best! Manage the *cause* of the hyphema first then worry about the blood!
- Keep the patient as quiet as possible; tranquilize if necessary; prevent self-trauma.
- Restrict head movement if the patient is cooperative.
- Small hemorrhages usually resolve without treatment.
- Mydriatics.
  □ Prevent synechiae but can occlude drainage angle.
  □ Use 1% atropine q6-8h.
- Miotics.
  □ May facilitate synechiae formation but may increase drainage and expose a larger iris surface to enhance fibrinolysis.
  □ Rarely used.
- Antiinflammatory drugs.
  □ Topical corticosteroids: 0.1% dexamethasone or 1% prednisolone acetate, q4-6h, *not* hydrocortisone
  □ Systemic corticosteroids at standard antiinflammatory dosage
  □ NSAIDs usually are not recommended because they can predispose the patient to rebleeding. NSAIDs are used, however, to manage hyphema secondary to ERU.

- Measure intraocular pressure 2-3 times a day; secondary glaucoma is a common sequela.
  □ Topical β-blockers (e.g., timolol maleate) and carbonic anhydrase inhibitors (dorzolamide) can be used q8-12h if glaucoma develops (CoSopt contains both agents in one bottle).
  □ Surgical intervention usually is contraindicated.
  □ Intracameral (within the anterior chamber of the eye) administration of tissue plasminogen activator can be used as an aid to clot dissolution but has limited effect on large clots.

Prognosis
- Varies depending on the amount of blood and the etiologic factor
- Nonclotted blood may be resorbed in 5-10 days, clotted blood in 15-30 or more days.
- Hyphema occupying more than one-half the anterior chamber has a poor prognosis.
- Recurring hyphema has a poor prognosis.
- Possible sequelae include synechiae, cataracts, blindness, glaucoma, and phthisis bulbi.

LENS LUXATION
- Rarely an emergency among horses because most cases are secondary to anterior uveitis (see p. 470).

UVEITIS
- Along with corneal ulcers, uveitis is the most common ocular problem in horses and is the leading cause of blindness. The disorder usually is nongranulomatous anterior uveitis with the inflammation confined to the iris, ciliary body, and anterior and posterior chambers. Some individuals, however, may have primary choroiditis and peripapillary optic neuritis.
- Uveitis can have many causes. Some are obvious, such as trauma, but most remain elusive, as is the case in any species. Equine *recurrent* uveitis (ERU), however, has a *strong* association with previous or current infection with one or more serovars (serotypes) of *Leptospira interrogans.*
- ERU also is called iridocyclitis, moon blindness, and periodic ophthalmia.
- Uveitis most commonly occurs among horses older than 15 years and among Appaloosas.
- Unfortunately, many cases of equine uveitis do not manifest as emergencies when they really are. Rapid and prolonged treatment may prevent future recurrences and tragic long-term sequelae.
- The horse's uveal tissue has a profound ability to become inflamed after seemingly mild ocular insults. This, combined with the uveitic syndrome among horses that occurs after *Leptospira* infection, makes this group of diseases a therapeutic challenge.
- The risk of loss of vision due to uveitis is high. Sight is reduced in the acute period, and sight-threatening sequelae of inflammation are common. The sequelae include:
  □ Corneal decompensation and edema

- ☐ Glaucoma
- ☐ Cataracts
- ☐ Vitreal opacities, hemorrhage, and liquefaction
- ☐ Retinal detachment
- In many cases the eye being examined in an "emergency" has likely had subclinical disease for days to weeks; therefore treatment results are poorer than expected.
- ➤ ■ *All* cases necessitate aggressive initial therapy (q1-2h topically); therefore, use of a transpalpebral lavage system (see p. 117) may be beneficial.

Etiology

- The most common known causative agent is *Leptospira* organisms.
- Any number of bacterial agents that cause septicemia can cause uveitis (e.g., *Rhodococcus equi, Salmonella,* and *Escherichia coli*), as can borreliosis, intraocular parasites, and some viruses (EHV, EVA, influenza).
  - ☐ Most common in neonatal foals and usually is bilateral
- Trauma
- Immune mediated
- Lens induced
- Neoplasia, particularly lymphosarcoma

Clinical Signs

- **Examine *both* eyes!**
- Complete examination often necessitates heavy sedation, eyelid akinesia, topical anesthesia, and pupil dilation.

ACUTE SIGNS

- Pain, lacrimation, blepharospasm, photophobia
- Hyperemia of the conjunctiva and scleral vascular engorgement
- Intraocular pressure is reduced (<15 mm Hg)
- Corneal changes
  - ☐ Edema: Mild and focal to severe and diffuse
  - ☐ Keratic precipitates may be present on the endothelial surface (whitish dots coalescing to greasy yellowish-white plaques)
  - ☐ May have early corneal vascular ingrowth from the limbus
- Anterior chamber findings
  - ☐ *Aqueous flare is a hallmark of anterior uveitis!*

  Flare results from the presence of protein and cells in the normal hypocellular and protein-poor aqueous humor. Flare usually is subtle and is assessed in a *totally dark room* with a *focal dot or slit of light directed into the eye at an angle* from the examiner's line of view.
  More severe cases have fibrin, hypopyon, or hyphema in the anterior chamber.

  - ☐ Pupil
    - ☐ *Miotic!*
    - ☐ Dilates slowly, if at all, with 1% tropicamide
  - ☐ Iris changes
  May be swollen with loss of the fine surface architecture of the normal iris
  The iris color may be dulled to profoundly abnormal in light-colored irises (blue irises turn yellowish-green).

Corpora nigra may be swollen with rounded, rather than normal, spiculated, contours.

The iris is slow to respond to mydriatic agents.

□ Fundus findings: The fundus is often poorly seen because of anterior segment inflammation.

Examination is facilitated by the use of indirect ophthalmoscopy, which is much more effective in penetrating hazy media.

The vitreous humor contains cellular infiltrate, liquefaction, and "floaters."

Possible choroiditis, retinal edema, and focal to diffuse nonrhegmatogenous retinal detachment

Peripapillary yellowish "rays" of retinal detachment are seen in many cases

CHRONIC SIGNS

- Corneal changes
  □ Diffuse edema, fibrosis
  □ Fibrovascular ingrowth from the limbus, focal or diffuse
  □ Focal to multifocal superficial erosions
  □ Iris changes if glaucoma has occurred
- Iris changes
  □ Posterior synechia: Focal to diffuse with resultant dyscoria (abnormality of the shape of the pupil)
  □ Loss of corpora nigra
  □ Hyperpigmented (some patients have chronic depigmentation)
  □ Preiridal fibrous membrane
  □ Abnormal surface neovascular changes (rubeosis iridis) in some instances
- Lens changes
  □ Cataract
  □ Lens luxation
- Other findings possible
  □ Complete vitreal liquefaction
  □ Secondary glaucoma
  □ Retinal detachment with or without vitreous degeneration and traction bands
  □ Retinal and optic nerve degeneration and atrophy
  □ Blindness
  □ Phthisis bulbi

Diagnosis

- CBC and chemistry profile
- Serologic assays with paired samples if possible
  □ Leptospirosis titers: Serovars *pomona, bratislava, autumnalis grippotyphosa, hardjo, icterohaemorrhagiae, canicola* and as many others as the laboratory can test.

  Results may be difficult to interpret because many horses have positive titers and no clinical disease.

  □ Borreliosis
  □ Brucellosis
  □ Toxoplasmosis
  □ Others

- Conjunctival biopsy if *Onchocerca* infestation is suspected (rare).
- Aqueous and vitreous samples may be of great value for serologic assay, polymerase chain reaction analysis, dark-field analysis, and culture.

Treatment

- Aggressive, prolonged medical management of acute uveitis reduces the incidence of secondary complications. Treatment should *not* be discontinued prematurely but should continue on a tapering schedule for 4-6 weeks *beyond the time when there is no evidence of aqueous flare and the eye looks normal.* Lifelong treatment may be necessary.
- Chronically painful, blind eyes should be enucleated, or an evisceration-implant procedure should be performed.
- *Manage the cause, if known! The cause is usually not discovered in cases of ERU.*

Medications: One from Each Category during Acute Flare-ups
CORTICOSTEROIDS

- Topically, subconjunctivally, or systemically, corticosteroids are the basis of therapy in most cases if *no* corneal ulcer is present (systemic corticosteroids may be used in the presence of a corneal ulcer).
- Topical 1% prednisolone acetate (*not* succinate) solution is the steroid of choice; 0.1% dexamethasone ointment also is highly effective. Hydrocortisone is *not* effective.
  - Either medication is administered q1-4h in the acute period and tapered *slowly* over weeks or months as signs diminish.
  - Subconjunctival steroids administered under the *bulbar* conjunctiva (*not* palpebral conjunctiva) may be used but *only* when the cornea is healthy, not currently ulcerated or with irregular epithelium (ulcer may be imminent). They do *not* substitute for topical agents but merely supplement them.

  Methylprednisolone acetate, 10 to 30 mg every 2 weeks.
  Triamcinolone, 10 to 20 mg every 2 weeks, used with caution because it can cause laminitis.

- Systemic corticosteroids can be used at standard antiinflammatory dosages but *not in conjunction with systemic NSAIDs.*

MYDRIATIC AGENTS

- Topical 1% atropine solution is the preferred mydriatic.
  - 1-2 drops or a small spray q6-8h to effect (every few hours in acute flare-ups to every few days as inflammation subsides)
  - Monitor for colic (see pp. 188, 456).
- Tropicamide (Mydriacyl) can be used q2-3h
- 2.5%-10% phenylephrine can be added (atropine therapy is maintained) if the pupil does not dilate. This therapy is of questionable efficacy in the care of equine patients.

TOPICAL NSAIDS

- Flurbiprofen, diclofenac, and ketorolac are available in any human pharmacy.
- These agents seem to be very beneficial in some cases and of no apparent benefit in others.

- May be the only antiinflammatory option if the corneal integrity is in question, precluding the use of topical corticosteroids. NSAIDs should be used with caution because they can induce melting corneal ulcer (Guidera et al, 2001).
- May be used in combination with topical corticosteroids

CYCLOSPORINE
- Cyclosporine q8-12h may be useful in some cases but is of no benefit in others. Intraocular penetration after topical administration is poor, but some clinicians report that the drug does seem to decrease recurrences. However, this is generally not the clinical experience of others. The drug is no longer commercially available in ophthalmic formulation.

SYSTEMIC NSAIDS
- Phenylbutazone, 2.2-4.4 mg/kg *or*
- Flunixin meglumine, 0.5-1.0 mg/kg, not longer than 1-2 weeks. This is the drug of choice to use in all acute cases.
- Aspirin, 20-25 mg/kg per day PO. This is a good choice for long-term maintenance *not* for acute flare-ups.

Continue all medications 10-14 days *beyond the time when clinical signs have resolved*, and only then begin a slow taper. Continue topical corticosteroids q12h for 4-6 additional weeks. Before discontinuing them, carefully examine the eye for signs of uveitis and then reexamine them weekly for 1 month. Advise the owner to examine the eye daily with a penlight for signs of inflammation (redness, mild cloudiness, miosis in dim light) and to request reexamination immediately if abnormalities develop.

SYSTEMIC ANTIBIOTICS
- Should be administered in all cases of uveitis secondary to systemic disease and in any case suspected to be associated with *Leptospira* infection.

EXPERIMENTAL TREATMENTS
- Intravitreal, subconjunctival, or subscleral implantation of slow-release cyclosporine devices has been reported to be beneficial (Gilger et al, 2000) as has pars plana vitrectomy (Fruhauf et al, 1998). Refer to these references for additional information.

GLAUCOMA
Acute, primary glaucoma is rare among horses, but it does occur. Most cases of glaucoma are chronic, insidious sequelae of ERU. Glaucoma and ERU are most common among horses older than 15 years and specifically Appaloosas.

Etiology
Most cases are secondary glaucoma associated with:

- Chronic ERU (anterior uveitis, moon blindness, iridocyclitis) possibly because of:
  - Filtration angle obstruction by inflammatory debris
  - Angle fibrosis
  - Angle collapse (from iris bombe, chronic inflammation, and adhesions)
  - Postinflammatory fibrovascular pupil obstruction or obstruction of iris absorption of aqueous humor

□ Posterior synechiae
- Trauma
- Acute anterior displacement of a luxated lens (the usual cause of lens luxation is trauma or chronic uveitis)
- Anterior vitreal prolapse
- Tumors

Clinical Signs
- *Elevated intraocular pressure is the hallmark of the disease!*
  □ Pressure should be assessed by means of applanation tonometry (Tonopen, widely available in the United States). Normal value: 15 to 28 mm Hg with Tonopen. The examination should be performed before auriculopalpebral nerve block and sedation if possible.
  □ Refer if necessary.
- Other signs vary. In many cases the disease is not diagnosed until it is chronic, acute clinical signs having been absent or missed.
- Sight is variable. Horses can continue to see for a protracted period after the onset of elevated intraocular pressure (IOP). This is unlike dogs, who usually lose their sight after 36-48 hours of elevated IOP.
- Pain is variable. Some individuals seem normal, whereas others manifest exquisite pain.
- Lacrimation, photophobia, blepharospasm, and small convulsive jerking movements of the head during rest may be present or absent.
- Hyperemia of the conjunctiva and episcleral vein engorgement are occasionally present but not to the degree seen in canines.
- Corneal changes:
  □ Edema: Mild, focal to severe, diffuse
  □ Linear white lines or bands of mild to moderate edema traversing the cornea or branching in any direction. These striae usually are a *chronic* change caused by breaks in Descemet's membrane and disruption of adjacent endothelial cell function.
  □ Focal to diffuse superficial ulcers if corneal edema is severe
- Pupil
  □ Midposition to slightly dilated but may be normal
  □ Slowly responsive to unresponsive to bright light stimulus
  □ Be sure to check direct and indirect responses to light.
- Iris
  □ Normal in an acute, primary case (rare)
  □ Usually an abnormal dark chocolate brown or a darker color than normal for the eye (a change caused by uveitis)
  □ Corpora nigra absent or abnormally smooth in contour because of previous bouts of inflammation and fibrosis
- Lens
  □ If glaucoma is secondary to anterior lens luxation the lens (often cataractous) is readily seen in the anterior chamber. If corneal edema prevents examination of the anterior chamber, ultrasound examination is indicated.
  □ Posterior lens luxation can occur.
- Fundus
  □ Optic and retinal atrophy may be present.

- □ Optic nerve cupping is variably present.
- The eye may be slightly to grossly enlarged (buphthalmic, hydrophthalmic). This is a chronic sign.

Diagnosis
- Measure the intraocular pressure by means of applanation.
  - □ The patient is tranquilized, and topical anesthetic is applied to both eyes.
  - □ The eyelids are held open with *pressure on the bony rim.* Make sure that finger pressure is *not* transmitted to the globe.
  - □ Normal intraocular pressure for a horse is approximately 15 25 mm Hg.
- If tonometry is not available, gross assessment of intraocular pressure is made by means of gently rocking the index and middle fingers alternately back and forth on the dorsal portion of the globe, through the closed eyelid. Use the patient's other eye or the examiner's eye as a control. In these cases, immediate referral to a specialist for confirmation is recommended.

Treatment
- The insidious nature of glaucoma among horses means that many cases are hopeless from the onset, and treatment is often unrewarding.
- The condition frequently slowly progresses despite medical treatment.
- Medical management: *Aggressive medical management should be reserved for eyes that **still have vision.*** Individuals with acute disease, and some with chronic disease, may show improvement in the short term.
- Choose one drug per category:
  - ◻ Topical *corticosteroids* (0.1% dexamethasone or 1% prednisolone acetate) q4-6h. The cornea is stained before therapy. Topical corticosteroids generally are not used if there is evidence of corneal epithelial loss.
  - □ Ophthalmic β-*adrenergic antagonists* such as timolol maleate, 1-2 drops of 0.5% solution q12h or in combination with topical carbonic anhydrase inhibitors (CoSopt) q12h
  - ◻ Oral carbonic inhibitors (acetazolamide, 1-3 mg/kg PO q6h). Monitor serum K+ level during treatment.
  - □ 1% atropine, q6-8h, then to effect.
    - □ Contraindicated in most species, but in the care of horses, atropine is a mainstay of glaucoma therapy.
    - ◻ Enhances uveoscleral outflow of aqueous humor and is beneficial in most cases; however, *measure IOP q12h in the first few days of treatment.* A few patients have pressure spikes during atropine treatment.
    - □ Contraindicated if anterior lens luxation is present.
  - □ Systemic NSAIDs at standard doses.
- Surgical management.
  - □ Referral to specialists for laser cycloablation or cryocycloablation. Reserve these procedures for sighted eyes.
  - □ Either procedure works well in some cases and can provide good, long-term control of IOP.
  - □ Unfortunately, many cases have dramatic postoperative elevations in IOP that destroy any remaining vision.
  - □ Blind eyes should be enucleated, or an intraocular silicone prosthesis should be implanted.

REFERENCES

Andrew SE, Brooks DE, Smith PJ et al: Posterior lamellar keratoplasty for treatment of deep stromal abscesses in nine horses, *Vet Ophthalmol* 3:99-103, 2000.

Andrew SE, Brooks DE, Biros DJ et al: Equine ulcerative keratomycosis: visual outcome and ocular survival in 39 cases, *Equine Vet J* 30:109-116, 1998.

Faber NA. Detection of Leptospira spp in the aqueous humor of horses with naturally acquired recurrent uveitis, *J Clin Microbiol* 38:2731-2733, 2000.

Fruhauf B et al: Surgical management of equine recurrent uveitis with single port pars plana vitrectomy, *Vet Ophthalmol* 1:137-151, 1998.

Gilger BC et al: Long-term effect on the equine eye of an intravitreal device used for sustained release of cyclosporine, *Vet Ophthalmol* 3:105-110, 2000.

Grahn BH, Cullen CL: Equine phacoclastic uveitis: the clinical manifestations, light microscopic findings, and therapy of 7 cases, *Can Vet J* 41:376-382, 2000.

Guidera AC, Luchs JI, Udell IJ: Keratitis, ulceration, and perforation associated with topical nonsteroidal antiinflammatory drugs, *Ophthalmology* 108: 936-944, 2001.

Matthews AG: Nonulcerative keratopathies in the horse, *Equine Vet Educ* 12:271-278, 2000 (tutorial article).

Romeike A, Brugmann M, Drommer W: Immunohistochemical studies in equine recurrent uveitis (ERU), *Vet Pathol* 35:515-526, 1998.

Wollanke, B, Rohrbach BW, Gerhards H. Serum and vitreous humor antibody titers in and isolation of *Leptospira interrogans* from horses with recurrent uveitis, *J Am Vet Med Assoc* 219:795-799, 2001.

---

42 Reproductive System

Robert B. Hillman, James A. Orsini, Thomas J. Divers, and Donald H. Schlafer

STALLION BREEDING INJURIES
Paraphimosis

The inability to retract the penis into the sheath occurs most frequently after trauma sustained while the stallion is attempting to breed an uncooperative mare. Other factors that result in paraphimosis include:

- Large lesions of the glans penis
- Edema of the prepuce after castration
- Myelitis
- Spinal injuries
- Viral infection
- Physical exhaustion
- Inanition
- Paralysis of the retractor muscles after tranquilization

Physical examination includes evaluation of the sensation of the penis and prepuce and of the stallion's ability to move the penis. Institute therapy as soon as possible to limit formation of edema, cellulitis, hematoma, thrombosis, and gangrenous necrosis of dependent structures.

Treatment
- Manage the inciting cause when possible.
- Prevent further trauma to the penis and prepuce.

REPRODUCTIVE

- □ Clean the penis and prepuce with mild disinfectants, rinse, and dry thoroughly by blotting gently with nonirritating substance.
- □ Liberally apply a lanolin-based antibiotic cream to the entire penis and prepuce. Petroleum jelly also can be used. Repeat cleaning and local treatment daily.
- □ Avoid exposure to freezing temperatures because edematous tissues are highly susceptible to additional damage by frostbite.
- Reduce swelling:
  - □ With acute trauma, use cooling techniques (e.g., cold water showers, applying a plastic sleeve filled with crushed ice or snow).
  - □ After the acute phase, gently massage with alternating cold and hot showers. Consider placing an air splint on the distal end of the penis and inflating it for a maximum of 15-20 minutes.
  - □ Swelling also can be reduced by covering the penis with an elastic bandage beginning at the distal end of the penis and wrapping proximally. The bandage is left in place for 15-20 minutes.
- Administer nonsteroidal antiinflammatory drugs (NSAIDs):
  - □ Flunixin meglumine, 1 mg/kg IV or IM q12-24h
  - □ Phenylbutazone, 2.2 mg/kg PO q12-24h
- Administer prophylactic antibiotics to prevent infection and abscess formation. Use either:
  - □ A combination of potassium penicillin, 22,000 U/kg IV q6h

or

Procaine penicillin, 22,000 U/kg IM q12h

and

Gentamicin, 6.6 mg/kg IV or IM q24h (Use gentamicin only if creatinine concentration is normal, stallion is urinating, and hydration is assured.)

  - □ Ceftiofur, 3.0 mg/kg IV or IM q12h
- Administer a diuretic:
  - □ Furosemide, 1 mg/kg IM
- Provide support:
  - □ Support of the penis and prepuce is very important to avoid additional vascular impairment and increased edema. Place a support around the penis and prepuce to hold the penis in the sheath.
  - □ Use nylon mesh attached by rubber tubing or gauze (Fig. 42–1). This material allows urination without retaining moisture and does not chafe the skin.
- Daily cleaning and treatment of the penis and sheath, combined with massage, are required.
- Once the swelling is reduced sufficiently to return the penis to the prepuce, retain the penis with a purse-string suture at the preputial orifice, or fabricate a retention device from a 500-ml narrow-neck plastic bottle.
  - □ Remove the bottom of the plastic bottle, pad the edges with tape, and place the bottle over the end of the penis with the urethral process at the neck of the bottle.
  - □ Hold the bottle in place with rubber tubing or gauze attached to the neck and tied in a pattern similar to that used for the nylon mesh.

Penile Hematoma

Most hematomas are caused by damage to the erect penis by direct kicks from unreceptive mares or trauma during collection. Superficial vessels of the penis and

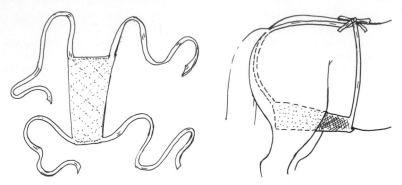

FIGURE 42-1. Support placed around the penis and prepuce to hold the penis in the sheath.

prepuce or, less commonly, small leaks in the corpus cavernosum are the source of the hematoma.

► Swelling may be rapidly progressive and can result in paraphimosis.

Treatment

Early treatment is important to prevent permanent dysfunction.

- Control swelling
  - □ Ice packs or cold hydrotherapy for at least 30 minutes a minimum of three times daily
- Antibiotics for 7-10 days. Use either:
  - □ A combination of potassium penicillin, 22,000 U/kg IV q6h

or
Procaine penicillin, 22,000 U/kg IM q12h
and
Gentamicin, 6.6 mg/kg IV or IM q24h (use gentamicin only if creatinine concentration is normal, stallion is urinating, and hydration is assured)

  - □ Ceftiofur, 3.0 mg/kg IV/IM q12h
- NSAIDs
  - □ Flunixin meglumine, 1 mg/kg IV or IM q12-24h
  - □ Phenylbutazone, 2.2 mg/kg PO q12-24h
- Diuretics
  - □ Furosemide, 1 mg/kg IM according to circumstances (PRN)
- Supportive care of the penis and prepuce
  - □ See earlier, Paraphimosis.
  - □ Check frequently.
  - □ Clean and lubricate often.
- Management
  - □ Keep the stallion isolated from any exposure to mares in estrus.
- Surgery
  - □ If vessels have to be ligated or if the tunics of the penis are ruptured (recognized by continued enlargement of the hematoma), refer to a surgical facility for repair as soon as possible.

□ In less complicated cases, delay surgery for 7-10 days to allow the hematoma to organize.

Prognosis

Early and appropriate therapy is critical to prevent secondary reproductive dysfunction, such as fibrosis that can cause deviation of the penis, thermal damage to the testes, nerve damage, or paraphimosis. The prognosis for return to function is better assessed after 3 weeks of rest by exposing the stallion to a mare and performing a complete reproductive examination.

Paralysis of the Retractor Muscle after Tranquilization
Treatment

- Administer 8 mg/450 kg benztropine mesylate (Cogentin) IV slowly as soon as possible after the causative drug, and immediately institute conservative therapy as described earlier.

Large Lesions of the Glans Penis

- Carcinoma of the penis usually requires referral for phallectomy.
- Cutaneous habronemiasis occurs primarily in warm months as granulomatous growths on the urethral process, but they can involve the glans, prepuce, and scrotum. Biopsy is needed to confirm this diagnosis and to eliminate the possibility of a more serious primary lesion, such as squamous cell carcinoma. Oral administration of ivermectin, 0.2 mg/kg, and corticosteroids, dexamethasone powder, 5 mg/450 kg PO, often results in rapid reduction in the size of the lesion. Supportive therapy as described earlier is indicated.

Paraphimosis Secondary to Inanition or Debility

- Provide dietary supplementation and perform a complete physical examination to eliminate the other causes of hypoproteinemia (parasitism, bad teeth, chronic disease).
- Maintain supportive therapy, combined with mild exercise, for a long period until the edematous swelling of the penis and prepuce is resolved and the penis returns to its normal position.
- Protect the individual from exposure to freezing temperatures to prevent additional damage.

Penile dysfunction is a common sequela. Treatment failure leaves the penis insensitive and cold to the touch. Thrombi form within the cavernous spaces, and the tissues fibrose. These tissues are prone to continued trauma and excoriation if left untreated. If the paraphimosis is permanent, refer the patient for phallopexy after castration.

NOTE: Continued service of some stallions has been accomplished through conscientious supportive care and retraining the stallion to ejaculate with manual assistance or the modified use of an artificial vagina. This is not appropriate treatment of all affected stallions. To be successful, the stallion must possess appropriate breeding behavior and penile sensation, and all personnel must be dedicated to the care, handling, and retraining of the stallion.

Prognosis

Varies with the initiating cause but is generally regarded as poor to fair.

OTHER REPRODUCTIVE INJURIES
Ruptured Corpus Spongiosum

The corpus spongiosum is rarely damaged in a breeding stallion housed alone but can be injured by kicks sustained a few centimeters below the anus in stallions that are turned out with a band of mares or other horses. Hematoma formation in this area can have disastrous complications, including obstruction of the urethra, with consequent rupture of the urinary bladder and death.

Diagnosis

- Based on history of trauma to the region and identification of the hematoma, which is evident as a painful, fluctuant swelling below the anus.
- Investigate integrity of the bladder by means of rectal examination if the patient tolerates it, but this procedure often is quite painful. If examination is not possible, use abdominocentesis to diagnose uroperitoneum following rupture of the urinary bladder (see Chapter 44, p. 536).
- Catheterization often is difficult because it is painful to pass the catheter beyond the hematoma.

Treatment

- Administer immediate therapy for controlling inflammation and preventing potentially fatal sequelae while stabilizing the patient for transport to a referral surgery center.
- Antiinflammatory drugs:
  - Corticosteroid: Dexamethasone, 0.05-2.0 mg/kg IV
  - Flunixin meglumine, 1 mg/kg IV q12-24h, provides analgesia as well.
- Hydrotherapy
  - Ice packs or cold water hosing for a minimum of 30 minutes at a time.

Prognosis

Poor for return to service.

Abrasions and Lacerations

Trauma to the skin of the penis and prepuce can be caused by mare tail hairs, breeding stitches, stallion rings, artificial vaginas, kicks, whips, or lead ropes that strike an erect penis (as in disciplining of show and racing stallions to discourage arousal at inappropriate times) or by breeding mares through a wire fence. Because of the vascularity of this region, open wounds in the penis and prepuce bleed profusely.

▶ *As with other traumatic injuries to the penis and prepuce, early treatment is essential to prevent sequelae that can interfere with reproductive performance.*

Diagnosis

- Perform a careful physical examination; this involves thoroughly cleaning the wound to recognize involved structures.
- Identify subtle lesions that may interfere with breeding performance or precipitate more serious problems (e.g., trauma involving the urethra, inflammation near the scrotum).

Treatment

- Clean the wound gently to remove debris and blood, rinse, and dry thoroughly.
- Apply a lanolin-based cream with an antibiotic such as tetracycline to the entire penis to prevent dryness and infection.
- Reduce swelling.
  □ Low-pressure cold hydrotherapy
  □ Ice packs
- Support the penis and prepuce as soon as possible if paraphimosis develops (see paraphimosis, p. 472).

Testicular Trauma

- Thermal damage to spermatogenic cells within the testicles is an added complication of testicular injury.
- Emergency care is to manage the primary injury and protect the testicular parenchyma from inflammatory hyperthermia and subsequent testicular degeneration and atrophy.
- As with trauma to other external genitalia, testicular trauma can result in paraphimosis.

Diagnosis
PHYSICAL EXAMINATION
- Unilateral or bilateral heat, pain, or swelling (swelling may be minimal because the tunica albuginea is not elastic)

ULTRASONOGRAPHY
- May identify hematoma formation (anechoic or hypoechoic regions) or fibrosis (hyperechoic) that indicates previous injury

Treatment
- Reduce swelling with ice packs or cold hydrotherapy.
- Antiinflammatory drugs:
  □ Flunixin meglumine, 1 mg/kg IV or IM q12-24h
- Antibiotics, use either:
  □ A combination of potassium penicillin, 22,000 U/kg IV q6h

or
Procaine penicillin, 22,000 U/kg IM q12h
and
Gentamicin, 6.6 mg/kg IV or IM q24h (use gentamicin only if creatinine concentration is normal, stallion is urinating, and hydration is assured)

  □ Ceftiofur, 3.0 mg/kg IV/IM q12h
- Prophylactic hemicastration to protect the unaffected testicle in unilateral injuries.
- Sexual rest for a minimum of 3-6 weeks.

POSTCASTRATION COMPLICATIONS
Immediate Complications
Hemorrhage
ETIOLOGY
- Improperly applied emasculator

- *Reversing emasculator*
- Testicular vessels insufficiently crushed because scrotal skin included in emasculator

SIGNS
- Blood dripping for several minutes after surgery is not unusual.

| **CAUTION:** Continuous bleeding for 15-30 minutes.

- Testicular artery is the usual source.

TREATMENT
- Hold *anesthetized* cord and reapply crushing forceps or emasculator.
- Reanesthetize patient, if needed, to crush end of cord safely.
- Tightly pack sterile gauze into the inguinal canal, and close the scrotum with sutures or towel clamps.
- *Leave packing in place for a minimum of 24 hours.*
- Topical coagulants are of uncertain value and are not recommended.

Evisceration

- *Uncommon, possibly fatal.*
- Standardbreds and Tennessee Walking Horses are more commonly affected.
- Generally occurs within hours after castration but can occur days later.
- *Immediately anesthetize* to minimize contamination and damage to prolapsed intestine.
- Administer intravenous fluids, hypertonic saline solution, 4 ml/kg IV, to minimize hypotension.
- Clean, irrigate, and replace prolapsed intestine.
- Ligate spermatic cord and vaginal tunic proximally.
- Close superficial inguinal ring or pack it with sterile gauze for 24-48 hours.
- Start parenteral administration of broad-spectrum antimicrobial agents and fluid therapy along with NSAIDs.
- Refer to surgical facility if resection of devitalized intestine is needed.
- Prolapse of the greater omentum through the scrotal incision after castration generally is not an immediate emergency but signals potential evisceration.

Delayed Complications

- Edema is the most common complication
  - □ Treatment: Open the incision, begin hydrotherapy and antimicrobial agents
- Funiculitis: Inflammation of the spermatic cord
- Infection: *Clostridium* organisms
- Peritonitis
- Penile injury
- Hydrocele

MARE REPRODUCTIVE EMERGENCIES: DYSTOCIA

Because of severe abdominal press (straining) and early detachment of the placenta, dystocia in a mare is life-threatening for both the mare and the fetus and requires immediate obstetric assistance. Before the arrival of the obstetrician, advise the owner to keep the mare walking to reduce straining. Placing a nasogastric tube in the trachea so the glottis cannot close also reduces the ability of the mare to generate an abdominal press.

Perform obstetric manipulations in an area large enough to allow a thorough examination and management of corrective maneuvers to a standing or recumbent mare.

▶ | **NOTE:** Avoid use of stocks if possible. Restraint should be the minimum required to ensure the safety of the clinician while not alarming the mare. Frequently, a holder standing at the head on the same side as the obstetrician is all that is required. A nose twitch can be used if necessary. In rare instances, use of a rope side line may be indicated to control the mare's rear legs, but the danger exists of the mare becoming entangled. Use drugs (tranquilizers or anesthetics) with *caution* if the fetus is alive, because they sedate the fetus and the mare.

Obtain a complete history while disinfecting the perineal region and performing a genital examination.

▶ Remember: *Be clean, be gentle, and use lots of lubrication!*

Treatment

Once a diagnosis is made and a plan of action formulated, it may be necessary to administer epidural anesthesia, 2% lidocaine, 5-8 ml (see Chapter 33, p. 125). If the required manipulation is simple, do not perform epidural anesthesia because the mare can assist the delivery once the corrective action is performed. Nearly all manipulations to correct the abnormalities in presentation, posture, or position necessitate some repulsion of the fetus to gain working room. Standing the mare with her hindquarters elevated assists corrections.

- Reduce straining by:
  - Keeping the mare walking (but this complicates manipulations)
  - Placing a nasogastric tube in the trachea
  - Pulling out the tongue to prevent closing the glottis, or
  - Administering epidural anesthesia
- If initial manipulations are unsuccessful, induce general anesthesia with xylazine, 0.5-1.0 mg/kg, and ketamine, 2.2 mg/kg, to stop the straining, and allow elevation of the rear quarters to provide more room for repositioning of the fetus.
- While the mare is anesthetized, a hoist may be used to elevate the rear quarters. If this is to occur:
  - Insert an intravenous catheter and administer guaifenesin (formerly called glyceryl guaiacolate), 100 mg/kg IV total, as a 5% solution, 50 g/L, to prevent struggling.
  - After administering the guaifenesin, monitor respiratory and cardiac effects closely because of the weight of the pregnant mare's organs on her diaphragm.
- If practical, administer oxygen intranasally to the mare at 15 L/min (see Chapter 12, p. 64). If the foal's head is in the pelvis, oxygen can be administered to the foal as long as doing so does not impede manipulations to deliver.

Common Causes of Dystocia and Corrective Measures
Fetotomy equipment should be up-to-date and in good repair
- Thygesen fetotome

- Wire saw
- Wire saw sounding wire
- Wire saw leader
- Handgrips for the wire saw
- Double-jointed Krey Schottler hook
- Obstetric snare
- Eye hooks
- Three obstetric chains (60 inches [150 cm])
- Obstetric chain handles
- Lubricant (J-lube), stomach pump, and nasogastric tube

RETENTION OF HEAD AND NECK
- Secure the head with eye hooks (dead foal only) or a head snare before repelling the body to allow for more room to extend the head and neck.
- If repositioning is unsuccessful and a live fetus exists, cesarean section is indicated.
- If the fetus is dead, partial fetotomy (transection of the neck) saves time and reduces trauma resulting from extensive manipulation.

CARPAL FLEXION
- Repel the fetus and extend the leg while pushing the carpus in a dorsolateral direction and bringing the flexed fetlock in a ventral and medial direction, guarding the hoof to prevent uterine trauma.
- If the fetus is dead, it may be less traumatic and more time saving to perform a partial fetotomy (transect the leg through the carpus, leaving part of the carpus on the forearm to allow putting on of chains for traction).

SHOULDER FLEXION
- Elevate the shoulder to produce carpal flexion and proceed as described earlier. This maneuver is difficult, so if both legs are involved and the fetus is alive, cesarean section is indicated if the correction cannot be accomplished after anesthetizing the mare and lifting the hindquarters.

FOOT-NAPE POSTURE
- Can result in third-degree perineal laceration if not corrected as the leg extends dorsally when the elbow contacts the pelvic brim as the mare strains.
- Repel the fetus, shift the legs to a position under the head, and apply traction.

FLEXED HOCK POSITION
- Repel the fetus, push the hock in the dorsolateral direction while bringing the flexed fetlock in a medioventral direction, guarding the hoof and extend the leg. Repeat on second leg and apply traction.
- If the fetus is dead, partial fetotomy (cutting through the hock just below the point of the hock) usually saves time and injury to the reproductive tract.

BREECH POSITION (BILATERAL HIP FLEXION)
- Repel the fetus and position the legs in a bilateral flexed hock position and proceed as described earlier. Completely extending one leg before flexing both hocks allows the fetus to enter the mare's pelvic canal , making it very difficult to flex the second hock.

TRANSVERSE PRESENTATION

- If the fetus is alive, cesarean section is advised.
- With a small fetus in a dorsotransverse position (back of fetus presented to the cervix), it may be possible to repel the anterior portion of the fetus and grasp the base of the tail to produce a bilateral flexed hip position and proceed as described earlier.
- A transverse ventral presentation is best resolved with cesarean section. Must be differentiated from twins.

TWINS

- The presence of twins must be differentiated from a transverse ventral presentation, which can be difficult, because the clinician may not be able to reach far enough to touch the abdomen.
- Repel one foal while extracting the other one. If both continue to pull into the pelvis, suspect a transverse presentation. Check the orientation of the feet.

Notes on Fetotomy

- Fetotomy is indicated if the fetus is dead and the procedure results in reduction of time, effort, and trauma during delivery. Fetotomy in horses is complicated by the mare's strong tenesmus and the fragile nature of the equine reproductive tract. The procedure is best performed by an experienced clinician using specialized equipment. Extensive or prolonged fetotomy frequently causes injury to the cervix or uterus that results in subfertility or infertility.
- The mare should be well restrained with the hindquarters elevated. Epidural anesthesia should be administered to diminish abdominal straining (see p. 125). Tranquilizing the mare with a combination of xylazine, 0.15 mg/kg, and acepromazine, 0.04 mg/kg IV, decreases contractions.
- Make transverse and oblique cuts by introducing the head of the fully threaded fetotome to its desired position in the dorsum of the genital tract and then advancing the wire around the part to be removed. Make cuts keeping the head of the fetotome in the hollow of the hand and maintaining finger contact with the fetus at all times.
- Keep the number of incisions to the minimum needed to deliver the fetus without extensive trauma to the mare's reproductive tract.
- Transect flexed extremities through the joints (avoid cutting long bones) by advancing the wire from a partially threaded fetotome with a wire saw leader around the limb or neck. Slide the wire saw through the second tube of the fetotome, and adapt the fetotome to the fetal part to be sectioned. Solid fixation is important. It is necessary to cut through the flexed joint, leaving part of the carpus or tarsus on the fetus so that traction can be applied without the chains slipping off. Check the wire after each cut to make sure none of the strands is broken, because broken strands can traumatize the endometrium or cause the wire saw to break during subsequent cuts. Minimize entrance to and maneuvering in the genital tract to the minimum needed to perform the fetotomy to prevent trauma and contamination. *Remember: Be clean, be gentle, and use lots of lubrication.*

Treatment after Dystocia and Fetotomy

- Involution of the uterus is delayed after fetotomy. Use oxytocin to aid in involution, 20 IU/450-kg mare IV, IM, or SQ q2h.

- Use systemic antibiotics because of the increased incidence of retained placenta and endometritis after fetotomy, particularly if the uterus is atonic. Use either:
  - Potassium penicillin, 22,000 U/kg IV q6h, or procaine penicillin, 22,000 U/kg IM q12h, and gentamicin, 6.6 mg/kg q24h (use gentamicin only if creatinine concentration is normal, mare is urinating, and hydration is normal)

or

  - Ceftiofur, 3.0 mg/kg IV or IM q12h, and metronidazole, 15 mg/kg PO q8h
- Flushing the uterus with 2-4 L of physiologic saline solution and infusing the uterus with a chemotherapeutic agent (e.g., 2.0 g oxytetracycline in 100-200 ml saline solution) is recommended if there is no response to oxytocin.

Postfoaling Colic

Mares frequently exhibit mild colic after delivery of a foal because the uterus contracts to expel the placenta. Walking the mare for 10 minutes or more frequently resolves the problem. If colic persists or becomes more severe, check the mare for a ruptured uterine artery or a gastrointestinal problem, such as ruptured cecum or rupture of another organ.

UTERINE TORSION

- Usually occurs in mares from 8.5 months of gestation to term.
- No known predilections, and often no known cause, can be determined.
- Less than 50% of cases of torsion occur at parturition.

Diagnosis
CLINICAL SIGNS
- Colic in the third trimester
- Discomfort that is mild in most cases and usually is temporarily responsive to analgesics
- Depression, pawing, flank watching, kicking, rolling
- Pain proportional to the degree of torsion and the involvement of the gastrointestinal tract

PHYSICAL EXAMINATION
- Normal to slightly increased temperature, pulse, respirations
- Normal or decreased gastrointestinal sounds

RECTAL EXAMINATION
- Carefully palpate the uterine wall to identify uterine tears or ruptures.
- Carefully palpate other abdominal structures to recognize any concurrent or associated gastrointestinal involvement.
- The broad ligaments are tightly pulled downward on one side.
- Asymmetry of the broad ligaments indicates the direction of the torsion (this often is not easy to determine).
  - Clockwise (from rear): Right tighter than left, left crosses over top of uterus
  - Counterclockwise (from rear): Left tighter than right, right crosses over top of uterus

Nonsurgical Treatment
- Manipulation per vagina at term
  - When diagnosed at term, 80% of cases of uterine torsion can be corrected by vaginal manipulation.

> **CAUTION:** In late gestation with partial torsion, traction applied to the foal can cause uterine rupture that can result in fatal hemorrhage in the mare or peritonitis. *Correct the torsion first!*

  - Keep the mare standing! (*Do not use sedatives;* use epidural anesthesia [see p. 125] to minimize straining.)
  - Elevate the mare's hindquarters (stand her on a ramp or hill).
  - Try to pass through the cervix (if torsion is less than 270 degrees).
  - Manually correct the torsion.

  Grasp the fetus as far in as possible (upper forearm or body).
  Rock back and forth and gain momentum to assist derotation (may have to repeat to complete derotation).

  - After derotation, the mare should spontaneously begin second-stage labor.

  Labor may be delayed because of decreased uterine contractility caused by edema or vascular congestion.
  Induce parturition if necessary with 20-40 IU oxytocin.

- Rolling with plank in the flank (Fig. 42–2.)
  - Can be performed on preterm torsion but should be avoided at term due to the increased risk of uterine rupture.
  - Anesthetize the mare (see Chapter 56, p. 757).

  Drop the mare in lateral recumbency on the side to which the torsion is directed.

  - Place a board (3-4 m long by 20-30 cm wide) across the recumbent mare's upper paralumbar fossa (see Fig. 42–2).
  - Have an assistant kneel on the board.
  - Roll the mare *slowly* to reduce the risk of rupture; for example:

  Diagnosis: Clockwise torsion (torsion is to the right); counterclockwise torsion (torsion is to the left)
  Treatment: Lay the mare down in right lateral recumbency and rotate her clockwise. Lay the mare down in left lateral recumbency and rotate her counterclockwise.

  - Assess progress with successive rectal examinations.
  - Repeat if necessary.

Surgical Treatment
- Although preterm torsion can be surgically corrected on the farm, a mare with torsion diagnosed at term should be referred to a surgical facility as soon as possible because cesarean section may be needed (see colic in the late-term pregnant mare, p. 245).
- Insert a nasotracheal tube to prevent the glottis closure required for abdominal press.

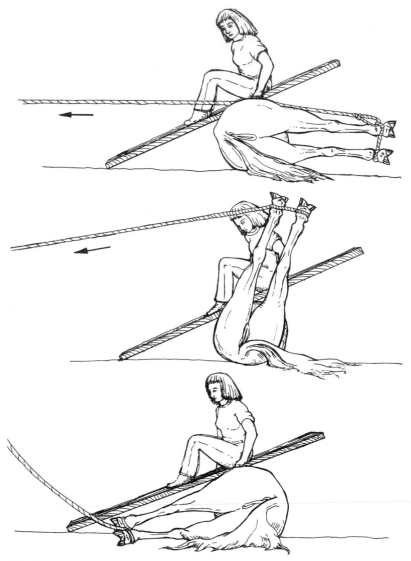

FIGURE 42-2. Rolling with plank on the flank.

- Perform the operation through a flank incision with the mare standing (preferred).
- Make the incision on the side toward which the torsion has occurred, and gently lift the gravid uterus back into normal position.

Prognosis

FOR CURRENT PREGNANCY
- Nonsurgical correction: 85% success rate
- Surgical correction: 73% success rate

COMPLICATIONS
- Premature placental separation that results in death or abortion
- Necrosis and rupture of the uterine wall
- Peritonitis
- Endotoxic shock
- Recurrence of torsion in the same pregnancy

FOR FUTURE PREGNANCIES
- Good for the mare to conceive and carry another pregnancy.
  Worsens with:
  - Cesarean section
  - Uterine rupture
  - Torsion in late gestation
  - Extensive torsion
  - Delay in diagnosis and treatment

Uterine Rupture

- In the peripartum period, uterine rupture is most often caused by mutation or fetotomy
- Earlier in gestation, rupture can be caused by violent intrapartum movement or can occur as a sequela to hydrops or uterine torsion.

Diagnosis

HISTORY
- Moderate to severe abdominal pain during the third trimester or within hours to 3 days after foaling

CLINICAL SIGNS
- The mare may show no pain after rupture until signs of peritonitis develop.
- Exsanguination may occur, but external bleeding is rare.

PREPARTUM RECTAL EXAMINATION
- Try to identify the uterus and the fetus.
- The fetus may not be palpable if it has slipped down into the abdomen.
- The uterus may still be twisted or feel corrugated and thick as involution begins immediately.
- If the tear is small and dorsal, rectal examination may help identify localized peritonitis by the presence of fibrin on the uterine surface and in the peritoneal aspirate.

ABDOMINOCENTESIS
- Large volumes of clear to blood-tinged fluid are obtained at several sites. If peritonitis is present, white blood cells and debris are plentiful.

ULTRASONOGRAPHY
- Transabdominal ultrasonography is performed to identify the fetus in the abdomen.
- Transrectal ultrasonography usually is unrewarding.

LAPAROTOMY
- Laparotomy is the only means by which a definitive diagnosis can be made if the lesion cannot be reached with a careful endometrial digital examination.

Treatment
POSTPARTUM
- Refer to surgical hospital for ventral midline laparotomy (see p. 245).
- Administer fluids and antibiotics.

PREPARTUM
- Refer to a surgical hospital for ventral midline laparotomy.
- Per vagina. If the fetus can be extracted through the vagina and the tear is small, dorsal, and close to the cervix, the uterus sometimes can be sutured through the vagina and cervix.

HYDROPS OF FETAL MEMBRANES
Definition
- *Hydramnion:* Hydramnios or hydrops of the amnion
- *Hydrallantois:* Hydrops allantois
- Excess fluid accumulation (hydrops) in either the allantoic or the amniotic cavity is not a common occurrence in mares but can lead to the mare's death if not diagnosed and managed quickly. Hydramnion occurs most often in pregnancies with congenitally abnormal foals, and hydrallantois is caused by an abnormal chorioallantois. The location of the fluid can be determined clinically but does not alter the therapeutic regimen.

Diagnosis
HISTORY
- Normal pregnancy until 7.5-11 months of gestation

CLINICAL SIGNS
- Increased uterine fluid over 10-14 days
  - Hydrallantois accumulates fluid more rapidly.
  - Abdominal distention
  - Abdominal discomfort
  - Difficulty in walking
  - Difficulty in breathing
  - Recumbency if condition is severe enough

PHYSICAL EXAMINATION
- Distention of the uterus
- Inability to palpate the fetus
- Complications:
  - Severe ventral edema

- Abdominal pain
- Rupture of the abdominal muscles
- Rupture of the prepubic tendon
- Inguinal herniation
- Uterine rupture

Treatment

INDUCE ABORTION: FLUID THERAPY

- Provide intravenous fluids as the uterine fluid is removed to prevent cardiovascular collapse. The hydrops often contains 30-50 gallons (114-189 L) of fluid. Hypertonic saline solution (5%-7%) with or without hetastarch is a good choice.
- Induce abortion by means of gradual dilation of the cervix over 15-20 minutes.
- Drain fetal fluids slowly.
- Forced extraction of the fetus is often necessary because uterine inertia usually is present.

INDUCE PARTURITION

- Induction of parturition with oxytocin, 20-40 IU, is effective in some but not all cases. Oxytocin may be useful if the fetus is near term.
- Treatment with 20-mg dexamethasone 24 hours before induction helps mature the fetal lungs in a fetus close to term.
- Administer fluid therapy as described above.

FOLLOW-UP CARE

- Uterine involution usually occurs normally.
- Provide follow-up therapy with ultrasound examination and repeated drainage if necessary.

Prognosis

The prognosis for future reproductive performance varies depending on uterine involution. Because most cases of hydramnion are caused by congenitally abnormal foals, it is recommended that the mare be rebred to a different stallion.

Induction of Parturition

Induction of parturition is being successfully used in many practices, but it is not without risk. Before induction, each mare must be carefully evaluated to ensure fetal maturity to avoid delivery of a premature foal that demands prolonged neonatal intensive care with its extensive commitment of time and expense. When the proper preinduction criteria are strictly followed, an essentially normal birth occurs, and a healthy foal is delivered.

If it becomes necessary to induce a mare before term, neonatal intensive care facilities, equipment, and personnel must be available if the foal is to survive. Induction of parturition requires professional assistance at delivery.

Indications for Induction at Term

- History of premature placental separation
- Previous delayed parturition due to uterine atony
- Injury or tear at previous foaling

- Previous production of an icteric foal (neonatal isoerythrolysis). Induction is performed to prevent ingestion of colostrum until it can be checked for compatibility with the newborn foal's blood
- Teaching and research investigation
- Placentitis or placental thickening unresponsive to medical treatment that results in abnormal heart rate and movement

Indications for Induction before Term (Requires Neonatal Intensive Care!)

- Preparturient colic
- Excessive ventral edema with impending rupture of the prepubic tendon
- Hydrops of the amnion
- Severe injury to mare (e.g., fracture)
- Imminent death of mare
- Severe placental dysfunction unresponsive to treatment and resulting in deterioration of the foal

Induction Criteria

- Length of gestation, minimum of 330 days (shorter for Miniature Horse)
- Enlarged udder with teats distended with colostrum
- Relaxation of sacrosciatic ligaments
- Electrolyte changes in colostrum indicated by test strips for increased calcium content
  - Predict-a-Foal test (Animal Health Care Products, Chino, CA)
  - Sofchek teat strips (Environmental Test Systems, Elkhart, IN)
  - Titrets calcium hardness test kit (CHEMetrics, Inc., Calverton, VA)

Induction Protocol

- Oxytocin, 20-40 IU IM, 2.5-10 IU IV, repeated every 15-20 minutes until delivery completed, or 40-100 IU IV in 1 L of saline solution over 30-60 minutes for an approximately 450-kg mare. Foaling usually is finished within 60 minutes with any of these protocols.
- Once induction is started, monitor delivery until concluded.

Complications

- *Premature placental separation.* Occasionally the red, velvetlike allantochorion with its cervical star appears at the vulvar lips. *Open the membrane immediately to allow passage of the amnion containing the fetus.* If the allantochorion is not ruptured, the membrane separates from the endometrium, resulting in the birth of a severely hypoxic or possibly dead foal.
- *Malpresentation of the fetus.* In rare instances the foal presents with malalignment. If delivery does not appear to be progressing normally (no sign of the amnion with the feet present) by 20-30 minutes after administration of oxytocin, and clean exploration of the reproductive tract reveals malalignment, correction usually is easily performed before strong abdominal contractions begin that force the fetus into the pelvic canal.
- *Delivery of a premature foal.* If induction criteria are strictly followed, premature delivery is rare. If parturition must be induced before term, this must be anticipated.

- *Neonatal maladjustment syndrome* (see p. 555).

VAGINAL AND VESTIBULAR BLEEDING
Postpartum Hemorrhage
- Bleeding due to trauma from foaling is seldom life threatening, even with third-degree perineal lacerations.

Treatment
- Tetanus toxoid
- Medical neglect: Most vaginal and vestibular bleeding requires no treatment.
- Profuse hemorrhage.
  - If possible, ligate the affected vessel.
  - Pack vagina and vestibule with a large tampon or ice packs (tampons can be made of rolled cotton secured with umbilical tape).
  - Cover tampon with petroleum jelly or an oil-based antibiotic preparation (mastitis preparations work well).
- Hematoma: *Do not drain.*
  - May be drained at a later date, after the vessel has clotted and the hematoma has organized.
  - May cause difficulty in defecating. Continue laxative diets (bran, mineral oil, or both) until the hematoma resolves or is drained.
  - Antibiotics for large hematomas.

Hemorrhage during Late Pregnancy
Bleeding late in pregnancy of older mares often is caused by the presence of varicose veins at the vulvovaginal junction.

- In most cases, hemorrhage is minimal and is best managed with benign neglect.
- If hemorrhage is persistent and voluminous, the affected vessel may have to be ligated.
- Bleeding from varicose veins must be differentiated from bleeding from the cervix, which can signal an impending abortion.

Vaginal Bleeding after Natural Service
- Minimal hemorrhage in maiden mares may result from perforation of a persistent hymen, does not require treatment, and must be differentiated from vaginal rupture.
- Vaginal rupture may occur when a small mare is bred to a large stallion.
- *Clinical signs* include mild to moderate bleeding, tenesmus in rare instances, and bulging small intestine from the vulvar lips.

Diagnosis
- Perform careful speculum examination of the vagina. A tube speculum may provide a satisfactory view of the injury, but a Caslick speculum is preferred for more complete evaluation of the injury.
- A careful, clean (sterile gloves and lubrication) digital examination can help determine whether the peritoneal cavity is penetrated.

- Peritoneal aspiration may reveal the presence of peritonitis or spermatozoa.

Treatment
WOUND NOT ENTERING THE PERITONEAL CAVITY
- Gentle lavage with sterile saline solution
- Infusion of a local antibiotic (e.g., nitrofurazone [Furacin])
- Tetanus booster
- If tenesmus is present:
  □ Flunixin meglumine, 1.0 mg/kg q12-24h IV or IM
  □ Epidural anesthesia: 5-8 ml 2% lidocaine (see p. 125)
- Systemic antibiotics for at least 1 week. Use either:
  □ A combination of potassium penicillin, 22,000 U/kg IV q6h

  or
  Procaine penicillin, 22,000 U/kg IM q12h
  and
  Gentamicin, 6.6 mg/kg q24h (use gentamicin only if creatinine concentration is normal, mare is urinating, and hydration is assured)
  or
  Ceftiofur, 3.0 mg/kg IV or IM q12h
  and
  Metronidazole for vaginal anaerobes, 15 mg/kg PO q8h

WOUND ENTERING THE PERITONEAL CAVITY
- Tetanus booster
- Local and systemic antibiotics (as described)
- Peritoneal lavage with large volume of sterile physiologic saline solution (PSS)
- Wash herniated intestines with sterile saline solution, and replace the intestine through the laceration.

NOTE: If extensive trauma to the herniated small intestine or gross contamination of the peritoneal cavity has occurred, refer the mare for surgery. In this case, treatment consists of cleaning and replacing the herniated intestine and in the interim suturing the vulvar lips closed for transport to the referral center. If the mare is showing signs of shock (depression, cold extremities, elevated heart rate, pale mucous membranes) administer intravenous fluids before shipment.

After surgery or whenever there has been perforation of the abdominal cavity through the vagina, it is recommended that the mare be cross-tied for at least 5 days to prevent lying down.

ARTERIAL RUPTURE (UTERINE ARTERY, EXTERNAL ILIAC ARTERY)
- More common among older mares and multiparous mares
- Usually occurs after parturition and leads to sudden death
- Once the mare has a history of periparturient hemorrhage, she is more likely to bleed in future pregnancies.
- Bleeding can occur into the abdomen or into the broad ligament.

Diagnosis
CLINICAL SIGNS
- Colic, sweating, increased heart rate, anemia, death

- Can occur anytime from 30 minutes to several weeks post partum

| **NOTE:** Clinical signs may be masked soon after parturition by postpartum colic.

RECTAL EXAMINATION
- Hematoma in the broad ligament or uterine wall may be palpable per rectum and usually is painful.

Treatment
NONSURGICAL
- Keep the mare quiet.
- Administer a small dose of acepromazine, 0.01-0.02 mg/kg, only if the patient is anxious. A key principle in survival is production of "permissive hypotension." Although crystalloids and colloids, including hemoglobin (Oxyglobin), are indicated, every effort should be made to keep the systolic blood pressure between 70 and 90 mm Hg until it is clear the bleeding has stopped.
- If the mare is very weak it is recommended to move the foal to a neighboring stall.
- Administer blood transfusion or plasma therapy (see p. 336). Autotransfusion is possible (see p. 336).
- Oxytocin, 20 IU IM every 30 minutes
- Oxytocin decreases bleeding from the myometrium and intraluminal bleeding only. *It does not affect bleeding from the external iliac or uterine artery; do not administer oxytocin if a hematoma is present in the broad ligament.*
- Analgesic: Flunixin meglumine, 1 mg/kg IV or IM q12-24h

SURGICAL
- Surgical correction is unlikely to be successful because of acute and rapidly ongoing bleeding.

ANTIBIOTICS
- Administer ceftiofur or penicillin-gentamicin, and metronidazole for large hematoma of the vagina or broad ligament.

INTRAVENOUS FLUIDS
- Administer fluids if the mare is hypotensive (document increased heart rate, poor pulse quality, and cold extremities, or systolic blood pressure less than 80 mm Hg measured with an indirect blood pressure cuff—tail is the easiest site). Do not administer hypertonic saline solution unless the mare's condition is rapidly deteriorating!
- Aminocaproic acid (Amicar), 10-20 mg/kg, is administered slowly IV in the fluids or by means of slow infusion if fluids are not being administered.

| **NOTE:** Iliac artery rupture is a common sequela to a displaced pelvic fracture. Progressive swelling in a rear limb usually is present.

Prognosis
Poor with any treatment if there is uncontrolled bleeding into the abdominal cavity.

Retained Placenta
- Placenta is normally expelled within 1½ hours of foaling; retention longer than 3 hours is considered abnormal.

REPRODUCTIVE

- Institute treatment immediately to prevent serious complications, which include metritis, septicemia, laminitis, and death.

Signs

Protrusion of the fetal membranes from the vulva is the most obvious sign of retained placenta and alerts the clinician to the possibility of the complications described. However, the same complications can result from undetected retention of a small piece (tip of the horn) of placental tissue. This underscores the need for careful examination of all fetal membranes after foaling so that appropriate therapy can be instituted immediately if a portion of the placenta is retained.

Treatment

- If the membranes protrude from the vulva and extend below the hocks, they can stimulate kicking, which endangers the foal. Tie the membranes in a knot above the hocks. Do not cut the exposed placenta because the weight assists in the cleaning technique.
- Administer oxytocin using one of the following protocols:
  - 20-40 units as a bolus IM
  - It is generally recommended to administer 20 units IM 3 hours post partum and to repeat the dosage with another 20 units every 1-1½ hours for three additional injections if necessary.
  - 10-100 units of oxytocin in 1 L of saline solution administered slowly IV over 30-60 minutes
- If the retained membranes are not expelled by 12 hours after foaling, broaden the treatment to include:
  - Systemic antibiotics (ceftiofur, 3.0 mg/kg IM or IV q12h, or penicillin, 22,000 U/kg IV q6h, or procaine penicillin, 22,000 U/kg IM q12h, and gentamicin, 6.6 mg/kg q24h) (only if hydration is normal and mare is urinating)
  - NSAIDs (flunixin meglumine, 0.3 mg/kg q8h)
  - Infusion of the allantochorionic space with 10-12 L of 1%-2% povidone-iodine solution through a nasogastric tube and tying closed the opening of the fetal membranes. Distention of the uterus, cervix, and vagina stimulates release of endogenous oxytocin, which additionally stimulates uterine contractions. Distention of the uterine wall also allows the uterine crypts to release the fetal villi. With this technique, the membranes usually are passed within 30 minutes.
- If fetal membranes are still retained after this treatment, continue systemic antibiotics and NSAIDs until the membranes are passed. Gentle manual removal can be attempted but should never exceed 10 minutes. Successful techniques include:
  - Gentle tension on the protruding membranes
  - Carefully sliding the hand between the chorion and the endometrium massaging to free the membrane.
  - Twisting the exposed fetal membranes to form a tight cord. This technique sometimes is combined successfully with the slow intravenous administration of oxytocin described previously.
- Tetanus toxoid

| **NOTE:** Monitor for signs of laminitis (see p. 368).

| **CAUTION:** Occasionally, oxytocin has been reported to cause an intussusception of the uterus and persistent colic. The uterine intussusception can be palpated at rectal examination and corrected by means of intrauterine control using an empty, sterile bottle (e.g. wine bottle).

Acute Septic Metritis

- In most cases, acute septic metritis occurs when there is extensive trauma and resulting contamination of the reproductive tract during a difficult dystocia.
- The incidence increases when corrective manipulations take a long time, excessive force is used for extraction, or a lengthy fetotomy is needed.
- Retention of the fetal membrane, if untreated, can result in septic metritis.

Signs

- Signs of septicemia include increased temperature, pulse, and respirations, anorexia, injected mucous membranes, dehydration, and perhaps beginning signs of shock (cold extremities, and so on).
- Vaginal discharge usually is not copious in mares, but a thin, watery discharge with a variable smell (sweet to putrid depending on the organisms involved) may be seen. The vaginal walls are inflamed.
- Rectal examination reveals an enlarged, usually thin-walled uterus distended with fluid.

Treatment

- Systemic antibiotics as dictated by culture and sensitivity. Penicillin, gentamicin, and metronidazole can be used until laboratory results are reported.
- Flunixin meglumine, 0.3 mg/kg IV or IM q8h.
- Intravenous fluids to correct dehydration and shock.
- Uterine lavage with large volumes of warm saline solution.
- Oxytocin, 10 units after uterine lavage.

Uterine Lavage Technique

- Place 1 or 2 L of warm (45°C-47°C) saline solution in a plastic sleeve knotted just above the hand to prevent the fluid from running down into the fingers. Wrap the tail and disinfect the perineal region before carefully passing a catheter through the cervix. While placing the catheter, cover the exposed end to prevent aspiration of air into the uterus.
- With the catheter in position (6-8 inches [15-20 cm] within the uterus), place the exposed end inside the sleeve containing the saline solution. Clamp the sleeve tightly around the end of the catheter, invert it, and elevate the sleeve to allow the saline solution to run into the uterus. When the saline infusion is almost completed *but before it is finished*, lower the sleeve below the level of the uterus. The saline solution and uterine contents siphon back into the sleeve. If a clear plastic sleeve is used, it is easy to examine evacuated uterine contents.
- Lavage is repeated until the recovered fluid is acceptably clear. The uterus then can be treated locally with the appropriate antibiotics.
- Because fluid may continue to accumulate with toxemia, careful monitoring is needed until the infection is controlled. Removal of the toxic uterine fluid

should resolve systemic signs. Lack of improvement demands repeated flushing and continued treatment.

EARLY THERAPY FOR LAMINITIS see (p. 368)
- Soft footing
- Comfortable caudal foot support
- Aspirin, 90 grains (5.4 g)/450-kg horse PO q48h
- Antibiotics and fluid therapy
- Pentoxifylline, 8.4 mg/kg PO q12h
- Nitroglycerine cream, topically, q12h
- Flunixin meglumine, 0.3 mg/kg q8h

VENTRAL RUPTURE

Ventral rupture includes rupture of the prepubic tendon or of the abdominal muscles. It occurs most often in late gestation. Although any breed is affected, there is a higher incidence among draft breeds. Individuals at higher risk include older mares, sedentary mares in which extensive ventral edema develops several weeks before anticipated foaling (because of decreased muscle tone), and mares with hydrops or twins. In many cases no identifiable predisposing factors or causes are found.

Diagnosis
- Definitive diagnosis can be made only at postmortem examination.

Clinical Signs
- Abdominal pain: Can be differentiated from other causes of colic by the presence of increased pain on palpation of the caudal abdomen
- Reluctance to walk
- Dependent abdomen or discrete bulge of the ventrolateral abdomen
- *Thick* plaques of ventral edema that do not decrease with exercise. Plaques are from the increased pressure of the uterus on the caudal epigastric and caudal superficial epigastric veins or from trauma to the muscles.
- Elevation of the tuber ischii; this occurs when the prepubic tendon ruptures and the udder moves cranially.
- Blood in the milk is caused by rupture of vessels.

Treatment
- Repair of abdominal muscle ruptures (see p. 245) is difficult and is performed only if the cause (hydrops or external trauma) is unlikely to recur.
- Extensive edema or hydrops with or without rupture of the prepubic tendon:
  - *If gestation is more than 330 days,* induce parturition with oxytocin, 20 units/450-kg mare IM, or as drip, 20-100 units over 30-60 minutes.
  - Pretreat with 20 mg dexamethasone 24 hours before induction to hasten fetal lung maturity.
  - If gestation is less than 330 days, and the mare's condition is stable:
    - Using a belly band or wrap with wide adhesive tape, support the abdomen until parturition is safely induced.
  - Older mares with extensive ventral edema:

Evaluate dietary protein.
Check teeth and deworming.
Encourage daily mild exercise to reduce edema.

Uterine Prolapse

In the rare instances in which uterine prolapse occurs, prompt treatment is needed to prevent additional injury, shock, and even death of the mare. Before arrival, advise the owner to restrain the mare and if possible cover the prolapsed uterus in a moistened sheet or towel to avoid further trauma or dehydration of tissues. Elevating the uterus serves to decrease edema.

Treatment

- Sedate the mare as needed.

CAUTION: Large doses of some tranquilizers (acepromazine) can enhance signs of shock.

- Administer epidural anesthesia, 1 ml 2% lidocaine/75 kg or 0.25 mg xylazine/kg mixed in 8-10 ml saline solution.
- Clean and replace the uterus. Use large volumes of warm, mild antiseptic solution to cleanse the endometrial surface thoroughly. Before attempting replacement, carefully palpate to confirm that the bladder is not within the prolapsed uterus. The presence of a distended bladder requires drainage before replacement. This can sometimes be done by passing a soft rubber stallion catheter through the urethra. If this is not possible, empty the bladder by placing a 2-inch (5-cm), 14-gauge needle through the uterine wall into the bladder and apply gentle pressure.
- Replace by applying firm, gentle pressure with the flat of the hand and the fingers closed or using a clenched fist. Apply pressure first near the cervix and gradually work the everted uterus back through the cervix. It is important to gently work all sides evenly, being careful to use a flat surface (flat of hand) to prevent poking holes through the uterus. Having an assistant elevate the everted uterus on a tray or sling assists replacement. Once the uterus is passed through the cervix, it is important to be sure the tips of the horns are not inverted. If an arm is not long enough to reach the tip of the uterine horn, grasp an empty, clean wine bottle by the neck and carefully extend the flat base of the bottle to the tip of the horn.
- Once the uterus is replaced, flush with 2-3 L of warm saline solution a minimum of two times (see acute septic metritis, p. 493) for siphoning technique). Then place 2 g of tetracycline powder in the uterus.
- Systemic treatment includes oxytocin, 20 units IM, to involute the uterus and systemic antibiotics (ceftiofur or a combination of penicillin and gentamicin) and flunixin meglumine, 0.30 mg/kg; tetanus toxoid; and other recommended treatments (see p. 368) to prevent metritis and laminitis.

MASTITIS

Clinical Signs

- Swollen udder, usually unilaterally (possible for only one lobe to be involved)
- Pain on udder palpation

- Ventral edema
- Fever
- Depression
- Anorexia
- Only one half of clinical cases are found in lactating mares, and one fourth of clinical cases have signs within 8 weeks of weaning.

Diagnosis
Based on gross examination and culture of the milk for Gram stain. Collect milk in a sterile vial after swabbing the teat with alcohol. *Streptococcus zooepidemicus* frequently is the cause.

▶ An aseptic cause of mastitis is avocado poisoning.

Treatment
- Administer 10 units of oxytocin if the mare is not pregnant, and strip the gland frequently using lubricant. Hot pack the gland several times per day.
- Administer penicillin if small, Gram-positive organisms are cultured. Administer trimethoprim-sulfadiazine or gentamicin if Gram-negative rods are cultured. Confirm with sensitivity testing as soon as possible.
- Intramammary infusions q12h-q24h or after milking with a commercial bovine preparation.
- Flunixin meglumine, 0.25 mg/kg q8h if the mare has systemic illness.

Prognosis
Usually very good. Mares do not commonly have a recurrence after a single incident.

AGALACTIA
- Occasionally observed in a mare in any geographic region; most common where fescue pasture is contaminated with the fungus *Acremonium coenophialum*
- In addition to agalactia, mares grazing infested pasture may have a prolonged gestational length, increased incidence of stillbirths and retained placenta, increased placental thickness, and decreased prolactin and progesterone concentrations.
- Agalactia is an emergency because foal death occurs from sepsis if prompt treatment is not provided.

Treatment of Foal
- Two liters of a high-quality colostrum (specific gravity, 1.080 or more) if foal is younger than 24 hours. Administer colostrum in a smaller amount if the foal is older than 24 hours, to provide immunoglobulin A (IgA).
- Administer 1-2 L of equine plasma IV to all foals born to agalactic mares unless the colostrum can be given within 2-3 hours after birth and IgG determinations 14-18 hours after birth show an adequate serum IgG level (>800 mg/dl).
- Feed foal appropriately and keep warm and dry (see p. 769).
- Administer antibiotics, such as ceftiofur, 3.0-4.0 mg/kg IV q8-12h, if the foal is several hours old when found.
- Administer sucralfate, 1 g PO q6h.
- Provide routine postnatal care:
  - Perform a clinical examination.

- □ Dip navel with 1% chlorhexidine or 2% iodine.
- □ Administer an enema with *soft* rubber tubing and warm water, adding a small amount of Ivory or green soap.

Treatment of Mare

- Administer domperidone, 1.1 mg/kg PO q24h, a dopamine receptor antagonist that does not cross the blood-brain barrier and is effective in many cases. The drug is not Food and Drug Administration (FDA) approved for use in the horse; information is available through D. L. Cross, Department of Animal Dairy and Veterinary Sciences, Clemson University, Clemson, SC 29631; (864) 656-5155.
- An alternative is perphenazine, 0.3-0.5 mg/kg PO q12h, which is available through local pharmacies.
- Manage any factors that cause agalactia, such as malnutrition, water deprivation, and concurrent illness.

FOAL REJECTION

Occurs primarily in primiparous mares; more common in certain families or breeds. The Arabian breed appears to be overrepresented.

Treatment

- Rule out medical conditions that cause a painful udder. If no udder abnormality is present, gently restrain the mare with *low*-dose acepromazine, 10 mg/450-kg mare. Feed the mare grain during the bonding process to encourage the mare to allow the foal to nurse. Hand-milking the mare and feeding the foal by bottle held under the mare's udder reinforces a positive experience for the mare and foal. Avoid painful restraint of the mare if possible, although a twitch can be used if other methods fail. After tranquilizing the mare, place the mare in stocks to prevent sideways movement.
- A final approach, although more risky, is to place the mare and foal in a large paddock with other horses to promote maternal behavior in the mare. Watch closely and continuously! Proper attention to the foal regarding adequate serum antibody titers and nutrition is important during the adjustment period.
- If these treatments are unsuccessful in a few days, the foal should be bonded with a nursemare or fed as an orphan. Nursemare farms are listed in Box 42-1.

ABORTION

- It is important to establish the cause of abortion whenever possible to plan appropriate preventive measures.
- Isolate the aborting mare and prevent other pregnant mares from contacting the area where the abortion occurred as well as from the aborted fetus or placenta.

Submission of Samples to a Diagnostic Laboratory
WHEN POSSIBLE SUBMIT
- Entire fetus
- Entire placenta
- Serum sample from mare
- Complete history

BOX 42-1. Nursemare Directory

ALABAMA
Magnolia Farms
Christi Parsons
PO Box 33
Odenville, AL 35120

INDIANA
Fairview Equine Center
Thomas W. Arens
PO Box 745
Westfield, IN 46074-0745
(317) 877-0338

For-rest Hill Farm
6250E 550N
Lafayette, IN 47905-9762

KENTUCKY
Robin and Archie Borns
Nicholasville, KY 40340
(859) 272-1835
(859) 229-1750

Brumback's in Kent
(606) 824-6954
(606) 824-6334

C & G Partnership
PO Box 177
Soldier, KY 41173
(606) 286-2367

Charles Davis and Cynthiana Kent
(859) 234-6479

Horse Play Farm
PO Box 52
Paris, KY 40361
(606) 987-3399

Legacy Land
Gail Curtsinger
1820 Clintonville Rd.
Winchester, KY 40391
(859) 745-6122

John Porter
Morehead, KY 40351
(606) 784-2823

Mountain View Farms
PO Box 89
Ezel, KY 41425
(606) 725-5635

Pinecrest Farms
PO Box 276
Millersburg, KY 40348
(606) 484-2281

Roseberry's Nurse Mares
Tammy and Don Roseberry
PO Box 162
Butler, KY 41006
(859) 472-5421

Walton Hills
319 Walnut Street
Carlisle, KY 40311
(606) 289-5273

MARYLAND
Pouska Farms
Kathleen (Dolly) Pouska
2720 Biggs Highway
North East, MD 21901
(410) 658-5062

MICHIGAN
Goose Creek Ranch
995 61st Street
Pullman, MI 49450-9778
(616) 236-5918

MISSOURI
Box LT Morab & Cattle Ranch
RR3, Box 235
Ava, MO 65608-9553
(417) 683-4426

NEW YORK
North Slope Farm
PO Box 4
Trout Creek, NY 13847-0004
(607) 865-7926
(607) 865-7927

The Nursemare Farm
Debra Pease
PO Box 60
Claverack, NY 12513

Sandy Kistner Nurse Mare Service
Warwick, NY 10990
(845) 988-5265

TEXAS
Sherwood's Farm and Equine Nursery
345 Woelke Road
Sequin, TX 78155
(830) 303-5444

WASHINGTON
Blue Ribbon Farms
Buckley, WA 98321
(253) 862-9076

Continued

BOX 42-1 Nursemare Directory *Continued*

El Dorado Farm
Enumclaw, WA 98022
(360) 825-7526

Puget Sound Reproductive Center
17028 Trombley Road
Snohomish, WA 98290
(360) 568-7455

CANADA
AA Arabians
Sheila Clarkson
RR#4
Orangeville, ONT 19W 2Z1
(519) 941-4387

Carson Farms
RR#2
Listowel, ONT N4W 3G8
(519) 291-2049

Cyberfoal 2000
Peter Hurst
Site 30, Box 11, RR8
Calgary, Alberta T2J 2T9
(403) 931-3840

Colostrum bank available at some sites.
Reprinted with permission from *The Horse Source* and *THEHORSE.COM, 2/27/01.* Both are part of *The Blood Horse,* Inc. Additions and deletions are made based upon the most current available information. Telephone numbers or current operations status may change.

SAMPLES TO SUBMIT WHEN IMPOSSIBLE TO DELIVER WHOLE FETUS
- Note fetal and placental abnormalities.
- Measure crown-rump distance
- Determine fetal and placental weights.
- Carefully collect a 2-inch by 3-inch (5 by 7.5-cm) piece of lung, adrenal gland, and kidney and three pieces of placenta. Be sure to include any pieces from any abnormal areas. Place each tissue specimen in a separate plastic bag and label clearly.
  - 5 ml of fetal heart blood
  - 5 ml of sterile stomach contents
  - A 0.25-inch (0.6-cm)-thick section of tissue placed in formalin solution for histopathologic examination
  - Liver, lung, kidney, adrenal gland, placenta, heart, thymus, spleen, small intestine, and brain. Pack samples in a cooler and send by overnight carrier with a complete history.

History Should Include
- Owner's name and address
- Veterinarian's name and address

MARE HISTORY
- Identification
- Breeding history (date, artificial insemination or natural)
- Foaling history
- Vaccinations
- Clinical illness and treatment during pregnancy. Feeding program, including any recent changes. Abnormalities in aborted fetus and placenta.

HERD HISTORY

- Number of mares on farm (resident and nonresident)
- Number of foals
- Number of nonbreeding performance horses
- Other species on farm
- Number of previous abortions and stage of abortion
- Foal problems
- Housing
- Contact with new or transient animals
- Clinical illness in herd in last 6 months
- Vaccination program
- Nutritional program including pasture plants and mineral supplements
- A second maternal serum sample should be submitted 2 weeks after abortion.

REFERENCES

Stallion Breeding Injuries

Varner DD et al: *Diseases and management of breeding stallions,* St. Louis, 1991, Mosby.

Wilson DV, Nickels FA, Williams MA: Pharmacologic treatment of priapism in two horses, *J Am Vet Med Assoc* 199:1183-1184, 1991.

Dystocia

Vandeplassche M: Dystocia. In McKinnon AO, Voss JL, editors: *Equine reproduction,* Philadelphia, 1993, Lea & Febiger.

Uterine Torsion: Nonsurgical

Wichtel JJ, Reinertson EL, Clark TL: Nonsurgical treatment of uterine torsion in seven mares, *J Am Vet Med Assoc* 193:337-338, 1988.

Uterine Torsion: Surgical

Pascoe JR, Meagher DM, Wheat JD: Surgical management of uterine torsion in the mare: a review of 26 cases, *J Am Vet Med Assoc* 179:351-354, 1981.

Arterial Rupture

McKinnon AO, Voss JL: *Equine reproduction,* Philadelphia, 1993, Lea & Febiger.

Mastitis

McCue PM, Wilson DW: Equine mastitis: a review of 28 cases, *Equine Vet J* 21:351-353, 1989.

Foal Rejection

Houpt KA: Foal rejection and other behavior problems in the postpartum period, *Comp Contin Educ* 6:S144-S150, 1984.

43 Respiratory System

Thomas L. Seahorn and Thomas J. Divers

REPRODUCTIVE

Emergencies of the respiratory system are generally diseases causing respiratory distress, however in some cases the disease can be life threatening without producing distress, such as pleuropneumonia, and therefore is treated as an emergency.

The initial diagnostic goal when evaluating a patient with respiratory distress is to determine whether the problem is an upper respiratory disorder (obstruction) or a lower respiratory problem (e.g., pulmonary edema, bronchoconstriction, pneumothorax). The presence of upper respiratory disease, including tracheitis, usually can be determined on the basis of the noise the patient is making when breathing, especially on inspiration. The presence of lower respiratory disease causing respiratory distress usually can be determined by means of auscultation of the thorax. Inspiratory dyspnea often is more pronounced than expiratory dyspnea with upper airway obstruction, whereas the reverse is true with lower airway obstruction, such as heaves.

The presence of life-threatening respiratory infection without respiratory distress that necessitates emergency care, such as pleuropneumonia or aspiration pneumonia, usually can be determined with the history, auscultation of the thorax, and routine diagnostic procedures, such as ultrasonography and tracheal aspiration.

RESPIRATORY DISTRESS WITH RESPIRATORY NOISE, AIRWAY OBSTRUCTION

- *Labored breathing* usually producing *noise.*
- The list of differential diagnoses is long so perform a complete physical examination with ancillary diagnostic equipment to identify clinical features that narrow the possible causes.
- *Remember that acute respiratory obstruction often is rapidly progressive for three reasons:*
  - The primary disease process, such as edema, often is progressive.
  - Constant turbulence of airflow against the compromised airway leads to increased edema.
  - Increased negative pleural pressure caused by increased effort against an obstructed airway may lead to pulmonary edema.
- Consider any acute respiratory noise an emergency.

Laryngeal Obstruction

Nasotracheal intubation can be difficult to perform on a distressed patient. In most cases, tracheotomy is preferred. If the instruments to perform the tracheotomy are not readily available, attempt nasotracheal intubation! If the patient collapses, perform nasotracheal intubation because it is faster. Secondary pulmonary edema is a common occurrence with acute severe upper airway obstruction; routinely administer furosemide in these cases.

Laryngeal Edema: Anaphylaxis

The cause often is unknown, but it can be an *anaphylactic reaction* (see Chapter 36, p. 308) to vaccine antigens and can accompany *purpura hemorrhagica* (see p. 304).

DIAGNOSIS
- Endoscopic examination is the best diagnostic tool. Edema and collapse of the tissues around the larynx are seen. *Avoid tranquilization if possible.*
- Administer acepromazine, 0.02-0.04 mg/kg IV, and butorphanol, 0.01-0.02 mg/kg IV, for sedation if necessary to better examine the larynx endoscopically.
- Do not administer acepromazine if systemic anaphylaxis is a possibility.
- Do not use xylazine because it increases upper airway resistance.

TREATMENT
- If laryngeal edema is caused by an **anaphylactic** reaction, administer **epinephrine**, 3-7 ml/450-kg adult (1:1000 as packaged), administer **slowly IV**. If time permits, dilute in 20-30 ml of 0.9% saline solution. Similar doses of epinephrine may be administered IM or SQ in less severe cases. If respiratory stridor is found, suggesting 80% or more compromise of the airflow, pass a nasotracheal tube to prevent further obstruction and the need for tracheotomy.
- If laryngeal edema is severe, perform tracheotomy (see p. 67).
- If pulmonary edema has developed (crackles on auscultation or froth at the nostril), *begin* furosemide therapy, 1 mg/kg IV, and see p. 511.
- Dexamethasone, 0.1-0.2 mg/kg IV bolus; dimethyl sulfoxide (DMSO), 1 g/kg IV in 3 L of 0.9% saline solution may also be administered.
- For systemic anaphylaxis, administer both crystalloid and colloid fluids because affected individuals are hypotensive.
- Intranasal or intratracheal oxygen.

PROGNOSIS
Generally good but the condition may persist for several days or recur.

Arytenoid Chondritis

In most cases, the chondritis has been present for an extended time period, and the obstruction may be acute. If noise is apparent at rest, there is probably 80% or more compromise of the airway.

DIAGNOSIS
- Endoscopic examination

Treatment
- Tracheotomy (see p. 67 for procedure)
- Surgical removal (arytenoidectomy) of the diseased cartilage

Hypocalcemia
- Hypocalcemic patients can have laryngeal paresis and consequently laryngeal obstruction.

DIAGNOSIS
- History is important, such as lactation in a mare, however idiopathic cases have occurred not associated with lactation.

- Other clinical signs: *Trismus of facial muscles, thumps, and trembling.*
- Confirm all presumptive cases by measuring serum calcium levels. Serum calcium concentration usually is less than 6.5 mg/dl in adults with severe clinical signs. Profuse sweating, hypochloremia, and resultant alkalosis further exacerbate hypocalcemia.

Treatment

- Calcium borogluconate, 11 g *slowly IV* over 20 minutes to an adult (450 kg) while monitoring heart rate and rhythm
- *Do not administer subcutaneously!*

| **NOTE:** Calcium borogluconate is safer than calcium chloride.

- If clinical signs do not abate, a second treatment may be required. Administer additional calcium diluted with polyionic fluids at a slower rate.

Acute Guttural Pouch Empyema

- Often associated with *Streptococcus equi* infection.

DIAGNOSIS

- Endoscopic examination of pharynx, larynx, and guttural pouch
- Ultrasound examination: Fluid within guttural pouch
- Radiographic findings of a fluid line in the guttural pouches
- Nasal discharge
- Swelling and pain behind ramus of mandible

TREATMENT

- Tracheotomy is rarely needed.
- Appropriate antibiotic (penicillin), administered both systematically and through an indwelling catheter in the guttural pouch that serves to improve drainage.
- Pass a Chambers catheter into the guttural pouch for drainage and lavage with 1 L of *nonirritating* polyionic fluid (warm saline solution with potassium penicillin), after administering acepromazine, 0.02 mg/kg IV, and butorphanol, 0.01 mg/kg IV, for sedation. If the respiratory obstruction is not severe, substitute xylazine for the acepromazine to lower the head during the flushing procedure and improve drainage.

Laryngeal Spasms or Temporary Paresis

Frequent postanesthetic complication and therefore a problem at referral centers performing general anesthesia. Commonly occurs after removal of the endotracheal tube during recovery. Pulmonary edema quickly follows the obstruction and is a factor in the prognosis. More common among adults with laryngeal paresis, such as draft breeds.

TREATMENT

- Tracheotomy (see p. 67) or pass a nasotracheal tube
- Furosemide, 1 mg/kg IV
- DMSO, 1 g/kg IV in 3 L of 0.9% saline solution, plus dexamethasone, 0.1-0.2 mg/kg, in cases of pulmonary edema
- Oxygen

Proximal Esophageal Choke

On rare occasions can cause respiratory distress if the obstruction is in the proximal esophagus.

DIAGNOSIS
- Endoscopic examination.
- Dorsally collapsed larynx.
- Feed material may be seen at the esophageal opening or immediately on entering the esophagus.

TREATMENT
- Pass a nasogastric tube to relieve the esophageal obstruction. If intubation is unsuccessful, perform tracheotomy.

Pyrrolizidine Alkaloid Toxicity

Acute laryngeal paralysis is rare in cases of pyrrolizidine alkaloid poisoning. Clinical and biochemical evidence of liver disease is present.

TREATMENT
- Tracheotomy relieves respiratory distress, but the prognosis is poor because of the potential for liver failure.

Strangles with Involvement of the Retropharyngeal Lymph Nodes in Foals

Obstruction usually is caused by septic lymphadenopathy. In most cases, there is not a "mature" abscess to be drained. *These cases are difficult to manage*, although the prognosis for survival is good. Dysphagia may be a presenting symptom.

DIAGNOSIS
- History and clinical signs

TREATMENT
- Tracheotomy (see p. 67)

> **NOTE:** Expect a purulent discharge from the tracheotomy site with a soft-tissue reaction around the area.

- Drain the lymph node if an abscess is present. Ultrasound examination may be helpful in determining whether there is an abscessed lymph node. Often a well-developed abscess, "ripe for draining," is not present. Endoscopy of the guttural pouch may reveal a "bulging" abscess on the floor of the guttural pouch. If this is the clinical finding, the abscess may be incised and drained using a surgical laser. Endoscopy should not be performed unless there is adequate airflow.
  - Anatomy is complicated: Use ultrasound guidance to identify the abscess, although this often is not possible.
  - A 12-gauge teat cannula inserted through a stab incision into the lymph node may drain the abscess.

> **NOTE:** With or without drainage, laryngeal paralysis or dysfunction often is seen at endoscopic examination months later.

- Endoscopic-guided surgery using a laser to drain a lymph node(s) into the guttural pouch
- Penicillin: Clinical improvement may take 1 week or more. Penicillin, 44,000 U/kg q6h IV, is preferred in the initial stages of treatment to speed the recovery. If a tracheotomy is performed, place the intravenous catheter as far from the tracheotomy site as possible. If aspiration occurs, broader-spectrum antibiotics are indicated.

Idiopathic Laryngeal Paralysis in Foals
HISTORY
- A young foal with stertorous breathing with no other physical abnormalities

DIAGNOSIS
- Endoscopy
- Rule out other causes in young foals:
  - Hyperkalemic periodic paralysis (HYPP) in Quarter Horses with "Impressive" breeding homozygous for the defective gene. There should be both laryngeal and pharyngeal collapse with HYPP. Does not usually cause clinical signs in newborn foals.
  - Transient displacement of the soft palate in newborn foals. Milk reflux is more of a problem than respiratory obstruction, although affected foals may make a noise when handled.
  - Selenium deficiency also can cause collapse of the airways and respiratory noise with distress in very young foals. Consider this in areas (primarily northern United States and Canada) known to be selenium-deficient. Administer selenium *IM (not IV)* if a deficiency is suspected.

TREATMENT
Tracheotomy: For immediate relief (see p. 67)

PROGNOSIS
- Very poor for idiopathic cases: Most cases have little improvement.
- For other differential diagnoses: Good.

Hyperkalemic Periodic Paralysis
Airway obstruction occurs in homozygously affected foals. A loud fluttering sound may be made during episodes and a persistent noise after treatment. Most cases do not necessitate tracheotomy and can be managed medically. Stressful events such as weaning or excitement may precipitate onset or worsening of clinical signs.

DIAGNOSIS
- Young Quarter Horse foals usually (<5 months).
- Endoscopically, there is collapse of the soft palate, pharynx, and larynx. Do *not* use xylazine for sedation because doing so increases upper airway resistance.
- Direct descendant of Impressive on both sides of lineage.
- Confirm homozygous status for the defective gene by DNA means of evaluation:
  - *Collect*: 1 EDTA tube (5-10 ml) of blood labeled with the patient's name. Do not freeze or separate.
  - *Send to*: Veterinary Genetic Laboratory/HYPP Test, School of Veterinary Medicine, University of California, Davis, CA 95616-8744.

CLINICAL CHEMISTRY FINDING
- Serum potassium value often is normal; slight elevations are found in some foals. Some patients have an elevated creatine kinase value, but this finding is not uniform.

TREATMENT
- 50 ml of 50% dextrose IV if hyperkalemia is present. Do not use if the patient has collapsed and is believed to have suffered hypoxic brain damage. The high concentration of dextrose can aggravate central nervous system (CNS) intracellular acidosis as the dextrose is metabolized anaerobically to lactic acid. The benefit of glucose is to stimulate insulin release and move potassium intracellularly. Insulin level is elevated within 5 minutes after glucose infusion and causes an immediate intracellular shift.
- 1 mEq/kg 7.5% or 8.4% $NaHCO_3$ IV over 5-10 minutes to shift potassium intracellularly. Dextrose, 0.5 g/kg IV, may be preferred in place of $NaHCO_3$ because $NaHCO_3$ decreases the level of ionized calcium, which has a "cellular protective" activity against hyperkalemia. $NaHCO_3$ may contribute to respiratory acidosis. Paradoxic CNS acidosis may be caused by the administration of $NaHCO_3$ although evidence of this phenomenon is not strong in the horse.
- Acetazolamide, 2.2 mg/kg PO q12h.
- Remove alfalfa hay, molasses, and electrolyte supplement.

Selenium Deficiency
Can cause a variety of signs in foals and adults. In young (sometimes newborn) foals, pharyngeal and laryngeal paresis results in respiratory noise or milk reflux.

DIAGNOSIS
- Geographic location and clinical signs (may be involvement of the skeletal muscles resulting in weakness, abnormal gait, and so on)
- Serum creatine kinase values are variable but if elevated should arouse suspicion. Collect blood for measurement of selenium (<10 mg/dl supports the diagnosis).

TREATMENT
- IM injection of selenium (*not IV*). Repeat in 3 days.

Tracheal Collapse
May be caused by trauma or a progressively enlarging mass (e.g., hematoma, thyroid cyst, abscess) dorsal to the trachea. Most common in *adults* (usually older than 10 years). Miniature horses and Shetland ponies. The collapse generally occurs throughout the cervical and thoracic area. *S equi* or *Rhodococcus equi* abscesses also can collapse the trachea at the thoracic inlet in individuals 6 months to 1 year of age.

CLINICAL SIGNS
- Respiratory noise
- Respiratory distress
- Cyanosis

DIAGNOSIS
- Confirmed at endoscopic examination of the upper airway and trachea. Provide intranasal oxygen during the endoscopic examination. The edges of the flattened

trachea may be palpated in the jugular furrow in some cases. Radiography or ultrasonography is useful in cases resulting from an impinging mass, especially a mass at the thoracic inlet.

TREATMENT
- The extent of the collapse in Miniature horses and Shetland ponies makes repair difficult. If the collapse is in only a single area of the neck, extraluminal prosthetic devices can be implanted to increase tracheal diameter. Surgically drain or incise the compressing masses.
- A rare cause of tracheal collapse is a mediastinal abscess or tumor (e.g., *S equi* abscess) or severe pneumomediastinum. The diagnosis is based on radiographic, endoscopic, or ultrasound examination. Treatment requires *both* tracheotomy and placement of an endotracheal tube through the tracheotomy site and passed beyond the site of the obstruction. Drainage of a cranial thoracic abscess can be performed with ultrasound guidance. It may be necessary to anesthetize the foal with a short-acting anesthetic to move the leg far enough forward to place the drainage tube.

Tracheal or Bronchial Foreign Body
In rare instances, horses inhale foreign bodies such as sticks or twigs down the trachea, and the object lodges in a primary bronchus. This results in acute onset of coughing with variable respiratory distress.

DIAGNOSIS
- Endoscopic examination

TREATMENT
- Removal by means of endoscopy is difficult. Referral and a surgical approach for removal of the foreign body may be required.

Epiglottitis
- May cause a respiratory noise and on *rare* occasions produce respiratory distress similar to croup in humans. In horses, tracheotomy is rarely needed for epiglottitis.
- Treatment with throat spray (dexamethasone [Furacin]), systemic antibiotics, and nonsteroidal antiinflammatory drugs (NSAIDs) is recommended.

Guttural Pouch Tympany
- In foals, this can cause a respiratory noise and predispose the foal to pneumonia, however it rarely causes respiratory distress.

Nasal Obstruction
For respiratory distress to occur, both nares must be compromised. The most common causes of acute, bilateral nasal obstruction are

- Trauma, including foreign bodies
- Anaphylaxis
- Snake bite
- Acute obstruction of the jugular vein, along with low head carriage (depression or tranquilization)

- Some chronic diseases of the nasal cavity, such as neoplasia or granuloma, occasionally cause acute onset of respiratory distress

Trauma to the Nasal Cavity

Trauma to the nasal cavity can occur when a healthy horse runs into an object in the field or when a patient with cerebral disease engages in continuous head pressing. It also occurs in severely depressed individuals that keep their heads lowered and frequently have a gastric tube inserted.

Management of Blunt Trauma (Injury to the Nose)

- *Keep affected individual as quiet as possible* and *do not use xylazine or any tranquilizer that causes lowering of the head* or an increase in upper airway resistance.
- Apply ice packs to the external nasal surface.
- Spray lidocaine with epinephrine (25 ml in each nostril for an adult) into the nasal cavity. Phenylephrine spray (10%) also can be used.
- If progressive nasal swelling is expected, secure a small tube (9- to 15-mm diameter, 4- to 8-cm length) by suturing to the nostril to help maintain a patent nasal airway. This is easier than performing tracheotomy, however nasal mucosal necrosis can result from the pressure of the tube.
- Tracheotomy may be needed in some cases.
- Try to keep the head level or elevated. If the affected individual safely tolerates it, the head should be tied in an elevated position.
- Begin administration of antibiotics (e.g., penicillin).
- Suture any wounds.
- Administer tetanus toxoid.

Thrombosis of Jugular Veins

Bilateral thrombosis of the jugular veins occurs in severely ill patients receiving medications, especially hypertonic fluids or acidic or alkaline drugs, through the jugular vein. Unfortunately, many of these patients are depressed and hold their heads lower than normal because of the primary disease. Progressive nasal edema can result. With medical treatment, tracheotomy can be avoided if the patient can maintain its head in a normal position.

TREATMENT

- Medical treatment is primarily antiedema therapy (e.g., furosemide 1 mg/kg IV slowly). Administer further intravenous treatments through the lateral thoracic vein or cephalic vein.
- If one jugular vein is patent with a catheter in place, remove the catheter and place it elsewhere (e.g., lateral thoracic vein) if possible.
- Begin aspirin, 60-120 grains (3.9-7.8 g)/450-kg adult PO, along with pentoxifylline, 8.4 mg/kg PO q12h. Give aspirin every 2-3 days for its antiplatelet effect. Pentoxifylline has both antiplatelet aggregation and anticytokine effects, in addition to making red blood cells more deformable.
- If hypoproteinemia is compounding the problem, administer plasma (2-10 L), fresh or fresh frozen, or hetastarch (2-10 ml/kg). Consider cost and expected benefit. If plasma is administered, add 100 U heparin to the plasma to stimulate antithrombin III activity before administration.

Bee Sting

Bee stings or vaccine reactions can produce acute severe nasal edema.

TREATMENT
- Cold compresses
- Antihistamines, such as doxylamine succinate, 0.5 mg/kg *slowly IV*
- Dexamethasone if the edema is progressive and severe: 0.1-0.2 mg/kg q24h IV
- Epinephrine, 3-5 ml of 1:1000 solution IV to a 450 kg adult, if the swelling is rapidly progressive or if there are signs of systemic hypotension (tachycardia, poor pulse quality)
- Tracheotomy if needed (see p. 67)
- Keep the head level or elevated

Snake Bite
- Venomous snakes may bite horses and cause severe tissue necrosis.
- The nose is a common site for a bite, and severe swelling results.
- Swelling is marked with rattlesnake bites.

DIAGNOSIS AND CLINICAL SIGNS
- The swelling is initially warm, then becomes cool as the skin becomes necrotic. Shaving the area may be needed to identify the fang marks. The most frequent sequelae:
  - Airway obstruction when bitten on the nose
  - Severe cellulitis often associated with infections with *Clostridium* organisms
  - Hemolytic anemia rarely occurs
- Severe systemic effects from the venom are not common in adults. In foals, systemic effects include hypotension and shock, which should be managed appropriately with *intravenous fluids,* inotropic or pressor drugs (e.g., dopamine, 5-10 µg/kg per minute, or dobutamine, 5-15 µg/kg per minute, or norepinephrine, 0.02-0.1 µg/kg per minute), or both fluids and drugs. Remember that foals do not have as dramatic an increase in blood pressure in response to pressor drugs as do adults. Change in heart rate should be monitored in foals receiving β- and α-agonist combination drugs. More than a 40% increase in heart rate is a signal to slow the rate of drug administration.

TREATMENT
- If the airway becomes obstructed, perform tracheotomy (see p. 67).
- If the nose is bitten and airway obstruction has not developed, keep the head level or elevated to minimize severe swelling. Pass a nasotracheal tube, shortened stomach tube, or syringe case and leave it in place to prevent airway obstruction.
- Flunixin meglumine is administered to decrease inflammation and diminish systemic effects caused by proinflammatory prostanoids. It has little effect on platelet function.
- Administer penicillin in all cases, 22,000-44,000 U/kg, preferably IV q6h, or 22,000 U/kg IM q12h.
- Metronidazole, 15 mg/kg q8h PO, and gentamicin, 6.6 mg/kg IV q24h (if hypotension is absent or minimal dehydration). Penicillin can be added to the treatment to improve anaerobic coverage. Substitute ceftiofur, 3.0 mg/kg IV or IM q12h, or gentamicin if hydration and renal function are a concern.
- Tetanus toxoid for adults or toxoid and antitoxin in foals.
- If hypotensive therapy is needed: Administer fluids, including hypertonic saline solution, plasma, and finally pressor drugs, if the fluids do not correct the hypotension (see Systemic Shock, p. 615).

- Antivenin (equine origin) is not recommended unless administered within first 8 hours of the bite. It may benefit foals bitten by coral snakes.

RESPIRATORY DISTRESS WITHOUT NOISE
Pneumothorax

Severity depends largely on the inciting cause and the completeness of the mediastinum. Inflammatory causes, such as pneumonia, rarely result in bilateral pneumothorax, whereas traumatic pneumothorax can be unilateral or bilateral. Idiopathic pneumothorax (no evidence of trauma but probable lung rupture) often is bilateral or causes such a marked increase in intrapleural pressure on the affected side that the opposite side is compromised.

Traumatic Pneumothorax

If the mediastinum is complete, the pneumothorax is unilateral. The patient has a rapid respiratory rate but its condition remains stable. If pneumothorax is bilateral, signs are more severe and respiratory distress is progressive.

DIAGNOSIS
- The patient exhibits signs of respiratory distress (flared nostrils and increased respiratory rate).
- Auscultation reveals little or no dorsal movement of air (either bilaterally or unilaterally).
- Confirm findings with radiographs (the dorsal lung margin can be seen) or ultrasonography (air echo that does not move with respiration; see p. 33).
- Perform diagnostic aspiration with a 3.5-inch (8.8 cm) needle or catheter with stylet. Attach a short extension tube to the needle or catheter, place 3-5 ml of sterile saline solution into the tube, and hold the tube proximally as the needle is advanced into the dorsal thorax (usual depth 2 inches [5 cm]). If pneumothorax is present, the saline "bubbles" back up as the thorax is entered and the air is forced out. If negative pressure is still present, the saline solution is sucked into the thorax.

TREATMENT
- Administer intranasal oxygen, 10-20 ml/kg per minute through a nasopharyngeal tube. Even with unilateral pneumothorax, the other side of the lung can be physically compromised caused by the positive pressure on the mediastinum.
- Close any wounds and suture as soon as possible unless internal pneumothorax is also possible .
- Remove the air in the thorax after the wounds are closed. Use an 18-gauge needle or a 4-inch (10 cm) teat cannula.
- Start broad-spectrum antibiotic therapy for all forms of externally induced pneumothorax: Potassium penicillin, 44,000 U/kg q6h IV, and gentamicin, 6.6 mg/kg IV q24h, or ceftiofur, 3.0 mg/kg IV q12h.
- Administer analgesics.

Pneumothorax Secondary to Pneumonia

Generally unilateral because the mediastinum usually is complete with inflammatory disease. Alveoli may rupture in severe pneumonia, or air leaks into one side of the chest from a chest drain, resulting in pneumothorax. Unilateral pneumothorax in patients with pneumonia can cause severe respiratory distress because the pneumothorax is compounded by bilateral lung disease, and the pressure of the tension pneumothorax forces the mediastinum to the opposite side.

TREATMENT
- Replace leaking chest valve if a problem.
- Place a 3.5-inch (8.8 cm), 16-gauge IV catheter **high** in the 13th intercostal space. As soon as the chest is entered, pull the stylet back ¼ inch (0.6 cm). Using a 60-ml syringe and three-way stopcock or vacuum pump (*make certain the pump is set on suction*), aspirate the air.

Idiopathic Pneumothorax
Affected individuals have no evidence of external trauma nor do they have pneumonia. They often have bilateral pneumothorax or bilateral compromise, are in severe respiratory distress, and may die acutely. Tension pneumothorax is suspected in these cases.

TREATMENT
- Bilateral: With severe respiratory distress, decompress the thorax as described and place a one-way chest tube Heimlich valve **high** on the chest wall. *This must be done quickly!* Affected patients have tension pneumothorax; therefore an incision into the thorax may reduce internal thoracic pressure.
- Unilateral: If the patient's condition is stable, there is no need to suction the thorax unless pressure in the hemithorax is compromising the opposite side of the thorax.

Pneumomediastinum
Commonly found radiographically after tracheal aspiration but rarely necessitates treatment. Tracheal perforation (most often from kicks) or severe axillary wounds occasionally result in pressure pneumomediastinum, which can severely affect preload (venous return) to the heart and cause life-threatening hypotension with respiratory distress. The diagnosis is confirmed radiographically and endoscopically.

TREATMENT
- *Tracheal perforation:* Endoscopic examination of the trachea reveals the point of perforation. Perform repair through a ventral cervical incision with the patient standing. Do not close the skin incision.
- *Axillary wound:* Cross-tie the patient to decrease movement, and pack the wound to prevent more air from entering the wound.
- In both situations, administer intranasal oxygen, 10-20 ml/kg per minute, and administer fluids to improve venous return and cardiac preload. In severe cases of tracheal perforation, surgery is needed.

Pulmonary Edema
Acute pulmonary edema frequently arises from conditions that increase pulmonary vascular pressure, such as left-sided *heart failure,* or that alter the *permeability* of the *pulmonary vascular endothelium,* such as *endotoxic shock, purpura hemorrhagica, adverse drug reactions,* or *anaphylaxis.* Other causes of pulmonary edema include:

- Smoke inhalation
- Neurogenic—pulmonary edema may accompany head trauma
- Iatrogenic overzealous administration of intravenous fluids in recumbent neonates or adults with anuric acute renal failure

Pulmonary edema usually occurs with acute problems and rarely is observed in hypoproteinemic patients with glomerulopathy or protein-losing enteropathy despite the presence of severe subcutaneous edema.

Diagnosis
- Physical examination and the presence of a preexisting disease such as acute heart failure, endotoxic shock, or anaphylaxis.

Treatment
- Manage the primary disease.
- Reduce edema.
- Provide oxygen support until adequate ventilation is restored.
  NOTE: If anxiety is present, sedate with diazepam, 0.05-0.2 mg/kg IV or IM.

Pulmonary Edema Secondary to Endotoxic Shock/Systemic Inflammatory Response Syndrome*
TREATMENT
- Low-dose flunixin meglumine, 0.1-0.2 mg/kg IV; DMSO, 1 g/kg IV diluted in 3 L of 0.9% saline solution or 5% dextrose; dexamethasone, 0.25 mg/kg IV bolus.
- Furosemide, 1 mg/kg IV (monitor systemic blood pressure because it can lower cardiac output).
- Intranasal oxygen, 10-15 L/min per 450-kg adult.
- Pentoxifylline, 8.4 mg/kg PO q8-12h.
- Cardiac output usually is low; manage with plasma and dobutamine, 2-10 µg/kg per minute. Use of steroids is controversial.
- Hypertonic saline solution is the fluid of choice when intravenous fluids are needed in the management of pulmonary edema and hypotension.

Pulmonary Edema Secondary to Heart Failure
TREATMENT
- Digoxin, 1 mg IV/450-kg adult
- Furosemide, 1 mg/kg IV
- Intranasal oxygen, 10-15 L/min
- Arterial vasodilator to decrease afterload (e.g., hydralazine, see p. 172)

Pulmonary Edema Secondary to Anaphylaxis (Adverse Drug Reaction)
TREATMENT
- Epinephrine, 3-5 ml for adults, diluted in 20-30 ml of saline solution and administered slowly IV or in less severe cases, IM or SQ
- Dexamethasone, 0.1-0.2 mg/kg IV bolus
- Furosemide, 1 mg/kg IV

---

*A shocklike syndrome similar to endotoxic shock and which can be initiated by any inflammatory disorder.

- Intranasal oxygen, 10-20 ml/kg per minute
- Intravenous plasma or synthetic colloid (hetastarch)

Purpura Hemorrhagica
- Rarely causes acute pulmonary edema

TREATMENT
- Dexamethasone, 0.1-0.2 mg/kg IV
- Furosemide, 1 mg/kg IV q24h
- Intranasal oxygen

Fluid Therapy in Patients at High Risk of Development of Pulmonary Edema
- High-risk patients include:
  - Septic foals
  - Septic and recumbent foals
  - Equine endotoxic shock
  - Generalized anaphylactic diseases causing rapid protein loss
  - Fluid therapy for hypovolemia is required for many of these patients.
- Hypertonic saline solution initially, 4-8 ml/kg, to improve cardiac output and blood pressure and to decrease pulmonary arterial pressures
- Oncotic plasma expanders, equine plasma, or hetastarch may decrease lung fluid volume and are recommended, but these agents are expensive.

Airway Obstruction
TREATMENT
- Perform immediate tracheotomy or pass a nasotracheal tube.
- Furosemide, 1 mg/kg IV.

Smoke Inhalation

Horses may be seriously affected or die of smoke inhalation in a barn fire. They can die without skin burns. Three pulmonary consequences can occur in association with smoke inhalation:

- Carbon monoxide poisoning: Immediate
- Pulmonary edema: Hours later
- Pneumonia: Hours to days later

Smoke inhalation and pulmonary edema are the immediate primary concerns when affected individuals are examined after a fire.

Diagnosis and Clinical Findings
RESPIRATORY SIGNS FOLLOWING SMOKE EXPOSURE
- Coughing
- Labored breathing
- Polypnea
- Frothy exudate

Other Clinical Findings
- Tachycardia

- Widespread wheezes and crackles
- Cyanosis

TREATMENT
- Manage pulmonary, laryngeal, or pharyngeal edema.

  | **NOTE:** If skin burns are present, avoid corticosteroids! (see Pulmonary Edema, p. 511.)

- Prevent airway obstruction from fibrin debris: Suctioning through an endoscope is preferred. (Suction should be performed in multiple, brief [<20second] pulses because prolonged, continual suction causes hypoxemia.)
- Perform tracheotomy *only* if life-threatening laryngeal edema is occurring. Tracheotomy prevents the patient from removing necrotic casts from the lower airway by coughing.
- Oxygen therapy: Humidified, 10-15 L/min for adults, administered intranasally or through tracheotomy; continue oxygen during suctioning!
- Alleviate bronchoconstriction:
  □ Clenbuterol, 0.8-1.6 mg/kg IV or PO q12h (may be nebulized: 10 ml containing 0.03 mg/ml)

  or

  □ Atropine, 0.014-0.02 mg/kg IV *once or twice only* (7 mg/450-kg adult) or glycopyrrolate (0.0022 mg/kg IV q 8h)
- Prophylactic therapy for shock. Despite the presence of pulmonary edema, fluid therapy is needed to maintain tissue perfusion. Fluid therapy is essential for patients receiving furosemide to manage pulmonary edema.
  □ Polyionic fluids to prevent shock: Maintenance rate, 1-2 L/h (adult). Add KCl (20-40 mEq/L) if renal function is normal and if serum potassium value is normal or low.
  □ *Plasma*, 1-2 L with antiendotoxin antibodies. Larger volume in severe cases or synthetic colloids, such as hetastarch.
  □ NSAIDs: Flunixin meglumine, 0.25 mg/kg q8h *or* ketoprofen, 1 mg/kg q12h
- Therapy for sepsis: Administer *broad-spectrum bactericidal antibiotics* to patients believed to be in a septic state (fever or the presence of intracellular bacteria on examination of tracheal sputum). If deep burns exist on the body or if tracheotomy is performed, administer antibiotics:
  □ Ceftiofur, 3 mg/kg q12h

  or

  □ Penicillin, 22,000 IU/kg IV q6h, and amikacin, 15-25 mg/kg IV q24h *or* enrofloxacin, 7.5 mg/kg PO q24h *or* 5 mg/kg IV q12-24 h

  and

  □ Metronidazole, 15 mg/kg PO q8h.

Chronic Obstructive Pulmonary Disease, Chronic Recurrent Airway Obstruction

Horses with heaves often experience respiratory distress after exposure to allergens or an infectious agent. Airways of affected patients appear to be hyperactive to particulate matter (e.g., dust, mold spores, noxious fumes, and even high humidity), predisposing the individual to respiratory crises despite good management. Increased mucus production and decreased lung function provide the ideal environment for secondary infections, which frequently trigger episodes of respiratory distress. Fever of 39.5°C-40°C (103°F-104°F) often is present in patients with bacterial bronchitis and heaves.

Diagnosis

- Clinical findings
- Auscultation: Fine crackles and wheezes usually are heard over most lung fields. The lungs sometimes are abnormally quiet (especially ventrally) in severe episodes. This sign is confused with ventral consolidation (pneumonia) or pleural effusion, but horses with pleuropneumonia infrequently have respiratory distress, and when they do, they usually have signs of sepsis (injected, discolored mucous membranes, severe depression, and commonly a hemorrhagic or fetid discharge from the nostrils).
- Response to treatment often is a useful diagnostic test if heaves is thought to be the problem. A marked response to a single injection of atropine supports the diagnosis.
- Tracheal sputum examination: The sample can be collected through an endoscope for both culture and cytologic examination.* It is important that the procedure be performed rapidly to prevent flow of oropharyngeal fluid down the trachea and contamination of the sample. *If the patient is in severe respiratory distress, do not perform a transtracheal wash (TTW) because severe pneumomediastinum can occur.*
- Sedation may be needed for the endoscopic procedure: Xylazine, 0.3 mg/kg IV, and butorphanol, 0.01 mg/kg IV.

Treatment

- Atropine, 0.014-0.02 mg/kg (7-10 mg IV/450-kg adult), for immediate relief unless severe tachycardia (>80 beats/min) is present.

NOTE: Atropine decreases intestinal motility, so advise owners to monitor for signs of colic, although colic is unusual when this dosage is used once.

- Corticosteroids
  □ Dexamethasone, 0.02-0.06 mg/kg PO or parenterally q24h until a clinical response is seen.
- Antibiotics: If there is a fever or if bacterial bronchitis is suspected as the underlying cause of heaves: Ceftiofur, 3 mg/kg q12h.
- Glycopyrrolate; 0.005 mg/kg IV, IM, or SQ q8-12h, can be used instead of atropine but is not as effective. Higher dosages may result in gastrointestinal atony, gas distention, or small-colon impactions in some patients.
- Clenbuterol 0.8-1.6 mg/kg IV or PO q12h

CAUTION: If the patient has a high heart rate (>80 beats/min), do not administer atropine or glycopyrrolate. Be cautious when administering other bronchodilators to patients with severe tachycardia.

---

*An Endoscopic Microbiology Aspiration Catheter (Mila International, Florence, KY 41042) can be used if culture is needed. A sterile polyethylene 205 tubing with an adapter (Intramedic and Intramedic Luer Stud Adapter. Becton Dickinson, Parsippany, NJ 07054) also works well for sample collection for cytologic examination and culture.

- Intranasal oxygen: 10-15 L/min through a nasopharyngeal catheter sutured at the nostril. Bubble the oxygen through warm water if possible.
- Use nebulization as additional therapy, or use "puffers" (meter-dosed inhalers) in chronic cases (see Chapter 52, p. 663). *These should not be used solely for therapy in acute severe cases.* For severe respiratory distress, use nebulization with an ultrasonic nebulizer or other type of nebulizer that delivers particles of 0.5 μm or smaller. A combination that is useful is 250 mg aminophylline, 1-2.5 ml 10% acetylcysteine, and 2.5-5.0 mg albuterol (for inhalation), in addition to one of the following antibiotics: Ceftiofur, 1-2 ml; amikacin (preservative free), 1 ml; tobramycin (preservative free, 300 mg). The solution can be mixed with a saline solution to prepare a 30-ml volume. Clenbuterol (10 ml containing 0.03 mg/ml) and/or, ipratropium bromide (250 μg [12 puffs]), and beclomethasone (1-2 μg/kg [10-20 puffs]) or fluticasone (1-2 mg) may be delivered with an aeromask, or albuterol, 720 μg [8 puffs])aerosolized with Torpex.*
- Furosemide, 1.0 mg/kg IV or IM, improves lung function but generally without noticeable clinical improvement.
- *Do not use NSAIDs to treat patients with heaves* unless another disease necessitates use of these drugs. NSAIDs can decrease the level of prostaglandin E_2 and its bronchodilatory effect.
- Maintain adequate hydration because dehydration thickens the mucous plugs in the airways. Provide fresh, clean water and electrolyte and glucose supplementation. In some cases it may be necessary to administer fluids through a nasogastric tube or intravenously.
- Move the patient to an area with fewer irritants!

Prognosis

Good in most cases. However, satisfactory clinical improvement may require 3-5 days. Do not expect improvement in horses with heaves and concurrent bacterial bronchitis until corticosteroid therapy is added to the antimicrobial therapy. Some older patients with a prolonged history of heaves with severe parenchymal disease may not respond to this treatment, especially if they are not responsive to a test dose of atropine. Radiographs are recommended.

Management

- Management of heaves involves minimizing contact with allergens by changing feeds (generally best to prevent hay exposure) and bedding (newspaper can be used) so that the mold count and dust are decreased.
- Most affected individuals should be kept outside 24 hours a day if possible. If not, it is best to move them to the end of the barn (or an area with the best ventilation) and outside at haying time and during bedding change.
- In the southeastern United States, some individuals exhibit respiratory signs of heaves while at pasture (pasture-associated heaves) and may improve within 24 hours if they are simply housed in a barn.
- Intradermal skin testing and radioallergosorbent testing (RAST) may be used in the hope of identifying the allergen. RAST appears more reliable for detecting the allergen. Perform both tests if desensitization is considered.

---

*Torpex. Boehringer Ingelheim, Vetmedica Inc., St. Joseph, MO 64506.

NOTE: On the rare occasion, a 3- to 6-month-old foal recovering from "typical" foal pneumonia develops "heavy" signs. A transtracheal aspirate may reveal *Aspergillus sp.* and no bacteria. Treatment with bronchodilators and occasionally corticosteroids is required.

Viral (or Postviral) Respiratory Distress Syndrome

- Most often seen in *young adults* and rarely foals exposed to viral infections of the upper respiratory tract. The incidence among horses with viral upper respiratory infections is low.
- Affected individuals initially have a fever (often as high as 41.4°C [106°F]) associated with the viral infection and within 1-3 days experience severe tachypnea with labored breathing.
- The pathophysiologic mechanism of the syndrome is undetermined and is believed to be an overreactive airway triggered by the virus or irritant. This syndrome is distinctly different from pleuropneumonia (see p. 522), which results in severe weight loss and marked ventral ultrasonographic and/or radiographic abnormalities.

Diagnosis

- History: Includes recent arrival from a sale barn or recent exposure (show) to a large group of young horses.
- Fever as high as 41.4°C.
- Auscultation: Wheezes and crackles are heard but are less dramatic than the clinical signs; lung sounds are quiet for the effort expended in breathing.
- Transtracheal aspirate usually is nonseptic, although bacteria, e.g., *Pasteurella* organisms, and fungi, e.g., *Aspergillus* are occasionally cultured.
- Most individuals affected are not toxic, and they have a normal appetite but labored breathing.
- Affected individuals may look like patients with heaves, but the age (foals and young adults) and history are different.
- Radiographs and ultrasonography show abnormalities (e.g., interstitial pattern or alveolar edema and roughening of the pleura), but the abnormalities are not severe!

Treatment

- Bronchodilators:
  - Clenbuterol, 0.8-1.6 µg/kg PO q12h for 2-3 days (make sure potassium intake is adequate because β-adrenergic drugs can decrease serum potassium concentration)

  and

  - Glycopyrrolate, 5 mg/450-kg adult SQ q8h for 2-3 days
- Intranasal oxygen: 10-20 ml/kg per minute continuously
- Antimicrobial therapy: Ceftiofur, 3.0 mg/kg, for bacterial infections, especially when *Pasteurella* organisms are cultured

Prognosis

Despite respiratory distress for 3-6 days, the prognosis is good. *In rare cases, such as when a horse has not been vaccinated or a mule has not been previously exposed to influenza, rapid progression to death may result* from the influenza virus infection.

Rhodococcus equi Pneumonia in Foals

Generally affects foals between 2 weeks and 3 months of age and rarely horses older than 4 months. Manifests as acute respiratory distress. *R. equi* infection must be differentiated from bronchointerstitial pneumonia of viral or unknown causation, because it also results in respiratory distress in nursing foals.

Diagnosis

- The age of the foal (2 weeks to 4 months)
- A history of previous *R. equi* infection on the farm
- Swollen joints without severe lameness in approximately 25% of affected horses
- Geographic location (increased prevalence in some areas of the country, e.g., dry, dusty, warm areas)
- Season: Most commonly affects foals in the late spring
- Clinical presentation: Acute respiratory distress, high fever, and minimal cough
- Auscultation:
  □ Harsh lung sounds are heard diffusely, except for the caudal tip, which is generally loud but normal.
  □ Lung sounds often are less musical than with other bacterial infections.
- Tracheal aspiration: Use the least traumatic method of collection: Percutaneous TTW with an Intracath or similar catheter (see p. 2). Insertion of an Intracath does not require local anesthesia or an incision and therefore is less stressful. If sedation is needed, use 5 mg of diazepam or 0.5 mg/kg xylazine.

NOTE: This method of tracheal aspiration is more expensive than other diagnostic methods. Culture and *Gram stain* the aspirate. *R. equi* organisms are small, pleomorphic, Gram-positive rods (see Chapter 6, p. 17).

- Chest radiographs: Use standard units and a 400-speed film or screen combination, and 80 kilovolt (peak) [kV(p)] at 20 mA 0.2- to 0.3-second nongrid. *R. equi* infection often produces a "white out" of the lungs, except for the caudal tips of the diaphragmatic lung lobes, which remain black. Many *R. equi* abscesses can be seen ultrasonographically (see p. 56).

Treatment

- Antibiotics:
  □ Clarithromycin, 7.5 mg/kg PO q12h, *and* rifampin, 5 mg/kg PO q12h

  or

  □ Azithromycin, 10 mg/kg PO q24h for 5-10 days and then every other day and rifampin, 5 mg/kg PO q 12 h

NOTE: Some foals are in severe respiratory distress, so compliance by owners is important to ensure that the entire dosage is swallowed!

  □ Vancomycin, 5-7 mg/kg diluted and administered slowly IV q8-12 h, if the foal is unable to swallow oral medications.
- Trimethoprim-sulfamethoxazole, 20 mg/kg PO q12h should be added if *Pneumocystis carinii* infection is suspected
- If additional aerobic bacteria are observed on gram stain, ceftiofur should be added to the *Rhodococcus* therapy
- Intranasal oxygen, 10-20 ml/kg per minute continuously (see Chapter 12, p. 64)

- Intravenous fluid therapy: Polyionic fluids may be required at a maintenance rate of 40 ml/kg IV over 24 hours if dehydration is present and foals are unable to nurse. DMSO, 1 g/kg slowly IV diluted in 1 L of 0.9% saline solution, is useful in acute, severe cases.
- β_2-specific bronchodilators: Clenbuterol, 1.6 µg/kg PO q12h. *Do not use* aminophylline; it rarely is efficacious, there is risk of drug interaction with erythromycin, and toxic levels of aminophylline can cause seizures in foals.
- Ulcer prophylaxis: Ranitidine, 6.6 mg/kg PO q8h, and sucralfate, 1-2 g q6-8h; do not combine or administer sucralfate simultaneously with orally administered antibiotics, bronchodilators or H_2/proton pump blockers.
- Intranasal oxygen

NOTE: On hot days, some foals receiving erythromycin experience high fevers (41.1°C-43.4°C [106°F-110°F]). Cool with alcohol or cold water bath, and fans, place in the shade, and administer dipyrone, 10 ml IV. Keep indoors on hot days.

Acute Bacterial Pneumonia and Respiratory Distress in Foals Due to Etiologic Agents Other than *Rhodococcus equi*

Common in neonatal foals (see Sepsis, p. 552) and rare in older foals. Fever and respiratory distress in a nursing foal and a radiographic cranioventral pattern of disease or pleural effusion are compatible with bacterial pneumonia. Age, tracheal wash, farm history, and so on, are important in ruling out *R. equi* infection in 2-week to 4-month-old foals.

Diagnosis and Clinical Findings

- Auscultation of the chest varies; crackles and wheezes or a "consolidated bronchial tone sound" are frequently heard cranioventrally. Pleural effusion and occasionally quiet bronchial sounds are heard ventrally on auscultation.
- Clinical pathology: Results of a leukogram that generally support sepsis; toxic neutrophils with a left shift; and elevated fibrinogen value.
- Tracheal wash: Perform TTW and submit sputum for aerobic and anaerobic culture and Gram stain. The most common organisms are Gram-negative rods, e.g., *Pasteurella* organisms, *Escherichia coli*, and occasionally anaerobic organisms.
- Thoracocentesis: *only if* ultrasound findings indicate pleural effusion *and* the fluid is believed to contribute to respiratory distress or when an etiologic agent is not isolated with TTW. Butorphanol, 0.025 mg/kg IM, or diazepam, 5 mg IV, can be administered before the procedure.
- Radiography: A chest radiograph may be needed to rule out *R. equi* infection and diffuse bronchointerstitial pneumonitis.
  - A radiographic pattern suggesting abscessation and diffuse involvement of the lung is characteristic of *R. equi* infection. Multiple joint swellings, marked neutrophilia, and thrombocytosis indicate the presence of *R. equi* infection.
  - Acute interstitial pneumonia, viral or idiopathic, is ruled out by the presence of a lower fibrinogen value, less responsive leukogram, more diffuse disease pattern at clinical and radiographic examination, and the absence of pathogenic bacteria in tracheal aspirate.

Treatment

- Broad-spectrum antibiotics:

RESPIRATORY

- □ Ticarcillin/clavulanic acid, 44-50 mg/kg IV q6h

  or

- □ Ceftiofur, 3-5 mg/kg IV q8-12h
- □ Amikacin should be added for the synergistic benefit and improved Gram-negative spectrum if renal function is normal and the foal is receiving IV fluids.
- □ Metronidazole, 15 mg/kg PO q12h for foals younger than 3 weeks and q8h for older foals, only if anaerobic organisms are seen at TTW or if *E. coli* or *Enterobacter* organisms are cultured. The latter finding may indicate increased risk of an anaerobic organism also being present.
- Intranasal oxygen, 10-20 ml/kg per minute
- Antiulcer prophylaxis:
  - □ Ranitidine, 6.6 mg/kg q8h PO or 1.5 mg/kg IV q8h or other H$_2$ blocker
  - □ Sucralfate, 1-2 g q6-12h PO 60 minutes before ranitidine.
  - □ Remove pleural fluid using diazepam (Valium) for sedation and adequate restraint; use a teat cannula and 60-ml syringe with a three-way stopcock. The fluid often is bright red.

Respiratory Distress in Newborn Foals

This may occur because of severe birth asphyxia, prematurity, meconium aspiration, fractured ribs, and/or sepsis. Management and treatment is often complex and the specifics are presented beginning on p. 552. Begin oxygen immediately!

Bronchointerstitial Pneumonia in Foals

Bronchointerstitial pneumonia is a primary rule-out for *R. equi* infection affecting the same age or *older* foal and is of unknown etiology. It causes severe respiratory distress with a high fever, *usually affecting one horse on a farm*. Consider this disease when a patient with suspected *R. equi* infection has negative results for *R. equi* on tracheal aspiration. The prognosis for these foals is fair with corticosteroid treatment. If not treated with corticosteroids, most of the affected individuals have respiratory distress for 3-5 days before dying. Some may survive. The cause of the syndrome is unknown; it may be toxic, immunologic, or a nonbacterial infection.

Diagnosis
CLINICAL PRESENTATION
- Respiratory distress: Tachypnea and cyanosis
- Frequently bright, alert, and nursing
- High fever: 38.9°C-41.7°C (102°F-107°F)
- No severe inflammatory changes on leukogram
- Several weeks of age
- *R. equi* negative
- No intracellular bacteria in tracheal aspirate

RADIOGRAPHIC FINDINGS
- Diffuse disease, with or without a nodular pattern
- No abscesses

Treatment

- Corticosteroids: Dexamethasone, 0.4-0.8 mg/kg IV or IM q12h for 2 days, followed by a tapering dosage (*only if R. equi* infection is believed unlikely on the basis of age and no *R. equi* organisms are found at TTW)
- Improvement should be seen within 48 hours after corticosteroids are started.
- Intranasal oxygen: 5 L/min continuously.

| **CAUTION:** Small oxygen tanks may last for 1-2 hours only.

- Antibiotics: Ceftiofur, 3.0 mg/kg IV q12h
- Bronchodilators:
  - Clenbuterol, 0.8-1.6 µg/kg PO q12h
  - Nebulization: See pp. 516, 663. The higher dosage of acetylcysteine should be used because this agent is a glutathione (antioxidant) donor.
- DMSO, 1 g/kg IV, diluted in 1 L of isotonic fluid and balanced polyionic fluids to maintain hydration. *Do not* administer sodium bicarbonate because this may increase the respiratory rate and even decrease blood pH if there are severe alveolar ventilation-perfusion abnormalities.
- Ulcer prophylaxis medication:
  - Sucralfate, 1-2 g PO q6-8h preferred

  or

  - Ranitidine, 6.6 mg/kg PO q8h or 1.5 mg/kg IV q8h, or other H_2–proton pump blocker
- *Thermoregulatory control:*
  - Alcohol or cold water bath and fan
  - Dipyrone, 5-10 ml three to four times daily if needed

ACUTE RESPIRATORY DISTRESS IN FOALS AFTER ANTHELMINTIC TREATMENT

Although this complication is rare, nursing or weanling foals may develop respiratory distress 1-3 days after administration of an anthelmintic. This is believed to be a result of the death of a large number of ascarid or strongyle larvae in the lungs.

Diagnosis

- History of receiving an anthelmintic, often for the first time
- Signs of respiratory distress within 48 hours after anthelmintic treatment
- Clinical signs:
  - Labored breathing
  - Tachypnea
  - Coughing
  - Nasal discharge
  - Body temperature ranging from normal to 39.8°C (102.5°F)
- Auscultation:
  - Wheezes heard over lung fields bilaterally
- Transtracheal wash:
  - Usually nonseptic
  - Cellular reaction may be a mixture of neutrophils and eosinophils.

Treatment

- Corticosteroids, *single dose only:* Dexamethasone, 0.1 mg/kg; usually marked improvement seen
- Antibiotics:
  - Trimethoprim-sulfamethoxazole, 20 mg/kg PO q12h

    and/or

  - Procaine penicillin, 22,000 U/kg IM q12h

    or

  - Ceftiofur alone, 3.0 mg/kg IV q12h

Prognosis

Good

PLEUROPNEUMONIA AND SEPTIC PLEURITIS

- Although the disease process may be present for several days, *consider pleuro-pneumonia in an adult an emergency!*
- Unlike most forms of pneumonia in foals, pleuropneumonia in an adult is commonly complicated by anaerobic infection, which is associated with a greater risk of necrosis and infarction of the lung.
- ▶ *Pleuropneumonia is the most common cause of infectious pleural effusion in the horse* (Table 43–1).

Clinical Signs

- Usually most severe in the midventral right lung, and abnormal lung sounds usually are more prominent in this area. Other clinical signs include forelimb or sternal edema, *low-grade colic,* pleurodynia, laminitis, fever, and anorexia.

Diagnosis

- *The odor of the sample obtained by means of TTW or thoracocentesis can be important in management!* A fetid odor indicates the presence of anaerobic bacteria, *worsens the prognosis, and increases the cost of treatment.* Air echoes within the pleural fluid may also indicate the presence of anaerobic infection. (See also p. 52.) Discuss this finding with the owner!

TABLE 43–1. Signs and Physical Findings of Pleuropneumonia

	Clinical Signs	Auscultation Findings
Acute	Respiratory distress, cough (usually soft), red to dark brown exudate at nostril, severe depression	Crackles and in some areas wheezes, increased ventral bronchial sounds if effusion is minimal
Subacute to chronic	Weight loss, soft cough, poor performance, normal to increased respiratory rate	Pleural effusion, no ventral lung sounds, normal to loud dorsal sounds, radiating heart sounds, normal to increased respiratory rate

- Transtracheal aspiration (*preferred over bronchoalveolar lavage*). Use a BBL Vacutainer, Columbia broth with sodium polystyrene sulfonate (SPS) and increased cysteine (Becton-Dickinson, Cockeysville, MD). Submit for both *aerobic* and *anaerobic* culture.
- Thoracocentesis: Indicated if there is the suspicion of pleural effusion (decreased ventral lung sounds and radiating heart sounds). Ultrasonographic findings confirm the presence of fluid.
- Quick method (for culture only). Requires 18-gauge, 1.5- to 3.5-inch (3.75- to 8.9-cm) needle. Aerobic-anaerobic culture medium (BBL Vacutainer, Columbia broth with SPS and increased cysteine, Becton-Dickinson, Cockeysville, MD).
- Indwelling chest drain: Indicated if a large volume of fluid is present or if the effusion is flocculent and fetid (the same site as the thoracocentesis is preferred if the site is ventral enough to provide adequate drainage).
  - Requires a blunt-tipped 24F trocar catheter (Deknatel, Howmedica, Inc., Floral Park, NY); one-way valve (make a latex condom into a one-way valve by opening the closed end and attaching the other end to the catheter with tape).

PROTOCOL (see p. 72)
- Pass the blunt-tipped 24F trocar catheter 4-6 cm through a stab incision.
- Remove the trocar and manipulate the catheter to obtain the best flow rate.
- Attach the one-way valve to the catheter to prevent pneumothorax. Tape the condom over the end of the tube with the cut end distal and place a purse-string suture around the catheter to hold it in place.
- Determine the site for the thoracocatheter using ultrasound examination.

Treatment
- *Manage all cases of adult pleuropneumonia aggressively.*
- Start broad-spectrum antibiotics immediately.

OPTION 1
- Penicillin, 44,000 U/kg q6h IV

  and

- Gentamicin,* once-daily treatment with 6.6 mg/kg IV

  and

- Metronidazole, 15 mg/kg PO q6-8h

OPTION 2
- If decreased renal function or if cost of option 1 is prohibitive:
  - Ceftiofur, 3 mg/kg IV or IM q12h

  and

  - Metronidazole, 15 mg/kg PO q6-8h

---

*Serum creatinine concentration must be monitored during treatment. If azotemia is present, administer fluids or use Option 2. Monitoring peak and trough gentamicin levels is the best method to prevent renal toxicity associated with aminoglycoside usage.

RESPIRATORY

Supportive Therapy for Concurrent Toxemia

- Adults with abnormal mucous membrane color, toxic-appearing neutrophils or bands, and tachycardia:
  - □ Intravenous therapy with polyionic fluid
  - □ Flunixin meglumine, 0.25 mg/kg q8h IV or IM
  - □ J5 hyperimmune plasma, 2 L IV
  - □ Prophylaxis for laminitis:
    - □ Pentoxifylline,* 8.4 mg/kg PO q12h

  and/or

    - □ Aspirin,* 11-20 mg/kg (90 grains [6 g]/450 kg adult) PO q48h
    - □ Intranasal oxygen, 10-20 ml/kg per minute
    - □ Nitroglycerine cream applied over digital arteries

Prognosis

Prognosis for survival is generally good in acute cases unless severe tachypnea, severe polypnea, toxemia, and hemorrhagic-fetid nasal exudate are present. These findings support the presence of infarction and a poorer prognosis. In patients with pulmonary infarction, rib resection ultimately may be needed to improve recovery.

ASPIRATION PNEUMONIA

Aspiration pneumonia is common among horses. Chronic aspiration caused by a mechanical or neurologic condition of the pharynx or larynx is generally not an emergency. Acute aspiration results from esophageal choke, iatrogenic causes, or meconium aspiration in foals. In rare instances, horses spontaneously reflux gastric contents because of anterior enteritis, small-bowel obstruction, or gastric dilatation.

Occasionally, horses have severe respiratory distress after aspirating a large volume of material. Severe respiratory distress may be caused by misdirected gastric tubes and meconium aspiration in foals. *This is an emergency.*

Iatrogenic Aspiration Pneumonia
Diagnosis

- History of coughing and distress after tubing
- Auscultation of the trachea and lungs reveals a loud fluttering sound with crackles and wheezes hours later; ingesta seen at the nostrils.
- Tracheal endoscopic examination.
- Percutaneous TTW preferred over endoscopic aspiration to eliminate any possible confusion over contamination from the endoscope.

Treatment

- Corticosteroids: Dexamethasone, 0.1-0.2 mg/kg q24h on day 1 and 0.05-0.1 mg/kg on day 2.

| **NOTE:** Corticosteroids are for chemical aspiration only.

---

*These are believed useful in preventing thrombosis of pulmonary vessels.

- DMSO, 1 g/kg diluted in 3 L of saline solution and administered over 30-60 minutes.
- Antibiotics:
  - Penicillin, 44,000 U/kg IV q6h

  and

  - Gentamicin, 6.6-8.8 mg/kg IV q24h

| **CAUTION:** Monitor renal function and provide intravenous fluids if needed.

  and

  - Metronidazole, 15-25 mg/kg PO q6-8h

  or

  - Ceftiofur, 3.0 mg/kg IV q12h

  and

  - Metronidazole, 15-25 mg/kg PO q6-8h

ADJUNCT SUPPORTIVE TREATMENT

- Intranasal oxygen: 10-20 ml/kg per minute continuously. Place a soft rubber tube in the nasopharynx, suture it to the false nostril, and administer humidified oxygen from a portable tank.
- Flunixin meglumine, 0.25-1.1 mg/kg, or phenylbutazone, 2.2-4.4 mg/kg IV or PO after discontinuing corticosteroid therapy.
- Aspirate the lower airway by infusing warm sterile saline solution followed by suction if aspiration occurred within a "window" of 30 minutes. If the suction is forceful using a pump, it should be for brief periods of <20 seconds, with simultaneously administered oxygen.

NOTE: In rare instances distress occurs despite proper nasogastric tubing and administration of oral medication. These episodes of reflux esophageal spasm or esophageal or gastric irritation are alarming because the immediate concern is aspiration pneumonia or gastric rupture; however, within 30-60 minutes, the patient is normal.

NOTE: Almost all adults with choke have some aspiration pneumonia. Ultrasound examination of the chest 24-48 hours after the onset of choke generally reveals moderate to marked pleural abnormalities. In most cases, recovery is excellent regardless of these findings.

Meconium Aspiration in Foals

Diagnosis

Based primarily on the history. Commonly seen with fetal (in utero) diarrhea and stress associated with a colicky mare. Affected foals typically are born with brown-stained amniotic fluid. Foals with this history should be presumed to have aspirated meconium and generally show respiratory distress in the first few days of life.

Treatment

- Corticosteroids: Dexamethasone, 0.1-0.2 mg/kg IV q24h on day 1, 0.05-0.1 mg/kg on day 2. Use of corticosteroids is controversial, but in the newborn, a decreased pulmonary inflammatory response may be necessary to prevent hypoxia and reversion to fetal circulation through pulmonary hypertension.

- Broad-spectrum antibiotics:
  □ Ticarcillin-clavulanate (Timentin), 44-50 mg/kg IV q6h and amikacin, 18 mg/kg IV q24h

  or

  □ Ceftiofur, 3.0 mg/kg IV q12h and amikacin as an alternative
- *If severe*, administer intranasal oxygen at 5 L/min (see Chapter 12, p. 64), and DMSO, 1 g/kg diluted in saline solution.
- Perform tracheal suction if a fluttering sound is heard at auscultation of the trachea. Pass a catheter down the trachea, infuse 10 ml of saline solution, and aspirate using a 60-ml syringe. Repeat several times if aspirated material is retrieved. Oxygen should be administered simultaneously, and aspiration kept brief to prevent further oxygen debt.

ADDITIONAL CAUSES OF RESPIRATORY DISTRESS

- Diaphragmatic hernia (see p. 219)
- Botulism (see Chapter 40, p. 400)
- Fractured ribs (foals) (see Chapter 45, p. 550)
- Internal respiratory failure caused by hemolysis or intoxication.

EPISTAXIS

Epistaxis caused by head trauma rarely necessitates emergency treatment unless the nares are obstructed. Tracheotomy is then required. Conditions causing epistaxis that can be life threatening and necessitate emergency evaluation and therapy are:

- Guttural pouch mycosis
- Thrombocytopenia
- Rupture of the longus capitis muscle

Guttural Pouch Mycosis

Bleeding may be the only clinical sign in adults with guttural pouch mycosis; bleeding and neurologic signs rarely occur simultaneously. In some cases, yellow exudate is seen at the nostril before bleeding is observed. Middle-aged or older pastured horses are most commonly affected. Owners report finding blood on the stall wall or on the nose before major bleeding occurs. The bleeding is generally unilateral unless major bleeding happens.

Diagnosis

- A tentative diagnosis is based on history; endoscopic examination is needed for a definitive diagnosis.
- Endoscopic examination: Unless there is evidence of hypotension, elevated heart rate, pale mucous membranes, or slow capillary refill time, sedation facilitates the passage of the endoscope. Use of a guidewire passed through the biopsy channel assists in entering the pouch. An alternative is to pass a Chambers

catheter on the opposite side of the endoscope to elevate the guttural pouch flap. The lesion, often a yellowish-green, diphtheritic membrane with clot formation, is most commonly found dorsally in the medial or lateral compartment.

Treatment

- Once the diagnosis is confirmed, surgery is needed as soon as possible.
- If blood loss is severe, blood transfusion (see Chapter 37, p. 336) and polyionic fluids are needed to stabilize the patient's condition. Hypertonic saline usually is not administered unless hypovolemic shock is clinically evident.
- If sedation is needed to transport the patient, use diazepam, 0.05 mg/kg IV.
- If the bleeding is uncontrollable and life threatening, ligation of the common carotid artery on the affected side is helpful even though some bleeding continues.

NOTE: Ligation of the common carotid artery can result in severe neurologic signs and blindness.

Epistaxis Due to Thrombocytopenia

Can be a severe problem and require emergency treatment (see p. 336).

Rupture of the Longus Capitis Muscle

Can mimic severe guttural pouch hemorrhage and is differentiated at endoscopic examination. Treatment is symptomatic: Keep the affected individual quiet; administer fluids and blood transfusion and maintain a patent airway.

Ethmoid Hematoma

The initial clinical sign usually is a unilateral blood-tinged nasal discharge. With progression of the hematoma, respiratory noise from partial airway obstruction develops.

Diagnosis

- Endoscopic examination usually reveals a dark reddish-black or even greenish discolored mass in the ethmoid turbinate region. Radiographs are helpful in identifying masses in the paranasal sinuses.

Treatment

- Laser surgery or cryosurgery is generally recommended for large lesions, although intralesion injections with 4% formalin via endoscope can be effective for smaller lesions. **Rarely, an adverse event, including acute death, may occur immediately after the formalin injection.** If the cribriform plate is necrotic the formalin may enter the calvarium and brain. CT can be used before the injection to determine if the cribriform is intact. Large ethmoid hematomas require excision of the mass via paranasal sinus surgery. Autologous blood transfusion (collection in CDP 10 days before surgery) should be considered.

Exercise-Induced Pulmonary Hemorrhage

Rarely is the bleeding so severe that it results in respiratory distress and death. In some cases of acute death, bleeding is within the thoracic cavity.

Nasal Masses

Rarely are nasal masses (e.g., tumor, granuloma) a cause for emergency treatment; however, they are some of the most common causes of epistaxis and upper respiratory noise and obstruction.

REFERENCES

Respiratory Distress with Noise

Altmaier K, Morris EA: Dorsal displacement of the soft palate in neonatal foals, *Equine Vet J* 25:329-332, 1993.

Mair TS, Lane JG: The differential diagnoses of sudden-onset respiratory distress, *Equine Vet Educ* 8:131-136, 1996.

Traub-Dargatz JL et al: Respiratory stridor associated with polymyopathy suspected to be periodic paralysis in four Quarterhorse foals, *J Am Vet Med Assoc* 201:83-85, 1992.

Bronchointerstitial Pneumonia in Foals

Lakritz J, Wilson D, Berry CR et al: Bronchointerstitial pneumonia and respiratory distress in young horses: clinical, clinicopathologic, radiographic, and pathologic findings in 23 cases (1984-1989), *J Vet Intern Med* 7:277-288, 1993.

Pleuropneumonia

Carr EA, Carlson GP, Wilson WD, Reed DH: Acute hemorrhagic pulmonary infarction and necrotizing pneumonia in horses: 21 cases (1967-1993), *J Am Vet Med Assoc* 210:1774-1778, 1997.

Racklyeft DJ, Love DN: Bacterial infection of the lower respiratory tract in 34 horses, *Aust Vet J* 78:549-559, 2000.

Pneumothorax

Boy MG, Sweeney CR: Pneumothorax in horses: 40 cases (1980–1997), *J Am Vet Med Assoc* 216:1955-1959, 2000.

Aerosol Therapy

Lekeux P, Duvivier D: Aerosol therapy. Available at: www.ivis.org. Document BO331.1101, Nov 13, 2001.

44 Urinary System

Thomas J. Divers

Primary urinary tract emergencies in the horse are uncommon; however, when they do occur, the disease can be life threatening if not properly diagnosed and treated. The most common urinary system emergencies are acute renal failure, discolored urine, lower urinary tract obstruction, and ruptured bladder in the foal and occasionally in the adult.

ACUTE RENAL FAILURE

Acute renal failure (ARF) usually results from nephrotoxic causes or vasomotor nephropathy (e.g., ischemic causes). The most common pathologic finding is acute tubular necrosis.

Nephrotoxic Causes

- Consider aminoglycoside nephrotoxicity if a patient becomes *depressed* while being treated with aminoglycosides or a few days after therapy is discontinued.
- Aminoglycoside-induced renal failure *usually* results in polyuric renal failure and is typically responsive to treatment if diagnosed early.
- Tetracycline-induced renal failure may occur if 20 mg/kg per day or greater is administered (foals appear more resistant to toxic effects but may occasionally be affected) or may occur with normally recommended dosages in dehydrated horses.

Diagnosis

- History, physical examination, laboratory findings.

Laboratory Findings

- Azotemia, isosthenuria, hyponatremia, hypochloremia.
- Azotemia in the horse is best determined by means of measurement of serum creatinine.
  - In some cases of ARF, especially those with diarrhea, the blood urea nitrogen (BUN) value may remain normal or be mildly elevated, but the creatinine value is markedly elevated.
  - The presence of prerenal azotemia is best determined by clinical examination, urinalysis, and time required for serum creatinine concentration to return to normal after fluid therapy is started (most prerenal azotemia is corrected within 36 hours after initiation of fluid therapy). The upper range for creatinine from *prerenal azotemia* is generally *7-8 mg/dl*. A BUN to creatinine ratio >20 suggests a prerenal component.
  - Suspect renal azotemia if the BUN to creatinine ratio is <10, serum potassium concentration is elevated, urine specific gravity is 1.006-1.012 despite large volumes of intravenous fluid therapy, and creatinine concentration does not decline or declines slowly over several days after fluid therapy is started.
  - Newborn foals sporadically may have a serum creatinine concentration in the 5-8 mg/dl range (and sometimes higher) without other evidence of renal

dysfunction. This is most common in foals born to mares with placental dysfunction. The creatinine concentration generally returns to normal in these patients within 2 days. Some Quarter Horses have a normal serum creatinine concentration of 2.4 mg/dl.

- Serum potassium and calcium values typically are normal or low with ARF, but the potassium concentration may be high if the renal failure is oliguric. The finding of hyperkalemia in a patient with ARF suggests a more guarded prognosis because it indicates oliguric or anuric renal failure.

Treatment

- *General treatment* (see next page)
- Specific treatment: Peritoneal or pleural dialysis may be useful in reducing toxic agents, but the results are variable. This procedure is *rarely* needed.
- Dialysis protocol:
  □ Monitor electrolyte status.
  □ Administer warm lactated Ringer's solution with 1.5% dextrose for peritoneal dialysis.
  □ If no cardiopulmonary abnormalities are identified, dialysis may be administered at 40 ml/kg. After 30-60 minutes, drain fluid. At least 70% of the fluid should be recovered. With repeated dialysis, nearly 100% of the fluid should be retrieved.
  □ In foals, the omentum often interferes with this procedure, making peritoneal dialysis difficult.
  □ Hemodialysis: A health care company is available for on-site dialysis. Contact Dr. Thornhill by fax at (630) 896-8594.

| **NOTE:** The jugular veins must be patent and in good health.

Pigment Nephropathy

- Most common after a severe tying-up episode or several milder episodes
- Grossly discolored urine is not a prerequisite for myositis-induced ARF.
- Hemolysis is less likely to result in renal failure than is myopathy, although individuals with hemolysis and disseminated intravascular coagulation are at risk of ARF.
- Depression caused by uremia occurs 3-7 days after the tying-up episode or hemolytic crisis.
- Aspartate aminotransferase (AST) measurement helps confirm previous myopathy.

Vasomotor Nephropathy

- Any condition predisposing to hypotension or release of endogenous pressor agents potentiates hemodynamic-mediated ARF.
- Causes:
  □ Acute blood loss, severe intravascular volume deficits, septic shock, thrombotic episodes, coagulopathy, and acute heart failure, including pericarditis.
- Vasomotor nephropathy can cause severe renal failure without accompanying histologic findings. Diffuse renal cortical or medullary necrosis occasionally occurs.
- Acute glomerulopathy is rare in horses but can occur with purpura hemorrhagica or other systemic vascular diseases.

Diagnosis
- History, physical examination, clinical signs

Laboratory Findings
- Elevated serum creatinine value with concurrent low urine specific gravity (<1.020), hematuria, hypochloremia, hyponatremia.
- The rare case of acute glomerulopathy may cause gross hematuria and marked proteinuria.
- Hyperkalemia suggests primary intrinsic renal failure as opposed to prerenal azotemia.

General Treatment Principles for Acute Renal Failure

- Fluid replacement for volume deficits and electrolyte and acid-base correction! Hypertonic saline solution followed by 0.9% saline solution is the preferred initial fluid therapy in most cases. Potassium (20 mEq/L) is added after it is clear that the patient is polyuric!
- Monitor serum sodium, chloride, potassium, and bicarbonate levels and correct any abnormalities.
- Assess the character of ARF: Polyuric (excessive excretion of urine) versus oliguric (diminished urine excretion).
  - Monitor blood pressure to assess adequacy of volume replacement. If blood pressure remains low despite volume replacement, administer hypertonic saline solution to restore blood pressure and help assure adequate glomerular filtration pressure. The systolic arterial pressure must be at least 90 mm Hg and ideally 110 mm Hg. This can be monitored with a Dynamap or other monitoring device. The measurements may be only an estimate of the true blood pressure. The cuff (bladder) width should be approximately 25%-45% the tail circumference for the most accurate mean measurement.
  - Determine whether the patient has oliguric or polyuric renal failure. If oliguric renal failure is suspected, monitor the packed cell volume, plasma protein concentration, and central venous pressure (CVP).
  - To measure CVP, insert a 24-inch (60-cm) Intracath (Becton-Dickinson) catheter into the jugular vein and into the anterior vena cava. Use a manometer with a baseline at the level of the right atrium. Normal CVP is <8-10 cm water. In foals, measurement can be done with a 20-cm Mila catheter. Determination of CVP in a recumbent foal is difficult and probably inaccurate, however accuracy is improved by placing the foal in a sternal recumbency for the measurement.
- Once volume deficits are corrected and systemic blood pressure restored, manage **oliguric** renal failure with **dopamine**, 3-7 µg/kg per minute IV continuously, and furosemide, 1-2 mg/kg q2h for four treatments. Blood pressure should not rise above normal values (mean value, 110-120 mm Hg) during the infusion. Dobutamine, 5 mg/kg per minute, may be administered if the CVP is normal and blood pressure is low normal. Controversy exists among clinicians regarding the proven efficacy of dopamine in ARF in humans and some other species. Many still recommend its use in the care of horses with oliguric or anuric ARF.
  - Discontinue dopamine within 24-48 hours and furosemide immediately if therapy is successful in converting oliguria to polyuria.

- □ Continue to monitor urine output. If oliguria reoccurs, repeat dopamine and furosemide.
- □ Furosemide therapy alone is contraindicated in the management of rhabdomyolysis-induced renal failure.
- □ Mannitol, 0.5-1.0 g/kg IV, may be used in combination with furosemide in acute *oliguric* renal failure.
- □ Do not use mannitol if the patient is anuric.
- □ Administer aminophylline, 0.5 mg/kg, to improve glomerular filtration rate in premature or septic foals with respiratory distress and renal failure.
- □ *Refractory* hypotension* and anuria in foals should be managed with norepinephrine 0.1-1.0 μg/kg per minute.
- **Polyuric** ARF:
  - □ Administer 40-80 ml/kg per day polyionic fluids (usually 0.9% saline solution with 20 mEq/L potassium chloride) IV until a precipitous drop in serum creatinine concentration occurs.
  - □ Continue with intravenous fluids at 40-60 ml/kg a day for the next several days until creatinine concentration has returned to normal.
  - □ Furosemide and dopamine should not be used in polyuric states.
  - □ If sedation is required, use small doses of xylazine, because it can increase urine production.
  - □ If the patient is anorexic, 50-100 g of dextrose/L is added to the intravenous fluids for calories.
  - □ Acute glomerulopathy is managed as described above with therapy for the systemic condition, such as steroids for vasculitis.

ACUTE SEPTIC NEPHRITIS

Acute septic nephritis is rare in horses other than *Actinobacillus equuli* nephritis in foals. These foals usually are younger than 7 days (most are 2-4 days old), and many are found dead in the pasture without obvious clinical signs. Overwhelming bacteremia and endotoxemia are the primary concerns with *A. equuli* rather than renal failure. Most infected foals have a low serum immunoglobulin G (IgG) concentration. Gram-negative enteric bacteria and *Streptococcal zooepidemicus* may occasionally cause acute bilateral septic nephritis in adults. Treatment should include intravenous fluids and antibiotics. Initial antibiotic therapy, pending microbiology results of urine culture and sensitivity, is either ceftiofur, 4 mg/kg IV q12h or TMP/S 20 mg/kg IV q12h.

Leptospira interrogans serogroup *pomona* can cause ARF and hematuria in horses. Fever, leukocytosis, and pyuria without microscopically detectable bacteriuria should raise the index of suspicion for *L. pomona*. Serum titers are very high for *L. pomona* and the other serotypes. Treatment includes intravenous fluids as recommended for other causes of ARF. Also administer penicillin, 22,000 U/kg IV q6h.

RENAL TUBULAR ACIDOSIS

Type I renal tubular acidosis (RTA) may occasionally cause acute and severe depression in horses related to unusually low blood pH. This type of RTA occurs

---

*With adequate fluid therapy and high CVP but low arterial pressure.

usually, although intermittently, in adults and may be preceded by drug therapy for another condition, renal injury, or there may be no predisposing cause.

Diagnosis

The diagnosis is based upon the presence of a severe metabolic acidosis and hyperchloremia with a neutral to alkaline urine pH.

Treatment

Sodium bicarbonate, administered intravenously and orally (up to 100 g PO q12h), with supplemental potassium chloride.

DISCOLORED URINE

Discolored urine results from bilirubinuria (see p. 316), hemoglobinuria (see p. 326), myoglobinuria, pyuria, or hematuria (Table 44–1). *The color and consistency of normal adult urine vary widely because of the amount of mucus in the urine.* The urine of some horses normally contains pigments that cause a reddish-brown discoloration best seen in urine-stained snow.

Hematuria

Recognized blood clots or uniform red discolored urine without blood clots. Most frequent causes:

- Urethral hemorrhage: Habronemiasis, calculi, idiopathic (male proximal dorsal urethral hemorrhage), urethritis, neoplasia (squamous cell carcinoma most common)
- Bladder: Calculi, cystitis, neoplasia, amorphous debris, bleeding diathesis (warfarin toxicity), blister beetle toxicity
- Kidney: Calculi, trauma, nephritis, vascular anomaly, parasite migration (strongyle or *Halicephalobus deletrix*), neoplasia, glomerulopathy, papillary necrosis, blister beetle, and leptospirosis

Diagnosis

- Signalment, age, duration of hematuria, and the time during urination when hematuria is most pronounced are helpful. Examples:
  - Hematuria after exercise suggests cystic calculi.
  - Hematuria only at the beginning of urination indicates a urethral lesion.
  - Hematuria uniformly throughout urination implicates a bladder lesion or more likely bleeding from the kidney.
  - Hematuria only at the end of urination suggests bladder hemorrhage or proximal urethral syndrome in adult males.
- If discolored urine is recognized but clots are not seen, hemoglobinuria, bilirubinuria, or myoglobinuria must be ruled out.
  - Differentiate using urine dipstick evaluation, packed cell volume, plasma protein, color of plasma, color of mucous membranes, serum chemistry (e.g., creatine kinase, AST, γ-glutamyl transferase), conjugated bilirubin, and urine sediment examination (presence of red blood cells). A few patients with normal urine produce reddish-brown spots in snow after urination. This is believed to be caused by metabolized plant pigment that does not discolor urine but discolors snow.

TABLE 44-1. Differential Diagnosis of Discolored Urine

	Hematuria	Hemoglobinuria	Drugs	Bilirubinuria	Myoglobinuria
Urine color*	Red, bright, or dark	Pink (also red or dark red)	Any color, (e.g. orange), rifampin	Dark brown (green foam when shaken in a tube)	Brown to red to black
Consistency	Occasional clumps of blood are seen, and the discoloration is not uniform	Consistent discoloration	Consistent discoloration	Consistent discoloration	Consistent discoloration
Plasma color	Normal	Usually pink	Variable	Icteric	Usually normal unless anuric
Urine dipstick: blood	Almost always positive for both hemolyzed and non-hemolyzed blood	Consistently strongly positive for hemolyzed blood	Negative	Negative unless secondary renal disease with hemolysis or hematuria	Consistently strongly positive for hemolyzed blood
Sediment and cytologic features of urine	RBCs and ghost cells	Pigment casts and some secondary RBCs due to tubular disease	Normal	Normal to few RBCs if renal disease	Pigment casts, RBCs due to tubular disease
Laboratory tests	Variable PCV and protein; MCV may be increased; creatinine is increased if both kidneys sufficiently diseased	Low PCV; normal to high protein; MCV may be increased; increased unconjugated bilirubin	No change	Increased liver enzymes and bilirubin (both conjugated and unconjugated)	Increased creatine kinase; any increase in serum creatinine is a reflection of glomerular filtration rate.

RBCs, Red blood cells; *PCV*, packed cell volume; *MCV*, mean corpuscular volume.
*Never use this alone for diagnosis.

□ Confirm the origin of hematuria with a physical examination: Examine the urethra (after tranquilization in males); palpate the urethra, bladder, ureters, and left kidney. Perform an endoscopic examination, ultrasonography, or both. A 1-m endoscope usually is adequate to examine the bladder even in some males. After disinfecting the instrument, tranquilize the patient to attain penile relaxation, and gently pass the scope retrograde by way of the urethra after *lightly* lubricating the *outside* of the scope with sterile K-Y jelly. The mucous membrane of the urethra is generally pale white to pink, although a few small red foci are normal. *Minimal* dilation with air is needed in some cases to move the mucosa away from the tip of the scope. Excessive air causes the patent to strain, and the urethral mucosa becomes hyperemic. In very rare cases, fatal air embolism occurs. The presence of hyperemia and tortuous vessels in the urethra near the opening of the accessory sex glands is sufficient to confirm the diagnosis of idiopathic urethral hemorrhage in adult males. Hyperemia throughout the urethra is more consistent with urethritis or endoscopy irritation. Once the endoscope is in the bladder, the ureteral openings can be seen.

Treatment

Emergency treatment is rarely required unless clots are causing urinary obstruction, or rupture of the kidney has occurred, resulting in life-threatening hemorrhage or colic. Management of life-threatening hemoglobinuria, myoglobinuria, and bilirubinuria is discussed with hemolytic anemia (see p. 326), rhabdomyolysis, and liver failure (see p. 316).

OBSTRUCTION OF THE LOWER URINARY TRACT

Clinical Signs

- Hematuria, pollakiuria (frequent urination), dysuria (painful or difficult urination), and tenesmus (ineffectual and painful straining in urinating) are common. Dribbling of small amounts of urine and signs of colic, agitation, and sweating also occur. Stranguria (slow and painful discharge of urine) is most commonly a result of lower urinary tract obstruction and may be caused by acute lower urinary tract infections or neurologic disorders, such as herpes myelitis.

General Information

- Usually caused by urethral calculi or calculi at the trigone of the bladder that prevent normal urine voiding
- Rarely caused by blood clots
- Urethral obstruction is more common in males and rarely occurs in individuals younger than 1 year
- Urethral obstruction can be caused by severe preputial trauma or cellulitis (see Chapter 42, p. 476).

Diagnosis

- Rectal examination.
  □ Enlarged bladder (patients with abdominal or intestinal pain also may have bladder distention).

URINARY

- Cystic calculi can generally be palpated during rectal examination and be seen at rectal ultrasound examination (7.5-MHz rectal probe).
- In males, urethral calculi are frequently palpated percutaneously a few inches below the anus in the perineum.
- In males, the urethra seems painful to palpation, and pulsations or swelling of the urethra is detected.
- Passing a urethral catheter (stallion catheter) after tranquilization is helpful.
- Ultrasonography of the perineal region and urethra with a 7.5-MHz scanner can depict calculi and urethral swelling.
- Urethral endoscopy is used although it generally is not necessary.

Laboratory Findings
- Unless bladder rupture is suspected (see next section), laboratory tests routinely are unnecessary.

Treatment
- Surgical removal of the stone. In mares, this procedure can often be performed manually with epidural (lidocaine and xylazine) anesthesia.
- In some cases, the stone can be accidentally forced back into the bladder by a urethral catheter.
- Follow-up examination of the urinary tract is important to determine bladder function (rectal examination), presence of other stones (ultrasound examination of the urinary tract), urinary tract infection (culture and urinalysis), and renal function (measurement of serum creatinine).

RUPTURED BLADDER

Most cases of ruptured bladder occur in young male foals within the first few days of life (average, 4 days), although it can occur in adults as a result of urinary calculi or in foaling mares. Rupture of the bladder or urachus causing uroperitoneum occurs in older foals with urachal abscess, ischemia of the apex of the bladder, prolonged recumbency (e.g., premature foals, botulism, central nervous system disturbances), or from abdominal trauma.

If the urachus ruptures, a substantial accumulation of subcutaneous urine causes severe stranguria, subcutaneous swelling, colic, and distress. Differentiate the subcutaneous swelling from hematoma or septic cellulitis by means of aspiration and cytologic examination. If urine is confirmed, prompt surgical removal of the urachus is required.

Ruptured Bladder in Foals
Clinical Signs
- Usually diagnosed within the first 2-3 days of life in otherwise healthy foals and is most common in males. In these cases, the rupture most likely occurs during delivery.
- May also occur anytime during the first 2 weeks in septic and specifically recumbent foals. Recumbent neonatal foals should have an indwelling urinary catheter placed to monitor urine output and prevent bladder rupture. Catheterization of fillies is difficult however it is most easily achieved with Cook, 8, 10 or 12 Fr;

55-cm Foley catheter.* In recumbent foals, rupture of the urachus may be as common as rupture of the bladder. There is no sex predilection in this group of foals.

- Stranguria, dysuria, depression, bilaterally symmetric ventral abdominal distention
- Stranguria and dysuria are often misinterpreted as rectal tenesmus. With tenesmus, the rear limbs are positioned farther under the body than in stranguria or dysuria.

Diagnosis

- History: Generally young males and can occur in females
- Clinical signs
- Laboratory findings
- *Hyponatremia, hypochloremia, hyperkalemia, azotemia*
- Ratio of peritoneal fluid creatinine concentration to serum creatinine concentration >2:1 confirms the diagnosis of uroperitoneum. With large amounts of peritoneal fluid, as in uroperitoneum, it is preferable to perform abdominocentesis with an 18-gauge needle. A teat cannula creates a large defect in the abdominal wall, and if surgery is not performed within a few hours, urine leaks through the abdominal wall defect into the subcutaneous tissues. The history, clinical, ultrasound, and serum laboratory findings are so characteristic that peritoneal fluid evaluation generally is not necessary! Peritoneal fluid creatinine determinations using point of care equipment, e.g., I-Stat, may be inaccurate.

Treatment

- Correct acid-base and electrolyte abnormalities before surgery.
  - Administer 0.9% saline solution with 5% glucose IV.
  - Avoid exogenous insulin therapy (to drive potassium into cells) for hyperkalemia. If significant electrocardiographic abnormalities (QRS complexes without P waves) are recognized, administer 100 ml of 50% dextrose with 0.5 g calcium borogluconate to increase the endogenous insulin level and protect the myocardium.
  - If severe hyperkalemia and abdominal distention are present, remove abdominal fluid before anesthesia. If drainage is performed several hours before surgery, subcutaneous leakage of abdominal fluid occurs if the intraperitoneal catheter is removed.

Surgery

- Usually successful if performed within the first 5 days of life. The surgery generally is not an urgent emergency; electrolyte abnormalities are corrected, and in some cases, such as severe distention or hyperkalemia, the abdominal fluid can be removed before surgery.
- Induction of anesthesia is best performed by mask induction with isoflurane or sevoflurane.
- A second operation sometimes is needed if urine continues to leak from the bladder.

---

*Cook Australia, 12 Electronics Street, Eight Mile Plains, Queensland 4113 Australia; 0 61 7 3841 1188; fax 0 61 7 3841 1288; www.cookgroup.com.

□ It is occasionally advantageous to place an indwelling urethral catheter at surgery for the first 24 hours postoperatively, particularly in foals that have chronic bladder distention before rupture due to other problems, such as maladjustment syndrome, prematurity, and sepsis.

In Older Nursing Foals

Ruptured bladder occurs without warning in 4- to 10-week-old foals. The apex of the bladder is necrotic, resulting in rupture. Affected foals are depressed, have abdominal distention, and may or may *not* have the classic electrolyte abnormalities of hyponatremia, hypochloremia, and hyperkalemia that occur in younger individuals. Diagnosis is confirmed with ultrasound examination and comparison of urine to blood creatinine concentrations. Treatment is similar to that of younger patients, except the urachus and apex of the bladder are removed.

Ruptured Bladder in Adults

- Unusual in adult for causes other than urethral calculi.
  □ Can occur after foaling.

Clinical Signs

- Difficult to diagnose from clinical signs alone. Depression and anorexia 2 days after rupture may be the only signs seen. Stranguria may be present.

Diagnosis

- Peripheral blood sample:
  □ Azotemia
  □ Hyponatremia
  □ Hypochloremia
- Abdominal ultrasonography: Large volume of slightly echogenic fluid
- Abdominocentesis:
  □ Peritoneal fluid creatinine-plasma creatinine ratio >2:1
  □ Identification of calcium carbonate crystals
- Endoscopy of the bladder is indicated to determine the extent of the tear. The endoscope should be properly disinfected and the vaginal area appropriately cleaned before the procedure.

Treatment

- Surgical repair: Not needed immediately.
  □ Small dorsal tears may not necessitate surgery.
- Drainage of peritoneal fluid. Use an indwelling mushroom catheter:
  □ Place the catheter at the ventral most aspect of the midline.
  □ Clip and aseptically prepare the site after local anesthesia is administered.
  □ Make a stab incision with a #20 blade through the skin into the linea alba.
  □ Introduce a 4-inch (10-cm) cannula; confirm the presence of fluid.
  □ Use a bitch catheter to help direct mushroom catheter into the opening made by the cannula.
  □ Suture the skin around the mushroom catheter after removing the bitch catheter. Apply antiseptic cream and keep catheter end clean when it is not draining; use a small syringe to prevent ascending contamination.

- Intravenous fluids: Polyionic fluids at maintenance or slightly higher rate
- Antimicrobial therapy: Trimethoprim-sulfamethoxazole, 20 mg/kg PO q12-24h. Metronidazole 15 mg/kg PO q8h should be added if endoscopy or catheterization is performed.
- Heparin: 100 IU/kg SQ q12h with the goal of reducing abdominal adhesions.

PROLAPSE OF THE BLADDER

Prolapse of the bladder can occur as eversion of the bladder or in association with a prolapsed or torn vagina. Eversion of the bladder through the urethra occurs in females with severe straining. The mucosal surface of the bladder is obvious, and the ureteral opening may be seen. The ureters may still be patent.

Treatment

- Epidural anesthesia is performed. For a 450-kg mare, 5-7 ml of 2% lidocaine or 80 mg of xylazine diluted with 8 ml of sterile saline is administered with an 18-gauge, 1.5-inch (3.8-cm) needle (see p. 125).
- Clean the bladder with sterile saline solution and perform an examination to rule out intestinal involvement in the herniated bladder. If a part of the bladder is necrotic, debride and suture it.
- Use gentle consistent pressure on the bladder to attempt to return the everted bladder to the abdomen either with or without sphincterotomy. This is generally difficult because of bladder swelling; general anesthesia and abdominal laparotomy may be required. Return the bladder to its normal position with sphincterotomy and laparotomy; use the ligaments of the bladder as a guide for inverting the bladder through the urethra. Infuse 1 L of warm saline solution into the bladder to ensure repositioning and to check for tears. Leave a Foley catheter with the cuff inflated with saline solution in the bladder for 24 hours, and administer prophylactic antibiotics. To replace a bladder that has prolapsed through a vaginal tear, it may be necessary to remove the urine by aspiration before the bladder can be returned.

RUPTURED URETER(S)

Rupture of one or both ureters may uncommonly occur in newborn foals and even more uncommonly in post foaling mares. In foals (both males and females), signs may not be seen for 3-5 days. Serum creatinine is elevated and electrolyte abnormalities, similar to those seen with a ruptured bladder, may occur. Ultrasound examination of the abdomen, including the retroperitoneal space, and radiographic contrast studies may be needed to confirm the diagnosis. Surgical repair with temporary placement of ureteral catheter(s) is the treatment of choice in most cases.

ACUTE URINARY INCONTINENCE ASSOCIATED WITH FOALING

Acute urinary incontinence can be caused by damage to the bladder muscle or, more commonly, damage to the urethral sphincter during foaling. If the urethral sphincter is lacerated, it is sutured after a Foley catheter is placed in the bladder. If the sphincter is injured but not lacerated, treatment includes

- Phenylpropanolamine, 1-2 mg/kg PO q12h
- Systemic antimicrobials, such as trimethoprim-sulfamethoxazole

If the bladder wall (detrusor muscle) is damaged and the bladder is enlarged with no physical obstruction of the urethra, as in upper motor neuron bladder that frequently occurs with herpes myelitis, treat with:

- Bethanechol, 0.03-0.05 mg/kg SQ q8h or 0.16 mg/kg PO q8h
- Phenoxybenzamine, 0.4 mg/kg PO q6h

REFERENCES

Aleman MR et al: Renal tubular acidosis in horses (1980-1999), *J Vet Intern Med* 15:136-143, 2001.

Voss ED, Taylor DS, Slovis NM: Use of a temporary indwelling ureteral stent catheter in a mare with a traumatic ureteral tear, *J Am Vet Med Assoc* 214:1523-1526, 1999.

Neonatology

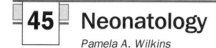

45 Neonatology

Pamela A. Wilkins

PHYSICAL EXAMINATION OF THE NEWBORN FOAL

Healthy, term foals are precocious neonates that can stand and nurse from the udder within 2 hours of delivery. Vital signs change dramatically within the first 24 hours of life (Table 45–1).

- At 20 minutes of age, a normal, healthy foal has an effective suckle reflex, can sit sternally without assistance, and attempts to rise.
- A finger inserted in the ear or nostril results in a head shake and a grimace reflex.
- Thoracolumbar stimulation performed by briskly running the thumb and forefingers down either side of the foal's thoracolumbar spine elicits attempts to rise characterized by throwing the front legs forward, lifting the head and neck upward, and trying to push off with the hindlimbs.
- The foal's heart rate at this age approaches 100 beats/min, and the respiratory rate averages between 40 and 60 breaths/min.
- A newborn foal that displays generalized hypotonia and an inability to rise, sit sternally, or suckle may be suffering from:
  - □ Peripartum asphyxia
  - □ In utero–acquired septicemia
  - □ Prematurity or dysmaturity
- A thorough history of peripartum events and careful examination of the foal and placenta help differentiate these conditions

TABLE 45–1. Neonatal Vital Signs during the First 24 Hours

	Age		
Parameter	**<10 Minutes**	**≤12 Hours**	**24 Hours**
Heart rate (beats/min)	<60	100-200	80-100
Respiratory rate (breaths/min)	40-60	20-40	20-40
Body temperature (°F/°C)	99-102/37-39	99-102/37-39	99-102/37-39

We recognize and appreciate the contribution and original work of Wendy E. Vaala, VMD, in the first edition, on which this chapter is based.

Placenta

A history of premature separation of placental membranes, prolonged delivery or dystocia, and meconium staining of the foal are periparturient events associated with neonatal asphyxia. A maternal history of prepartum purulent vaginal discharge, precocious udder development and lactation, or evidence of abnormal discoloration of the placenta, particularly in the area of the cervical star, increases the index of suspicion for placentitis and in utero sepsis. A normal placenta weighs approximately 10% to 11% of the foal's birth weight. Evaluate unusually heavy (or light) placentas by means of gross and light microscopic examination. Peracute cases of placentitis may produce only generalized edema without obvious areas of infection. Small placentas with large areas of abnormal villus formation have been associated with neonatal dysmaturity. Therefore histopathologic examination of the placenta is strongly recommended if a neonate shows early signs of doing poorly.

Prematurity

Foals from abnormally long gestations can have signs of prematurity. The term *dysmaturity* rather than *prematurity* may be more appropriate in these cases. Unusually short (<320 days) or abnormally long (>360 days) gestation has been associated with the birth of foals with signs of prematurity, including:

- Small body size
- Fine, silky hair coat
- Generalized weakness
- Increased passive range of limb motion
- Flexor tendon and periarticular ligament laxity
- Incomplete cuboidal bone ossification
- Domed forehead
- Floppy ears
- Inability to regulate body temperature

Some foals born after a prolonged gestation have slightly different clinical features, characterized by a large frame with poor muscle development, erupted incisors, and long hair coats. The physiologic findings may be similar to those of dysmature foals, but the foals are considered "postmature."

Mucous Membranes and Sclera

- The mucous membranes of a healthy neonate are pale pink with a capillary refill time of <2 seconds. Pale mucous membranes suggest the presence of anemia. Pale yellow mucous membranes suggest the presence of neonatal isoerythrolysis.
- Gray or slightly blue mucous membranes indicate shock, poor peripheral perfusion, or hypoxemia. Cyanosis appears only if the PaO_2 is <35-40 mm Hg, even if the packed cell volume (PCV) is within the normal range. Tissue damage begins when PaO_2 is <60 mm Hg.
- Do not rely on mucous membrane color to diagnose hypoxemia.
- Increased respiratory rate and effort can be clinical signs of pulmonary or cardiac disease. Of these two signs, *increased effort is the most reliable,* because foals with central respiratory depression due to hypoxia, hypothermia,

hypoglycemia, or hypocalcemia may not have an appropriate increase in respiratory rate in response to the pathologic changes in the lung.

- Hyperemic, injected mucous membranes and hyperemic coronary bands may indicate sepsis or systemic inflammatory response syndrome (SIRS). Petechiae on oral mucous membranes or inside the pinnae also are associated with sepsis and SIRS. Icteric mucous membranes are observed with hemolysis, sepsis, equine herpesvirus (EHV-1) infection, and liver disease.

NOTE: It is important to differentiate large- and small vessel injection. Small-vessel injection imparts a generalized, bright red appearance to the mucous membranes and suggests more severe disease.

- The sclera should be white with only faint vessels apparent. Marked injection is indicative of septicemia. Prominent scleral hemorrhages can be observed after birth trauma.

Cardiovascular System

The *cardiac rhythm* of a neonate should be regular. However, nonpathologic sinus arrhythmia may be present for a few hours post partum. *Heart rate* averages between 70 and 100 beats/min during the first week of life.

Bradycardia

- Bradycardia is associated with severe:
  - Hypoglycemia: Use a stallside dextrometer, available in most human pharmacies, to diagnose diabetes (see p. 629).
  - Hypothermia: Carefully rewarm the foal.
  - Hyperkalemia: Most common with anuric renal failure or ruptured bladder but also occurs with massive tissue damage secondary to hypoxia, asphyxia, or muscular diseases such as white muscle disease (see p. 408).
  - Asphyxia: Perhaps the *most common cause* of bradycardia is hypoxemia. Many foals respond readily to increased oxygen in the inspired air, administered by means of intranasal insufflation, flow-by oxygen, or nasotracheal intubation and ventilation.

Tachycardia

- Tachycardia occurs with:
  - Sepsis: Fever often is absent at examination
  - Hypovolemia
  - Hypoxemia
  - Anemia
  - Pain: Abdominal or musculoskeletal in origin
  - Stress
  - Hypocalcemia: Occurs with severe asphyxia

Murmurs

Murmurs associated with patent ductus arteriosus (PDA) may persist for several days after birth. The typical PDA murmur is a continuous machinery murmur or a holosystolic murmur heard loudest over the left side of the base of the heart. Soft, blowing murmurs usually are associated with blood flow and are exacerbated by anemia.

> **NOTE:** Persistent murmurs, murmurs present for more than 5-7 days after birth that do not resolve, or murmurs associated with exercise intolerance or hypoxemia may be caused by persistent PDA, patent foramen ovale, ventricular septal defect, or another congenital heart anomaly and should be investigated further.

Peripheral Pulses

Peripheral pulses should be easy to palpate. The great metatarsal artery is the easiest site to use. Bounding, hyperkinetic pulses are associated with early stages of compensated sepsis. Weak, thready pulses indicate cardiovascular collapse and shock.

Respiratory System

The resting *respiratory rate* of a newborn foal averages between 20 and 40 breaths/min. Because foals have a thin chest wall and a relatively rapid respiratory rate, thoracic auscultation often shows air movement throughout the chest even when there is lung disease, especially diffuse interstitial disease. Moist end-expiratory crackles are commonly heard after birth as the foal expands its lungs. Unusually quiet lung sounds auscultated immediately after birth are compatible with incomplete alveolar inflation and lung atelectasis. Marked areas of ventral dullness on auscultation and percussion indicate areas of consolidation, atelectasis, or pleural effusion. Breathing effort should be minimal once the lung liquid has been reabsorbed, which takes several hours. Areas of dorsal dullness when the foal is in sternal recumbency suggest pneumothorax.

Respiratory distress
- Respiratory distress is exacerbated by recumbency and characterized by:
  □ Nostril flare
  □ Expiratory grunting
  □ Rib retraction
  □ Increased abdominal effort
  □ Paradoxic respiration (chest wall collapses during inspiration)

Apnea
- Apnea and unusually slow or irregular respirations are abnormal and have been associated with:
  □ Hypoglycemia
  □ Hypothermia
  □ Central respiratory depression secondary to asphyxia: Probably the most common cause in neonatal intensive care units
  □ Prematurity

Diagnostic Tests

Thoracic radiography and ultrasonography help identify pulmonary consolidation, abscessation, and pleural effusion. Arterial blood gas analysis is the most accurate assessment of pulmonary function. These samples are most easily collected from the metatarsal artery or the decubital artery (Fig. 45–1). The artery can be used for repeated sampling. A small, subcutaneous, intradermal bleb of 2% lidocaine (without epinephrine) makes collection easier for foals hypersensitive to arterial puncture.

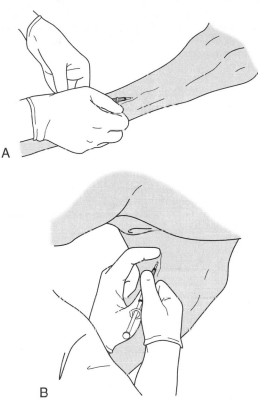

FIGURE 45-1. Arterial blood gas samples are most easily collected from **A,** the metatarsal artery or **B,** the decubital artery.

Abdominal Examination

Abdominal Auscultation

- Should show bilateral borborygmi. Ingestion of colostrum and the act of suckling itself enhance gastrointestinal (GI) motility and passage of meconium and manure.

Meconium

The first manure a foal passes, meconium, is composed of cellular debris, intestinal secretions, and amniotic fluid ingested by the fetus. It is dark, blackish-brown, or gray and is firm, pellet-like, or pasty. All meconium should be passed within 24 hours of birth and is followed by softer, tan "milk feces." Absence of manure passage can be associated with:

- Atresia coli: This problem is suggested by lack of fecal staining in enema fluid
- Meconium impaction
- Ileus
- Intestinal obstruction

Because of the foal's thin body wall, distention of the small or large intestine results in visible, generalized abdominal enlargement. Simultaneous auscultation or percussion of tympany indicates the presence of a gas-distended viscus. Tight, tympanic, dorsally distributed distention is compatible with gas accumulation. Turgid, ventrally distributed, pendulous distention can be seen with uroperitoneum and peritoneal effusion.

Causes of Colic (with or without Abdominal Distention)

- Meconium or fecal impaction: The impaction usually can be found by means of digital examination, although abdominal radiography or ultrasonography may be needed to find more proximal impaction.
- Enteritis (see Chapter 35, p. 188)
- Ileus (see p. 188)
- Intussusception (see p. 42): May be found with ultrasound
- Gastroduodenal ulceration: Classic signs of this problem in older foals include rolling onto the back, sialorrhea or ptyalism, and odontoprisis (grinding teeth).
- Peritonitis: Differential diagnoses include ruptured duodenal or gastric ulcer, enteritis, and urachal abscess.
- Intestinal volvulus: Severe pain that can progress to depression
- Uroperitoneum: Increased amount of free fluid on sonogram; peritoneal creatinine concentration at least two times serum creatinine concentration (see Chapter 44, p. 537)

Diagnostic Aids

NASOGASTRIC INTUBATION

- Performed to check for reflux. *Reflux* is associated with ileus due to ischemic hypoxic intestinal damage, peritonitis, or enteritis or obstruction due to intussusception, impaction, volvulus, or duodenal stricture. The presence of occult blood–positive reflux is associated with hypoxic intestinal damage and enteritis caused by *Clostridium* organisms and occasionally *Salmonella* organisms. If severe gastric distention is present, passage of the tube beyond the cardia may be difficult. Lidocaine applied to the nasogastric tube or injected down the tube helps relax the esophagus and facilitate entry into the stomach. Use the largest-diameter tube that can be passed in cases in which the presence of reflux is suspected but no fluid is obtained.

ABDOMINAL RADIOGRAPHY

- Can be used to determine the location, but not necessarily the cause, of gas or fluid distention. Gaseous distention of the small intestine characterized by gas-fluid interfaces within the lumen can be found in foals with ileus due to enteritis, peritonitis, hypoxic GI damage, and small-intestinal obstruction (see p. 239). Concurrent large bowel distension is frequently associated with ileus due to hypoxia or enteritis. Primary large-bowel distention occurs with obstruction due to meconium retention, volvulus, or displacement.
- Radiographic settings on portable and stationary machines vary a great deal and depend on the model and brand of the unit, cassettes, film-screen combinations, and focal distance. Consultation with a radiologist or radiologic technician is recommended for guidelines.

CONTRAST STUDIES

- Barium enema radiographic examination (barium mixed with warm water and administered by gravity flow through a cuffed Foley catheter inserted in the

rectum) helps identify meconium impaction and may help with the diagnosis of atresia.
- Upper GI contrast radiography is used to document the delayed gastric emptying and prolonged transit time that occur with ileus, obstruction, and gastroduodenal ulcer disease.
- Contrast radiography of the upper GI tract is performed by administering 5 ml/kg barium sulfate suspension through a nasogastric tube. Serial radiographs are obtained 10, 20, 30, and 60 minutes and 2 and 4 hours after administration of the contrast agent. Contrast radiography is used to find GI obstruction and ulceration. Normal findings are:
  - Barium begins leaving the stomach immediately and is gone after 1.5-2 hours.
  - The cecum fills by 2 hours.
  - The transverse colon fills by 3 hours.

TRANSABDOMINAL ULTRASONOGRAPHY (see p. 40)
- Allows evaluation of:
  - Small-intestinal motility
  - Bowel wall thickness
  - Degree of gastric or small- or large-intestinal distention
  - Volume and character of peritoneal fluid

Healthy foals have flaccid, motile, fluid-filled loops of small intestine with a wall <0.3 mm thick and minimal amounts of peritoneal fluid. Round, fluid-distended loops of bowel can be seen with ileus, enteritis, and small-bowel obstructive disease. Enteritis results in a generalized increase in bowel wall thickness and edema. Severe hypoxic-ischemic bowel disease can produce focal increases in bowel wall thickness with or without intramural gas accumulation (i.e., intestinalis pneumatosis). Small-intestinal intussusception has a doughnut-shaped pattern caused by the telescoping of one segment of bowel into another. The presence of an excessive volume of clear, nonechogenic peritoneal fluid is compatible with uroperitoneum. An increase in peritoneal fluid echogenicity is associated with increased cellularity, as in peritonitis, hemoperitoneum or ruptured abdominal viscus.

ABDOMINOCENTESIS
- Used to obtain peritoneal fluid for analysis and cytologic examination. The procedure is best performed by means of sterile technique and ultrasound guidance with a 20-gauge needle or a teat cannula.

> **CAUTION:** *Use care in performing abdominocentesis with a teat cannula: Omental herniation can result. Needles can also penetrate the intestine.*

- The finding of peritoneal fluid with an increased nucleated cell count and protein concentration is consistent with peritonitis. Peritoneal fluid with a creatinine concentration greater than twice serum creatinine concentration establishes the diagnosis of uroperitoneum. If there is distended intestine, abdominocentesis can result in bowel perforation and peritonitis.

GASTROSCOPY
- Used to document gastric ulceration. Also used to evaluate duodenal ulceration if the duodenum is entered. Withhold food and drink for a minimum of 3-6 hours before gastroscopy to ensure adequate gastric emptying.

➤ □ It is important that the stomach of the foal not be excessively filled with gas during the examination, because this exacerbates colic. Try to remove all gas before withdrawing the endoscope from the stomach.

Urogenital System
Urination

- *Time to first urination* is approximately 8-12 hours, fillies taking slightly longer than colts to void for the first time. Because of a persistent frenulum, some colts do not drop the penis to urinate for the first week after birth. The specific gravity of the first urine produced usually is >1.035. Observe urination closely to be certain the foal does not have a *patent urachus,* in which case urine drips from the umbilicus.
- Healthy, well-hydrated foals urinate frequently, often after nursing. *Urine specific gravity* is low in nursing foals (1.001-1.010) because of the high-volume liquid diet. Foals with peripartum asphyxia may have oliguria due to decreased renal blood flow and urine production. Dysuria can be observed with uroperitoneum, urachitis, patent urachus, or urachal diverticulum.
- *Uroperitoneum due to a bladder or urachal defect* most likely occurs post partum in association with congenital weakness of an area in the bladder wall, poor blood flow to certain areas of the bladder, cystitis, umbilical remnant infection, or improper lifting of recumbent foals with an underlying compromise to bladder integrity. Signs include:
  □ Decreased urination
  □ Straining to urinate
  □ Pendulous, fluid-filled abdominal distention
  □ Mild abdominal malaise and depression
- Large amounts of free fluid on a sonogram, peritoneal fluid creatinine concentration at least two times serum creatinine concentration. Rupture of a ureter or urachus (subcutaneous or intraabdominal) causes postrenal azotemia.

Umbilicus

- Examine the *umbilical stump* for signs of infection characterized by thickening or abnormal discharge. Transabdominal ultrasonography is used to measure internal umbilical remnants. Normal diameter in foals 3-7 days of age is as follows:
  □ Umbilical vein at external stump, <1 cm
  □ Umbilical vein at liver, <1 cm
  □ Umbilical artery at bladder, <1 cm
  □ Umbilical arteries and urachus, <2.5 cm
- Palpate the umbilicus, inguinal region, and scrotum (in colts) for congenital hernia. The testes may not be descended at birth.

Ophthalmic Examination

- *A pupillary light response* is present and is more sluggish than in an adult.
- A consistent menace response often is not present until 2-3 weeks of age.
- Ventral medial strabismus is common.
- Examine the foal's eyes for corneal cloudiness, congenital cataracts, microphthalmia, or entropion.
- Ophthalmic examination may show a persistent hyaloid artery remnant coursing from the optic disk to spread on the posterior lens capsule, often resembling

a spider's web. This is not an abnormality and should disappear with time. Suture lines frequently can be seen in the center of the lens.

- Examine the retina for signs of detachment and hemorrhage. Scleral hemorrhage can be associated with sepsis, disseminated intravascular coagulation, or suspected birth trauma.

Neurologic Evaluation

Healthy foals are bright, alert, and very responsive to touch and sound. While being restrained in a standing position, foals often alternate between periods of hyperactivity and struggling and episodes of sudden, complete relaxation (flopping). Foals should stand with an erect, angular head and neck carriage and a basewide stance in front. Their gait is exaggerated. *Limb reflexes* are increased. When recumbent, foals have strong resting extensor tone and a crossed extensor reflex that exists for as long as 1 month. Foals normally spend approximately 50% of their time sleeping. When sound asleep, normal foals may be extremely difficult to arouse and may exhibit rapid eye movement, limb twitching, and irregular breathing patterns.

Neurologic Disease

► The most common cause of neurologic disease among newborn foals is peripartum hypoxic damage. *Hypoxic-ischemic encephalopathy (neonatal encephalopathy)* can produce:

- Loss of menace response, central blindness
- Fixed, dilated pupils
- Nystagmus
- "Jittery" behavior
- Seizure activity ranging from grand mal clonic seizures to tonic posturing, extensor rigidity, and focal seizures
- Stuporous attitude, hypotonia
- Abnormal respiratory patterns
- Coma
- Failure to locate udder, loss of ability to recognize dam
- Barking noise or other abnormal vocalizations
- Dysphagia
- Dysuria
- Wandering

Causes of Neonatal Seizures

- Hepatoencephalopathy: Unusual
- Congenital malformations: Rare
- Head trauma: Cerebrospinal fluid (CSF) aspiration may be indicated. Treat with mannitol unless there is severe bleeding, as suggested by CSF fluid. Dexamethasone, 2-4 mg/kg, may be helpful early in the course. Dimethyl sulfoxide (DMSO), 1 g/kg IV diluted in 1 L of lactated Ringer's solution q12 or 24h may be beneficial.
- Neonatal encephalopathy: Administer oxygen and improve cardiac function, polyionic crystalloids, colloids (plasma), dextrose in water (5%-20%) and positive inotropic agents (e.g., dobutamine, 2-10 µg/kg per minute), to normalize arterial pressure with hypoxia or head trauma. Magnesium may have some benefit in reducing reperfusion injury (see p. 603).

- Meningitis: Antimicrobial therapy and other supportive therapy. *Halicephalobus gingivalis* nematode infection (older nomenclature: *Halicephalobus deletrix, Micronema deletrix)* has been documented as a cause of CNS disease in foals younger than 3 weeks.
- Hypoglycemia: See p. 558.
- Hypocalcemia: Administer 10% calcium gluconate, 1-2 ml/kg, and Ca^{2+}, 9-18 mg/kg, slowly IV over 5-10 minutes. Slow or stop infusion if bradycardia develops. Follow with a maintenance infusion of calcium: 10% calcium gluconate, 5 ml/kg per day.
- Hyponatremia: Hypertonic saline solution, 1 ml/kg repeated-dose administration every 15 minutes until serum Na^+ concentration is >125 mEq/L *but <135 mEq/L only if hyponatremia has been present for less than 12 hours and you are positive of this finding.*
- Toxins: For example, aminophylline.

Musculoskeletal System

- Examine the *musculoskeletal system*, including mandible, limbs, and ribs, for fractures due to birth trauma. Fractured ribs often are difficult to detect but frequently produce a clicking sound on auscultation, heard in synchrony with respiration. Keep foals with fractured ribs quiet, generally with the affected side down. Foals normally have a mild carpal and fetlock valgus conformation in front; fetlock varus is more common behind. Examine limbs for more severe angular and flexural deformities. Palpate joints and physis for signs of swelling and heat (see Chapter 39, p. 343).

Dysmaturity, Prematurity

- Musculoskeletal signs:
  - □ Increased passive range of joint motion
  - □ Periarticular ligament and flexor tendon laxity
  - □ Incomplete cuboidal bone ossification (see p. 385) (detectable only on radiographs) of carpus and tarsus. If severe, restrict exercise and provide assistance as the foal attempts to stand.

Severe Flexor Tendon Laxity

- Treatment includes:
  - □ Controlled exercise
  - □ Shoes with heel extension
  - □ "Light" protective wraps if weight bearing results in trauma to heel bulbs and fetlock

Septic Arthritis Signs

- Lameness
- Fever: Variable
- Painful, warm joint effusion frequently accompanied by marked leukocytosis and hyperfibrinogenemia.
- Treat with joint lavage using balanced electrolyte solution with 10-20 g DMSO added to 1 L, and systemic antimicrobials. Small volumes of an antimicrobial (amikacin, <1 ml, or 250 mg per joint) can be instilled in the joint after lavage, but monitor total dose. If two or more joints are treated, the total daily dose of

amikacin should be reevaluated and altered as required on the basis of peak and trough kinetics.

Septic Osteomyelitis

- Variable lameness
- Fever
- Painful swelling over physis or epiphysis proximal to joint, with or without sympathetic joint effusion
- Radiographic evidence of periosteal osteolytic and proliferative changes.
- Leukocytosis and hyperfibrinogenemia usually accompany the condition.
- Treat with long-term antimicrobial therapy; aspirate physis for culture and sensitivity; use nonsteroidal drugs conservatively to provide analgesia and decrease inflammation. Support unaffected limbs. The need for long-term nonsteroidal analgesia should prompt prophylaxis for gastric and duodenal ulcer disease in the care of these patients.

Limb Contracture

- Can involve proximal (carpus, tarsus) or more distal (fetlocks, pasterns) joints. Tendon contracture has been associated with in utero malpositioning, toxins, and neonatal hypothyroidism. Therapy for *contracted tendons* includes physical therapy, systemic analgesics, splinting, casting, controlled exercise to prevent extensor tendon rupture, and oxytetracycline, 1-3 g IV q24-36h for a maximum of three doses. Measure serum creatinine concentration before and after treatment.

> **CAUTION:** *Acute oliguric renal failure has been reported to occur after this treatment.*

- Casting and splinting have been associated with exacerbation of lateral laxity, promote rub and pressure sore development, and should be used with care.

Nursing Behavior

A healthy foal *consumes between 10% and 20% of its body weight in milk daily* with an average weight gain of 1-3 pounds (0.45-1.35 kg) per day. Foals nurse at least several times an hour. Udder distention in the mare is one of the earliest signs of a "fading foal" that is no longer nursing effectively. Milk dripping from a foal's nose after nursing may be the result of:

- Cleft palate: Although it has to be ruled out, cleft palate is one of the least common causes of dysphagia among foals!
- Subepiglottic cyst.
- Dorsal displacement of the soft palate.
- Generalized weakness due to sepsis, dysmaturity, peripartum hypoxia.
- Dysphagia associated with perinatal asphyxial syndrome (PAS).
- White muscle disease.
- Esophageal pooling of milk.

Catheterization and Blood Sampling

The jugular vein is the most common site for venipuncture in an awake, active foal. In more depressed foals, the saphenous and cephalic veins can be used. Sites for arterial blood gas sampling include the lateral metatarsal (first choice), decubital, transverse facial, facial, and less frequently, the brachial artery (see Fig. 45–1).

GENERALIZED WEAKNESS, LOSS OF SUCKLE

▶ The most common causes of weakness and reluctance to suckle among newborn foals are:

- Sepsis
- Peripartum asphyxia
- Prematurity, dysmaturity

Sepsis

▶ The leading cause of neonatal foal morbidity and mortality. Most commonly associated with Gram-negative bacterial infection and endotoxemia. The clinical signs associated with sepsis are the result of unbalanced stimulation of the immune system after exposure to microbial toxins. During sepsis release of endogenous proinflammatory and antiinflammatory mediators (e.g., tumor necrosis factor and interleukins 1, 2, and 6) precipitate a cascade of metabolic and hemodynamic changes that can finally result in multiple organ system failure. As septic shock advances, the patient dies of a combination of cardiopulmonary failure, generalized coagulopathy, disruption of metabolic pathways, and loss of vascular endothelial integrity.

The organisms most commonly associated with foal sepsis include *Escherichia coli, Actinobacillus, Pasteurella, Klebsiella, Salmonella,* and *Streptococcus.* Viral pathogens such as EHV-1 and equine arteritis virus also can produce sepsis-like syndromes (SIRS), as can tissue damage associated with PAS.

Clinical Signs and Diagnosis

- The clinical signs observed with sepsis depend on the integrity of the host's immune system, the duration of illness, and severity of the insult.

SIGNS DURING EARLY HYPERDYNAMIC PHASES OF SEPSIS

- Lethargy
- Loss of suckle
- Hyperemic, injected mucous membranes and sclera
- Hyperemic coronary bands
- Petechiae inside pinnae and on oral mucosa
- Decreased capillary refill time
- Tachycardia, increased cardiac output, hyperkinetic bounding pulses
- Tachypnea
- Variable body temperature
- Extremities that often remain warm to the touch
- Responsiveness on the part of the foal

SIGNS DURING ADVANCED UNCOMPENSATED SEPTIC SHOCK

- Depression
- Profound weakness, recumbency
- Dehydration
- Hypotension unresponsive to fluid support

- Decreased cardiac output, tachycardia, cold extremities, thready peripheral pulses
- Prolonged capillary refill time
- Oliguria
- Hypothermia
- Respiratory compromise: Tachypnea, dyspnea, hypoxemia, cyanosis

LOCALIZED SITES OF INFECTION: SPECIFIC SIGNS
- **Pneumonia, pleuritis:** Tachypnea, dyspnea, fever, abnormal lung sounds, ventral dullness, and friction rubs with pleural effusion
- **Meningitis:** Seizures, stupor, opisthotonos
- **Hepatitis:** Icterus
- **Nephritis:** Variable urine production, proteinuria, hematuria
- **Peritonitis, enteritis:** Colic, ileus, diarrhea, abdominal distention
- **Synovitis:** Painful, warm joint distention, lameness, fever
- **Physeal, epiphyseal osteomyelitis:** Variable joint distention, localized pain over epiphysis or physis, lameness, fever
- **Uveitis:** Blepharospasm, miosis, hypopyon, epiphora
- **Omphalitis:** Variable enlargement of umbilical remnant, umbilical discharge, fever

Clinical Pathology
- **Leukopenia,** neutropenia (white blood cell count, <5000/µl; neutrophils, <4000/µl), elevated band neutrophil count (bands, >50-100/µl). Neutrophils show toxic changes.
- **Plasma fibrinogen** concentration may be normal with acute sepsis. Fibrinogen increases in response to inflammation over 12-24 hours. Hyperfibrinogenemia in a newborn foal indicates chronicity and suggests the presence of in utero infection.
- **Hemoconcentration** due to hypovolemia.
- **Hypoglycemia** (glucose, <60 mg/dl): Depletion of reserves or loss of control over glucose homeostasis.
- **Hypogammaglobulinemia** due to failure to absorb colostral antibodies or increased protein catabolism due to sepsis. Normal foals have a serum immunoglobulin G concentration ([IgG]) >800 mg/dl. Partial failure of passive transfer (FPT): [IgG] between 200 and 800 mg/dl. Complete FPT: [IgG] <200 mg/dl.
- **Hyperbilirubinemia** due to a combination of sepsis-associated hemolysis; abnormal hepatic function.
- **Lipemia** resulting in opalescent serum due to impaired lipid clearance.
- **Azotemia:** Increased creatinine or blood urea nitrogen value associated with dehydration, renal ischemia, and direct renal damage.
- **Hypoxemia:** PaO_2 <60 mm Hg associated with ventilation-perfusion mismatching, pulmonary hypertension, or reduced cardiac output. May occur in combination with respiratory acidosis.
- **Metabolic acidosis:** Arterial pH, <7.35; HCO_3, <23 mEq/L due to poor peripheral perfusion and anaerobic metabolism. An increase in lactate level in these cases may contribute to the observed acidemia.

Cultures for Diagnosis
- Blood, synovial fluid, cerebrospinal fluid, peritoneal fluid, urine. Tracheal aspiration, although useful in the evaluation of foals with pneumonia, often is too stressful to perform on septic neonates with severe respiratory distress.

Radiographs

- Obtain thoracic radiographs with the foal in lateral recumbency and the forelegs pulled forward to improve evaluation of the cranioventral lung fields. Obtain thoracic radiographs with the foal standing when possible. It may be desirable to image both sides of the thorax.
  - **Bacterial bronchopneumonia** commonly is associated with an alveolar pattern and air bronchograms in the cranioventral and caudoventral lung fields (Fig. 45–2). Acute bacterial pneumonia also can present as diffuse interstitial disease.
  - **Viral pneumonia** can be characterized by a diffuse interstitial pattern (Fig. 45–3).
  - **Aspiration pneumonia** is associated with caudoventral and cranioventral infiltrates.
  - **Surfactant deficiency** and **hyaline membrane** formation produce a diffuse, ground-glass appearance of the lung with prominent air bronchograms. This radiographic appearance also has been seen in foals with viral pneumonia (Fig. 45–4). The ground-glass appearance can be mimicked in lateral thoracic radiographs of foals with hemothorax.
- Serial *radiographs of swollen joints or painful physes* at a minimum of 5-day intervals are recommended to detect signs of articular damage and osteomyelitis.

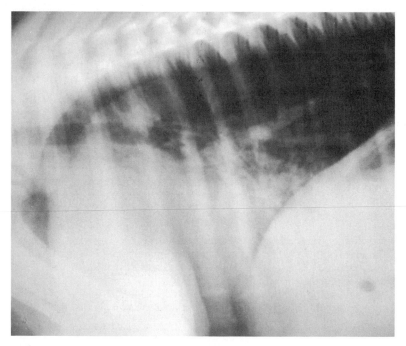

FIGURE 45–2. Recumbent lateral thoracic radiograph of a foal with bacterial pneumonia. The radiograph shows marked alveolar infiltrate involving the caudal and ventral lung fields. This finding is compatible with consolidation secondary to bronchopneumonia.

- Plain abdominal radiographs can help identify the location of gas distention. Ileus associated with *enteritis* or *peritonitis* is associated with generalized mild to moderate distention of the small and large intestines.

OTHER DIFFERENTIAL DIAGNOSES OF GENERALIZED WEAKNESS
- **Neonatal encephalopathy (formerly known as neonatal maladjustment syndrome):** Behavior changes, loss of suckle and dam recognition, seizures.
- **Neonatal isoerythrolysis:** Icterus, hemolysis, anemia, hemoglobinuria.
- **Ruptured bladder:** Abdominal distention, dysuria, hyponatremia, hypochloremia, hyperkalemia, azotemia.
- **Meconium impaction:** Colic, straining to defecate, tail flagging.
- **Prematurity, dysmaturity:** Small body size, silky hair coat, tendon and joint laxity, domed forehead, floppy ears.
- **Syndrome of inappropriate antidiuretic hormone (ADH) secretion (SIADH):** Foals 12-48 hours of age with decreased urine volume, concentrated urine, hyponatremia, and hypochloremia. Serum creatinine concentration can be variable. The foals gain excessive weight consuming a milk diet owing to retention of free water within the vascular space.

These foals are *not* in renal failure, and the treatment of choice is fluid and milk restriction with monitoring of urine output, urine specific gravity, and serum electrolyte values. Clinical signs are associated with electrolyte disturbances (hyponatremia), which can be severe. The key to diagnosis is concentrated urine and weight gain.

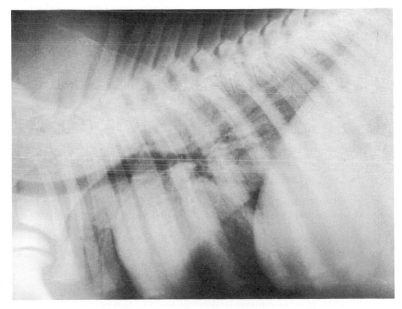

FIGURE 45-3. Recumbent lateral thoracic radiograph of a 24-hour-old foal. The pregnancy was complicated by severe bacterial placentitis. Radiograph shows an interstitial pattern most pronounced in the caudodorsal lung fields.

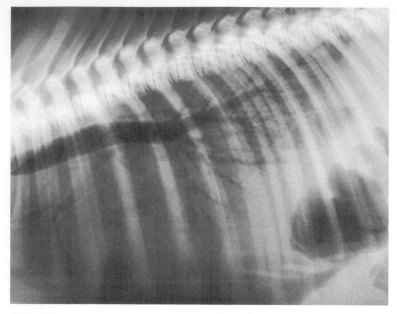

FIGURE 45-4. Recumbent lateral thoracic radiograph of a premature foal. Cesarean section was performed at 322 days of gestation. A diffuse alveolar pattern in all lung fields is compatible with diffuse pulmonary atelectasis.

- **Tyzzer's disease: 8-42 days of age,** icterus, markedly increased concentration of hepatocellular enzymes.

General Therapy for Septicemia
CARDIOVASCULAR SUPPORT: FLUID THERAPY
- Crystalloids, 20 ml/kg over 20 minutes, to manage severe hypovolemia and hypotension. Balanced electrolyte solutions are optimal for rapid volume expansion.

    NOTE: Dextrose-containing fluids alone are not indicated for rapid volume expansion. This crystalloid dose can be repeated as necessary.

    The foal should be reevaluated after each bolus and before administration of the next. The goal is volume resuscitation but not overhydration or overloading with sodium.

- Maintenance rate is 5% dextrose calculated as follows:
    - 100 ml/kg per day for the first 10 kg body weight
    - 50 ml/kg per day for the second 10 kg body weight
    - 20-25 ml/kg per day for the remainder of body weight
    - This provides the volume needed for a recumbent foal not consuming a milk diet for maintenance. If the foal is not receiving milk or total parenteral nutrition (TPN) as an energy source, this rate, or the dextrose concentration, can be adjusted to provide 4-8 mg/kg per minute until dextrose needs are met.

- Monitor blood pressure, central venous pressure (goal, 2-6 cm water), urine output, heart rate, peripheral pulses, and respiratory function. There is no "magic" number for mean blood pressure in foals, but a mean pressure between 45 and 50 mm Hg usually is adequate if the pulse pressure difference is >30-40 mm Hg.
- Plasma may be needed to maintain oncotic pressure and intravascular fluid volume. Minimum volume to administer is 20 ml/kg over 60 minutes. One liter of plasma provides the equivalent sodium load of a normal milk diet in a normal foal in a single day.
- Volume expansion alone usually is sufficient to correct mild to moderate metabolic acidosis. Severe metabolic acidosis may necessitate bicarbonate supplementation, but be aware that for each milliequivalent of bicarbonate administered, a milliequivalent of sodium also is administered. Prefer isotonic (1.3%) solutions (150 mEq $NaHCO_3$/L).

> Bicarbonate should not be administered to patients in cardiac arrest or that need considerable resuscitation efforts (see p. 598). Ensure adequate ventilation before administering bicarbonate. *Avoid* rapid infusion: It is unnecessary and may induce respiratory or paradoxic CNS acidosis.

Sepsis-induced hypotension can be difficult to manage, because some foals may be less responsive to adrenergic drugs. This may be simply a function of how they manifest sepsis or may be associated with developmental age. **Treatment** recommendations include:

- Isotonic fluids as indicated earlier.
- **Dopamine:** 2-10 μg/kg per minute continuous infusion. Low doses stimulate dopaminergic receptors and may improve renal blood flow. Moderate doses stimulate α-adrenergic receptors and support cardiac function. High doses (>10-12 μg/kg per minute) produce α- and β-adrenergic effects with tachycardia (if heart rate increases more than 50%, therapy should be slowed), increase blood pressure, and reduce splanchnic perfusion and urine output. Titrate the dose for each patient. Larger doses of dopamine can induce pulmonary venoconstriction, which can exacerbate pulmonary hypertension.
- **Dobutamine:** 2-15 μg/kg per minute continuous infusion. Used to treat patients with adequate volume expansion as a β-adrenergic, inotropic agent to improve cardiac output and oxygen delivery. Titrate dose to effect. Discontinue if severe tachycardia develops (>50% increase).
- **Vasopressin:** 2-10 μg/kg per minute. At this low dose, vasopressin provides support for adrenergic pressors, particularly in septic patients, without inducing renal effects.
- For unresponsive moderate to severe hypotension:
  - **Norepinephrine:** 0.1-3.0 μg/kg per minute
  - **Epinephrine:** 0.1-1.0 μg/kg per minute. Expect measured lactate concentration to increase substantially when this drug is used.
  - **Phenylephrine:** 1-20 μg/kg per minute. Although this pressor almost always increases measured pressure, the generalized vasoconstriction produced may be counterproductive in the treatment of the patient.

Combinations of the foregoing treatments are commonly used, and good first-choice combinations include dopamine and dobutamine, dobutamine and vasopressin, and dobutamine and norepinephrine.

RESPIRATORY SUPPORT

The aim of therapy is to minimize ventilation-perfusion mismatching.

- **Cautious fluid therapy** to maintain adequate left ventricular and atrial pressure to promote more uniform lung perfusion.
- **Frequent repositioning** of foal to reduce dependent lung atelectasis. Encourage sternal recumbency.
- **Intranasal (IN) humidified oxygen therapy** to manage hypoxemia (PaO_2, <70 mm Hg; SaO_2, <90%) if ventilation is adequate. Use oxygen flow of 2-10 L/min. The provided FIO_2 is quite unpredictable and depends greatly on the minute volume. Administered through a cannula positioned in the nasal passage with the end of the cannula at the level of the medial canthus of the foal's eye. Tape or suture nasal cannula in place. Oxygen tubes in both nostrils can be used to increase FIO_2.
- **Mechanical positive-pressure ventilation** (PPV) to prevent alveolar collapse, reduce respiratory muscle fatigue, and address increased oxygen consumption associated with sepsis. Positive end-expiratory pressure (**PEEP**) (4-8 cm water) and pressure support (8-16 mm Hg) may be needed. **PPV** is indicated if IN oxygen therapy alone fails to correct hypoxemia or if $PaCO_2$ is >65 mm Hg and is unresponsive to respiratory stimulants and is not associated with metabolic alkalosis. Peak airway pressure should be kept at a minimum level and less than 30 cm water to prevent barotrauma. Increased $PaCO_2$ can be tolerated (permissive hypercapnia) as long as pH is acceptable and there are no signs of carbon dioxide narcosis or deleterious cardiovascular effects. FIO_2 should be kept as low as is practical. Prolonged FIO_2 at >50% may result in oxygen toxicity.
- **Caffeine** administration is used to manage abnormally slow respiratory rate, hypoventilation, and respiratory acidosis secondary to central respiratory center depression. Administer 10 mg/kg PO or per rectum as a loading dose, followed by 2.5-3 mg/kg PO once or twice daily as a maintenance dose. Therapeutic trough serum concentration is 5-25 µg/ml. Toxicity (CNS signs) is associated with concentrations greater than 40-50 µg/ml.

NUTRITIONAL SUPPORT

- **Hypoglycemia** is managed initially with a glucose infusion best administered as a constant infusion of 5% or 10% solution at a rate of 4-8 mg/kg per minute.

NOTE: At this rate, a 50-kg foal would receive 120-240 ml of 10% dextrose per hour.

▶ *Do not give foals bolus infusions of 50% dextrose!*

- **Caloric requirements:** A healthy foal consumes 10%-20% of its body weight daily in milk, which equals 100-120 kcal/kg per day. Sepsis and fever are assumed to increase caloric requirements to 150 kcal/kg per day, although this may not be true in all cases. Many ill foals gain weight on 10% body weight equivalent feeding(~54 kcal/kg per day).
- **Enteral feeding:** Use mare's milk, foal milk replacer, or goat's milk.

NOTE: The goal is 10%-20% of body weight per day in milk administered in small volumes every 2-3 hours. If GI function is questionable, begin enteral feedings cautiously at 5%-10% of the foal's body weight per day. Supplement with parenteral nutrition if <10% of body weight in milk is fed daily for 2 consecutive days.

➤ | **CAUTION:** *Never feed a cold foal!*

- **Parenteral nutrition:** Solutions are hypertonic and must be administered continuously through large peripheral veins and long catheters (>5 inches [12.5 cm] long) at precise flow rates. Use an infusion pump, dial-a-flow regulator, or a Buretrol solution set to administer TPN. Test blood for hyperglycemia and hypoglycemia, and check urine for glucosuria to help regulate the amount of glucose delivered. Monitor serum for lipemia. Monitor PCV and total protein for signs of dehydration. The presence of persistent hyperglycemia suggests loss of control of glucose regulation and does *not necessarily indicate* that too much glucose is being administered. In these cases, insulin can be administered as a continuous infusion at 0.0125-0.2 U/kg per hour. Use regular insulin and pretreat all lines because insulin adsorbs to plastic. Changes in insulin and glucose rates should be made slowly and over many hours (~4 h). Target blood glucose concentrations to remain between 80 and 180 mg/dl.
  - □ **To make insulin infusion:** Place 15 U **regular** insulin in a 100- to 150-ml *glass* container of sterile 0.9% saline solution. Begin infusion at 2-4 ml/h. Increase at 4-hour intervals by 2 ml/h until desired blood glucose concentration is reached. Measure blood glucose concentration frequently to ensure hypoglycemia is not present. When the foal's condition appears to be stable, discontinue insulin infusion gradually, frequently checking glucose level.
  - □ **Components of parenteral nutrition:**

    50% dextrose
    8.5% or 10% amino acids
    10% or 20% lipids

  - □ Daily caloric requirements should be met primarily by lipids and glucose. Lipids should contribute approximately 50% nonprotein calories. To ensure the amino acids are used for structural protein and not catabolized for energy, the ratio of nonprotein calories to grams of nitrogen should be maintained between 100 and 200.
  - □ **Caloric density:**

    Lipids, 9-11 kcal/g
    Carbohydrate (glucose), 3.4 kcal/g
    Protein (amino acids), 4.0 kcal/g

  - □ **Starting formula** for parenteral nutrition:

    10 g/kg per day of dextrose
    2 g/kg per day of amino acids
    1 g/kg per day of lipids
    5-10 ml/d of multivitamins
    Add trace minerals if the foal needs prolonged parenteral nutritional support
    Potassium chloride can be added to the parenteral formula

  - □ When first starting TPN, begin at one-fourth the desired flow rate. Check blood for lipemia and blood and urine for hyperglycemia (blood glucose level, >180 mg/dl) at 3- to 4-hour intervals and increase flow rate by one fourth until the final rate is achieved. **Sample calculation for 50-kg foal:**

    Dextrose: 10 g/kg per day = 500 g = 1 L of 50% dextrose
    Amino acids: 2 g/kg per day = 100 g = 1 L of 10% amino acids

Lipids: 1 g/kg per day = 50 g = 0.5 L of 10% lipids
Total volume: 2.5 L of TPN administered over 24 hours at 140 ml/h

- Begin TPN at 35 ml/h. Slowly increase the rate every 3-4 hours by 35 ml until 140 ml/h is reached.

ANTIMICROBIAL THERAPY

Broad-spectrum, bactericidal antimicrobials are indicated. Administer for a minimum of 10-14 days provided no localized areas of infection develop. Specific sites of infection (e.g., pneumonia, meningitis, arthritis and osteomyelitis) necessitate prolonged antimicrobial therapy. Penicillin and aminoglycoside antimicrobials are a popular combination that provides coverage against Gram-positive and Gram-negative aerobes and anaerobes. Antimicrobial dosages:

- Penicillin: 22,000-44,000 U/kg IV q6h.
- Amikacin: 25-30 mg/kg IV q24h combined with therapeutic drug monitoring. Peak concentrations at 30 minutes should be >60 µg/dl and 23-hour trough concentration should be <2 µg/dl.
- Gentamicin: 6.6 mg/kg IV q24h. Thought to be potentially more nephrotoxic than amikacin in very young foals; use cautiously only in well-hydrated foals. Many Gram-negative organisms may be resistant to gentamicin.
- Ceftiofur sodium: 2-10 mg/kg IV q6-8h; less nephrotoxic; must be administered frequently if IV route is used: 2-5 mg/kg IM q12h.
- Ticarcillin/clavulanic acid: 50-100 mg/kg IV q6h; less nephrotoxic.
- Trimethoprim-sulfonamide: 25-35 mg/kg PO or IV q12h; do not use with uncertain GI function. Many Gram-negative organisms may be resistant.
- Third-generation cephalosporins if meningitis is suspected: Cefotaxime, 50 mg/kg IV q6-8h.
- Imipenem–cilastatin sodium: Broadest-spectrum β-lactam bactericidal antimicrobial. A recommended dose is 15 mg/kg slowly IV q6h.

NOTE: Imipenem–cilastatin sodium is expensive, and seizure has been reported as an adverse effect.

- Fluconazole for fungal infections: 8.8 mg/kg PO q24h loading dose, 4.4 mg/kg PO q24h maintenance dose.

IMMUNE SYSTEM SUPPORT: COLOSTRUM ADMINISTRATION

- Feed only foals with normal cardiovascular status and body temperature.
- Ideally, foals should receive approximately 1 L of colostrum with a specific gravity >1.060 administered in three to four feedings during the first 8-10 hours of life. This dose is equivalent to 1 g IgG per kilogram body weight.

PLASMA TRANSFUSION

- Use plasma to manage FPT to provide opsonins, to improve immune response, to support oncotic pressure and defend intravascular fluid volume.
- Administer hyperimmune plasma from donors negative for A and Q antigens and antibodies.
- If orally administered, serum-derived commercial IgG products are used. They should be mixed with colostrum to improve absorption. The same dose of 1 g IgG per kilogram body weight is recommended. Absorption of these products can be erratic and foals should be reevaluated after administration of these products.

- Foals older than 18 hours or foals with GI dysfunction may be unable to absorb sufficient colostral antibodies and need plasma transfusion.
- **Minimum plasma volume** to administer: **20 ml/kg.** The volume of plasma required to manage FPT depends on the [IgG] in the recipient's blood and donor's plasma. Because of sepsis-induced protein catabolism, septic foals need a larger volume of plasma than do healthy foals to increase serum [IgG] to the same level. Administer sufficient plasma to increase serum [IgG] above 800 mg/dl for septicemia. Recheck serum and blood [IgG] every few days during treatment to ensure concentrations remain adequate.
- **Sources of commercial plasma: [IgG] ≥ 2500 mg/dl**

HiGamm Equi	Polymune Plus	Immuno-Glo
Lake Immunogenics	Veterinary Dynamics, Inc.	Mg Biologics
348 Berg Road	P.O. Box 2406	1721 Y Ave
Ontario, NY 14519	Chino, CA 91708-2406	Ames, IA 50014
(800) 648-9990	(800) 654-9743	(515) 769-2340

General Nursing Care

- **Provide warmth**, using heating pads, warm fluids, radiant warmers, forced hot air blankets, and fluid jacket warmers (Intratherm, a warm intravenous fluid pouch, and Safe and Warm reusable instant heat measuring 7-9 inches [17.5-22.5 cm], from Safe and Warm Inc., Boulder City, NV 89005; [800] 421-3237).
- **Maintain sternal recumbency** as much as possible. Frequent repositioning helps prevent decubitus sores and dependent lung atelectasis.
- Apply **sterile ocular lubricant** to eyes of foals that spend most of their time in lateral recumbency to prevent exposure keratitis and ulceration.
- **Antiulcer medication** can be administered if desired. Gastroduodenal ulcers in these patients are most likely associated with GI hypoperfusion. Critically ill foals have an alkaline gastric milieu and a blunted response to inhibitors of acid production, thus the use of histamine$_2$ (H_2) antagonists and proton pump inhibitors may be of little use in the care of these patients. Omeprazole (GastroGard) has not been evaluated for safety in the treatment of foals younger than 30 days, however it is routinely used clinically.
  - **Ranitidine**, 6.6 mg/kg PO q8h, 1.5 mg/kg IV q8h, and/or
  - **Sucralfate**, 1-2 g/45 kg PO q6h

Peripartum Asphyxia (Neonatal Maladjustment Syndrome)

Asphyxia can result from any periparturient event that impairs or disrupts utero-placental perfusion or umbilical blood flow. Asphyxia produces multiple organ system damage in addition to the more commonly recognized behavioral and neurologic deficits.

The following are periparturient events associated with fetal or neonatal asphyxia:

- Dystocia: Supply more oxygen through an intranasal or nasotracheal tube for the mare to help reduce fetal hypoxia
- Induced delivery: Cervical dilatation is a prerequisite for induction to reduce the risk of dystocia
- Cesarean section

- Premature placental separation
- Placentitis: Fetal membranes greater than 11% of foal's body weight
- Severe placental edema: Uteroplacental thickness greater than 2 cm
- In utero meconium passage with or without postpartum meconium aspiration
- Twinning
- Severe maternal illness, especially with hypoxia
- Abnormally prolonged gestation
- Pregnancy complicated by reduced fetal fluid volume increases risk of umbilical cord compression during labor and suggests the presence of chronic placental dysfunction

Diagnosis

Peripartum asphyxia produces a wide range of clinical signs. Asphyxia induces a critical *redistribution of cardiac output*. The result is preferential blood flow to the heart, brain, and adrenal glands and decreased perfusion of the lungs, GI tract, spleen, liver, kidneys, skin, and muscles. Diagnosis is based primarily on clinical signs.

SIGNS ASSOCIATED WITH SPECIFIC ORGAN INJURY

- **Hypoxic ischemic encephalopathy (neonatal encephalopathy):** Loss of suckle, loss of dam recognition, apnea, hypotonia, anisocoria, sluggish pupillary light reflex, dilated pupils, depression, tonic posturing (preference for lying in extensor posture with occasional pedaling limb movements, hyperesthesia, focal or grand mal seizures, and coma).
- **Renal tubular necrosis:** Oliguria, anuria, generalized edema with fluid or sodium overload.
- **Ischemic enterocolitis:** Colic, ileus, abdominal distention, gastric reflux, diarrhea (possibly bloody).
- **Meconium aspiration, pulmonary hypertension, or surfactant dysfunction:** Respiratory distress, tachypnea, dyspnea, rib retractions, apnea.
- **Cardiac dysfunction due to myocardial infarction and persistent fetal circulation:** Arrhythmia, tachycardia, murmurs, generalized edema, hypotension.
- **Hepatocellular necrosis, biliary stasis:** Icterus.
- **Adrenal gland necrosis:** Weakness, hypotension.
- **Parathyroid necrosis:** Lipemia, seizures.

BIOCHEMICAL ABNORMALITIES

- Vary widely depending on the severity of specific organ injury
  - **CNS:** Increased blood-brain barrier permeability, increased CSF protein
  - **Renal:** Proteinuria, increased urinary value of gamma-glutamyl transferase, azotemia, hyponatremia, hypochloremia, increased fractional sodium excretion
  - **GI:** Occult blood–positive reflux or diarrhea
  - **Respiratory:** Hypoxemia, hypercapnia, respiratory acidosis
  - **Cardiac:** Hypoxemia, increased values of myocardial enzymes, tachycardia or bradycardia
  - **Hepatic:** Increased values of hepatocellular and biliary enzymes, hyperbilirubinemia

□ **Endocrine:** Hypocortisolemia, hypocalcemia, hypoinsulinemia, or peripheral insulin resistance resulting in poor control of blood glucose, SIADH (see p. 555)

OTHER DIAGNOSTIC AIDS

- **Abdominal ultrasonography or radiography** (recommended technique: 85 kilovolt (peak) [kV(p)]/20 mAs) to assess for intramural gas accumulation, generalized intestinal distention, thickening of bowel wall; associated with necrotizing enterocolitis.
- **Thoracic radiographs** (65-75 kV(p)/5-8 mAs) to detect diffuse lung atelectasis; decreased pulmonary vascular pattern secondary to pulmonary hypertension and persistent pulmonary hypertension of the neonate (PPHN). Normal findings on thoracic radiographs do not exclude the presence of respiratory abnormalities.
- **Echocardiography** to assess for patent foramen ovale, patient ductus arteriosus, and pulmonary hypertension associated with persistent fetal circulation.

Therapy
CENTRAL NERVOUS SYSTEM DISTURBANCES

- Administer **diazepam**, 0.11-0.44 mg/kg IV, for immediate seizure control; effect is short lived; repetitive doses contribute to respiratory depression. For severe or persistent seizure activity, use **phenobarbital**, 2-10 mg/kg IV q8-12h; monitor serum values (15-40 µg/ml). Higher doses can produce respiratory depression and hypotension.
- **Magnesium infusion:** Magnesium is thought to play a role in ameliorating secondary neuronal cell death after hypoxic-ischemic insults to the CNS. It has effects on calcium channels, N-methyl-D-aspartate receptors and vascular reactivity. The loading dose is 50 mg/kg for 1 hour and is followed by 25 mg/kg per hour. Using sterile technique, remove 20 ml from a 100-ml bag of 0.9% saline solution. Replace that volume with 20 ml 50% magnesium sulfate. For the average 50-kg foal, begin constant rate infusion (CRI) at 25 ml/h for 1 hour, then decrease to 12.5 ml/h.
- **Avoid xylazine** for sedation unless it is the only drug available. Xylazine causes transient hypertension, exacerbates existing CNS hemorrhage, and contributes to respiratory depression and reduced GI motility.
- **Avoid acepromazine**, because it lowers seizure threshold and produces hypotension.
- **To reduce cerebral edema:** Administer **DMSO**, 0.5-1.0 g/kg slowly as 10%-20% solution over 1 hour; IV **mannitol**, 0.25-1.0 mg/kg as 20% solution over 10-20 minutes; and an osmotic diuretic. May exacerbate cerebral hemorrhage. Questions remain as to the location of any edema that develops in neonatal encephalopathy. If edema has a role in the pathophysiology of this syndrome, most current evidence suggests that any edema is intracellular, not interstitial; therefore the use of osmotic diuretics is unwarranted in most cases. Some clinicians never use DMSO or mannitol in the management of cerebral edema and report no change in outcome. Others report that the antioxidant properties, with or without antiedema, of mannitol are of clinical benefit.
- **Protect from self-trauma:** Wrap legs. Apply a soft head helmet (Velcro foam leg wraps and helmet available at [702] 851-1217). Pad walls and provide soft bedding. Apply ocular lubricant to reduce risk of traumatic corneal ulceration.

- Keep the patient's head low during resuscitation. Keep the head elevated 30 degrees when the patient is in lateral recumbency, if cerebral injury is suspected, and after successful resuscitation.
- Do not overhydrate.

RENAL FAILURE
- **Monitor fluid in and urine out** to evaluate renal function and avoid overhydration.
- **Dopamine infusion**: 2-10 µg/kg per minute. Lower doses stimulate dopaminergic receptors and enhance urine output by natriuresis. Medium doses recruit β receptors and support cardiac function, which may further improve renal perfusion. Higher doses stimulate α receptors and result in decreased splanchnic blood flow, renal blood flow, and urine production. Titrate the dose to the individual patient. Recommend **bladder catheterization** to allow accurate assessment of urine production.
- **Furosemide:** Administer small amounts (0.25-0.5 mg/kg q30-60 min) during dopamine infusion to enhance diuresis, or begin continuous infusion (0.25-2.0 mg/kg per hour).

> **CAUTION:** If administering furosemide through the same intravenous line as dopamine, avoid prolonged mixing of solutions in the line by administering either dopamine or furosemide solution as close to the catheter port as possible. Protect furosemide solution from light by wrapping the line in paper or foil. *Although furosemide administration can result in diuresis, prolonged use is associated with electrolyte and acid-base disturbances. The use of either dopamine or furosemide in the management of oliguric renal failure does not control the underlying problem. Judicious use of intravenous fluid, including fluid restriction, is indicated in these cases. Close attention to matching "ins and outs" is important.*

- **Mannitol:** 0.5-1.0 mg/kg IV as 20% solution over 15 minutes; osmotic diuretic.
- **Dobutamine,** (2-15 µg/kg per minute): Use if cardiac dysfunction and secondary hypotension are contributing to poor renal perfusion; discontinue or reduce dosage if tachycardia develops.

COLIC, REFLUX, ABDOMINAL DISTENTION
- **Nasogastric decompression** to check for reflux. Discontinue or reduce the volume or frequency of enteral feeding if reflux is present.
- **Percutaneous large-bowel trocarization** if abdominal distention is severe and causing respiratory compromise and continuous colic. Use a 16-gauge, 3½-inch (8.75-cm) catheter-over-stylet attached to 30-inch (75-cm) extension set. Sedate foal if necessary to keep it quiet in lateral recumbency. Clip and surgically prepare a site over one or both paralumbar fossae at the point of maximal bowel distention. Infuse a small bleb of lidocaine at the puncture site. Using sterile technique, advance the catheter and stylet through the skin and body wall into distended viscus. Remove the stylet and connect the extension set. Place the free end of the extension set into a small beaker of sterile water to monitor gas-bubble production. Once bubbling stops, a small volume of antimicrobial (e.g., amikacin diluted 50:50 with sterile water) can be infused as the catheter is withdrawn. Broad-spectrum systemic antimicrobial therapy is recommended for 3-5 days after trocarization.

- **Prokinetic drugs** for GI dysmotility: *These drugs are not recommended for routine use, because they can cause additional GI problems, such as intussusception or worsening colic, or neurologic complications.*
  - **Erythromycin**, 1-2 mg/kg PO or as slow IV infusion q6h; observe for colic, diarrhea, and intussusception. Stimulates small- and large-intestinal motility.
  - **Metoclopramide**, 0.25-0.5 mg/kg as slow IV infusion or per rectum q6h; observe for excitement. Stimulates gastroduodenal motility. This drug is also available as a syrup and may be useful in the management of delayed gastric emptying associated with gastroduodenal ulceration in older foals.
  - **Cisapride**, 0.2-0.4 mg/kg q4-8h PO. Stimulates small- and large-intestinal motility. Motility is not necessarily coordinated or progressive, and signs of colic may worsen.
  - **Lidocaine**, 1-2 mg/kg slowly IV followed by 0.05 mg/kg per minute. The pharmacokinetics of this drug have not been studied in neonates, and neonates are more susceptible than are older horses to toxicity with this drug.

  NOTE: Use lidocaine with caution. It may have several advantages with respect to analgesic and antiendotoxic effects.

  - **Neostigmine:** 0.005-0.01 mg/kg IM or SQ; has been used successfully to evacuate "gas"-distended large intestine.
- **Antiulcer medication**: Foals with hypoxic or ischemic GI damage are at increased risk of GI ulcers due to poor GI perfusion and the primary disease process. Acid production is *not* the cause of the ulcers, and the gastric milieu is likely more alkaline than it is in normal foals; therefore H_2 antagonists and proton pump inhibitors may not be needed.
  - **Ranitidine**, 6.6 mg/kg PO q8h or 1.5 mg/kg IV q8h, to increase gastric pH
  - **Sucralfate**, 20-40 mg/kg PO q6h, as cytoprotective agent.
  - **Antacids,** such as Maalox or Di-Gel: 30-60 ml q3-4h. Most antacids have a very short half-life, produce minimal change in gastric pH, and may provide transient pain relief.
- **Broad-spectrum, bactericidal antimicrobials** to reduce the risk of sepsis secondary to translocation of luminal bacteria across compromised GI mucosa. Sucralfate also may decrease bacterial translocation.
- **Parenteral nutrition:** With mild GI compromise, reduce the volume or frequency of enteral feeding and support the foal with parenteral nutrition. In cases of severe asphyxia accompanied by hypothermia, hypotension, shock, or advanced prematurity, recommend delaying all enteral feeds and providing parenteral nutrition.

PERSISTENT PULMONARY HYPERTENSION OF THE NEONATE AND PULMONARY VASOCONSTRICTION

- Control **hypoxemia**, because it is a consistent stimulus for pulmonary vasoconstriction and provides a high concentration of oxygen, up to 100% oxygen delivered during mechanical ventilation if necessary.
  - Intranasal: Oxygen, 5-10 L/min. The FIO_2 achieved with IN oxygen cannot be predicted.
- Acidosis accentuates hypoxic pulmonary vasoconstriction. Correct any *existing acid-base imbalance*. Attempt to achieve pH of 7.4. Use of bicarbonate to correct

NEONATOLOGY

acidosis cannot be recommended if $PaCO_2$ is increased and the foal does not improve with mechanical ventilation with appropriate minute volumes.
- Consider pulmonary vasodilators if other techniques fail:
  □ **Tolazoline:** Infant dose, 1-2 mg/kg IV over 10 minutes; if there is a good clinical response with an increase in PaO_2, follow with IV infusion at 0.2 mg/kg per hour for each 1-mg/kg pulse-dose administered. Causes adrenergic blockade, peripheral vasodilatation, GI stimulation, and cardiac stimulation.

> **NOTE:** *Tolazoline therapy frequently results in severe tachycardia and hypotension due to the nonselective vasodilatation produced and is not considered a first-choice approach.*

  □ **Nitric oxide** (NO) is an important modulator of vascular tone needed to achieve neonatal circulatory patterns. Ventilation with NO in 100% oxygen reduces pulmonary vascular resistance. Inhalation of **5-40 ppm NO** has been effective in reversing hypoxic pulmonary vasoconstriction in foals. Approximately 5-9:1 ratio/O_2:NO.
  □ **Future directions** for management of PPHN include endothelin-1 receptor antagonists and specific phosphodiesterase inhibitors.
- **Monitor blood pressure.** Support cardiac function with dopamine and dobutamine if indicated.
- Correct hyperthermia if present: Remove covers, heating pads.

RESPIRATORY COMPROMISE

- **Mild hypoxemia** (PaO_2, 60-70 mm Hg, SaO_2, >90%): Increase periods of time foal spends in sternal or standing position; turn q2h if recumbent; stimulate periodic deep breathing to reinflate atelectatic lungs; administer humidified IN oxygen, 2-10 L/min.
- **Moderate to severe hypoxemia** (PaO_2, <60 mm Hg; SaO_2, <90%) accompanied by **hypercapnia** ($PaCO_2$, >70 mm Hg): If not improved by treatment with a respiratory stimulant (e.g., caffeine) or if respiratory acidosis is affecting pH and is *not* associated with metabolic alkalosis and is therefore compensatory, provide PPV. Intubate nasotracheally, using a 7-10-mm-diameter, 55-cm-long, cuffed, silicone nasotracheal tube.*
- Begin PPV with initial **tidal volume of 5-10 ml/kg** and **PEEP of 4-6 cm water.**
- Use an inspired oxygen concentration of 60%-80% and reevaluate arterial blood gas values within 30 minutes of initiating PPV. Adjust inspired oxygen concentration accordingly with the goal of rapidly reducing FIO_2 to <50% to minimize the risk of oxygen toxicity.
- Attempt to maintain peak airway pressures below 30-40 cm water to reduce barotrauma.
- Breath rate is determined by $PaCO_2$ and the foal's initial breathing rate; some increase in $PaCO_2$ is permissible and may be necessary to prevent barotrauma. Some foals respond best to pressure support only, with no mandatory machine driven breaths.
- If **meconium aspiration** has occurred, attempt to treat the foal with IN oxygen alone. PPV can predispose to alveolar rupture and pneumothorax in these cases. Do not perform prolonged suction without oxygen administration.

*Silicon nasotracheal tube. Bivona, Inc., Gary IN; (800) 348-6064.

- **Intratracheal surfactant** instillation may be beneficial if surfactant dysfunction is suspected owing to severe asphyxia, pulmonary hypoperfusion, sepsis, or meconium aspiration.
- **Apnea and irregular respiration:** May be caused by hypoxic-ischemic damage to central respiratory center, hypocalcemia, hypoglycemia, or hypothermia. Check body temperature and correct hypothermia if present. Correct hypoglycemia and/or hypocalcemia. If central respiratory depression is suspected, consider respiratory stimulants:
  - **Theophylline:** Loading dose of 5-6 mg/kg administered slowly IV q12h

    Therapeutic levels, 6-12 µg/L.

CAUTION: *Therapeutic and toxic levels are within a narrow range, and therefore this therapy cannot be recommended as a first choice.*

Signs of toxicity: Seizures, colic, hyperesthesia, tachycardia; death occurs at levels >20 µg/L.
Aminophylline, a precursor of theophylline, can be substituted; 1 mg aminophylline = 0.8 mg theophylline. Same warning as with theophylline.

  - **Caffeine** is the FIRST CHOICE: Loading dose of 10 mg/kg PO initially; maintenance dose of 2.5-3 mg/kg PO q12-24h.

    Therapeutic range, 5-20 µg/L; toxic level, >40 mg/L

  - If apnea persists, **PPV** may be needed.
  - *If* PaO_2 *does not have a threefold to fivefold increase with 100% oxygen after 3-4 hours of treatment, suspect the presence of a shunt, which is a poor prognostic indicator. Rule out PPHN by a trial with NO in the inspired gas.*

SECONDARY INFECTION
- **Evaluate serum [IgG].** If [IgG] is less than 800 mg/dl and the foal is younger than 18 hours and has a functional GI tract, administer good-quality **colostrum** (specific gravity, >1.060) enterally or administer plasma transfusion. If foal is older than 18 hours or has compromised GI function, administer **plasma**. Serum [IgG] should remain >800 mg/dl. Provide maintenance broad-spectrum antibiotics if GI compromise is suspected, if the foal has signs of sepsis, or serum [IgG] is less than 800 mg/dl.

Prognosis

Between 60% and 80% of foals suffering from peripartum asphyxia recover fully and mature into neurologically normal adults. A poor outcome is associated with severe, recurrent seizures that persist for more than 5 days post partum, severe hypotonia that progresses to coma, severe multiorgan system damage that includes unresponsive renal failure or hypotension, and the development of concurrent septicemia. **Dysmature** and **premature foals** exposed to **severe peripartum asphyxia** have a poorer outcome than do term foals.

Prematurity and Dysmaturity

Prematurity is defined as the condition of a foal born after a gestation period of less than 320 days. **Dysmaturity** is defined as the condition of a foal born after a normal or prolonged gestation period in which there are signs of underdevelopment. Dysmaturity is associated with abnormal uteroplacental function, which can result in delayed fetal growth and maturation when chronic and in varying degrees of fetal asphyxia when acute.

Clinical Signs

In addition to **generalized weakness** and **hypotonia**, the following signs are characteristic of dysmaturity and prematurity:

- Low birth weight; thin body condition
- Short, silky hair coat
- Floppy ears, soft muzzle, flexor tendon laxity, periarticular laxity
- Increased range of passive limb motion
- Domed forehead
- Absent or diminished suckle reflex, ineffective swallow reflex
- Time to nurse and stand delayed more than 3-4 hours post partum
- Hypothermia due to poor thermoregulation
- Intolerance of enteral feeding, colic, abdominal distention, diarrhea, reflux
- Respiratory distress due to lung immaturity or surfactant dysfunction
- Visceral wasting, "gaunt" abdomen

Laboratory Findings

- **Leukopenia:** White blood cell count, $<6.0\text{-}10^3$/ml; neutropenia with neutrophil to lymphocyte ratio <1.0
- **Hypoglycemia** due to insulin response that contributes to abnormal glucose homeostasis
- **Hypocortisolemia** and poor cortisol response to stress and exogenous corticotropin
- **Hypoxemia,** variable hypercapnia, and lower pH values due to lung immaturity
- **Hyponatremia** and hypochloremia associated with renal immaturity

Therapy

- Attempt to establish the cause of prematurity or dysmaturity. **Examine the placenta.** If evidence of placentitis is present, initiate broad-spectrum, bactericidal antibiotic therapy.
- Observe closely for signs of **respiratory distress** and progressive respiratory fatigue. Therapy depends on the degree of respiratory dysfunction:
  - PaO_2, <60 mm Hg; $PaCO_2$, <60 mm Hg: Initiate intranasal oxygen therapy, 3-10 L/min; increase time spent in sternal recumbency; monitor arterial blood gas values.
  - PaO_2, <60 mm Hg; $PaCO_2$, $>65\text{-}70$ mm Hg: Begin PPV with PEEP. Use PPV with tidal volumes of 5-10 ml/kg. Attempt to keep peak airway pressure $<30\text{-}40$ cm water and inspired oxygen concentration $<50\%$ to reduce risk of barotrauma and oxygen toxicity; PEEP at 4-8 cm water. Excessive PEEP reduces cardiac output and necessitates CRI of dobutamine. Insufficient PEEP may not increase functional residual volume as desired.
  - If a foal shows signs of advanced prematurity and signs of severe respiratory distress immediately post partum, consider intratracheal instillation of surfactant in addition to PPV. *This is uncommon:* most foals, unless born before 280 days of gestation, *do not* have primary surfactant deficiency.

HYPOTHERMIA
- Maintain carefully controlled environmental temperature if foal shows poor thermoregulation. Provide external warmth using warm water pads, radiant heaters, forced warm air blankets, warmed intravenous fluids, and insulated fluid jacket warmers.

SELF-TRAUMA
- Reduce risk of decubital sores by providing soft bedding (e.g., synthetic sheepskin) for recumbent foals.

METABOLIC DISTURBANCES
- Monitor serum electrolyte concentrations. Hyponatremia and hypochloremia are the most common disturbances associated with renal and endocrine immaturity.

NUTRITION
- Foals ideally should receive approximately 20%-25% of their body weight in milk each day. Begin enteral feedings cautiously at a rate of 10% body weight in milk divided into 10-12 feedings per day. If the foal cannot tolerate sufficient enteral nutritional support, supply additional calories using partial or complete parenteral nutrition.

INCOMPLETE CUBOIDAL BONE OSSIFICATION (see p. 385)
- Most premature and dysmature foals have varying degrees of incomplete cuboidal bone ossification. Obtain a radiograph of one carpus (anteroposterior view) and tarsus (lateral view) to evaluate the degree of ossification. If the foal is active but has minimal cuboidal bone ossification, attempt to keep the foal non–weight-bearing, allowing only very short periods of controlled standing (~5 min/h).

Sleeve casts should not be used because they exacerbate lateral-medial instability by inducing additional joint laxity. If only mild incomplete ossification exists, restrict exercise and use **corrective shoeing and foot trimming** as needed to maintain a proper weight-bearing axis (see p. 385).

EVALUATE SERUM IMMUNOGLOBULIN G CONCENTRATION
- Do this within 12 hours of birth. If [IgG] is <800 mg/dl, administer colostrum supplementation, plasma transfusion, or both.

SECONDARY BACTERIAL INFECTION
- Premature and dysmature foals are at increased risk of infection. Consider broad-spectrum, bactericidal antibiotic therapy until the foal is up and nursing normally.

COLIC
Signs of Colic in Newborn Foals
- Poor nursing behavior
- Rolling, treading
- Abdominal distention
- Teeth grinding
- Tachycardia, tachypnea

Common Causes

- **Meconium impaction**: Can generally be confirmed with abdominal palpation and digital examination. If the foal is very distended, abdominal radiography or ultrasonography may be necessary. Overzealous therapy for meconium impaction can result in colic.
- **Ileus** associated with GI hypoxia secondary to peripartum asphyxia or septic shock.
- **Intussusception**: Can be seen with ultrasonography, also may be associated with intestinal hypoxia and resultant dysmotility.
- **Enteritis/peritonitis**: Frequently *Clostridium* organisms and accompanying bacteremia.
- **Gastroduodenal ulceration: Uncommon as a primary cause of colic in the neonate (see p. 565), but may be a primary problem in the older foal.**
- **Intestinal volvulus: A true surgical emergency.** Diagnosis suspected on the basis of clinical signs of severe pain, reflux, and abdominal distention. Ultrasonographic evaluation of the abdomen can confirm the presence of multiple loops of turgid, distended small intestine with minimal motility.

Meconium Impaction

Meconium impaction is more common in colts than in fillies. In addition to colic, abdominal distention, and poor nursing behavior, affected foals may have **tenesmus, tail flagging**, and an **arched-back posture**. If obstruction is complete, abdominal distention can develop rapidly.

Diagnosis

- Palpation of firm meconium within the rectum and pelvic canal on **digital examination**
- A history of unsuccessful **straining to defecate**
- Firm fecal material within the pelvic inlet detected with abdominal palpation, plain radiography, or contrast radiography after a barium enema examination
- Sonographic detection of echogenic material within the distal colon and rectum

Therapy
WARM, SOAPY (IVORY SOAP) WATER, GRAVITY ENEMAS

- Use a soft urinary catheter or small feeding tube and enema bucket with 75-180 ml of the solutions. If repeated enemas are needed, alternate soapy water with warm water or water mixed with J-lube or rectal lubricant to minimize excessive mucosal irritation. Avoid dioctyl sodium sulfosuccinate (DSS) enemas because of irritation.

▶ Repeated enemas may lead to pathologic tenesmus.

RETENTION ENEMAS

- Use Mucomyst or powdered *N*-acetyl-L-cysteine. If Mucomyst is used, add 40 ml of 20% solution to 160 ml water to make a 4% solution. If using the powder, add 8 g of powder and 1½ tablespoon (~22.5 g) of sodium bicarbonate (baking soda) to 200 ml of water. Insert a lubricated Foley urinary catheter with a balloon tip approximately 2-4 inches (5-10 cm) into the rectum and inflate the balloon. Slowly infuse 4-6 oz (120-180 ml) of acetylcysteine solution into the rectum. Occlude the catheter end for a minimum of 15 minutes. Deflate the balloon and remove the catheter. The retention enema can be repeated several times.

ORAL LAXATIVES

- Proximal (high) impactions require oral laxatives in addition to enemas. The safest, least irritating laxative is **mineral oil** (120-160 ml), administered through a nasogastric tube. Mineral oil lubricates around the impaction and reduces the risk of complete obstruction, which can rapidly result in severe and painful gas accumulation and abdominal distention. *Milk of Magnesia* (60-120 ml) is an oral laxative that should be used conservatively.

*Castor oil or DSS administered orally is **not recommended*** owing to excessive mucosal irritation and increased risk of severe diarrhea and colic.

INTRAVENOUS FLUID THERAPY

- Useful in cases of refractory impaction. Dextrose supplementation is recommended if nursing behavior is curtailed because of increasing abdominal distention and colic.

PERCUTANEOUS BOWEL TROCARIZATION

- If severe abdominal distention develops before the impaction is resolved, consider the technique described under the heading Peripartum Asphyxia (see p. 561). Trocarization often provides immediate pain relief without excessive medication and allows time for medical therapy to work.

ANALGESICS AND SEDATIVES

- May be needed to prevent self-trauma in foals that are down and rolling.
- **Flunixin meglumine,** 0.5-1.0 mg/kg IV q24-36h; avoid repetitive doses because of its ulcerogenic potential *and effects on the kidney.*
- **Butorphanol,** 0.01-0.04 mg/kg IV. This is an excellent *first choice* and usually is highly effective. Can be repeated as necessary for several doses at 1- to 4-hour intervals.
- **Xylazine,** 0.1-0.5 mg/kg IV; use sparingly because of adverse effects on GI motility. Some debilitated neonatal foals experience marked ileus or respiratory compromise after use of this agent. Administering butorphanol and xylazine together decreases the dosage of xylazine needed.

Ileus

Decreased GI motility is associated with ischemic and hypoxic bowel damage secondary to septic shock or peripartum hypoxia. Beware that intussusception can develop as a result of the ileus or prokinetic drugs used to promote motility.

Clinical Signs

- Decreased or absent borborygmi
- Tympanitic abdominal distention
- Colic
- Gastric reflux (bloody or dark brown to black reflux suggests mucosal damage; consider administration of sucralfate in these cases)
- Diarrhea or constipation

Diagnosis

- Based on results of physical examination and supported by several diagnostic techniques:
  - □ **Transabdominal ultrasound** examination shows distended bowel, lack of propulsive motility. If **necrotizing enterocolitis** is present, ultrasound examination shows gas echoes within bowel walls.
  - □ **Abdominal radiographs** show generalized small- and large-bowel distention. **Pneumatosis intestinalis,** gas formation within the bowel wall, is observed with severe necrotizing enterocolitis.

Therapy

Depends on the underlying cause.

SEVERE HYPOXIC/ISCHEMIC GUT DAMAGE WITH SEVERE GASTRIC REFLUX, BLOODY DIARRHEA

- Intestinal rest, discontinue all enteral feeding until reflux and diarrhea resolve and borborygmi return. Severe cases may necessitate up to 7 days of *complete* intestinal rest. Small amounts of enteral food (milk or commercial isotonic, easily digested products) support enterocyte and enzyme production.
- Parenteral alimentation (see p. 559)
- Broad-spectrum, bactericidal antibiotics recommended (see p. 560)
- Sucralfate, 20-40 mg/kg PO q6h
- If a foal show signs of endotoxemia, consider administering 1 L of hyperimmune plasma to provide opsonins and immunoglobulins to support the immune system.
- Slowly reintroduce enteral feeding, beginning with small volumes of colostrum or fresh mare's milk.
- Complications associated with necrotizing enterocolitis include septicemia, intussusception, peritonitis, anemia, and stricture formation.
- Rule out *Clostridium perfringens* and *Clostridium difficile* infection (see Antibiotic-Induced Diarrhea, p. 252).

MILD TO MODERATE ILEUS, MILD COLIC ASSOCIATED WITH FEEDING, VARYING AMOUNTS OF REFLUX, AND INCONSISTENT MANURE PRODUCTION

- Decrease volume of enteral feedings temporarily and support with partial parenteral nutrition.
- Allow controlled exercise, short periods of turn out with dam in a small paddock.
- If constipation develops, treat with enemas, oral laxatives (mineral oil), and psyllium in small amounts and maintain hydration with oral or intravenous fluids.
- Administer oral probiotic agents: Commercial products or 2-3 oz (60-90 ml) of active culture yogurt PO q12-24h.

Intussusception

Colic due to intussusception may be mild to severe, depending on the location and duration of obstruction. Abdominal distention and reflux usually develop. The diagnosis often is made with transabdominal ultrasonography. Sonography shows "bull's-eye" target lesions that represent a cross-sectional view of intussuscepted bowel. Contrast radiography may help identify the location of obstruction.

Surgical resection is the only definitive treatment. Prognosis for survival is guarded to grave if multiple intussusceptions are found, if there are large sections of compromised bowel, or if peritonitis is severe. Postoperative complications include recurrent intussusception, stricture formation, and intraabdominal adhesions.

Enteritis (With or Without Peritonitis)

May be caused by a primary GI disorder or other systemic conditions, such as septicemia or peripartum hypoxia (see pp. 552 and 561).

Clinical Signs

- Colic
- Abdominal distention, reduced or absent borborygmi, tympany
- Diarrhea (blood, mucus)
- Variable temperature
- Injected sclera, hyperemic mucous membranes if enteritis is associated with endotoxemia
- Prolonged capillary refill time, dehydration
- Tachycardia

Possible Infectious Causes of Enteritis in Neonatal Foals

BACTERIAL

- *Salmonella* organisms can cause acute to peracute diarrhea accompanied by peritonitis and endotoxemia. Affected foals often are bacteremic and are at increased risk of development of septic osteomyelitis or arthritis.
- *E. coli* septicemia: *E. coli* isolates recovered from the blood of foals with diarrhea have *not* been shown definitively to be enteric pathogens; many foals with *E. coli* bacteremia also have enteritis.
- *Clostridium* organisms (*C. perfringens, C. sordellii, C. welchii, C. difficile*) can produce fetid diarrhea that is often bloody, particularly with *C. perfringens* infection. Affected foals often have septicemia.
- *Rhodococcus equi* infection is associated with chronic diarrhea, weight loss, and peritonitis in older foals (1-4 months of age) affected with the more common respiratory form of this disease.

VIRAL

- Although coronavirus, adenovirus, and parvovirus have been isolated from foals with diarrhea, rotavirus is the most common cause of viral diarrhea in neonatal foals. Rotavirus produces nonfetid, watery diarrhea that may be accompanied by fever and anorexia. There has been an increased incidence of gastroduodenal ulcer disease during some rotavirus endemics.

PARASITIC

- *Strongyloides westeri* nematode larvae have been associated with mild neonatal foal enteritis.

NUTRITIONAL

- *Overfeeding* can produce gastric distention, ileus, and diarrhea. If the gastric digestive and absorptive capacities are overwhelmed, a large, rapidly fermentable carbohydrate load reaches the colon, and the result is diarrhea.

NEONATOLOGY

- *Sudden diet changes* (e.g., changes from mare's milk to artificial replacer) can result in diarrhea.

OTHER
- *Enterocolitis* associated with hypoxic or ischemic intestinal damage (e.g., necrotizing enterocolitis) (see Peripartum Asphyxia, p. 561).
- *Foal heat diarrhea* is caused by physiologic changes occurring in the GI tract and usually results in self-limiting diarrhea that occurs between 5 and 14 days of age and lasts less than 5-7 days.

Diagnosis (General Guidelines)
- **Blood culture** if septicemia is suspected (e.g., *Salmonella, E. coli, Clostridium* organisms)
- **Fecal culture** for *Salmonella* and *Clostridium* organisms. Polymerase chain reaction can be used for *Salmonella* organisms, and toxin assays should be performed on *Clostridium* organisms (see p. 252).
- **Fecal flotation, direct smear.**
- **Rotavirus** test: Rotazyme (ELISA), Abbott Laboratories, North Chicago, IL; Rota Test (latex agglutination), Wampole Laboratories, Carter Wallace, Inc., Cranbury, NJ.
- **Abdominal radiography:** Enteritis, especially during the early stages, often is associated with varying degrees of ileus and generalized gas or fluid accumulation within the bowel lumen. Intramural gas accumulation *(pneumatosis intestinalis)* occurs with severe necrotizing enterocolitis. Pneumoperitoneum occurs with bowel rupture.
- **Transabdominal ultrasonography:** An increased volume of intraluminal fluid and bowel wall edema is present with enteritis. Peritonitis is associated with an increased volume of echogenic peritoneal fluid with or without fibrin tags. Intramural gas accumulation casts bright white echoes and is associated with hypoxic intestinal damage.
- **Hematology, chemistry:** Leukopenia and neutropenia are associated with endotoxemia. Secretory diarrhea usually results in hypochloremia, hyponatremia, varying degrees of metabolic acidosis, hemoconcentration, and variable potassium concentrations.
- **Abdominocentesis** if peritonitis is suspected. Peritoneal fluid contains increased protein concentration and nucleated cell count.

Therapy (General Guidelines)
- **Maintain hydration** using polyionic fluids. Monitor serum concentrations of electrolytes, glucose, and creatinine, acid-base balance, PCV, and total protein. If the foal is anorexic, administer parenteral alimentation.
- **Broad-spectrum, bactericidal, parenteral antimicrobial therapy** is recommended for foals with severe diarrhea and toxic mucous membranes, because of the increased risk of Gram-negative septicemia.
- **Intestinal protectants:** Bismuth subsalicylate (Corrective Suspension, Phoenix Pharmaceutical Inc., St. Joseph, MO 64506), 0.5-1 ml/kg PO q4-6h; kaolin and pectin, 4-8 ml/kg PO q12h
- **Nonsteroidal antiinflammatory drug therapy** is recommended if the foal shows signs of endotoxemia. A "low dose" of flunixin meglumine, 0.25 mg/kg IV q8-12h, is preferred.

> *Conservative use of this drug is advised owing to its ulcerogenic potential and its potential for disrupting normal renal function.*

- **Plasma** administration benefits foals with signs of endotoxemia and foals with FPT or hypoproteinemia.
- Consider **antiulcer medication:** Sucralfate, 20-40 mg/kg PO q6h.
- **Loperamide:** 4-16 mg PO q6h beginning with the low dose and increasing in 2-mg increments every 2-3 doses. Because it increases segmentation rate and slows transit time, loperamide may enhance toxin absorption in cases of acute, infectious enteritis. Therefore, its use should be reserved for foals that do not have signs of severe endotoxemia.
- Lidocaine may be useful for ileus and abdominal pain (see p. 565).

REFERENCES

Koterba AM, Drummond WH, Kosch PC: *Equine clinical neonatology,* ed 2, Philadelphia, 2003, Lea and Febiger.
Wilkins PA: Foal diseases. In Bayley WM, Reed SM, editors: *Equine internal medicine,* ed 2, Philadelphia, 2003, WB Saunders.

46 Perinatology
Jonathan E. Palmer

Pregnant mares are considered at high risk of a poor outcome when they have a history of problems during past pregnancies or have a new problem during the current pregnancy.

Classification of High-Risk Pregnancy
EXAMPLES OF RECURRENT PROBLEMS RESULTING IN CLASSIFICATION OF HIGH-RISK PREGNANCY
- Placentitis
- Premature placental separation
- Recurrent dystocia
- Premature termination of pregnancy
- Abortion
- Premature birth
- Prolonged pregnancies
- Uterine artery hemorrhage

EXAMPLES OF CURRENT PROBLEMS RESULTING IN CLASSIFICATION OF HIGH-RISK PREGNANCY
- Precocious udder development
- Placentitis
- Twin pregnancy
- Premature placental separation
- Over term relative to past gestations
- Musculoskeletal problems

- □ Fractures
- □ Laminitis
- □ Lameness
- Endotoxemia
  - □ Colic
  - □ Colitis
- Recent hypotension, hypoxemia
- Recent abdominal surgical incisions
- Development of body wall hernia
- Neurologic disease
  - □ Ataxia
  - □ Weakness
  - □ Seizures
- Hydrops allantois, amnion
- Pituitary hyperplasia
- Granulomatous disease
- Lymphosarcoma
- Melanoma in the pelvic canal
- Hypoparathyroidism
- Recent hemorrhage
- Innumerable other problems

Threats to Fetal Well-Being

The mare's problem should be viewed in terms of how it threatens fetal or neonatal well-being. After understanding the danger, devise a plan to minimize or eliminate the threat, and put it into action.

- The mother has total control of the fetal environment.
  - □ The fetus must receive everything from the mother.
  - □ There is no means for the fetus to directly communicate its changing needs to the mare.
- The fetus can compensate for some changes brought about because of disturbances in maternal homeostasis.
- Classification of threats to fetal well-being:
  - □ Lack of placental perfusion.
  - □ Lack of oxygen delivery.
  - □ Nutritional threats.
  - □ Placentitis, placental dysfunction.
  - □ Loss of fetal-maternal coordination of maturation.
  - □ Interaction with other fetuses (multiple pregnancy).
  - □ Iatrogenic factors.
    - □ Drugs or other substances given to the mother.
    - □ Early termination of pregnancy (e.g., induction).

LACK OF PLACENTAL PERFUSION

- Cardiac output during pregnancy increases 30%-50%.
  - □ 50% goes to the uterus.
  - □ The rest goes to the skin, gastrointestinal tract, and kidneys to compensate for the increased demands of pregnancy.
- During the last trimester, there are dramatic increases in blood flow to the placenta:
  - □ In parallel with fetal growth.

- The late-term fetus has a very high oxygen demand.
- There must be a high rate of placental perfusion to receive enough oxygen.
- Poor placental perfusion.
  - Can be only short-term compensation through redistribution of fetal blood flow.
  - The margin of safety in late pregnancy is small.
- Whenever maternal perfusion is compromised, placental circulation and oxygen delivery may be compromised; the result is a significant threat to the fetus.

▶ | Maternal hypovolemia must be managed aggressively.

LACK OF OXYGEN DELIVERY TO THE FETUS
- Causes of lack of oxygen delivery to the fetus:
  - Decreased placental perfusion
  - Maternal anemia
  - Maternal hypoxemia
- Survival of the fetus depends on efficient oxygen transport, determined by unique aspects of placentation or placental oxygen transport mechanisms.
- Placental gas transport is completely flow dependent, independent of diffusion.
  - There is no significant loss of transport in the face of a diffusion barrier.
  - The pattern of flow of maternal and fetal blood determines the efficacy of placental gas transport.
- In the horse, alignment of fetal and maternal vessels results in a countercurrent flow pattern.
  - The vessels are parallel to each other and the flows are opposite.
  - The venous side of the fetal capillary bed is aligned with the arterial side of the maternal capillary bed so that the gradient of oxygen and other nutrients is the highest possible.
  - The most efficient pattern for transfer of oxygen and nutrients and removal of waste products.
- Consequences of countercurrent flow pattern in the horse:
  - Changes in maternal PaO_2 significantly change fetal PO_2.
  - Maternal hypoxemia may have a profound effect on the fetus.
  - May predispose the foal to hypoxic ischemic asphyxial disease.
  - When maternal PaO_2 is increased with inhaled oxygen, umbilical PO_2 increases significantly, and the driving force increases, allowing more efficient transport.
- Supplementing the pregnant mare with intranasal oxygen (10-15 L/min).
  - Increases oxygen delivery to the fetus.
  - May help when there is fetal hypoxemia.
- Serious consideration should be given to blood transfusion therapy in the care of anemic mares to prevent fetal hypoxemia.
  - However, giving blood transfusions to a broodmare may predispose her to produce antibodies against blood groups resulting in neonatal isoerythrolysis in the future.

NUTRITIONAL THREATS TO FETAL WELL-BEING
- The mare's nutritional state may directly affect the fetus's well-being
- Chronic maternal malnutrition

- □ Lack of intake (because of lack of opportunity)
- □ Malabsorption
- □ Tumor cachexia
- □ Other conditions
- Acute fasting
  - □ For elective surgical procedures
  - □ When the mare has colic
  - □ Because of a capricious appetite of the late gestational mare
- 30-48 hours of complete fasting in the late-term mare
  - □ Decrease in glucose delivery
  - □ Rise in plasma free fatty acids
  - □ An associated increase in prostaglandin production in both maternal and fetal placenta

    Maternal and fetal placenta and fetal fluids contain a complex mix of prostaglandins, which seems to be important in maintaining pregnancy and may have a role in initiation of parturition

  - □ There is an increased risk of preterm delivery within 1 week of an anorexia episode; the foal often appears premature and not ready for delivery
- It is important to support the mare's nutritional needs at the end of gestation
  - □ Supplementation
  - □ Encouraged to stay on a high plane of nutrition
- Avoid acute fasting
  - □ If the mare has to be fasted or becomes completely anorexic

    Intravenous glucose supplementation (0.5-1 mg/kg per minute)
    Intravenous administration of glucose negates the changes in prostaglandins and greatly decreases the risk of early delivery

- When periodically anorexic mares are refractory to being encouraged to eat
  - □ Treatment with flunixin meglumine, 0.25 mg/kg q8h

PLACENTITIS AND PLACENTAL DYSFUNCTION
- Placental diseases that occur in late term pregnancy:
  - □ Premature placental separation
  - □ Placental infection
  - □ Noninfectious inflammation
  - □ Placental degeneration
  - □ Placental edema
  - □ Hydrops allantois, amnion
- Infectious placentitis
  - □ Ascending pathogens

    Bacteria
    Fungi

  - □ Hematogenous spread of pathogens

    Viruses
    Bacteria
    Ehrlichia
    Fungi

□ Percentage of placenta affected is not a predictor of the outcome of the pregnancy; a foal born with widespread placental lesions may be better off than a foal with a focal placental lesion

▶| The presence of placentitis, no matter how extensive, is predictive of a serious problem.

□ 80% of foals born with placentitis are abnormal
- Bacterial placentitis: All cases should be managed as such until proved otherwise
  □ Treatment

  Antimicrobial agents (trimethoprim-potentiated sulfonamides)
  An antiprostaglandin drug (flunixin meglumine)
  Hormone supplementation (altrenogest)

LOSS OF FETAL-MATERNAL COORDINATION OF READINESS FOR BIRTH
- Normal timing of parturition is decided cooperatively
  □ Maternal events
  □ Fetal events
  □ Placental events
  □ Dynamic interaction among these three distinct forces
- Loss of coordination results in
  □ A premature foal
  □ A dysmature foal
  □ A postmature foal

IATROGENIC FACTORS
- There are a large number of possible iatrogenic factors
- A major cause is poor timing of induction of delivery
  □ Timed based on the calendar and convenience
  ⊓ Timed based on emergency considerations for the mare
- Maternal drug therapy
  □ Affect the fetus in a variety of ways
  □ Tranquilizers and analgesics (e.g., detomidine, butorphanol), have immediate (<30 seconds) and profound effects on the fetal cardiovascular system
  □ Although drugs clearly indicated for the mare should be administered, the effect on the foal and possible alternative agents should be considered

PRESENCE OF TWINS
- The mare is somewhat unique in her inability to support multiple fetuses.
- The reason for this is not entirely clear.
- Twins compete with each other in ways detrimental to each other.
- One twin suffering from fetal distress may initiate early parturition.
- Twins increase the risk of dystocia.

IDIOPATHIC FACTORS
- Many foals born with hypoxic-ischemic asphyxial disease have no history of abnormalities occurring during gestation or parturition.
- Although it is easy to blame problems during parturition, most problems occur during the antepartum period.

Fetal Monitoring

EQUINE BIOPHYSICAL PROFILE (see Table 9–1)

- Collection of ultrasound-derived observations
  - Fetal heart rate
  - Fetal aortic diameter
  - Maximum fetal fluid depths
  - Uteroplacental contact
  - Uteroplacental thickness
  - Fetal activity
- Lacks sensitivity
  - Fetus with normal profile may have a life-threatening problem
- Lacks specificity
  - Extreme values are found in normal fetuses
- Information gathered about the placenta in conjunction with other critical information can be valuable

FETAL HEART RATE MONITORING

- Ultrasound technique
  - Measures the rate only by calculating the difference between two beats; therefore the results can be inaccurate
  - Long-term measurements are not generally recorded, and the results may be misleading
- Fetal electrocardiography (ECG)
  - Any ECG machine with recording capabilities works
  - Electrodes are placed at the lumbosacral junction on both flanks
  - Periodic recordings over a period of at least 10 minutes; telemetry is used to record sample readings 10-20 times every 24 hours
  - Important fetal heart rate values:

    Heart rate
    Occurrence of accelerations and decelerations
    Beat to beat variability
    Changes in complex polarity
    Presence of arrhythmias
    Fetal atrial fibrillation
    Premature contractions
    Extreme bradycardia (<40 beats/min)
    Persistent tachycardia
    Multiple distinct patterns suggest the presence of a twin

47 Foal Cardiopulmonary Resuscitation

Jonathan E. Palmer

OVERVIEW AND IMPORTANT FACTS

- Cardiopulmonary failure in foals is secondary to other systemic conditions.
  - Shock or respiratory failure, which are progressive and in early stages treatable, lead to bradycardia, which then deteriorates to asystole.
  - Unlike humans, in whom the principal cause of cardiopulmonary failure is coronary artery disease, ventricular fibrillation is not a common presenting arrhythmia.
- **The key to successful treatment is early recognition and management of the predisposing conditions.**
- A high-risk period is birth because neonates may fail the transition from fetal to neonatal physiology.
  - Prompt intervention is vital in these cases.

As important as early intervention is thorough preparation. At the moment of crisis there is no time to formulate a plan. Rather, one of several well-thought-out plans must be initiated once the nature of the crisis is recognized. It is most convenient to store airway equipment and emergency drugs in one or two grips that can easily be transported stallside (Boxes 47–1 and 47–2). These cases also should contain resuscitation flow sheets with drug dosages in terms of amounts in milliliters needed for the typical foal as shown in Table 47–1. It can be convenient to code drug vials with colored tape so that you can easily direct bystanders to retrieve the appropriate drugs for the attending clinician. In general, people are much more knowledgeable about proper techniques of cardiopulmonary resuscitation (CPR) than in the past, in part because of the efforts of the American Heart Association to teach basic life saving and in part due to the portrayal of realistic CPR scenes in popular television series. This can play an important role in resuscitation because with minimal prompting, bystanders can be enlisted to help. In the following discussion, techniques ranging from basic to advanced life support are outlined in an effort to prepare the practitioner to meet the challenge of the moment of crisis with tools that result in a successful outcome.

Humane Aspects of Cardiopulmonary Resuscitation

- Often it is mechanically possible to successfully resuscitate a foal but not humanely appropriate to do so.
- Most arrests in foals are secondary to progressive systemic disease.
  - If the underlying disease is incurable (relative to available facilities, technology, and skill) it is not in the best interest of the foal to attempt revival.
  - If the likely outcome is not as predictable, initiation of resuscitation efforts becomes a value judgment.
- Discussion about whether resuscitation is appropriate should take place before the moment of crisis.

BOX 47-1. Equipment Required for Resuscitation

---

1. SELF-INFLATING BAG-VALVE DEVICE
Adult size: 1600 ml
With O_2 reservoir bag: 2600 ml
Laerdal Silicone Resuscitator
Laerdal Medical Corp.
1 Labriola Court
Armonk, NY 10504
(800) 431-1055

2. SILICONE-CUFFED ENDOTRACHEAL TUBES
Sizes 7, 9 10, or 12 mm, 55 cm long
Several suppliers such as:
Air Vet (Bivona), Inc.
5425 Raines Road, Suite 3
Memphis, TN 38115
(800) 343-6237

Cook Veterinary Products
PO Box 489
Bloomington, IN 47402
(800) 826-2380

Rusch, Inc.
53 West 23rd Street
New York, NY 10010
(212) 675-5556

3. BUBBLE-JET HUMIDIFIER
Puritan Bennett Corp.
9410 Indian Creek, Pky #300
Shawnee Mission, KS 66225-5905
(913) 661-0444

4. INTRANASAL O_2 TUBING
A number of options/prefer:
16F Levin 127-cm tubing
Davol, Inc.
100 Sockanosset Crossroad
Cranston, RI 02920
(401) 463-7000

5. O_2 LINE
A number of options/prefer:
Clear vinyl tubing ⅜-inch ID,
½-inch OD (⅛-inch thick)
VWR Scientific
200 Center Square Road
Bridgeport, NJ 08014
(856) 467-3333

6. O_2 FLOW METERS
1- to 15-L range
Local medical supply company

7. O_2 TANK
With regulator adapted for humidifier
and flow meter
E-size tank (655 L)
Local medical gas company

GENERAL CARDIOPULMONARY RESUSCITATION
Causes of Cardiopulmonary Failure

Primary cardiac failure is an unusual cause of cardiac arrest in foals. Possible causes of primary cardiac failure:

- Hypoxic-ischemic myocardial damage
- Congenital cardiac defects
- Myocarditis
- Endocarditis with coronary artery embolism

Ventricular tachycardia or fibrillation, the expected consequences of primary cardiac failure, occur as the initial arrhythmia in only approximately 10% of pediatric cases of cardiopulmonary arrest.

Cardiopulmonary failure in foals usually occurs as the result of systemic disease. Systemic disease can cause secondary respiratory or cardiac failure, which leads to hypoxic acidosis. The hypoxic acidosis causes respiratory arrest followed by development of nonperfusing bradycardia and finally asystole. If

---

BOX 47-2. Useful Equipment for Resuscitation

1. COMPACT SUCTION UNIT
Laerdal Medical Corp.
1 Labriola Court
Armonk, NY 10504
(800) 431-1055

2. DEXTROMETER
ACCU CHECK III-Chemstrip bG
Boehringer Mannheim
9115 Hague Road
Indianapolis, IN 46250
(800) 858-8072

3. NONINVASIVE BLOOD PRESSURE MONITOR
Critikon, Inc.
5820 West Cypress, Suite B
Tampa, FL 33634
(813) 887-2000

4. INTRAVENOUS PUMPS
Gemini PC-1
IMED Corp.
9775 Businesspark Avenue
San Diego, CA 92131-1192
(800) 854-2033

5. INTRAVENOUS CATHETERS
Arrow International, Inc.
PO Box 12888
3000 Bemville Road
Reading, PA 19612
(610) 378 0131

6. HME FILTER (HEAT-MOISTURE EXCHANGE FILTER)
Provides heat and moisture to airway and filters bacteria and viruses
Pall Biomedical Products Corp.
Glen Cove, NY 11542
(800) 645-6578

7. BLOOD GAS ANALYZER
StatPal II- PPG Industries
Biomedical Systems Division
11077 Torrey Pines Road
La Jolla, CA 92037
(800) 369-3457

8. DEFIBILLATOR WITH ELECTROCARDIOGRAPH
Life Pak-10
Medtronic Physiocontrol Corp.
1181 Willows Road
Redmond, WA 98073-9706
(425) 867-4000
Automated external defibrillator currently being developed by a number of companies

9. ELECTROCARDIOGRAPH
Datascope Corp.
580 Winters Avenue
Paramus, NJ 07632
(800) 288-2121

---

resuscitation is begun before a nonperfusing cardiac rhythm develops, the likelihood of revival is good (survival rate as high as 50%). However, if resuscitation efforts are delayed until after development of asystole, less than a 10% survival rate is to be expected. Because the cause of arrest in most cases is systemic disease and the onset of arrest follows progressive respiratory and circulatory failure, with careful attention to development of signs, resuscitation can be begun before complete failure.

Common causes of cardiopulmonary arrest include:

- Perinatal hypoxia that leads to central respiratory center damage resulting in hypoventilation
- Primary lung disease leading to hypoventilation and hypoxia
- Septic shock
- Hypovolemia
- Metabolic acidosis
- Hyperkalemia (e.g., ruptured bladder)
- Vasovagal reflex
- Hypothermia

TABLE 47–1. Dosage (ml/kg) of Drugs Commonly Used in Cardiopulmonary Resuscitation

Drug	Supplied	Dose/kg	ml/kg	ml/20 kg	ml/30 kg	ml/40 kg	ml/50 kg	ml/60 kg	ml/70 kg
Epinephrine, low dose	1 mg/ml	0.01-0.02 mg	0.01-0.02	0.2-0.4/ 3-5 min	0.3-0.6/ 3-5 min	0.4-0.8/ 3-5 min	0.5-1/ 3-5 min	0.6-1.2/ 3-5 min	0.7-14/3-5 min
Epinephrine, high dose	1 mg/ml	0.1 mg	0.1	2/3-5 min	3/3-5 min	4/3-5 min	5/3-5 min	6/3-5 min	7/3-5 min
Vasopressin	20 U/ml	0.3-0.6 U	0.015-0.03	0.3-0.6	0.45-0.9	0.6-1.2	0.75-1.5	0.9-1.8	1-2
Lidocaine	2%	1.5 mg	0.075	1.6	2.25	3.0	3.75	4.5	5.25
Bretylium	20 mg/ml 50 mg/ml	5-10 mg, max 30-35 mg	0.1-0.2	Every 5 min, max 3.3 mg/kg 2-4/10 min	3-6/10 min	4-8/10 min	Every 5 minutes, max 3.3 mg/kg 5-10/10 min	6-12/10 min	7-14/10 min
Atropine	0.54 mg/ml	0.02 mg	0.037	0.8, max 2×	1.1, max 2×	1.5, max 2×	1.8, max 2×	2.2, max 2×	2.6, max 2×
CaCl	10%	20 mg	0.2	4	6	8	10	12	14
NaHCO$_3$	1 mEq/ml	0.5-1 mEq	0.5-1	10-20	15-30	20-40	25-50	30-60	35-70
MgSO$_4$	50%, 500 mg/ml	14-28 mg	0.028-0.056	0.6-1.1	0.8-1.7	1.1-2.2	1.4-2.8	1.7-3.4	2-4

> For the patient to be successfully revived, the underlying cause of arrest must be recognized and managed.

Recognition of Impending Failure

- Respiratory failure is marked by hypercapnia and hypoxia caused by inadequate ventilation.
- Foals with failure due to respiratory center damage secondary to peripartum asphyxia:
  - Do not sense the hypoxia or hypercapnia.
  - Have inadequate respiratory effort.
  - Have periods of apnea.
  - Have an apparently normal respiratory rate and minimal effort.
- **If there is a lack of responsiveness or loss of consciousness, respiratory failure should be assumed until disproved.**
- Failure secondary to intrinsic lung disease or airway obstruction results in progressive respiratory failure.
  - Signs of respiratory compensation that precede failure:
    - Increased respiratory rate (tachypnea)
    - Increased respiratory depth (hyperpnea)
    - Increased work of breathing
    - Nostril flare
    - Use of accessory respiratory muscles
    - Sinus tachycardia
- Respiratory compensation followed by what appears to be rapid improvement may in fact be fatigue or toxic effects of extreme hypercapnia and prolonged hypoxia preceding respiratory arrest.
- Uncontrolled shock (inadequate delivery of oxygen and metabolic substrates to tissues) leads to cardiopulmonary arrest.
  - Shock can occur with normal, decreased, or increased cardiac output and blood pressure.
  - Respiratory failure and shock may begin as distinct problems but progress in concert to cardiopulmonary failure.
  - There is a dynamic balance between oxygen content of blood and cardiac output.
  - If either decreases, the other must increase to ensure adequate oxygen delivery to the tissues.
  - Oxygen content can increase only marginally when the patient is breathing room air.
  - Any significant decrease in cardiac output results in decreased oxygen delivery unless oxygen content increases with an increase in the concentration of inspired oxygen with intranasal oxygen.
- **Cardiopulmonary failure leads inevitably to cardiopulmonary arrest.**
- Signs of cardiopulmonary failure:
  - Tachycardia
  - Depression (nonresponsiveness)
  - Oliguria
  - Hypotonia
  - Weak proximal pulse with weak or absent peripheral pulse
  - Prolonged capillary refill time

- Late ominous signs:
Bradycardia
Hypotension
Irregular respiratory pattern

Clinical Approach to Cardiopulmonary Resuscitation

See Figs. 47–1 and 47–2.

➤ - Establish an airway
- Begin ventilation
- Begin chest compressions
- Give epinephrine
- Determine the presence of cardiac arrhythmia and treat accordingly

Establishing an Airway

Mouth-to-Nose Ventilation (Fig. 47–3)

- Use when an endotracheal tube is not available.
- Can be effective, facilitated by the fact that foals are obligate nasal breathers.
- Technique:
  - □ Place the fingers of one hand just behind the patient's chin with the palm and thumb occluding the lower nostril.
  - □ Place the other hand on the poll so that the head can be maximally dorsiflexed and straighten the airway to decrease the possibility of aerophagia.
  - □ As an alternative, turn the head so that the poll is on the ground in maximal dorsiflexion, allowing the free hand to place pressure on the cricoid to ensure occlusion of the esophagus.
  - □ **Do not elevate the head** (doing so can further compromise cerebral circulation).
- As soon as an endotracheal tube is available, insert it, because the fractional inspired oxygen content (percentage inspired) is no better than 16%-18%.

Endotracheal Tube Placement

- Size (internal diameter): 9-mm endotracheal tube for the average Thoroughbred or Standardbred foal. Small foals (e.g., Arabians): 7-mm tube; large foals: 10- to 12-mm tube.
- Length: 55 cm so that full nasotracheal insertion places the cuff in the mid trachea.
- Sterile technique should be used whenever possible to avoid introduction of nosocomial pathogens, but because time is critical, the priority is rapid intubation and initiation of resuscitation.
- **Intubation technique:**
  - □ Nasotracheal intubation can be performed without assistance in cardiopulmonary failure, allowing others present to begin cardiac compressions, establish intravenous access, prepare appropriate drug dosages, and attach monitoring equipment.
  - □ Perform intubation with the patient in lateral recumbency so that cardiac compressions can begin without delay.
  - □ **Do not elevate the foal's head** (can further compromise cerebral blood flow).

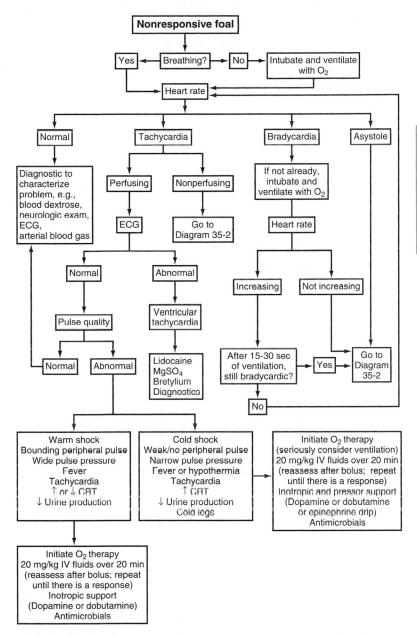

FIGURE 47–1. Nonresponsive foal algorithm. *ECG,* Electrocardiogram; *CRT,* capillary refill time.

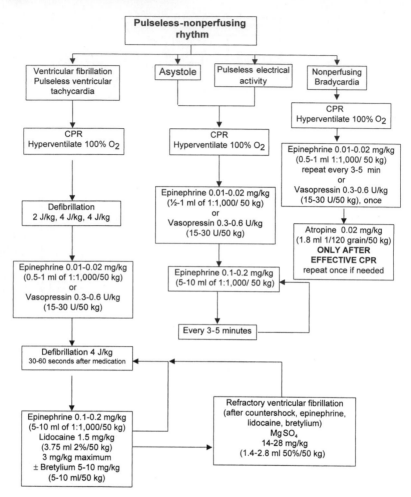

FIGURE 47–2. Cardiopulmonary resuscitation algorithm for foals.

- ▫ Dorsiflex the head to straighten the airway (Fig. 47–4).
- ▫ If an assistant is available, place one hand under the patient's chin, extending the head and neck, with the other pushing down on the poll to achieve dorsiflexion.
- ▪ Insert endotracheal tube through the nasal passage.
- ▫ The largest-diameter tube that passes through the nasal passage should be used.
- ▪ Once the tube reaches the level of the arytenoids, a rotating motion facilitates passage by allowing the beveled end to spread the arytenoids.
- ▪ Palpate the esophagus to ensure proper placement.
- ▫ Inadvertent inflation of the stomach is harmful.

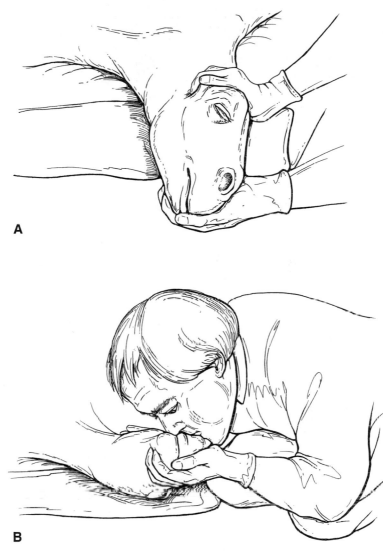

FIGURE 47–3. A, Position of foal's head for mouth-to-nose ventilation. **B,** Mouth-to-nose ventilation.

- Advance the endotracheal tube until only the adapter is evident at the nostril to minimize dead space.
- Secure with ties to a halter or around the poll.
- Inflate the cuff to ensure a tight seal (fill cuff until no air leak is heard during positive pressure ventilation).

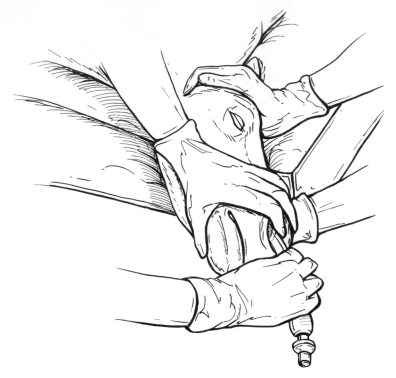

FIGURE 47–4. Placement of nasotracheal tube.

Ventilatory Aids

Anesthesia Bag

- Consists of a reservoir bag, an overflow port with pop-off valve, and a gas inflow port attached to an oxygen supply.
- Proper use of an anesthesia bag requires extensive training.

Demand Valve

- Requires a pressurized oxygen supply.
- Simple to use.
- **Prone to inducing barotrauma when** the operator is not trained or becomes distracted.

Self-Inflating Bag-Valve Device

- Of the three, the self-inflating bag-valve device is easiest to use, most versatile, and safest.
- Use a bag designed for human adult resuscitation (1600 ml with a 2600-ml oxygen reservoir bag).
- Operation
  - □ The bag fills via recoil drawing from the gas intake valve, oxygen input line or oxygen reservoir.

□ When the bag is compressed, the intake valve closes, and the patient outlet valve connected to the endotracheal tube opens to allow gas to flow to the patient.

□ During exhalation the patient outlet valve closes (to prevent rebreathing of exhaled gas on the next breath), and the exhalation valve near the patient connection opens.

□ The recoil of the bag draws gas into the bag for the next breath.

- An oxygen source is not needed.

□ The bag draws room air if no other gas source is available.

□ It is preferable to use a high concentration of oxygen during resuscitation, however resuscitation with room air can be quite effective.

- With an oxygen line attached:

□ The delivered oxygen concentration is between 30% and 80%.

□ With an oxygen reservoir bag and high flow (>15 L/min), oxygen concentration of 60% to 95% can be maintained.

The reservoir should be filled to maintain these high concentrations.

□ The flow needed to maintain the reservoir depends on the minute volume being delivered.

- If the self-inflating bag has a pop-off valve (usually set to 35-45 cm water to avoid barotrauma during normal ventilation), the valve needs to be easily occluded when low lung compliance, high airway resistance, an endotracheal tube obstructed by secretions or kinks, or the presence of pneumothorax make high airway pressure necessary.

Ventilation during Resuscitation

- Rate: Hyperventilate (40-60 breaths/min)
- Tidal volume: Estimated at 10 ml/kg
  □ Best gauged by means of careful observation of chest excursion to ensure proper ventilation.
- Auscultation of the lung fields after endotracheal placement to ensure even airflow can be helpful (occlusion of the main stem bronchi from overinsertion of the endotracheal tube is uncommon but possible).

CARDIOVASCULAR SUPPORT: ESTABLISHING CIRCULATION

▶ **Chest compressions should be initiated immediately if a nonperfusing cardiac rhythm is present. Do not delay until cardiac contractions stop.** The mechanism of blood flow during chest compression is not clear. The cardiac pump theory suggests that chest pressure causes cardiac compression, which propels blood while cardiac valves direct the blood flow forward. The thoracic pump theory suggests that the increased thoracic pressure caused by the compression propels the blood and that the venous valves direct it forward whereas noncompliant cardiac valves (as a result of myocardial rigor) make the cardiac contribution to blood flow minimal. There is evidence for both explanations.

Cardiac Compression (Fig. 47–5)

- Place the foal on a firm surface by removing any bedding.
- Position the foal with its withers against a wall so that it does not move during forceful compressions.

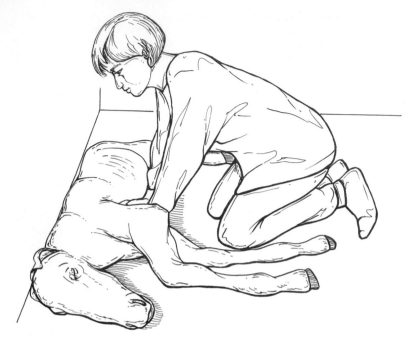

FIGURE 47–5. Cardiac compression.

- There is no difference in effectiveness of chest compressions from one side to the other.
- Time is important. It should not be wasted by repositioning the foal.
- Compression technique:
  □ Place the palm of the hand with the fist closed over the heart.
  □ Place the other hand to reinforce the compressing hand.
  □ The elbows should remain straight, and the motion for compression should originate from the waist (the upper body weight powering the compression results in increased endurance).
- Closed chest compression results in no more than 15% to 20% of normal cardiac output.
- To maximize cardiac output, half of the duty cycle should be compression and half relaxation.
  □ This is easiest to achieve with a rapid compression rate of 100-120 per minute.
  □ The resuscitator should not be overly ambitious in setting a rate. Too rapid a rate results in early operator fatigue.
- If an airway is secured, coordination between ventilation and chest compression is not needed.
  □ Cardiac output is enhanced by ventilation superimposed on chest compression.
  □ **Routine coordination of chest compression and ventilation** can result in increased cerebral pressure, which is clearly contraindicated in cases of hypoxic-ischemic encephalopathy and **should be avoided** in neonatal foals with possible perinatal hypoxia.

➤ Methods for measuring effectiveness of cardiac output:
- Feel a central arterial pulse.
- Monitor pupil size.
- Measure end-tidal carbon dioxide.

Central Arterial Pulse

- Traditional assessment of effectiveness of the chest compressions.
- Carotid or femoral artery.
- This can be difficult for several reasons:
  - Motion caused by chest compressions makes rapid location of the pulse difficult.
  - Skill and practice at locating the central arterial pulse are needed to make the judgment within seconds that there is an adequate pulse.
  - If someone talented enough to efficiently detect the presence of a pulse is available, it is likely their talent would be better used performing other vital tasks such as establishing a central intravenous line.

Pupil Size

- Preferable method, an indirect indication of adequate cerebral perfusion.
  - When perfusion of the head becomes inadequate (e.g., cardiac arrest), the pupils dilate widely.
  - When chest compression results in adequate perfusion to the head, the pupils assume a more neutral size.
- Pupil size can be monitored by the same person who is performing the chest compression.
- Chest compression technique should be adjusted as indicated by pupil size.

End-Tidal Carbon Dioxide (PETCO$_2$)

- The most effective measurement of cardiac output
- Best measured with a capnograph
  - When there is no cardiac output to the lungs, the PETCO$_2$ is 0 (alveoli are ventilated but not perfused)
  - If chest compression results in effective cardiac output and lung perfusion occurs, the PETCO$_2$ increases.
    - The more effective the chest compression in producing cardiac output, the higher is the PETCO$_2$.
    - Effective compressions result in a PETCO$_2$ of 12-18 mm Hg.
    - Manipulations during CPR that cause a change in PETCO$_2$ independent of cardiac output:
    - High-dose epinephrine therapy can cause a decrease in PETCO$_2$
    - Treatment with bicarbonate can increase PETCO$_2$ (buffering of acid in the central venous system results in a higher concentration of carbon dioxide in the blood delivered to the lungs).
  - Capnography results in immediate feedback to the resuscitator, allowing for beat to beat modification of technique and ensuring that the most effective cardiac output is achieved.

FOAL CPR

Complications of Chest Compression

- Rib fractures can result in:
  - Hemorrhage and possible hemothorax
  - Lung lacerations
  - Myocardial lacerations
  - Flail chest
  - Chest compression must be applied above the costochondral junction to produce effective cardiac output and decrease the risk of rib fractures.
  - The compliant nature of the ribs in neonatal foals makes fractures less likely.
- Pulmonary contusions
- Myocardial contusions

Vascular Access

▶ **Establishing vascular access is essential if the neonate does not respond immediately to ventilation and chest compression.** Because cardiopulmonary failure in neonates usually is secondary to other serious systemic disease, patients may already have an intravenous catheter. For those that do not, the jugular vein should be catheterized with whatever available materials the resuscitator believes results in the most rapid vascular access.

> **NOTE: It is contraindicated to give drugs by the intracardiac route.** The delivery of drugs is no more rapid than by the venous or intratracheal (IT) access route.

- Complications of intracardiac injections:
  - Interruption of chest compressions
  - Coronary artery laceration
  - Cardiac tamponade
  - Pneumothorax

DRUGS THAT CAN BE ADMINISTERED BY THE INTRATRACHEAL ROUTE

- Epinephrine (use high dose)
- Lidocaine
- Atropine
- Naloxone

Before vascular access is secured, some drugs can be given by the intratracheal route. Low volume, lipid-soluble drugs such as epinephrine, atropine, lidocaine, and naloxone can be absorbed if given by this route. To be absorbed, **the drug must be delivered beyond the endotracheal tube into the bronchial tree.** This can be accomplished by passing infusion tubing down the endotracheal tube and chasing the drug with fluids. However, this requires interruption of ventilation. An equally effective and more expedient method involves transtracheal injection of the drugs.

Transtracheal Injection of the Drugs

- Palpate the trachea to identify the level of the inflated cuff.
- Estimate the location of the end of the endotracheal tube.
- Inject the drug transtracheally below the tube, usually close to the thoracic inlet.
- Follow the injection with several large breaths.

Recent reports cast doubt on the reliability of absorption through the intratracheal route. This has led to the more frequent use of the intraosseous (IO) route for circulatory access (see Intraosseous Infusion Technique, p. 15).

Intraosseous Circulatory Access

- Substances injected into the bone marrow are absorbed almost immediately into the systemic circulation.
- The marrow cavity acts as a rigid vein; it does not collapse in the presence of hypovolemia or profound peripheral circulatory shock.
- The pharmacodynamics of intraosseous infused drugs approximate those of intravenous infusion.

DRUGS THAT CAN BE ADMINISTERED BY THE INTRAOSSEOUS ROUTE

- Fluids, glucose, sodium bicarbonate, calcium chloride
- Whole blood, plasma
- Resuscitation drugs: Epinephrine, lidocaine, atropine, dopamine, dobutamine, vasopressin
- Antimicrobials
- Other drugs: Phenobarbital, diazepam, butorphanol, insulin, mannitol

---

Intraosseous Needle Placement

- Most reliable entry point: Proximal tibia, on the midline of the anterior medial flat surface, 2-4 cm below the proximal tibial physis.
  - Care must be taken to be below the physis to make certain you enter the marrow cavity.
  - Others sites can be used; however, the absence of soft-tissue structures over the bone, ease of identification of the landmarks, flat entry surface, and simplicity of penetrating the marrow cavity make the tibial physis the preferred location.
  - This site is also away from areas used by other resuscitators, who are performing airway manipulations, jugular catheterization, and cardiac compression.
  - Stabilization after entry is more difficult at the proximal tibia than at other sites because of the medial location.
- If the patient is unconscious, it is unnecessary to use a local anesthetic, which speeds venous access.
- Aseptically prepare the site.
- A stab incision is not always necessary if the needle has not been used before.
- In mature newborn foals, standard intraosseous needles designed for adult humans can be used.
  - 12-gauge, 2.3-cm intraosseous infusion needle (Sur-Fast Intraosseous Infusion Needle, Cook Critical Care, Bloomington, IN 47402)
  - The needle handle provided facilitates entry into the bone.
- In premature foals, twins, and foals with intrauterine growth restriction with incomplete ossification:
  - 16- to 18-gauge needles may penetrate the cortex.
  - Use needles with stylets (spinal needles) because the lumen can become blocked with bone fragments.
  - Spinal needles are in danger of bending or breaking because of their length and narrow gauge.
  - Place the needle with a screw action directed distal at a slight angle (10-15 degrees from vertical) while applying a firm downward pressure until a loss of resistance is felt as the needle penetrates the marrow cavity.
- The needle should remain upright without support.

FOAL CPR

- Aspiration of bone marrow may be possible. If not, use a test infusion (by syringe) of saline solution.
  - □ Fluid should easily flow through the needle without resistance when flushed.
  - □ The ability to easily infuse fluids through conventional infusion tubing with no extravasation confirms correct placement.
- Secure the needle and infusion line so that the site can be examined for extravasation of fluids, indicating improper placement.
- Avoid placing the needle where the cortex has been unsuccessfully perforated or fractured. Failed attempts with cortical perforation requires moving to a new site.

COMPLICATIONS OF INTRAOSSEOUS INFUSION

- Extravasation into subcutaneous tissues
  - □ Incomplete insertion of needle
  - □ Overpenetration through opposite cortex
  - □ Poor insertion technique
  - □ Multiple cortical perforations
  - □ Dislodged needle

- Cellulitis associated with extravasation is uncommon.
- Osteomyelitis is rare.
- Growth plate injury does not occur.

DRUG THERAPY DURING RESUSCITATION (Table 47–1)
Epinephrine
Key Points
- Epinephrine is an endogenous catecholamine with both α- and β-adrenergic effects.
- α-Adrenergic effects:
  - □ Increase in systemic vascular resistance
  - □ Elevation of systolic and diastolic blood pressure
  - □ Decrease in perfusion of splanchnic, renal, mucosal, and dermal circulation
- β-Adrenergic effects:
  - □ Increase in myocardial contractility
  - □ Increase in heart rate
  - □ Relaxation of smooth muscle in bronchi
  - □ Relaxation of skeletal muscle vasculature

▶ The most important advance in the understanding of the mechanism of drug activity in CPR in the past 20 years is the insight into the importance of epinephrine in improving coronary perfusion pressure during cardiac arrest. During chest compression coronary blood flow is restricted to the diastolic period. *Diastolic aortic pressure determines coronary perfusion,* because during cardiac arrest there is no coronary capillary resistance and central venous pressure is low owing to minimal venous return. Epinephrine increases diastolic aortic pressure by simultaneously preventing runoff into peripheral tissues (by peripheral arterial constriction) and by increasing aortic tone. The combination of effective chest compression and the action of epinephrine results in a return of coronary perfusion, which is the most important step in resolving cardiac arrest no matter what the cause. **Without coronary perfusion there is no hope of return to normal cardiac rhythm.**

Indications

- Cardiac arrest regardless of underlying cause
  - Asystole
  - Idioventricular rhythms
  - Pulseless electrical activity
  - Symptomatic bradycardia nonresponsive to ventilation with oxygen
- Hypotension not related to volume depletion

EPINEPHRINE DOSE FOR PULSELESS CARDIAC ARREST

- Initial dose: 0.01-0.02 mg/kg IV or IO
- Subsequent doses and all intratracheal doses: 0.1 mg/kg IV or IO
- Dosing interval: Repeat every 3-5 minutes

Complications and Precautions

- Postresuscitation hypertension and tachyarrhythmia
- Increased cardiac oxygen demand and myocardial necrosis
- Inactivated when mixed with bicarbonate
- Several studies suggest that the high IV or IO dose (0.1 mg/kg) may not be beneficial and may be harmful. Its usefulness is not clearly established.

Vasopressin

Key Points

- The vasoconstrictor action is more potent than that of angiotensin II or norepinephrine.
- The pressor action is minimal in healthy individuals.
  - Baroreceptor-mediated bradycardia prevents a pressure increase.
- The pressor activity of vasopressin is marked in cardiac arrest.
  - Baroreceptor dysfunction
  - Autonomic failure

Indications

- As effective as epinephrine for ventricular fibrillation or pulseless ventricular tachycardia
- As effective as epinephrine as a vasoconstrictor
  - Fewer negative effects, so may be safer than epinephrine
  - Does not cause postresuscitation hypertension
- Can replace or be used in conjunction with epinephrine

Vasopressin Dose for Pulseless Cardiac Arrest
- Initial IV/IO dose: 0.3-0.6 U/kg
- Dosing interval: Effect lasts 10-20 minutes; repeated doses unnecessary

Complications and Precautions

- In healthy individuals (with intact baroreceptor response), bradycardia occurs with no change in blood pressure.

Fluids

Key Points

- Large volumes of fluids are important in treating hypovolemic or septic shock, which frequently leads to cardiac arrest.
- After cardiac arrest, **overzealous fluid administration is contraindicated**.
  - When hypovolemia leads to cardiac arrest, a nonperfusing rhythm develops, and the ineffective cardiac output resembles congestive heart failure.
  - With effective chest compressions, cardiac output is only 15% to 20% of normal.
  - If fluids are given rapidly, venous pressure increases and impedes coronary perfusion and return of a normal cardiac rhythm, despite effective chest compressions and high doses of epinephrine.
  - *If volume replacement is indicated because of severe dehydration, bolus administration is preferred rather than a continuous high flow rate.*
  - A moderate fluid rate should be used until spontaneous cardiac rhythm returns.
- Once a perfusing rhythm returns, increased fluid rates may be needed to help maintain cardiac output.
- Severe hypoglycemia can lead to cardiac arrest; however, **glucose-containing fluids should be avoided during resuscitation** unless a patient-side glucose determination indicates severe hypoglycemia.
  - Hyperglycemia and hyperosmolality, secondary to rapid glucose infusion, during resuscitation are associated with poor neurologic outcome in humans.

Sodium Bicarbonate

Key Points

- *The use of bicarbonate during cardiac arrest remains controversial.*
- Theoretical contraindications:
  - Sodium bicarbonate buffers acid by forming carbon dioxide eliminated by ventilation.
  - During resuscitation, carbon dioxide is not eliminated efficiently.
  - Carbon dioxide is highly soluble and moves across cell membranes quickly.

  Organic acids tend to accumulate in the blood during prolonged cardiac arrest.
  - Intracellular acidosis increases when bicarbonate buffers these organic acids, producing carbon dioxide, which reenters cells because, owing to capillary blood stasis, it is not carried away.
  - During CPR a venoarterial paradox develops.
    - Slow venous return produces severe venous hypercapnic acidemia.
    - Overventilation of the blood passing through the lungs causes arterial hypocapnic alkalemia.
    - The poorer the cardiac output, the more extreme is the venoarterial difference.
    - When there is a large venoarterial difference, administration of bicarbonate may exacerbate acidosis.
    - Myocardial acidosis is more marked than acidosis in other tissues.
    - Increased intracellular acidosis can result in considerable cardiac depression.
- **With poor cardiac output and coronary perfusion, the use of bicarbonate therapy is contraindicated.**

- Once efficient cardiac output is achieved, administration of bicarbonate may be helpful in returning the heart to a spontaneous perfusing rhythm.
  - If bicarbonate is administered to a patient being hyperventilated with 100% oxygen and who has effective cardiac output, it may reverse acidosis-induced cardiac depression.
  - It can also increase the effectiveness of epinephrine.
  - The combination of epinephrine and bicarbonate therapy under these circumstances can greatly improve recovery.
  - *Maintaining good cardiac output is critical for this effect.*

Indications
ABSOLUTE INDICATION
- Hyperkalemia (secondary to ruptured bladder)

PROBABLE INDICATIONS
- Preexisting metabolic acidosis leading to arrest
- Phenobarbital overdose

CONTROVERSIAL INDICATIONS
- Prolonged, nonresponsive arrest
- Aftermath of return to spontaneous circulation

CONTRAINDICATION
- Hypoxic lactic acidosis

SODIUM BICARBONATE DOSAGE
- 0.5-1 mEq/kg over 1-2 minutes
- Repeat once in 5-10 minutes if indicated

Potential Complications
- Significant cardiac depression secondary to increased intracellular carbon dioxide
- Hypernatremia with secondary cerebral hemorrhage.
- Hyperosmolality with secondary cerebral hemorrhage.
- Left shift of oxyhemoglobin saturation curve (less oxygen to tissues).
- **Bicarbonate and epinephrine cannot be given through the same intravenous line, because the epinephrine becomes inactivated.**

Atropine
Key Points
- Atropine is a parasympatholytic drug that accelerates sinus or atrial pacemakers and atrioventricular conduction.

Indications
- **Major indication: Vagally mediated bradycardia.**
- High vagal tone (except secondary to hypoxia) is an uncommon cause of bradycardia in neonatal foals.

- *Neonatal bradycardia is generally caused by hypoxia and should be managed with hyperventilation with 100% oxygen and epinephrine.*
  - □ Early treatment with atropine may exacerbate the hypoxic insult by increasing the heart rate; the result is higher oxygen demand of cardiac muscle in the face of inadequate oxygen delivery.
- Hypoxemia and hypercapnia result in stimulation of the carotid body and increase vagal tone with secondary bradycardia.
  - □ Hyperventilation can correct this form of vagally mediated bradycardia because lung inflation stimulates pulmonary receptors, which can override the carotid body stimulus.
  - □ If hyperventilation and epinephrine treatment do not result in resolution of the bradycardia, atropine therapy is indicated.
- Excessive vagal tone can be associated with gastrointestinal disease.
  - □ Extreme intestinal distention secondary to:

    Meconium impaction
    Necrotizing enterocolitis
    Bacterial enteritis (clostridiosis, salmonellosis).

  - □ Hypoglycemia often complicates this condition.
  - □ If hyperventilation with 100% oxygen, effective chest compressions, and repeated treatment with epinephrine does not resolve bradycardia, atropine is indicated.
- **In all cases of bradycardia, atropine should not be given before hyperventilation with 100% oxygen.**

ATROPINE DOSAGE

- 0.02 mg/kg IV or IO
- 0.04-0.06 mg/kg IT
- Repeat once in 5 minutes if indicated

Potential Complications
- Tachycardia
- Exacerbation of hypoxic insult due to an increase in the oxygen demand of cardiac muscle

Calcium
Key Points
- Calcium is essential for cardiac contraction.
- Calcium entry into myocardial cells induces actin-myosin coupling.
- Contraction is terminated when calcium is pumped out of the cell.
- Myocardial contractility is increased when calcium is infused intravenously into patients with normal cardiac function.
  - □ Calcium therapy during cardiac arrest can hasten cell death.
  - □ During cardiac arrest, calcium entry into the cell cytoplasm is believed to be the final common pathway of cell death.
  - □ Calcium channel blockers are protective during cardiopulmonary bypass.
- **Calcium is not recommended for management of asystole or pulseless electrical activity.**
  - □ Epinephrine is more useful than calcium.

Indications
- Hyperkalemia (secondary to ruptured bladder)
- Hypocalcemia
- Hypermagnesemia

CALCIUM CHLORIDE (CaCl) DOSE
- Elemental calcium, 5-7 mg/kg
- 10% CaCl, 0.2-0.25 ml/kg
- 10% calcium gluconate, 0.6-0.75 ml/kg

Potential Complications
- More rapid cell death in the presence of hypoxic damage.
- Rapid infusion results in bradycardia or cardiac standstill.

Defibrillation
Key Points
- The definitive management of ventricular fibrillation and pulseless ventricular tachycardia is *defibrillation*.
- **Defibrillation should not be used to manage asystole or bradyarrhythmia.**
- Ventilation with 100% oxygen and chest compressions should be continued until the moment of defibrillation.
- Defibrillation results in depolarization of a critical mass of myocardial cells to allow spontaneous organized myocardial depolarization to resume.
  - Defibrillation requires electrical current to pass through the heart.
  - The amount of current delivered to the heart depends on the energy delivered from the paddles and the transthoracic resistance.
  - There are numerous determinants of current flow through the heart.

Indications
- Ventricular fibrillation
- Pulseless ventricular tachycardia

DEFIBRILLATION DOSAGE
- Initial series of up to three rapid charges: 2 J/kg, 4 J/kg, 4 J/kg
- Subsequent defibrillations: 4 J/kg 30-60 seconds after treatment with epinephrine, lidocaine, or bretylium

---

Complications
- Defibrillation is potentially dangerous to the operator and other personnel.
  - No one should attempt defibrillation until they are trained both in the technique and with the defibrillator being used.
  - Improper placement of the paddles can cause serious burns.
- *Use of alcohol before defibrillation is a fire hazard.*

Lidocaine
Key Points
- Lidocaine suppresses ventricular arrhythmia by decreasing automaticity.

FOAL CPR

- Its local anesthetic properties suppress ventricular ectopy after myocardial infarction.
- It decreases conduction of reentrant pathways.
- It reduces the disparity in action potential duration between ischemic and normal tissue.
- It prolongs conduction and refractoriness in ischemic tissue.
- There is no experimental support for a major antifibrillatory effect, but lidocaine may prevent recurrence once conversion occurs.

Indications
- Ventricular fibrillation
- Ventricular tachycardia
- Prevent recurrence of ventricular fibrillation or ventricular tachycardia and wide-complex tachycardia, which usually are ventricular

---

LIDOCAINE DOSAGE

- Bolus dosage
  - Initial dose: 1.5 mg/kg IV
  - Repeat once in 5 minutes
  - 8-10 min later administer 0.5 mg/kg
- Intravenous infusion
  - 1 mg/kg loading dose
  - 20-50 µg/kg per minute
  - 60 × Body weight in kg = Mg of lidocaine added to 1000 ml of fluids
  - 20-50 ml/h results in a dose of 20-50 µg/kg per minute

Precautions
- Toxic effects
  - Neurologic signs
    - Depression
    - Paresthesia
    - Muscle twitching
    - Seizures
- Myocardial depression
- Circulatory depression

Bretylium Tosylate
Key Points
- Bretylium is an adrenergic neuronal blocker.
- It increases fibrillation threshold.
- It is synergistic with lidocaine.
- It has direct myocardial effects.
- It has biphasic adrenergic effects that cause hypertension followed by hypotension (in healthy individuals).
  - Bretylium initially releases norepinephrine from adrenergic nerve endings for approximately 20 minutes.
  - Subsequently it produces adrenergic blockade, which peaks at 45-60 minutes.
- The antiarrhythmic action is poorly understood.
- It increases action potential duration and effective refractory period.

Indications after Countershock, Epinephrine, and Lidocaine
- Ventricular fibrillation
- Ventricular tachycardia

BRETYLIUM TOSYLATE DOSAGE
- 5 mg/kg undiluted IV rapidly followed in 30-60 seconds by defibrillation
- If ventricular fibrillation persists, repeat with 10 mg/kg boluses
- Do not give more than a total of 35 mg/kg

Precautions
- Hypotension
- Hypertension
- Tachycardia

Magnesium Sulfate

Key Point
- Magnesium sulfate can be used in refractory fibrillation when countershock, epinephrine, lidocaine, and bretylium have failed.

Indications
- Hypomagnesemia
- Torsades de pointes

MAGNESIUM SULFATE (MgSO$_4$) DOSAGE
- 14-28 mg/kg diluted to 10 ml in 5% dextrose in water IV push

---

Precautions
- Hypotension
- Caution with renal failure

POSTRESUSCITATION TREATMENT
Goals
- To prevent secondary organ failure
- To allow transportation to a facility where intensive care can be delivered

Continued evaluation of cardiopulmonary function is vital, even if the foal is easily resuscitated and its condition initially appears stable. Foals often have recurrent episodes of hypoxia, hypercapnia, or cardiovascular instability. The underlying cause of cardiopulmonary failure must be recognized and managed. No matter what the original etiologic factor, if periods of hypoxia and hypotension go unrecognized and unmanaged, death is almost certain.

Guidelines for Postresuscitation Treatment
1. Search for and manage the underlying cause of cardiopulmonary failure.
2. Frequently assess cardiopulmonary function.
   - Signs of inadequate pulmonary function:
     □ Minimal and uneven chest excursions

- □ Inadequate or unequal breath sounds
- □ Increased respiratory effort (nasal flare, rib retraction)
- □ Paradoxic ventilation (increased diaphragmatic efforts at sucking the chest wall in on inspiration)
- Periodic arterial blood gas analysis
- Continuous electrocardiographic monitoring of heart rate and rhythm
- Evaluation of peripheral circulation and end-organ perfusion:
  - □ Skin temperature
  - □ Capillary refill time
  - □ Quality of distal pulses
  - □ Central nervous system responsiveness
  - □ Urine output
- Serial indirect blood pressure determinations
3. Administer humidified intranasal oxygen insufflation at 6-10 L/min.
4. Control hypothermia and maintain core temperature (if transporting, place the patient in a heated cab and not in a cold van).
5. Continue intravenous fluid therapy:
   - If the patient is in septic shock, once spontaneous circulation returns, initiate aggressive fluid therapy: 20 ml/kg boluses over 20 minutes with reassessment after each bolus administration.
   - Continue maintenance fluids after successful fluid resuscitation.
6. Provide pressor and inotropic support as needed (*must use intravenous infusion pump*) (Table 47–2):
   - Dopamine, 6-10 µg/kg per minute initially, titrate to effect to a maximum of 20 µg/kg per minute

TABLE 47–2. Relative Potency of Inotropes and Pressors

Drug	Infusion Rate*	α Effect (Pressor)	β Effect (Inotropic)	Use
Dopamine	1-5 µg/kg per min (dopaminergic effect)	+	+	First-line choice, good mixed α and β response
	5-15 µg/kg per min	++	++	
	10-20 µg/kg per min	+++	+++	
Dobutamine	2-20 µg/kg per min (high doses)	+ (++)	+++	Good β effects; add to dopamine for additional inotropic effect (limiting tachycardia)
Epinephrine	0.1-1 µg/kg per min (max 3 µg/kg per min)	+++	+++	Use if not responding to dopamine; good mixed α and β response
Norepinephrine	0.05-1 µg/kg per min (max 2 µg/kg per min)	+++	+	Primarily α effect; should be combined with a β drug
Phenylephrine	0.1-1 µg/kg per min	+++	0	Primarily α effect; should be combined with a β drug

*These rates serve as guidelines for treatment. The pharmacokinetics of these drugs are not consistent between patients and within the same foal over time. Therefore the dose must be titrated for the individual patient and adjusted over time.

- Dobutamine, 6-10 µg/kg per minute initially, titrate to effect up to 25 µg/kg per minute or higher (as high as 50 µg/kg per minute sometimes is required)

TO PREPARE DOPAMINE OR DOBUTAMINE INFUSION:

6 × Body weight in kg = mg of drug added to 100 ml of fluids
1 ml/h = 1 µg/kg per minute
Infuse 6-10 ml/h

- Epinephrine, 0.3 µg/kg per minute initially, titrate to effect up to 2 µg/kg per minute or higher
- Norepinephrine, 0.3 µg/kg per minute initially, titrate to effect up to 3 µg/kg per minute or higher

---

TO PREPARE EPINEPHRINE OR NOREPINEPHRINE INFUSION:

0.6 × Body weight in kg = mg of epinephrine or norepinephrine
added to 100 ml of fluids
1 ml/h = 0.1 µg/kg per minute

- In cases refractory to exogenous adrenergic agents, the use of low-dose vasopressin may be helpful (0.25-0.5 mU/kg per minute). Vasopressin may not only increase arterial blood pressure but also allow withdrawal of adrenergic agents.

TO PREPARE VASOPRESSIN INFUSION:

0.6 × Body weight in kg = Units of vasopressin added to 100 ml of
fluids
1 ml/h = 0.1 mU/kg per minute

- In cases that do not respond to traditional pressors, methylene blue therapy (0.5-2 mg/kg) may be useful. It blocks the action of nitric oxide, which is the local messenger causing active vasodilatation. Limited experience indicates this is a highly effective pressor when used to treat foals in endotoxic shock.

CAUTION· *The pressor response with this drug may be so effective that cardiac output decreases and perfusion fails.*

- Naloxone may be beneficial in blocking endorphin-mediated hypotension (hemorrhagic and septic shock). It also enhances myocardial sensitivity to β-adrenergic drugs.

▶ **Remember: The goal of pressor therapy is not to increase blood pressure but to increase and direct perfusion of tissues and maintain cardiac perfusion by maintaining diastolic pressure.** As blood pressure increases, afterload increases and cardiac output decreases. It is *counterproductive* to increase blood pressure at the expense of cardiac output. As blood pressure increases, more inotropic support of the heart is needed to concurrently support cardiac output. This is the reason mixed α and β support (dopamine, dobutamine, epinephrine) is useful.

7. When oxygenation is adequate, begin administration of glucose, 4 mg/kg per minute, to help clear metabolic acidosis. This is important because myocardial glycogen is generally depleted, and this step serves to prevent postasphyxia hypoglycemia. Monitor blood glucose level (stallside monitoring, as with a

glucometer, every 30 minutes until the result is stable) because the glucose infusion rate frequently must be adjusted to prevent hyperglycemia or hypoglycemia. If tolerated, the glucose infusion should be increased to 8 mg/kg per minute. The infusion rate occasionally must be greater than 8 mg/kg per minute to meet glucose demands.

BIRTH RESUSCITATION

Although most newborns make the transition from fetal life without incident, rapid recognition of the need to intervene is vital in achieving a successful outcome for those that do not (Fig. 47–6). The cause of cardiopulmonary failure at birth is readily evident. The lack of anticipation, however, can catch the attending clinician off guard. In a few cases, the risk to the foal may be clear (e.g., dysto-

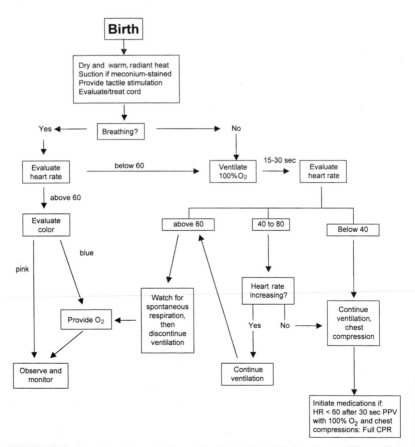

FIGURE 47-6. Overview of resuscitation of the foal at birth. *HR*, Heart rate; *PPV*, positive pressure ventilation; *CPR*, cardiopulmonary resuscitation.

cia or peripartum maternal disease). In others it is not. Even when attending what is expected to be a normal birth, the clinician must monitor the foal's progress and be prepared to intervene when indicated. *Birth resuscitation represents a special case of general resuscitation and necessitates modification of the approach.*

Fetal-Neonatal Transition

The fetus depends on the placenta for gas exchange. Compared with the newborn, the fetus is hypoxemic with a PaO_2 of 40 mm Hg in the umbilical vein. This does not imply tissue hypoxia because compensatory mechanisms allow for adequate delivery of oxygen to tissues. Hypoxemia is largely responsible for the pulmonary hypertension that ensures proper fetal blood flow.

Fetal Circulation

- Oxygen-rich blood returning from the placenta by way of the umbilical vein is directed to the heart and brain.
  - It bypasses the liver through the ductus venosus.
  - It travels to the right side of the heart through the posterior vena cava.
  - It enters the right atrium directly across from the foramen ovale. This blood tends to stream, flowing directly across the right atrium, through the foramen ovale. Oxygen-rich blood fills the left atrium.
  - Oxygen-rich blood is pumped by the left ventricle into the ascending aorta, which feeds:
    - The coronary arteries
    - The brachiocephalic artery
  - Ensuring that the heart and brain receive the most oxygen rich blood.
- Blood returning from the head and trunk is directed to the lower body and back to the placenta.
  - Blood from the anterior vena cava fills the right ventricle.
  - Because it enters the heart perpendicular to the foramen ovale and across from the tricuspid valve, blood flows into the right ventricle.
  - This blood is pumped into the pulmonary artery and is shunted through the ductus arteriosus to the descending aorta.
    - Hypoxemia-induced pulmonary hypertension ensures little pulmonary arterial flow.
    - Relative systemic hypotension, because the placental circulation accommodates 40% of the cardiac output, allows right to left shunting of the blood.
  - The descending aorta sends the blood to the lower body or back to the placenta.
  - Blood returning to the placenta has a PaO_2 of 15-25 mm Hg.

At Birth

- The result is an increase in systemic blood pressure.
- Vigorous breathing efforts at birth originate from central and peripheral chemoreceptors stimulated by:
  - The increase in systemic blood pressure
  - External stimuli
  - Progressive asphyxia if present

FOAL CPR

- There is a rapid decrease in pulmonary blood pressure with the first breath.
  - The first breath is accompanied by forceful expiration against a partially closed glottis; the result is effective distribution of air in the alveoli.
  - Adequate functional residual capacity is rapidly established.
  - Initial expansion of the lungs stimulates surfactant release, which allows further lung expansion.
  - Lung expansion is responsible for an initial decrease in pulmonary hypertension.
  - Ventilation with air results in a decrease in PCO_2 and an increase in pH and PO_2 in the lungs; the result is a dramatic decrease in pulmonary vascular resistance.
- Reversal of the relative pulmonary and systemic pressures results in closure of the foramen ovale and reversal of the shunting of blood through the ductus arteriosus.
  - The increase in oxygen flowing through the ductus arteriosus stimulates closure of the ductus arteriosus.

Unsuccessful Transition

- **If more than mild asphyxia occurs, the transition may be unsuccessful.**
- Moderate to severe asphyxia may result from:
  - Maternal systemic disease (colic, endotoxemia, hypotension, general anesthesia)
  - Placental disease (placentitis, premature placental separation)
  - Fetal disease (fetal infection, cord compression)
  - Intrapartum problems (dystocia, uterine inertia, premature placental separation).
- The fetus responds to asphyxia by reinforcing the fetal circulatory pattern. The neonate responds by reverting to the fetal pattern.
  - Increased hypoxemia and acidemia can increase pulmonary vascular vasoconstriction and result in the following chain of events:
    - Decrease in pulmonary blood flow
    - Decrease in left atrial return
    - Decrease in left atrial pressure
    - Increase in right to left shunting through the foramen ovale
  - In the fetus this process may be appropriate, because this would increase the amount of well-oxygenated blood (returning from the placenta) diverted to the heart and brain.
  - In a neonate without placental function, it makes the situation worse because the blood completely bypasses the lungs.

Development of Primary and Secondary Apnea

- Early, severe asphyxia can result in stimulation of the fetus to breathe while still *in utero*.
- If the resulting gasping activity does not correct the asphyxia, this activity stops, resulting in a period known as *primary apnea*.
- Within minutes a second spell of gasping activity (more irregular) occurs.
- If this second attempt to establish normal ventilation fails, the foal enters into a period of *secondary apnea*.
  - *Secondary apnea* **is irreversible unless resuscitation is initiated.**

- Asphyxia before birth may stimulate the foal to pass though these stages *in utero.*
  - It is difficult to determine how far the asphyxia has progressed at the time of delivery.
  - Foals who do not breathe at birth should be assumed to have secondary apnea and should be treated accordingly.

Birth Resuscitation Steps

Assessment

- *Initial assessment of the neonate should begin during presentation.*
- The peripheral pulse can be rapidly evaluated when the vaginal positioning of the foal is checked.
  - Relative heart rate and strength form a basis for monitoring the expected changes during this dynamic period.
  - This assessment only takes 5-10 seconds.
  - Calculating an accurate heart rate is unnecessary and counterproductive with the rapid changes occurring.
  - The apical pulse can be assessed as soon as the chest clears the birth canal.
- Bradycardia (heart rate of 40 beats/min or less) is expected during forceful contractions during passage through the birth canal.
- Transient, marked sinus arrhythmia commonly occurs when the first breaths are taken.
- Once the chest clears the birth canal, the heart rate rapidly increases.
- **Persistent bradycardia is an indication for rapid intervention.**
- Calculating a modified Apgar score (Table 47–3).
  - Helps determine the urgency and extent of intervention needed.
  - Waiting for the traditional 1-minute and 5-minute scores is inappropriate if severe *in utero* asphyxia has occurred.

  Resuscitation should be initiated before the 1-minute score is calculated for severely compromised neonates.

Clear the Airway

- Remove the membranes from the nostrils as soon as the nose is evident.
- If meconium staining is present and the foal is not yet active

TABLE 47–3. Apgar Score Modified for the Foal

Score	0	1	2
Heart rate	Absent	<60 beats/min irregular	>60 beats/min regular
Respiratory rate	Absent	Irregular	Regular
Muscle tone	Limp, lateral	Some flexion	Active, sternal
Reflex to nasal stimulation, ear tickle	No response	Grimace, weak ear flick	Sneeze or cough, ear flick, head shake

Score 7-8 = Normal.
Score 4-6 = Mild to moderate asphyxia: Stimulate, administer intranasal oxygen, ventilate.
Score 0-3 = Severe asphyxia: Begin cardiopulmonary resuscitation.

- □ Suction the nasal passages and nasopharynx.
- □ If this is rewarding and the foal is severely asphyxiated, suction the trachea.
  - □ Meconium is very difficult to suction because of its consistency.
  - □ Avoid overzealous suctioning because it can cause bradycardia and prolonged apnea.
  - □ Because suctioning removes the air in the lung, suctioning episodes should be limited to 10-15 seconds at a time with high flows of oxygen before and after each attempt.
- □ If the foal is vigorous and responsive, suctioning attempts are not beneficial.

Tactile Stimulation

- If spontaneous respiration and movement do not begin within seconds of birth, tactile stimulation is useful.
  - □ Rub the chest and head with a dry towel.
  - □ Stimulate the ear canal or nasal canal.
  - □ Gently compress the chest wall.
- **If spontaneous breathing efforts are not stimulated, intubate and ventilate immediately.**

Respiratory Support

- Apneic foals, foals that have an irregular, gasping respiratory pattern or remain bradycardic (<60 beats/min), need respiratory support.
  - □ If spontaneous respiratory efforts are present, give free-flow intranasal oxygen at a rate of 8-10 L/min.
  - □ If no spontaneous respiration is present, intubate and hyperventilate with 100% oxygen.
    - □ If oxygen is unavailable, use room air.
    - □ If ventilatory equipment is unavailable, use mouth-to-nose ventilation.

  Hyperventilation with 100% oxygen is the most important step in birth resuscitation.
  GOAL: To reverse persistent fetal circulation by inflating the lungs, delivering high oxygen concentration, and producing respiratory alkalosis. **Ninety percent of foals requiring birth resuscitation respond when ventilated.**

  - □ With the first delivered breath, give a prolonged inspiratory phase lasting about 5 seconds to ensure lung expansion.
  - □ Give a delivered breath rate of 40-60 per minute.
  - □ Gauge the depth by chest excursions.
  - □ Consistent volumes of lung fluid should be seen escaping from the nostril during both spontaneous and delivered ventilation.
- If the asphyxia is mild and short lived, after 30 seconds of ventilation with 100% oxygen, the heart rate should be >60 beats/min and soon approach 100 beats/min.
  - □ Watch for spontaneous respiration. Once present, extubate and begin administration of free-flow intranasal oxygen.
- If the asphyxia is advanced and myocardial damage is present, bradycardia persists and cardiovascular support should be initiated.

- The more advanced the asphyxia, the longer it is until spontaneous ventilation begins.

Cardiovascular Support
- Chest compressions should begin immediately if:
  - The foal remains bradycardic despite ventilation and a nonperfusing rhythm develops.
  - There is a nonperfusing rhythm or cardiac standstill at birth.
- If a perfusing, spontaneous cardiac rhythm does not develop within 30-60 seconds of initiation of chest compressions, begin drug therapy.

Thermal Management
- Birthing areas of foals usually are cold.
- A healthy foal has little trouble handling cold environmental temperatures.
- A foal with even mild asphyxia can have difficulty with thermal control.
  - Towel dry
  - Place the foal on dry bedding
  - Provide an external heat source
    - Heat lamp
    - Hot water bottles
    - Warm-water heating pads
    - Hot air blanket
    - If the foal is depressed and remains hypothermic, move it to a warm environment.

Drug Treatment
- As in all cases of cardiopulmonary failure, epinephrine should be given early and often.
- **Epinephrine is the most useful drug to manage cardiac failure secondary to birth asphyxia.**
- Follow the guidelines for general CPR (see p. 582), **except:**
- **Atropine** *should not be used to manage bradycardia in newborns.*
- The initial bradycardia stimulated by hypoxia is vagally mediated.
- Reasons not to use atropine:
  - Atropine-mediated reversal of early hypoxic bradycardia is purely symptomatic and does not control the underlying cause (hypoxia).
  - If the heart rate increases and hypoxia is not corrected, the myocardium goes further into oxygen debt.
  - This leads to an atropine-nonresponsive bradycardia due to hypoxic myocardial damage.
  - Managing the underlying cause, hypoxia, with ventilation with 100% oxygen, chest compressions, and epinephrine reverses bradycardia as rapidly as does atropine therapy and prevents further damage.
- **Doxapram** *is not used to treat apneic newborns.*
- Doxapram stimulates respiration in primary apnea.
- In secondary apnea, the respiratory center is nonresponsive to doxapram, and the drug increases the oxygen demand of the myocardium in the face of prolonged and severe hypoxia.
- Giving doxapram wastes valuable time.

- Ventilation (even if supplemental oxygen is not available) is as effective as doxapram in reversing primary apnea and is the only effective therapy during secondary apnea.
- **At birth it is impossible to differentiate primary from secondary apnea.**
- **Fluid therapy** *during resuscitation of a newborn foal should be administered conservatively.*
- The newborn is not volume depleted, unless bleeding has occurred (e.g., cord hemorrhage, fractured rib).
- Severe *in utero* asphyxia results in larger than normal vascular volume.
  - Fetal myocardial asphyxia causes decreased cardiac output resulting in less flow to the placenta.
  - With the aid of uterine contractions, the fetus still has good venous return from the placenta.
  - The result is higher than normal vascular volume in newborns with severe prepartum asphyxia.
  - The decrease in blood pressure is from effects of asphyxia on myocardial function.
- Fluid overloading can exacerbate a failing heart.
  - High fluid rates can decrease coronary perfusion.
- Patients in hemorrhagic shock benefit from a bolus of 20 ml/kg non–glucose-containing fluid if initial resuscitation attempts are not successful.
- Once spontaneous circulation is established and the foal is adequately oxygenated, treatment with glucose-containing fluids at a rate of 4 mg glucose per kilogram per minute is indicated.
  - Helps clear metabolic acidosis
  - Supports cardiac output because myocardial glycogen stores are depleted
  - Helps prevent postasphyxia hypoglycemia

Persistent Pulmonary Hypertension

- Despite successful return of spontaneous circulation, some foals retain the fetal circulation pattern with pulmonary hypertension and right to left shunting through the foramen ovale and patent ductus arteriosus.
- These foals benefit from:
  - Mechanical ventilation with 100% oxygen
  - Maintenance of arterial blood pH above 7.45-7.50 by

  A high respiratory rate to produce respiratory alkalosis

| **CAUTION:** Do not allow the $PaCO_2$ to fall below 30 mm Hg.

  - Bicarbonate administration to produce a metabolic alkalosis
- **The most effective management of persistent pulmonary hypertension is inhalation therapy with 5-20 ppm nitric oxide.**
  - Nitrous oxide causes pulmonary vasodilatation without affecting systemic blood pressure.
  - Limited clinical experience shows nitrous oxide to be effective in foals, even at low concentrations.

Neonatal Hypoxia

- Many foals may remain hypoxemic (PaO_2, <60 mm Hg) after birth.
  - Hypoxic-ischemic encephalopathy leading to general depression

- Central respiratory center damage
- Systemic hypoxic damage leading to hypotension
- Hypoxic lung damage
- Ventilation perfusion mismatching
- Primary lung disease
- Sepsis
- These foals are generally weak.
  - Encourage them to remain sternal.
  - Turn from side to side (on the sternum) every 2 hours.
- Administer nasal insufflation of moist oxygen at a rate of 4-10 L/min.
- Monitor $PaCO_2$ by arterial blood gases every 4-6 hours.

Neonatal Hypercapnia
Many foals with peripartum asphyxia suffer from hypoxic-ischemic encephalopathy resulting in depression of central respiratory receptors. Although these foals are good candidates for transient mechanical ventilation, some respond adequately to respiratory center stimulants such as caffeine.

Caffeine
- Dose
  - Oral loading dose of 10 mg/kg
  - Oral maintenance dose of 2.5 mg/kg
  - Serum half-life of caffeine in human neonates is highly variable, making the pharmacodynamics difficult to predict.
    - Therapeutic trough serum concentrations in human neonates are between 5 and 25 µg/ml
    - Toxic reactions in human neonates occur with plasma levels greater than 40 µg/ml.
    - Limited experience in foals indicates that trough blood levels range between 4 and 10 µg/ml.
- Treated foals have an elevated level of arousal and become more reactive to environmental stimuli.
- Adverse reactions:
  - Restlessness
  - Hyperactivity
  - Tachycardia
- Caffeine therapy fails if the hypercapnia is compensation for metabolic alkalosis and the pH is not low.
- Critically ill neonatal foals commonly have electrolyte imbalances, which result in metabolic alkalosis as explained by the strong ion difference theory.
- These foals have secondary hypercapnia in an effort to counteract the alkalosis.
- Manage this physiologic response by correcting the electrolyte abnormalities and not by manipulating the respiratory system with drugs or mechanical ventilation.

Respiratory Support during Dystocia
- During prolonged dystocia, foals die of asphyxia.
- This can be prevented if the foal's nose is accessible while it is in the birth canal.
- Place an endotracheal tube.

□ Take care to assure that the tube is in the trachea.
□ Use a capnograph to:
  □ Verify endotracheal tube placement
  □ Obtain information about the effectiveness of cardiac output
- Once the airway is secured and the foal is being ventilated, much of the urgency to correct the dystocia is gone, allowing for reassessment of the situation and more time for manipulation.
- If correction of the dystocia is further delayed, and the tongue is within reach, an arterial blood gas sample from the lingual artery is used to assess the effectiveness of ventilation.
- These are collectively termed *EXIT procedures* (extrauterine intrapartum treatment).

REFERENCES

The delivery room. In Fanaroff AA, Martin RJ, editors: *Neonatal-perinatal medicine: diseases of the fetus and infant,* ed 7, sect IV, St. Louis, 2001, Mosby.

Fisher DE, Paton JB: Resuscitation of the newborn infant. In Klaus MH, Fanaroff AA, editors: *Care of the high-risk neonate,* ed 5, Philadelphia, 2001, WB Saunders.

Gregory GA: Resuscitation of the newborn. In Grenvik A et al, editors: *Textbook of critical care,* ed 4, Philadelphia, 2000, WB Saunders.

Neonatal Resuscitation: Guidelines 2000 for Cardiopulmonary Resuscitation and Emergency Cardiovascular Care, International Consensus on Science, *Circulation* 102(suppl): I-343-I-357, 2000.

Peckham GJ: Resuscitation of the newborn. In Holbrook PR, editor: *Textbook of pediatric critical care,* Philadelphia 1993, WB Saunders.

Pediatric Advanced Life Support: Guidelines 2000 for Cardiopulmonary Resuscitation and Emergency Cardiovascular Care, International Consensus on Science, *Circulation* 102(suppl):I-291-I-342, 2000.

Zaritsky AL: Pediatric resuscitation. In Grenvik A et al, editors: *Textbook of critical care,* ed 4, Philadelphia, 2000, WB Saunders.

Shock and Temperature-Related Problems

48 — Shock and Systemic Inflammatory Response Syndrome

Thomas J. Divers

Shock: *Inadequate tissue oxygenation,* most often caused by *decreased perfusion*

Septic shock: Most commonly a result of bacteremia or endotoxemia, both of which are responsible for triggering a cascade of mediators that cause the cardiopulmonary and vascular changes of shock, most commonly due to enterocolitis, metritis, pleuropneumonia, clostridial or staphylococcal infection, and neonatal septicemia.

Systemic inflammatory response syndrome (SIRS): The systemic response associated with release of vasoactive and inflammatory mediators that cause shock. Initiated by:

- Bacteremia
- Endotoxemia
- Traumatic shock
- Hemolysis
- Anaphylactoid-like reactions
- Localized infections
- Hyperthermia
- Hypothermia
- Dehydration
- Hypotension
- Any organ injury that causes hypoxia and release of vasoactive or inflammatory mediators

Multiple organ dysfunction syndrome (MODS): Septic shock or SIRS that causes dysfunction of one or more organs such that clinical consequences or signs from this organ dysfunction become apparent. The most commonly involved organs in the horse are the:

- Heart and cardiovascular system: Weak pulses, bright red congested membranes that turn a purplish color
- Renal system: Depression from azotemia and electrolyte abnormalities
- Intestinal tract: Ileus, diarrhea, colic
- Lung: Pulmonary edema

615

- Coagulation system: Most commonly thrombosis
- Feet: Laminitis

In both **septic shock** and **SIRS**, inadequate tissue perfusion and oxygenation are mostly a result of:

- Intravascular fluid volume loss
- Hypotension
- Heart failure
- Maldistribution of blood flow
- Diminished oxygenation of hemoglobin

Early in the course of septic shock and SIRS, the predominant cause of inadequate tissue perfusion-oxygenation is *maldistribution of blood flow*, frequently followed by systemic hypotension.

- *Early* maldistribution of blood flow results from:
  □ Decrease in arteriovenous tone caused by endogenous release of β catecholamines and release of mediators such as nitric oxide, cytokines, and autocoids
- *Leaky vessels*, which result from:
  □ Arachidonic acid metabolism (cyclooxygenase II): Prostanoids and leukotrienes
  □ *Macrophage* procoagulant production
  □ *Neutrophil* and platelet adherence to vessels that causes release of inflammatory mediators, oxidative enzyme activity, and activation of proteases and other damaging enzymes such as matrix metalloproteinases
  □ Release of autocoids (e.g., histamine, endorphins)
  □ Microthrombosis: Platelet aggregation, exposure of subendothelial collagen, and release of tissue factor and anaphylatoxins.

Treatment is most successful during the early stage of shock and SIRS. This is frequently called the *hyperdynamic* phase of shock and is associated with left ventricular dilation, increased heart rate, increased cardiac output (mostly due to increased heart rate), and decreased vascular resistance. The mucous membranes are generally hyperemic during this phase.

- Later stages of shock are associated with:
  □ Decreased cardiac index, including myocardial depression
  □ Diminished β_1 and α response (inappropriate vasodilation)
  □ Systemic hypotension: Often refractory to most drugs
- Further *maldistribution* of blood flow:
  □ Shunts
  □ Sludging in capillaries
  □ Further increase in vascular permeability: Capillary leak syndrome
  □ Vascular obstruction
- Diminished cellular oxygenation and increased cellular acid production
- Free radical formation and cellular death
- MODS

At this stage:

- Extremities are cold.
- Peripheral pulse is weak.
- Mucous membranes are dark.

- Capillary refill is slow (>3 seconds).
- Mentality is altered.
- Petechiation may be present.
- Urine production is diminished or absent.

As a result of severe hypoxemia, the intestinal barrier is damaged, allowing systemic absorption of normal enteric endotoxin or bacterial translocation (from the intestine to blood and other organs). Diminished hepatic phagocytosis of endotoxin and bacteria further exacerbates the systemic demise.

In the horse, damage to the circulation of the intestines, lungs, kidneys, and feet is the most life-threatening injury associated with septic shock and SIRS.

MANAGEMENT OF SEPTIC SHOCK AND SYSTEMIC INFLAMMATORY RESPONSE SYNDROME

Reestablish tissue blood flow to *above normal values without causing tissue edema!*

Volume Support

- Crystalloids: Hypertonic saline solution, balanced electrolyte fluid, or both. Hypertonic saline solution has the advantage of causing a rapid increase in cardiac output and systemic arterial pressure with a decrease in pulmonary arterial pressure and briefly diminished vascular tone.
- Administer these fluids rapidly and *ideally* while measuring systemic arterial pressure and central venous pressure (see p. 620).
- Although more expensive, the ideal fluid therapy is a combination of crystalloids and colloids. *Colloids are particularly important in treating septic shock and SIRS because of the vessel leakage that occurs and the inability of crystalloids to remain in the intravascular bed longer than 1 hour.*
- Plasma and hetastarch are administered; *plasma is preferred* because it has:
  □ *Albumin*, comparable with synthetic colloids in maintaining oncotic pressure. Although synthetic colloids have a higher molecular weight, plasma has the advantage of being negatively charged, which helps to maintain cations in the intravascular bed.
  □ *Antithrombin III*, an important inhibitor of the coagulation cascade; *40 units of heparin per kilogram body weight is added to the plasma at least 10 minutes before administration.*
  □ Fibronectin enhances opsonization of endotoxin and prevents bacterial translocation.
  □ Proteins C and S serve to inactivate clotting factors and enhance fibrinolysis.
  □ α_2 Macroglobulin inhibits proteases.
  □ Antibodies against lipopolysaccharide or cytokines are of some benefit but are not as important as the other plasma factors in managing septic shock and SIRS.
- Hetastarch, 2-10 ml/kg, can be used immediately while plasma is thawing.

Pump Support

If fluid therapy alone is unsuccessful in supporting normal blood pressure, cardiac output, and perfusion, or when central venous pressure increases, use β_1-agonist therapy. **This agent should be used only if there is adequate preload. It is harmful to increase the rate of a less than full heart!**

- Dobutamine*: 2-15 μg/kg per minute diluted in saline solution, for β_1 activity
- Dopamine*: 2-15 μg/kg per minute diluted in saline solution; *low dose* stimulates renal dopaminergic receptors and increases renal blood flow; *middle dose* also stimulates β_1 receptors; *high dose* causes β_1 and α stimulation, which decreases renal perfusion.
- *One of the best general indicators of successful perfusion of most organs is the production of a large volume of urine.* If fluid therapy and β_1-agonist therapy are unsuccessful in urine production, administer norepinephrine (β and α agonist), 0.5-1.5 μg/kg per minute or vasopress in 0.25-1.0 μg/kg per minute.

Oxygen Therapy

- **Adequate** oxygen: Normal or *above normal.*
- Hemoglobin level: Maintain within normal range
  - Too low (<3-7 g/dl) indicates need for transfusion.
  - Too high (variable) indicates need for additional fluids.
- For most patients, insert an intranasal tube to administer humidified oxygen.
- For a septic foal in septic condition with respiratory distress, administer positive pressure ventilation with 50% or more oxygen concentration.
- For persistent hypoxemia and probable pulmonary arterial hypertension, nitric oxide may be mixed in the oxygen line at a 1:5-1:9 ratio.

NOTE: PaO_2 must be maintained at more than 70 mm Hg (PvO_2, >35 mm Hg; SvO_2, >50%; lactate, <4 mmol/L).

Antimicrobial Support

Broad-spectrum coverage for Gram-positive and Gram-negative aerobes and anaerobes (e.g., ticarcillin–clavulanic acid, with or without amikacin or penicillin, and amikacin or a third-generation cephalosporin with or without amikacin or imipenem).

Surgical Treatment

- Establish drainage, resect, and debride necrotic tissue.

Prostanoid Inhibitors

- Flunixin meglumine, 0.25 mg/kg q8h
- Aspirin is reported not to inhibit in vitro endotoxin-stimulated coagulation

Endotoxin Inhibitors

- Hyperimmune plasma, 2-4 ml/kg IV: The antibodies against the core lipopolysaccharide may be of some benefit and other constituents of the plasma of more certain value.

---

*Systolic blood pressure must be maintained at more than 70 mm Hg in adult horses. Variable depending on blood volume and tissue oxygen uptake.

SHOCK

- Polymyxin B, 1000-6000 units/kg IV over at least 15 minutes; can be repeated two or three times over 36 hours in *nonazotemic patients* and *individuals with adequate urine production*. Polymixin may neutralize some circulating endotoxin; unfortunately, the cytokine cascade is established before treatment is begun in most patients. Although it is a very popular (in vogue) treatment of horses, polymyxin B may be of little benefit unless pretreatment can be performed, has some risk (renal toxicity and neuromuscular weakness), and is rarely used in human medicine although laboratory experiments have been performed for more than 30 years.

Additional Therapy

- Steroids, 0.25 mg/kg dexamethasone: Most studies show little value; inhibits arachidonic acid metabolism and therefore is commonly used.
- Pentoxifylline, 8.4 mg/kg PO or IV q12h: Commonly used to inhibit platelet aggregation and cytokines; improves deformability of red blood cells.
- Oxygen free radical inhibitors:
  - Dimethyl sulfoxide (DMSO): Commonly used and of questionable benefit
  - Vitamin E
  - Allopurinol: Little indication for use in the horse
  - Carolina rinse: Contains several antioxidants and cell protectants and has been used experimentally in abdominal surgery; not commercially available
  - Antihistamines: Rarely used in the management of shock and unlikely beneficial once clinical signs are present
  - Furosemide: Used to decrease pulmonary arterial wedge pressure (pulmonary edema) but can cause systemic vasodilation and decreased cardiac output
  - Oral glutamine: Oral fluids with essential amino acids, including glutamine, are provided when the gastrointestinal tract is functional to support enterocyte function and to decrease endotoxin absorption and bacterial translocation
  - Sodium bicarbonate: Used only when blood pH <7.2. Controversial. Do not use with respiratory acidosis (increased $PaCO_2$, hypocalcemia, or hypokalemia).
  - Nitroglycerine: Used topically, as in coronary band digital artery, if blood pressure has returned to normal and hypoperfusion of the feet is suspected. Vasodilation can cause hypotension.
  - Magnesium sulfate ($MgSO_4$), 0.1-0.2 g/kg IV over 24 hours: May have some cellular protective effects.
  - Additional therapy for persistent hypotension when fluids or pump drugs have been unsuccessful is methylene blue, 0.5-2.0 mg/kg, to inhibit nitrous oxide; naloxone, 0.02 mg/kg, an opioid antagonist; 50% glucose (1 g/kg with insulin [0.5 IU/kg per hour]) plus potassium chloride, 40 mEq/L; oxyglobin, 10 ml/kg; or a combination of these agents.
  - Granulocyte colony-stimulating factor, 10 μg/kg IV q24h, has been given to some foals with severe neutropenic and septic shock and SIRS. There is generally a response (increased granulocyte count) except in herpes infection, although the benefit in survival is doubtful.
  - Oxyglobulin—to improve perfusion and oxygenation.

MONITORING DURING TREATMENT OF SEPTIC SHOCK AND SYSTEMIC INFLAMMATORY RESPONSE SYNDROME

- Heart rate
- Cardiac contractility: M mode may be used to roughly estimate this value. Contractility should be 30%-50%.

- Arterial pressure: Tail cuff or subjective digital pulse pressure. An arterial line can be established for recumbent foals (mean arterial pressure should be >70 mm Hg, ideally 120-130 mm Hg systolic).* The accuracy of the indirect monitoring of blood pressure using oscillometric measurements can vary depending on:
  - The bladder cuff width-to-tail circumference ratio (No ideal ratio is known; however, 0.33:0.55 is recommended.)
  - Anesthetized vs. nonanesthetized
  - The positional location of the cuff in relation to the level of the base of the heart
  - The standing patient's head position
- At best, the indirect measurement gives an acceptable mean pressure and an indication of trends when performed intermittently in the identical manner and on the same patient. An accurate heart rate on the monitor should be displayed when blood pressure measurements are computed.
- Plasma protein: 4.2 g/dl to maintain oncotic pressure and prevent edema formation. If, oncotic pressure should remain >18 mm Hg in adults and >15 mm Hg in foals.
- Packed cell volume: 30%-45%
- PaO_2: >100 mm Hg. In recumbent foals, pulse oximetry can be used on the tongue for frequent measurement of oxygen saturation. Saturation of ≥97% is assurance that PaO_2 is ≥70 mm Hg and can be used to reduce the number of arterial blood gas measurements needed.
- PvO_2: >40 mm Hg. Lower values indicate abnormal oxygen delivery or increased oxygen extraction.
- SvO_2: Saturation >50%.
- Central venous pressure: 5-15 cm water. Too low is an indication for increased fluid rate; too high is an indication for decreased fluid rate, pump therapy, and therapy for renal failure.
- Blood pH: Determine metabolic or respiratory component and treat accordingly.
- ▶ Anion gap: To detect increased unmeasured anions (*if plasma protein level has decreased, lactate may be high with a normal anion gap!*) and treat appropriately. Most commonly, increased numbers of unmeasured anions are associated with lactic acidosis or renal failure and metabolic acidosis. Blood lactate value can be measured with an I-Stat and should be <2 mmol/L.
- *Urine production: Should be normal or increased after administration of intravenous fluids has started.*
- Electrocardiogram: Control arrhythmia (see p. 134).
- Platelet count, neutrophil count, and neutrophil morphology: Prognostic and therapeutic indicators
- Mucous membrane color: Indicates perfusion quality and tissue oxygenation at that site

REFERENCES

Mario PL: *The ICU Book,* ed 2, Baltimore, 1998, Williams & Wilkins.
Shoemaker WC et al, editors: *Textbook of critical care,* ed 4, Philadelphia, 2000, WB Saunders.

---

*In foals mean arterial pressure >60 mm Hg may be acceptable.

49 Temperature-Related Problems

Thomas J. Divers

HEAT STROKE

Usually occurs in poorly conditioned horses that are overworked in hot and humid climates. However, it can occur in individuals confined to poorly ventilated areas during hot and humid weather; this especially is a problem during transportation. Heat stroke also infrequently occurs among foals treated with erythromycin.

Diagnosis

Early diagnosis is important for effective treatment. The diagnosis is based on the history and clinical signs. Heat stroke can trigger a systemic inflammatory response, disseminated intravascular coagulation, renal failure, and other forms of organ dysfunction.

Clinical Signs

- Poor sweating response
  □ Hot, dry skin signals the early onset of heat stroke.
- Tachycardia with or without arrhythmia
- Tachypnea
- Elevated rectal temperature (41°C-43°C [106°F-110°F])
- Prolonged capillary refill time, muddy mucous membranes
- Depression
  □ May progress to coma and death
- Weakness
  □ May progress to collapse or ataxia
- Decreased appetite, refusal to work, ileus

Treatment

- Decrease the body temperature:
  □ The more rapid the cooling, the better is the prognosis.
  □ Move the affected horse to a shaded, well-ventilated area (use fans if available).
  □ Apply cold water hydrotherapy (approximately 6°C [42.8°F]) to entire body. Use alcohol baths over the neck, thorax, and abdomen if cold water is not available. Do not use wet towels because the towel cover prevents convection.
  □ Antipyretic: Flunixin meglumine (Banamine), which also is useful for its antiendotoxin effect. **Many exhausted horses may have endotoxemia!**
- Restore blood volume.
  □ Use any (crystalloid) fluid, but 0.9% saline solution *with potassium chloride (KCl), 20-40 mEq/L,* is recommended. Fluids should be 16°C-21°C [60°F-70°F](see p. 623).
  □ Use hypertonic saline solution if the heart rate is very rapid and the capillary refill time is prolonged (≥5 seconds).
- Administer 2 L of hyperimmune plasma (antibodies against endotoxin) for more severe cases.

ANHYDROSIS

Anhydrosis usually affects exercising athletes. It also occurs among stabled horses subjected to hot and humid environments for long periods of time. The condition represents an *inability to sweat* in response to normal stimuli. The problem can develop acutely but generally develops gradually. A form of anhydrosis occurs among young, healthy foals with persistent tachypnea.

Diagnosis

CLINICAL SIGNS

- Failure to sweat with appropriate stimuli (heat, exercise).

NOTE: Some horses have patches of sweating under the mane or in the pectoral or perineal regions.

- Tachypnea (some pant), decreased exercise tolerance, rectal temperature higher than normal after exercise (>40°C [104°F])
- Respiratory rate higher than heart rate.

LESS COMMON CLINICAL SIGNS

- Depression, anorexia, weight loss, alopecia

EPINEPHRINE OR TERBUTALINE CHALLENGE

- 1:1000 and 1:10,000 epinephrine, 0.1 ml intradermally, both concentrations. Affected individuals have little or no response (local sweating) within 1 hour.

NOTE: Intravenous epinephrine exacerbates the problem and should be avoided.

- Terbutaline, 0.5 mg intradermal injection, also can be used.

Treatment

- Antipyretic agent, such as flunixin meglumine; cold water hydrotherapy; and shade, with a fan if possible.
- The only proven prevention is to move the affected horse to a more temperate climate.
- Provide electrolyte supplementation to all horses exercising in hot weather (One AC, an electrolyte supplement, can be obtained from MPCO, Phoenix, AZ).
- Clip body hair: Useful in the care of otherwise healthy foals with persistent tachypnea.

EXHAUSTIVE DISEASE SYNDROME

Multisystemic changes occur in horses subjected to either brief maximal- or longer submaximal-intensity exercise, especially during hot and humid weather. Problems develop in association with fluid and electrolyte losses, acid-base changes associated with exercise, and depletion of the body's energy stores.

Diagnosis

- Tachypnea* (>40 breaths/min after a 30-minute rest)
- Tachycardia* (>60 beats/min after a 30-minute rest)

---

*May see a transient inversion; respiratory rate may be higher than heart rate. This is more common in humid environments.

- Elevated rectal temperature (40°C-41°C [104°F-106°F])
- Dehydration (may have fluid deficits of 20-40 L) and a lack of interest in water or food, despite the severe dehydration are common findings. Fluid losses of 6%-10% of body weight in endurance athletes can lead to heat exhaustion.
- Severe depression, decreased pulse pressure, decreased jugular distention, prolonged capillary refill time
- *Continued sweating* at reduced rate
- Cardiac irregularities (e.g., ventricular tachycardia)
- Muscle cramps or spasms and/or myopathy
- Decreased or absent intestinal sounds, unless spasmodic colic develops
- Lack of anal tone
- Synchronous diaphragmatic flutter, often associated with ileus
- Central nervous system signs
- Loss of >7% body weight

Laboratory Findings

- Hypochloremia, hyponatremia, abnormally low ionized calcium value, azotemia, high packed cell volume, increased muscle and liver enzyme values, increased lactate result.
- Variable bicarbonate concentration: Normal or high with milder cases, low with severe cases.

Treatment

- Decrease body temperature.
  - Move the patient to a shaded, well-ventilated area.
  - Apply cold water hydrotherapy frequently to entire body.
- *Fluid therapy* goal for exhausted patients is to replace volume, correct electrolyte abnormalities, and provide a source of calories. To expedite rapid rehydration, use two catheters.
  - Lactated Ringer's solution and KCl, 20 mEq/L 10-20 L/h, in more severe cases with suspected acidemia.
  - 0.9% saline solution and KCl, 20 mEq/L 10-20 L/h, in less severe cases without acidemia.
  - *With* 5% dextrose, 2 L/h.

If urination does not occur after several liters of fluids have been administered, discontinue KCl. If urination is normal, KCl can be increased to 40 mEq/L.

- **Hypertonic saline solution should not be used to treat exhausted endurance horses because these individuals may have marked deficits of intracellular fluids.**
- If synchronous diaphragmatic flutter or intestinal atony is found at physical examination, administer 100-300 ml of 20% calcium borogluconate IV *slowly* over 30 minutes. *Discontinue administration if cardiac irregularities develop or worsen.*
- If evidence of organ failure or severe metabolic acidosis (pH <7.1) is seen, administer bicarbonate solution.

NOTE: *Bicarbonate is contraindicated if synchronous diaphragmatic flutter is present and is not routinely used in the care of exhausted horses.*

- Administer oral fluids as long as there is no intestinal dysfunction: 5-8 L of electrolyte solution q30min as needed.
- Electrolyte solution:

- ▫ 2 tbsp (37 g) sodium chloride
- ▫ 1 tbsp (18 g) KCl (Morton's Lite salt)
- ▫ 1 L water
- ▫ Amino acids, such as glutamine
- Discontinue if discomfort or gastric reflux develops.
- Do not use phenothiazine tranquilizers. These patients are at high risk of cardiovascular collapse and death.
- Flunixin meglumine, 1 mg/kg IV initially then 0.3 mg/kg q8h
- Administration of nonsteroidal antiinflammatory drugs without appropriate fluid replacement is not recommended.
- Hyperimmune plasma with antibodies against endotoxin, 2 L (exhausted athletes are at increased risk of endotoxemia).
- Antioxidants: Vitamin E, 7000 U PO per adult

Prognosis

Generally good if appropriate therapy is instituted early. However, multisystemic complications develop in some patients 2-4 days after an episode of exhaustion. These manifestations include:

- Myopathy
- Rapidly progressive laminitis
- Renal dysfunction
- Gastrointestinal ulceration
- Elevation in values of liver-derived enzymes and bilirubin

FROSTBITE

Rare among horses but can occur in debilitated patients or foals exposed to extreme cold.

Diagnosis

- Cold extremity with color change: White to deep purple (may be warm and red if recirculation has started).

Treatment

- Rewarm extremity.
  - ▫ Move affected individual to a heated area or at least out of the wind.
  - ▫ Apply warm, damp towels. Avoid rubbing, which damages frozen cells.
- Restore dermal microcirculation.
  - ▫ Antiprostaglandin: Flunixin meglumine IV
  - ▫ Pentoxifylline, 8.4 mg/kg PO q12h
  - ▫ Vasodilator: Acepromazine
  - ▫ Platelet aggregation inhibitor: Aspirin
- Local treatment:
  - ▫ Topical aloe vera gel three to four times per day
  - ▫ Nitroglycerin ointment (2%) is applied to small areas that are most severely affected. *Caution: this may worsen any systemic hypotension.*

| **NOTE:** Wear gloves when handling ointment.

- Antimicrobial agents if necrosis is expected
- Fluid therapy
  - Warm crystalloids and colloids. If plasma is used, add heparin 40 IU/kg to the plasma before administration, to activate antithrombin III.

Prognosis
Influencing factors:

- Time of exposure
- Temperature
- Wind chill
- Moisture on skin
- Circulatory status of patient
- Effectiveness of treatment

Some patients slough skin or hooves in the affected limbs, whereas others have no additional signs once the limb is rewarmed. Edema and failure to rewarm usually are poor prognostic indicators for the limb.

In cases of septicemia, especially in foals, a similar syndrome is caused by arterial thrombosis. It is believed due to compromised circulation; septicemic foals are at increased risk for frostbite than are other horses.

HEAT

P A R T
3

Laboratory Tests

50 | Emergency Measurement of Complete Blood Cell Count, Serum Chemistry Values, Blood Gases, and Body Fluids in Equine Practice

Thomas J. Divers and Fairfield T. Bain

POINT-OF-CARE EQUIPMENT

Complete blood cell count (CBC), blood chemistries, and blood gas analysis can be an important and, in some cases, an essential part of evaluating the emergency or critical care equine patient. Clinicians traditionally rely on and send blood samples to a dedicated clinical pathology laboratory for testing. There have been significant advances in the last 5 years, such that many diagnostic tests can be performed using portable, point-of-care equipment. More than half of laboratory blood tests performed on intensive care unit (ICU) and emergency equine patients at university hospitals are now performed using point-of-care equipment.

Advantages
- Immediate access, if cartridges are at room temperature*
- User-friendly equipment
- Small amounts of blood needed (often only 1-3 drops)
- Results within 30 seconds to 5 minutes

Disadvantages
- Quality control. This has periodically been a problem with some lot numbers of cartridges.
- Some values are consistently incorrect. With the i-STAT portable clinical analyzer, this has been a regular problem with only the hematocrit (Hct).
- Tests must be conducted at temperatures of approximately 18°C-30°C (64°F-86°F).

BLOOD GASES AND BLOOD CHEMISTRIES

Several portable, point-of-care analyzers are available.

i-STAT Portable Clinical Analyzer

The i-STAT is marketed by Heska ([800] 464-3752; www.heska.com). This system has been extensively used during the past several years with accurate and uniform results except for Hct, which is falsely low. Hct and plasma protein are best

---

*Store boxes of cartridges in the refrigerator, where the shelf life is 1-2 years. Most cartridges must be kept at room temperature for 4 hours before use. Therefore keep one or two of each test set at room temperature, if the shelf life is only 2 weeks.

measured with a microhematocrit centrifuge and a refractometer. A variety of cartridges are available for the i-STAT (approximate cost, $5-$10 each). The most useful test kits are:

- i-STAT 7$^+$: K$^+$, Na$^+$, intracellular Ca^{2+}, pH, PCO$_2$, PO$_2$, TCO$_2$, HCO$_3^-$, base excess (BE), SaO$_2$
- i-STAT 8$^+$: K$^+$, Na$^+$, Cl$^-$, pH, PCO$_2$, blood urea nitrogen (BUN), glucose, TCO$_2$, HCO$_3^-$, BE, anion gap
- i-STAT 4$^+$: pH, PCO$_2$, PO$_2$, lactate, HCO$_3^-$, TCO$_2$, SaO$_2$, BE
- i-STAT Crea: Creatinine

Blood is collected in heparinized syringes for measurement of blood gases and in a heparinized syringe or heparin tube for chemistry analysis. Results are displayed on the handheld machine within 1-3 minutes with printing and/or storage capability.

IRMA

Another popular point-of-care machine is the Immediate Response Mobile Analysis (IRMA), marketed by Philips Medical Systems (www3.medical.philips.com). The IRMA instrument is larger than the i-STAT, is portable, and operates similarly to the i-STAT.

Palm Lab

This instrument can be used to measure albumin, aspartate aminotransferase (AST), BUN, total Ca^{2+}, creatine kinase (CK), creatinine, γ-glutamyl transferase (GGT), glucose, Mg^{2+}, P$^+$, K$^+$, total bilirubin, immunoglobulin G (IgG), and fibrinogen for approximately $1-$7 per individual test. There also are panels (presurgical, kidney, liver [e.g., AST, GGT, CK]) that can be obtained for $3.50-$5.50 per panel. Unlike the tests performed with i-STAT and IRMA, tests performed with the Palm Lab* may require the addition of time reagents, and results are available in 5-15 minutes. **The Palm Lab can be used to test foal IgG.**

COMPLETE BLOOD COUNT

There are automated systems for determining *equine* total white blood cell count and differentials, red cell count and indices, and platelet count. One instrument is the Vet ABC-Diff Hematology Analyzer, marketed by Heska. This instrument requires only a 12-μl sample volume, and results are available in minutes. Differentials on fluid or identification of immature neutrophils, toxic neutrophils, *anaplasma Phagocytophilia* (see Color Plates 11 and 12) or neoplastic cells must be identified by microscopic examination. The diff-quick stain is the best method of staining cells for examination.

GLUCOSE

Glucose is rapidly measured with one of several stallside kits (glucometers). Assure Chromed Inc. ([800] 818-8877; www.chronimed.com) and Accu-Chek

---

*Palm Lab, Inc., Box 237, Newburg, WI 53060; (877) 725-6522; www.palmlab.com.

LAB TESTS

(Boehringer Mannheim Corp.; www.boehringer-mannheim.com) are two instruments recommended. Glucose can also be measured with the i-STAT.

URINALYSIS

Multistix, Bayer Corp., is used to identify leukocytes, protein (may have falsely elevated readings in some horses), pH, blood (hemoglobin or myoglobin), bilirubin, and glucose. A refractometer is used to determine specific gravity.

BLOOD GAS INTERPRETATION
Acidemia

Acid-Base Disorder	Primary Change	Compensatory Change
Respiratory acidosis, PCO_2 >46 mm Hg	↑PCO_2	↑HCO_3^-
Respiratory alkalosis, PCO_2 <36 mm Hg	↓PCO_2	↓HCO_3^-
Metabolic acidosis, HCO_3^- <22 Meq/L	↓HCO_3^-	↓PCO_2
Metabolic alkalosis, HCO_3^- >28 Meq/L	↑HCO_3^-	↑PCO_2

Respiratory Compensation for Metabolic Acid-Base Disturbances
- Prompt
- Often dramatic changes in PCO_2

Metabolic Compensation for Respiratory Acid-Base Disorders
- Hours to days.
- Dramatic changes in HCO_3^- not likely.
- A primary disorder (look at pH) with proper compensation has HCO_3^- and PCO_2 both changing in the same direction. The pH does not fully return to normal and may or may not be restored to a normal range.
- HCO_3^- and PCO_2 values moving in opposite directions is suggestive of a primary metabolic and respiratory disturbance.

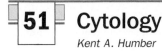

51 Cytology

Kent A. Humber

Cytologic evaluation provides useful information rapidly.

- Results are not always clear-cut.
  - □ Samples may not provide enough information for a diagnosis.
  - □ Biopsy and histopathologic examination may be needed for definitive diagnosis.
- Proficiency requires practice.
  - □ Duplicate slides can be kept and compared with the description and interpretation from the cytopathologist.

MANAGEMENT OF CYTOLOGIC SPECIMENS

- Interpretation of specimen is limited by the quality of the sample.
- Maximizing the probability of obtaining diagnostic information depends on interrelated procedures:
  - □ Obtaining the specimen
  - □ Preparation of the glass slides
  - □ Staining
  - □ Microscopic evaluation and interpretation

Obtaining the Specimen

Techniques for collection of peritoneal, thoracic, and synovial fluids, bronchoalveolar lavage (BAL), transtracheal wash (TTW), and cerebrospinal fluid (CSF) are discussed elsewhere (see Part 1, Procedures).

Preparation of Glass Slides

- Prepare as soon as practical after collection because cells are alive and continue to perform inherent "duties":
  - □ Neutrophils phagocytize contaminant bacteria, simulating a septic condition.
  - □ Macrophages phagocytize red blood cells, simulating previous hemorrhage.
- Use new, precleaned glass slides: Do not wash slides and reuse.
  - □ Residues alter cellular morphology and staining characteristics.

Staining

- Most common stains are the Romanowsky type (combinations of basic and acidic stains dissolved in methyl alcohol). Examples include Wright's stain, Giemsa Stain, and "quick" polychromatic stains.
- Polychromatic stains (e.g., Diff-Quik, Dip Stat, STAT III) are widely used in veterinary practice.
  - □ These stains do not undergo a metachromatic reaction, therefore some mast cell granules do not stain. The resulting misclassification of mast cells as macrophages leads to possible misdiagnosis of mast cell tumor.

LAB TESTS

631

- Follow the staining protocols recommended by the manufacturer, but make adaptations depending on the sample:
  - Thin smears and samples with lower total protein content require less time in the stain.
  - Thick smears and samples with higher protein content require more time in the stain.
- Slides can be restained if staining is insufficient in either the eosinophilic or basophilic tinctorial properties (omit the fixation step and immerse in the staining vat needed to correct the deficiency).
- These stains deteriorate with time and use.
  - A gradual decrease in staining quality indicates the need to replace the stain.
- The stains support bacterial and fungal growth; consistent presence of microorganisms indicates the need to change the stains rather than true septic conditions.
- Bacterial and fungal elements stain in a basophilic manner in Romanowsky-type stains. The shape and morphology of the bacteria are discernible, but Gram stain is necessary for further classification.
- New methylene blue stain is a basic dye taken up readily by nuclei, nucleoli, and mast cells. Eosinophil granules do not take up the dye. Erythrocytes do not stain and look like clear or pale blue circular areas.

Keys to Staining

- Follow staining protocols recommended by the manufacturer.
- Thin smears require less time in the stain.
- Thick smears require more time in the stain.
- Restain slides as needed to enhance tinctorial properties.
- Replace stain if deteriorated or contaminated with bacterial or fungal organisms.

Microscopic Evaluation

- Allow slide to dry in near-vertical position after staining.
- Remove the film of stain on the back (bottom) of the slide with an alcohol-moistened gauze sponge.
- Scan the smear with a 4×-10× objective to evaluate staining quality and look for localized areas of increased cellularity or unique staining features.
- Look for large objects such as crystals, foreign bodies, parasites, and fungal hyphae.
- Perform a detailed evaluation using oil-immersion objectives (50×-100×) to study nuclear and cytoplasmic morphology, the presence of cellular inclusions, and the presence and characteristics of microorganisms.

Keys to Microscopic Evaluation

- Scan smear using a 4×-10× objective.
- Perform a detailed evaluation using 50×-100× (oil immersion).

Interpretation

- A definitive diagnosis may not always be obtained; however, the general disease process (inflammation or neoplasia) is recognized quickly if a logical, methodical approach is used.
- A definitive diagnosis is not always necessary for immediate management of a case; preliminary findings may be used to direct further diagnostic efforts as well as initial therapeutic regimens.

► *Keys to Interpretation*

- Evaluate sample to identify the presence of a neoplastic versus an inflammatory process.
- The presence of inflammation does not exclude the presence of concurrent neoplasia.

INFLAMMATION

- For equine patients, most emergency cytologic evaluations are approached with the goal of identifying or ruling out an inflammatory process and, if an inflammatory process exists, identifying a causative microorganism.
- Inflammation may accompany neoplastic processes; the presence of inflammation does not exclude the concurrent presence of neoplasia.
- Inflammation can cause morphologic changes in cell populations that mimic neoplasia, and it may not be possible to rule out the presence of neoplasia before the inflammation is controlled with antimicrobial or antiinflammatory agents.
- Inflammation is identified by the presence of increased numbers of inflammatory cells:
  - Neutrophils
  - Eosinophils
  - Lymphocytes
  - Plasma cells
  - Macrophages
  - Giant cells
  - Mast cells (rare in horses)
  - Basophils (rare in horses)
- Inflammation is classified by terms implying the *duration* or the *type* of inflammation:

DURATION

- *Acute:* Neutrophils >70% of inflammatory cells
- *Subacute or chronic active:* 50%-70% neutrophils, 30%-50% macrophages
- *Chronic:* >50% macrophages

TYPE OF INFLAMMATION

- *Suppurative:* Neutrophils >85% of inflammatory cells
  - Septic or purulent: Presence of intracellular bacteria
- *Mononuclear:* Predominantly mononuclear cells without a significant suppurative component
- *Granulomatous:* Numerous epithelioid macrophages or giant cells
- *Eosinophilic:* Numerous eosinophils
- Inflammatory processes are not always "pure":
  - *Pyogranulomatous:* Suppurative or purulent process accompanied by granulomatous inflammation

► *Keys to Inflammation*

- *Acute:* >70% neutrophils
- *Subacute or chronic active:* 50%-70% neutrophils, 30%-50% macrophages
- *Chronic:* >50% macrophages
- *Suppurative:* >85% neutrophils
- *Septic (purulent):* Presence of intracellular bacteria

LAB TESTS

- *Mononuclear:* Predominantly mononuclear cells
- *Granulomatous:* Epithelioid macrophages or giant cells
- *Eosinophilic:* Eosinophils
- *Pyogranulomatous:* Suppurative or purulent accompanied by granulomatous inflammation

Submission of Cytologic Preparations and Samples for Interpretation

- Provide adequate history!
  - □ A cytopathologist who has a thorough understanding of the case is better able to provide meaningful information.
- Ascertain from the laboratory before submission the procedures for sample handling, fixation, number of slides required, packing, and shipping methods to maximize the likelihood of yielding useful information.
  - □ Generally, submit two to three air-dried, unfixed, unstained smears, along with two to three Romanowsky-stained smears (some tissues stain poorly when staining is delayed after preparation of the slides).
  - □ Submitting unstained smears allows cytopathologists to stain the slides with their preferred stain and provides slides for special stains.
  - □ Shattering of improperly packed slides during transport slows the diagnostic process or makes diagnosis impossible.
  - □ Simple cardboard mailers do not provide sufficient protection to prevent slide breakage if mailed in unpadded envelopes. Use bubble wrap, Styrofoam, or plastic slide holders.
  - □ Mark slides with the name of the client, date collected, and sample site. Pencil works well on the frosted area of slides. Use alcohol-resistant ink or another permanent labeling method on slides without frosted areas. Porous tape and adhesive labels are not adequate; they often are unreadable after staining.
  - □ Do not send slides in the same package as formalin-containing samples or in mailers previously used to ship formalin-containing samples.
  - □ Formalin vapors alter staining characteristics of cells and may make the slides unreadable.
  - □ Protect slides against moisture, which can cause cell lysis.
- Submit fluid samples in combination with glass slide smears prepared immediately after collection.
  - □ If the sample is low in cellularity, make direct smears as well as smears of concentrates of the sample in a manner similar to that used in preparing urine sediment.
  - □ Centrifuge the sample in a conical tube, discard the supernatant, and make a smear from the resuspended pellet. This preparation cannot be used to estimate nucleated cell count.
- Submit fluid samples in EDTA (lavender top) tubes to prevent clot formation. Also submit a sterile serum (red top) tube for possible microbiologic culture and sensitivity. If prolonged transit of a sample is anticipated, use a microbiologic transport system because bacterial growth eventually can occur in "sterile" red-topped tubes.

➤ Keys to Sample Submission

- Provide an adequate history!
- Verify with the laboratory the protocol for sample submission.
- Do not send slides in the same package as formalin-containing samples.
- Submit fluid samples in both EDTA (lavender top) and serum (red top) tubes.

PERITONEAL FLUID

- Normal peritoneal fluid is essentially a dialysate of plasma:
  - Low volume, cellularity, and total protein
  - Biochemical constituents are present in concentrations similar to those of plasma.
- Low-molecular-weight substances (e.g., glucose and urea) diffuse easily across the mesothelium and equilibrate quickly among plasma, interstitial fluid, and peritoneal fluid.
- High-molecular-weight substances (e.g., creatinine and most enzymes) are less readily diffusible and take more time for equilibration. Plasma proteins (very high-molecular-weight substances) are primarily limited to the vascular compartment.
- Normal peritoneal fluid contains a negligible amount of fibrinogen and therefore does not clot. Blood contamination, hemorrhage, or protein exudation is accompanied by increased fibrinogen content, and the sample may subsequently clot. Collect peritoneal fluid in an EDTA (lavender top) tube for cell count, total protein determination, and cytologic evaluation.

Cell Count and Cytologic Examination

Nucleated cell counts are performed in a manner similar to that used for blood: manual dilution with microscopic enumeration or automated cell counter.

- Normal cell count is fewer than 5000 nucleated cells per microliter.
- A nucleated cell count more than 10,000/μl is abnormal.
- Interpretation of cell counts of 5000-10,000 nucleated cells per microliter is not always clear-cut.
- Normal peritoneal fluid contains very few erythrocytes and negligible erythrophagocytosis (ingestion of erythrocytes by phagocytic cells).
- Normal leukocytes are present in peritoneal fluid (see Color Plate 13)
  - Neutrophils compose as much as 70% of the nucleated cell population, making fluid appear inflammatory to an inexperienced cytologist.
  - Large mononuclear cells and macrophages compose as much as 50% of the population. This group of cells includes nonreactive tissue macrophages of blood monocyte origin, activated macrophages, and mesothelial cells. The cells often are difficult to differentiate on the basis of morphologic features and are consequently grouped together and called *mononuclear phagocytes*.
  - Lymphocytes are present in small numbers. They have the same morphologic characteristics as lymphocytes found in blood. These cells recirculate into the bloodstream through the lymphatic lacunae in the diaphragm. Lymphoblasts are not present in normal peritoneal fluid, and their presence indicates the presence of neoplasia (lymphosarcoma).
  - Eosinophils: The presence of more than a rare eosinophil suggests the presence of parasites. Use further diagnostic procedures to rule out parasitic infection.
- Assessment of neutrophil morphology is very important in the cytologic evaluation of most samples, including peritoneal fluid. Neutrophils entering body cavities or tissues do not return to the bloodstream; therefore aging and cell death are normal events. These cells often are hypersegmented or display pyknosis, indicating senescent changes. Leukocytophagy (ingestion of leukocytes by phagocytic cells) may be detected.

LAB TESTS

▫ Bacterial cytotoxins damage inflammatory cells rapidly in vivo, particularly neutrophils. This acute cell injury causes cellular disruption and nuclear degeneration.

▫ Nuclear degeneration: Swollen, pale-staining nuclei (karyolysis), which may fragment (karyorrhexis)

▫ Karyolysis suggests the presence of sepsis; examine the smear carefully for the presence of microorganisms.

▫ When bacteria are present in peritoneal fluid, the prognosis is generally better with lower numbers of organisms that are highly phagocytized.

▫ When all bacteria have an identical morphology, it generally indicates abdominal abscessation (e.g., with *Streptococcus* organisms) and not intestinal leakage.

Interpretation of Peritoneal Fluid

NORMAL PERITONEAL FLUID

- Normal cell count is fewer than 5000 nucleated cells per microliter.
- Few erythrocytes and negligible erythrophagocytosis
- Neutrophils up to 70% of nucleated cell population
- Large mononuclear cells and macrophages up to 50% of nucleated cell population
- Small numbers of lymphocytes
- Rare eosinophils

ENTEROCENTESIS

- Accidental puncture of the intestine during abdominocentesis causes an inflammatory response in the peritoneal cavity but is usually without overt clinical signs or deleterious sequelae.
- The sample generally contains intestinal content and has a greenish-brown turbid appearance and a characteristic fermentative odor.
- Cytologic examination may show a population of relatively normal-appearing cells with large numbers of a mixed population of extracellular bacteria (cocci and rods) or very few nucleated cells with the bacterial population. The presence of cells is dictated by whether a volume of peritoneal fluid is obtained before enterocentesis and whether the viscus is entered immediately so that only gastrointestinal (GI) content is sampled.
  ▫ Protozoal organisms and plant material may be present, depending on the area of the GI tract entered.
  ▫ In cases in which only very few nucleated cells are present, consider the clinical findings to determine whether the sample is representative of enterocentesis or GI rupture.

GASTROINTESTINAL RUPTURE

- The site of rupture along the GI tract often influences the character of the fluid obtained at abdominocentesis (see Color Plate 14).
  ▫ Gastric and large-intestinal ruptures result in widespread contamination of the peritoneal cavity. The sample often is almost acellular; very few intact inflammatory cells can survive in such a hostile environment. Marked karyolytic degeneration usually is present, as are large numbers of a mixed population of bacteria.
  ▫ Small-intestinal and rectal ruptures usually result in less contamination of the peritoneal cavity because of the effectiveness of the omentum in isolating the affected intestine from the rest of the abdominal cavity.

SUPPURATIVE AND SEPTIC SUPPURATIVE INFLAMMATION

- Suppurative inflammation is diagnosed when the nucleated cell count and total protein content are elevated. The nucleated cell population is composed of high numbers of neutrophils.
- When intracellular bacteria are identified, the process is classified as septic suppurative inflammation. The neutrophils become "degenerate," and karyolytic and karyorrhectic changes are evident.
  - □ Normal neutrophil morphology does not exclude the possibility of a bacterial cause; if only small volumes of cytotoxins are produced by the microorganisms involved, cell morphology is not greatly affected.
  - □ Culture of the microorganism(s) and sensitivity testing for a variety of antimicrobial agents aids in formulating a specific therapeutic plan.

HEMORRHAGIC EFFUSION

- Hemorrhage can result from:
  - □ Iatrogenic contamination at the time of collection
  - □ Hemorrhagic diapedesis, usually from a compromised segment of the GI tract
  - □ Intraabdominal hemorrhage
  - □ Penetration of the spleen during abdominocentesis
- Recent hemorrhage into the peritoneal cavity or contamination of peritoneal fluid during sample collection may result in the finding of platelets at microscopic examination. Platelets are not usually seen if hemorrhage has occurred more than several hours previously.
- Macrophages "clean up" the erythrocytes in the abdominal cavity and display erythrocytophagy. Hemoglobin from the red blood cells is broken down and the iron conserved for new heme production (see Color Plate 15).
- Macrophages may contain iron pigment:
  - □ Hemosiderin: Refractile pigment, yellowish-green to dark brownish-black
  - □ Hematoidin crystals: Bright yellow and refractile
- The presence of erythrophagocytosis, hemosiderin pigment, or hematoidin crystals indicates previous hemorrhage. Differentiate pathologic process and iatrogenic causes.
- Packed cell volume and measurement of total protein content in the abdominal fluid are helpful in determining the amount of blood present in the fluid. It takes relatively few erythrocytes to impart a grossly red color to the fluid.

SEMINOPERITONEUM

- Vaginal perforation during breeding may result in septic or nonseptic inflammation, or seminoperitoneum. With seminoperitoneum, free sperm, neutrophils, and macrophages containing phagocytosed sperm heads may be found in the peritoneal fluid sample. Mild suppurative inflammation results from exposure of the peritoneum to seminal fluid.

UROPERITONEUM

- Rupture of the urinary bladder occurs most frequently among neonatal foals, although cases among adults have been described.
- Analysis of peritoneal fluid usually reveals an increased volume of clear, pale yellow fluid with low cell count and low specific gravity. Mild suppurative inflammation may be present owing to chemical irritation of the peritoneal surfaces.

- Calcium carbonate crystals may be identified during cytologic evaluation of fluid samples from adults.

NEOPLASIA

- Most cases involving neoplasia in the horse manifest as chronic symptoms (weight loss, weakness, and intermittent colic); however, tumors involving the GI tract have been reported to cause acute abdominal pain.
  - □ Neoplasms involving the GI tract include lymphosarcoma, squamous cell carcinoma, fibrosarcoma, adenocarcinoma, leiomyoma, leiomyosarcoma, myxosarcoma, lipoma, mesothelioma, intestinal carcinoid, and neurofibroma.
  - □ Intraabdominal tumors may not exfoliate cells into the peritoneal fluid; therefore the absence of neoplastic cells does not preclude a diagnosis of neoplasia. Positive findings of abdominocentesis result in a diagnosis of neoplasia approximately 40% of the time.
  - □ Tumors involving serosal surfaces, particularly those that cause erosion of serosal blood vessels, may cause bleeding into the abdominal cavity.
  - □ Inflammation secondary to tumor necrosis or infection results in peritonitis and the associated changes in peritoneal fluid.
  - □ Reactive mesothelial cells may be mistaken for neoplastic cells because of their highly pleomorphic appearance. This can result in difficult differentiation between a reactive or inflammatory process and neoplasia.

Incidental Findings

- Glove powder (talc) can be found in cytologic specimens whenever sterile technique is used for collection (see Color Plates 16 and 17). Microscopic examination shows large, round to hexagonal particles with a central fissure or nidus. The particles usually do not take up stain and are clear or slightly blue.
- Cornified squamous epithelial cells occasionally are found in samples in which a sterile preparation has been made before sampling. The cells typically are rolled up and appear as dark, deeply basophilic structures with ragged ends. These structures are commonly known as "keratin flakes" (see Color Plate 13).
- Microfilariae of *Setaria* organisms are occasionally found in peritoneal fluid samples (see Color Plate 18). The incidence is relatively low because of the widespread use of ivermectin anthelmintics.
- Lipemic peritoneal fluid occasionally is found in healthy foals.

➤ Keys to Peritoneal Fluid Interpretation

- Enterocentesis: "Normal" cells with extracellular bacterial organisms
- GI rupture: Paucity of intact cells, large numbers of bacteria
- Suppurative or septic inflammation: Neutrophils and intracellular bacteria
- Hemorrhagic effusion: Erythrocytes, platelets, erythrophagocytosis, hemosiderin, hematoidin
- Seminoperitoneum: Suppurative inflammation, free sperm, macrophages
- Uroperitoneum: Mild suppurative inflammation, calcium carbonate crystals (adults)
- Neoplasia: Differentiate from reactive mesothelial cells
- Incidental findings: Glove powder (talc), keratin flakes, *Setaria* microfilariae, lipemia

THORACIC FLUID

- Analysis is indicated when evidence of pleural effusion is obtained by means of auscultation, percussion, radiographic studies, or ultrasonographic evaluation.
- Normal pleural fluid is essentially a dialysate of plasma (as is abdominal fluid) with low cellularity and total protein concentration.
- Volume, cellularity, and biochemical composition of pleural fluid often reflect the pathophysiologic status of the visceral and parietal pleural surfaces.
- Effusions are noted in cases of:
  - Heart failure
  - Chronic hepatic disease
  - Hypoalbuminemia
  - Diaphragmatic hernia
  - Pleuropneumonia
  - Pulmonary abscessation
  - Thoracic abscessation
  - Thoracic or pleural neoplasia
  - Hemothorax
- Cell count, amount of total protein, and cellular makeup of thoracic fluid are essentially identical to those of peritoneal fluid. Interpretation of samples is performed in a manner similar to that of peritoneal fluid samples.
- Neoplasia involving the pleura often causes a uniform red color (hemorrhage) of peritoneal fluid. Septic pleuritis also may have a red color but is most commonly amber and hazy.

Normal Thoracic Fluid

- Normal cell count is fewer than 5000 nucleated cells per microliter
- Few erythrocytes and negligible erythrophagocytosis
- Neutrophils up to 70% of the nucleated cell population
- Large mononuclear cells and macrophages up to 50% of the nucleated cell population
- Small numbers of lymphocytes
- Rare eosinophils

SYNOVIAL FLUID

- Normal synovial fluid is a dialysate of plasma modified by the secretion of hyaluronic acid, glycoproteins, and macromolecules
- Synovial fluid functions:
  - Supply nutrition to articular cartilage, which is avascular
  - Lubricate the joint surfaces, limiting friction and wear between opposing articular cartilage surfaces

Cell Counts and Cytologic Examination

- Samples from the more commonly sampled joints usually contain fewer than 500 nucleated cells per microliter.
- Neutrophil count should not exceed 10% of the nucleated cell population unless there is obvious blood contamination of the sample.
- Most nucleated cells present in normal synovial fluid are lymphocytes and large mononuclear cells, which include monocytes, macrophages, and synovial lining cells (synoviocytes).

LAB TESTS

- Intact clumps of synovial lining cells are occasionally aspirated.
- The size and degree of cytoplasmic vacuolization in synovial fluid macrophages vary; some macrophages contain cytoplasmic metachromatic granules.
- Normal synovial fluid is essentially free of erythrocytes; however, almost all specimens contain some erythrocytes, commonly because of sample contamination with blood during the collection process. Erythrocytes also enter synovial fluid in a variety of disease processes involving the joint.

Interpretation of Synovial Fluid

NORMAL SYNOVIAL FLUID

- Normal cell count is fewer than 500 nucleated cells per microliter.
- Most nucleated cells are lymphocytes and large mononuclear cells.
- Neutrophils make up less than 10% of the nucleated cell population.

DEGENERATIVE AND TRAUMATIC JOINT DISEASE

- Typically fewer than 5000 nucleated cells per microliter, usually 1000-3000 cells per microliter.
- Mononuclear cells predominate. The extent of vacuolization in macrophages is of little diagnostic significance.
- Neutrophils usually are present as less than 10% of the nucleated cell population.
- It is difficult to differentiate acute traumatic injury with resultant hemorrhage from blood contamination during collection, particularly if there has been insufficient time for macrophages to phagocytize erythrocytes or break down hemoglobin into hemosiderin or hematoidin pigment.
- The presence of platelets or platelet clumps may be helpful in suggesting blood contamination.
  - □ The presence of erythrocytes phagocytized by macrophages suggests that the red blood cells were present in the fluid at collection.
- Cartilage fragments may be found in concentrated cytologic preparations with degenerative or traumatic joint disease; however, techniques for describing the severity of the joint disease on the basis of examination of the number and type of cartilage fragments have not gained wide acceptance.

INFLAMMATORY JOINT DISEASE

- Neutrophils usually are the predominant cell type.
- Two major groups of diseases classically respond with a neutrophilic (suppurative) inflammatory response:
  - □ Septic arthritis
  - □ Immune-mediated disease (e.g., rheumatoid arthritis and systemic lupus erythematosus)
- Septic arthritis should be the primary differential diagnosis when suppurative synovial fluid is obtained; immune-mediated arthritis is rare in horses.
- Noninfectious causes of neutrophilic inflammation include acute traumatic joint disease and chronic hemarthrosis.
- It is important to assess neutrophil morphology in synovial fluid samples:
  - □ Nuclear degeneration (karyolysis) is evident in cases of septic arthritis and can be more difficult to assess in synovial than in peritoneal or pleural fluid because of the presence of synovial fluid mucin, which can prevent neu-

trophils from flattening on a slide and therefore prevent true evaluation of nuclear morphology.
- □ Detecting bacteria in synovial fluid is more difficult than it is in other fluids. Bacteria often are rare and may be found either intracellularly in neutrophils or free in the fluid.
- Acute traumatic joint disease
  - □ Nucleated cell count usually is fewer than 5000/μl.
  - □ Mononuclear cells predominate.
  - □ An increased number of neutrophils may be present, making differentiation between sepsis and acute trauma difficult.
  - □ A nucleated cell count more than 30,000/μl is unlikely with acute traumatic injury.
  - □ Elevated cell counts secondary to trauma typically decrease within a few days to counts fewer than 5000 nucleated cells per microliter.
- Chronic hemorrhage.
  - □ Cellular response can vary but often is characterized by neutrophilia.
  - □ The presence of phagocytic cells displaying erythrocytophagy or containing iron pigment such as hemosiderin or hematoidin helps identify previous hemorrhage.
- In rare instances, synovial fluid has a nucleated cell count more than 5000/μl made up primarily of lymphocytes. Considerations include infection by *Mycoplasma* or *Borrelia burgdorferi* organisms.
- A single case of eosinophilic synovitis has been described with marked synovial hyperplasia and eosinophilic infiltration.

Keys to Synovial Fluid Interpretation

- *Degenerative and traumatic joint disease:* Fewer than 5000 nucleated cells per microliter, predominantly mononuclear cells, less than 10% neutrophils (neutrophil count may be higher in cases of acute traumatic joint disease).
- *Septic arthritis:* Neutrophils predominate; bacterial organisms may or may not be identified.
- *Immune-mediated arthritis:* Neutrophils predominate.
- *Chronic hemorrhage:* Often characterized by neutrophilia, erythrophagocytosis, hemosiderin, or hematoidin crystals.
- *Mycoplasma* or *Borrelia burgdorferi* infection: More than 5000 nucleated cells per microliter, predominantly lymphocytes.

BRONCHOALVEOLAR LAVAGE FLUID AND TRANSTRACHEAL ASPIRATE

- Techniques for collection of material by means of BAL or transtracheal aspiration are described on pp. 60-63.
- Protein determination is not routinely performed on these samples.
  - □ Samples are collected in saline solution and commonly contain only small amounts of protein, often in the form of mucus.
  - □ Samples from inflamed lungs also contain plasma proteins but are diluted by saline solution used during sample collection.
- Cell numbers often are low in samples because of dilution. It therefore is necessary to use methods to concentrate the cells present for microscopic evaluation.

□ Adding one or two drops of serum or commercially prepared bovine serum albumin before the slides are made helps preserve cells and yields better cellular morphology.
▪ Slides are stained with Romanowsky's stain. Additional stains may be helpful:
□ Gram stain: Identification and classification of bacteria.
□ Periodic acid–Schiff stain: Fungal organisms.
□ Perl's Iron Blue or Gomori's stain: Iron.

Microscopic Features
▪ Mucus appears as strands of flocculent material and stains pink to light blue with Romanowsky's stain.
▪ Curschmann spirals of mucus: Dark-staining tight spirals of mucus:
□ Do not overinterpret; these formations likely are the result of specific pH and protein concentrations and do not always represent inspissated mucus casts from small bronchi and bronchioles.
▪ Nucleated cells from the lower respiratory tract include epithelial cells and inflammatory cells:
□ Epithelial cells: Ciliated columnar epithelial cells (see Color Plate 19), nonciliated epithelial cells, goblet cells.
□ Inflammatory cells: Neutrophils, macrophages, eosinophils, lymphocytes, and mast cells.
▪ Erythrocytes are frequently present because of minor trauma to the epithelium during collection; however, they may be present because of hemorrhage into the respiratory tract.
▪ Other substances may be identified in samples:
□ Squamous epithelial cells from oral cavity or pharynx
□ Bacteria
□ Plant material
□ Pollen
□ Fungal elements
□ Starch granules from surgical gloves

Normal Cytologic Features
▪ Most nucleated cells in transtracheal aspirate or wash without lower respiratory disease are ciliated and nonciliated columnar epithelial cells and alveolar macrophages. Small numbers of neutrophils and lymphocytes may be present. A small amount of mucus usually is present.
▪ BAL samples contain predominantly macrophages and relatively few columnar epithelial cells. Small numbers of lymphocytes, epithelial cells, and neutrophils are present.

Interpretation of Bronchoalveolar Lavage Fluid and Transtracheal Aspirate
NORMAL BRONCHOALVEOLAR LAVAGE FLUID AND TRANSTRACHEAL ASPIRATE
▪ Samples often need to be concentrated because of low cellularity.
▪ Nucleated cell population includes epithelial and inflammatory cells.

OROPHARYNGEAL CONTAMINATION (see Color Plate 20)
▪ Contamination with material from the oropharyngeal cavity occurs occasionally during sample collection. Squamous epithelial cells and a mixed population of

predominantly extracellular bacteria often adhering to squamous epithelial cells are evidence of contamination.
- Evidence of oropharyngeal contamination also is found in samples obtained in cases of aspiration pneumonia.
  - Evidence of inflammation of the lower respiratory tract is present and should be considered in the interpretation.

ACUTE INFLAMMATION
- Suppurative inflammation characterized by a majority of neutrophils is one of the most common lesions detected at examination of the lower respiratory tract (see Color Plate 21).
  - Careful examination for the presence of intracellular bacterial microorganisms and of aerobic and anaerobic cultures of the sample is warranted.
  - Alveolar macrophages and columnar epithelial cells usually are present.
  - With chronic inflammation, the ratio of neutrophils to alveolar macrophages decreases, and binucleate and multinucleate macrophages appear.

CHRONIC OBSTRUCTIVE PULMONARY DISEASE
- Occurs because of hypersensitivity and hyperirritability of the lungs to inhaled irritants or allergens. Cytologic features (see Color Plate 22):
  - Increased amount of mucus.
  - Inflammation characterized by a predominance of neutrophils or a mixed neutrophil and macrophage exudate.
  - Hyperplastic ciliated respiratory epithelial cells and increased numbers of goblet cells may be present.
  - Eosinophils may be present in increased numbers, but this finding is not consistent; do not dismiss the diagnosis because of the absence of eosinophils.
  - A bacterial or fungal component may be present that usually is mild in relation to the degree of inflammation.

Eosinophilic Inflammation
- The presence of eosinophilic inflammation suggests hypersensitivity associated with allergic bronchitis or parasite migration:
  - *Dictyocaulus arnfieldi* in adults
  - *Parascaris equorum* in foals
- Eosinophilic inflammation usually is accompanied by marked alveolar macrophage proliferation.

SMOKE INHALATION
- Smoke inhalation usually is associated with a barn fire and causes severe injury to the respiratory tract.
- The upper respiratory tract is more vulnerable to the effects of heat, whereas the lower respiratory tract is affected by noxious gases and particles generated in the fire.
- The tracheal, bronchial, and bronchiolar epithelium may be destroyed or severely damaged; the result is edema and hemorrhage into the airways.
- Alveolar macrophages may be heavily laden with erythrocytes and carbon particles.
- The mucociliary clearance mechanism of the lungs is severely impaired, and secondary bacterial or fungal infection leads to an increase in the numbers of neutrophils and macrophages.

LAB TESTS

PREVIOUS HEMORRHAGE
- Causes
  - Exercise-induced pulmonary hemorrhage
  - Severe inflammation and necrosis of small blood vessels
  - Trauma, including previous aspiration procedures
  - Neoplasia
- Cytologic findings
  - Macrophages displaying erythrocytophagy or containing pigment compatible with hemosiderin or hematoidin. Special stains such as Perl's Iron Blue and Gomori's stains are useful in determining whether material present in macrophages contains iron.

SILICOSIS
- Silicosis or pneumoconiosis is best documented in the Monterey and Central Peninsula areas of California.
- Samples contain large numbers of macrophages; some contain cytoplasmic inclusions composed of pink crystalline material.
- Excessive mucus and increased numbers of neutrophils and hyperplastic epithelial cells are present.

NEOPLASIA
- Primary lung tumors are rare in horses. It is unlikely that BAL or transtracheal wash facilitates the diagnosis of primary or metastatic lung neoplasia.
- For neoplastic cells to be recovered in lower respiratory tract samples, the tumor must invade the bronchi or bronchioles in a central location in the lung to be collected using this technique.
- Pulmonary neoplasia has been diagnosed from BAL samples in humans; however, this does not appear to be a productive diagnostic procedure for equine patients.

▶ *Keys to Bronchoalveolar Lavage and Transtracheal Wash Interpretation*
- *Oropharyngeal contamination:* Squamous epithelial cells with adherent bacteria
- *Acute inflammation:* Neutrophils predominate, intracellular bacterial organisms present
- *Chronic inflammation:* Increased numbers of macrophages (some binucleate and multinucleate)
- *Chronic obstructive pulmonary disease:* Increased amount of mucus, hyperplastic respiratory epithelial cells, neutrophils, macrophages, eosinophils, and bacterial or fungal organisms
- *Eosinophilic inflammation:* Eosinophils, often accompanied by increased alveolar macrophage proliferation
- *Previous hemorrhage:* Erythrocytophagy, hemosiderin, or hematoidin
- *Silicosis:* Macrophages, some containing pink crystalline material, increased amount of mucus
- *Neoplasia:* Primary lung tumors rare; BAL is not a productive diagnostic procedure for pulmonary neoplasia in the equine patient

CEREBROSPINAL FLUID
- CSF is a low-protein ionic solution produced by secretory activity of the vascular choroid plexus cells, ventricular ependymal lining cells, and capillary endothelial cells of the brain.

- CSF sodium, chloride, and magnesium concentrations are greater than in plasma; however, concentrations of glucose and potassium are lower than in plasma.
- The osmolality of CSF is 6-7 mOsm/kg greater than that of plasma.
- CSF surrounds the central nervous system (CNS) to form an aqueous solution in which the brain and spinal cord are suspended.
  □ Protects the brain and spinal cord.
  □ Supplies nutrients to and removes metabolic waste products from the CNS.

Sample Collection
- Techniques for collection of CSF are described on pp. 120-121.
- Place the specimen in an EDTA (lavender top) tube and refrigerate it at 4°C to aid in cell preservation.
- Evaluate the sample as soon as possible after collection to eliminate changes resulting from cellular degeneration.

Sample Evaluation

COLOR
- Normal CSF is clear and colorless.
- Samples that are red or yellow should be centrifuged and reevaluated. Red discoloration caused by contamination with red blood cells clears with centrifugation. A red to brown to yellow color that does not clear with centrifugation suggests old hemorrhage. Yellow (xanthochromic) CSF usually is caused by disintegration of red blood cells within the subarachnoid space with resultant bilirubin formation.

TURBIDITY
- Increased nucleated cell counts usually cause turbidity. Perform total red blood cell and nucleated cell counts and a cytologic evaluation to determine the type of nucleated cells present.

COAGULATION
- Normal CSF does not coagulate. Coagulation can occur if trauma during collection leads to hemorrhage or if damage to barrier membranes has allowed fibrinogen to enter the CSF.

CELL COUNT
- Determine the nucleated cell count in undiluted CSF using a hemacytometer with a Neubauer ruling. Count the cells in all nine squares, and multiply the number of nucleated cells by 1.1 to determine the number of nucleated cells per microliter. Normal total nucleated cell count is 0-6/μl.

PROTEIN
- Total protein determination requires a dye-binding or turbidimetric procedure because of the milligram per deciliter concentrations normally present. Normal values are less than 80-100 mg/dl in adults and may be slightly higher (up to 180 mg/dl) in foals.

GLUCOSE
- Normal value is 60%-80% of serum concentration.
- Low CSF glucose concentration most often is associated with inflammation due to consumption by leukocytes or bacterial organisms.

CREATINE KINASE ISOENZYME (CK3 OR CK-BB)
- Normal value is <1 IU/L.
- CK isoenzyme measured in CSF is present in fat and dura mater. Although it may be increased from either neuronal cell damage or degeneration, enzyme value is not considered to be a reliable monitor of CNS disease.

Cytologic Examination
- Concentration techniques are necessary to prepare slides because of low cellularity. Cytocentrifugation is preferred. Centrifugation as in the preparation of urine sediment specimens can be used in the absence of a specialized cytocentrifuge.

Microscopic Features
- Red blood cells are absent.
- Most nucleated cells are small lymphocytes.
- Monocytes occasionally are present.
- Activated macrophages with vacuolization are not normally present.
- Neutrophils may be present but should be less than 10% of the nucleated cell population.

Interpretation of Cerebrospinal Fluid
NORMAL CEREBROSPINAL FLUID
- Clear and colorless
- 0-6 nucleated cells per microliter
- Small lymphocytes make up the majority of nucleated cells
- No nucleated cells are neutrophils
- Protein: 80-100 mg/dl (adult); up to 180 mg/dl (foals)
- Glucose: 60%-80% of serum concentration

BACTERIAL INFECTION
- White to amber to yellow; may be turbid
- Protein level and nucleated cell count are elevated
- Neutrophils are the predominant cell type
- Phagocytized bacteria may be present

VIRAL INFECTION
- Colorless to amber; may be clear or slightly turbid
- Protein level and nucleated cell count typically are elevated
- Nucleated cell population is made up primarily of small lymphocytes although this may vary with West Nile and Eastern encephalitis viral infections (see p. 413).

TRAUMA (HEMORRHAGE)
- Sample is red (recent hemorrhage) to yellow (xanthochromia, past hemorrhage).
- Protein level and nucleated cell count are mildly elevated.
- Macrophages displaying erythrocytophagy or containing iron pigments (hemosiderin or hematoidin) commonly are present.
- Neutrophils are present in increased numbers.

PROTOZOAL INFECTION

- Colorless to slightly yellow with no turbidity.
- Protein level and nucleated cell counts may be mildly elevated.
- Nucleated cell population consists of increased numbers of neutrophils, lymphocytes, and macrophages.
- CSF is abnormal in fewer than 30% of cases of equine protozoal myelitis.

▶ Keys to CSF Interpretation

- *Bacterial infection:* White, amber, or yellow; protein and nucleated cell count elevated; neutrophils predominate; bacterial organisms present
- *Viral infection:* Colorless to amber; may be clear or slightly turbid; protein and nucleated cell count elevated; small lymphocytes predominate in many cases
- *Trauma (hemorrhage):* Red to yellow (xanthochromic); protein and nucleated cell count mildly elevated; erythrocytophagy; hemosiderin, hematoidin, or both; increased number of neutrophils
- *Protozoal infection:* Colorless to slightly yellow; protein and nucleated cell counts may be slightly elevated; mixed inflammatory cell population normal in most cases

REFERENCES

Cowell RL, Tyler RD: *Diagnostic cytology and hematology of the horse,* ed 2, St. Louis, 2002, Mosby.

Kobluk CN, Ames TR, Geor RJ, editors: *The horse: diseases and clinical management,* Philadelphia, 1995, WB Saunders.

Meyer DJ: The management of cytology specimens, *Compend Contin Educ* 9:10-17, 1987.

Meyer DJ, Coles EH, Rich LJ: *Veterinary laboratory medicine: interpretation and diagnosis,* Philadelphia, 1992, WB Saunders.

Ziemer EL: Cytologic analysis of large-animal body fluids, *Vet Med* June 574-583, 1989.

LAB TESTS

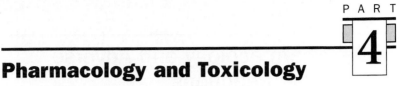

Pharmacology and Toxicology

52 Pharmacology and Adverse Drug Reactions

PHARMACOLOGY

Thomas J. Divers and J. Edward Kirker

This chapter provides answers to frequently asked questions regarding drugs used to manage equine emergencies.

ANTIMICROBIALS

β-Lactam Drugs (Penicillins, Cephalosporins, Carbapenems, Monobactams)

- Stability: When reconstituted, most β-lactam drugs are stable for 12-24 hours at room temperature (use sodium ampicillin and ticarcillin within 1 hour), 3-7 days when refrigerated (best), and 30 days frozen (−20°C [−4°F]). Some precipitate may be present at cold temperatures; if the drug goes back into solution after warming in water, it can be used.
- Incompatibility: Do not mix in the same syringe or solution with aminoglycosides.
- Orally administered penicillin V and cephalosporins: Poorly absorbed in horses older than 1 month and may cause diarrhea. Rarely indicated in equine practice.
- β-Lactam drugs generally are synergistic when combined with aminoglycosides in the patient.
- Activity of β-lactam drugs against anaerobic infection: Effective against many anaerobic agents (*Clostridium* and *Fusobacterium* organisms) but generally are *not* effective in the management of *Bacteroides fragilis* infection.

PROCAINE PENICILLIN
- Heating may increase procaine reactions.
- Repeated injection in the same muscle mass increases the risk of a procaine reaction.
- Dosages larger than 10,000 units/kg are poorly absorbed.

AMPICILLIN SODIUM
- Slightly less stable than penicillin salts after reconstitution (48 hours refrigerated). Use sterile water or saline solution, not dextrose.
- A wide range of dosages is used in the treatment of horses; the recommended dosage is 15 mg/kg IV q6-8h.

CEFTIOFUR
- Has been used for several years in horses intramuscularly and intravenously. There are a few reports of diarrhea occurring after use of ceftiofur. In intensive care facilities, adverse effects of ceftiofur are surprisingly uncommon.
- Autoimmune hemolytic anemia has rarely occurred.

650

- ❑ A dosage of two to five times the package insert recommendation is frequently used to treat critically ill patients (e.g., septic foals, patients with pleuro-pneumonia) with few adverse reactions.
- ❑ High intramuscular doses are irritating.
- ❑ Like most cephalosporins, ceftiofur can be given concurrently with aminoglycosides, but do not mix these agents in same syringe.
- ❑ Reconstituted solution can be used for up to 7 days if refrigerated.
- ❑ Dosages higher than labeled recommendations are frequently used to treat critical care patients, up to 8 mg/kg q8h IV.

TICARCILLIN-CLAVULANATE
- An acceptable drug for bacteremia in foals, either alone or combined with amikacin
- Irritating if administered intramuscularly
- Does not have the same spectrum as imipenem or some third and fourth generation cephalosporins

CEFAZOLIN SODIUM
- A first-generation cephalosporin that has been frequently used to treat horses, 11 mg/kg IV q6-12h
- Excellent spectrum of activity against most Gram-positive bacteria
- Enteric streptococci, *B. fragilis* organisms, and some staphylococci may be resistant

CEFADROXIL
- A first-generation cephalosporin
- Can be given orally to foals, but after 2-4 weeks of age the bioavailability is very low
- 10 mg/kg PO q12h to foals younger than 4 weeks

CEPHALOTHIN
- A first-generation cephalosporin
- 20 mg/kg IV q6h

"Newer" β-Lactam Antimicrobials
CEFOTAXIME
- A third-generation cephalosporin
- Achieves higher levels in cerebrospinal fluid (CSF) than do most other cephalosporins
- 20-30 mg/kg IV q6h

CEFEPIME
- A fourth-generation cephalosporin
- 11 mg/kg IV q8h

CEFOPERAZONE
- Third-generation cephalosporin used to control life-threatening bacteremia
- Dosage: 30 mg/kg IV q8h
- Like most third-generation cephalosporins, cefoperazone has retained activity similar to that of first-generation cephalosporins against Gram-positive organisms but has extended activity against many Gram-negative organisms

PHARMACOLOGY

- One of the only cephalosporins routinely effective against *Pseudomonas* organisms
- Has the potential to produce a bleeding disorder similar to that reported among foals treated with moxalactam
- In foals with severe liver disease or cholestasis, serum levels may progressively increase

CARBAPENEM GROUP: IMIPENEM/CILASTATIN
- Do not use with other β-lactam drugs (may antagonize activity)
- Can be used with amikacin
- Administer in intravenous fluids (e.g., saline solution), 15 mg/kg IV q4-8h
- Single most effective antibiotic for treating the septic foal

ZOSYN (PIPERACILLIN SODIUM AND TAZOBACTAM) INJECTABLE
- Tazobactam is a β-lactamase inhibitor and has no antibacterial activity.
- 2.25-g vial contains 2 g piperacillin, 0.25 g tazobactam.
- 3.37-5 g vial contains 3 g piperacillin and 0.75 g tazobactam.
- 4.5-g vial contains 4 g piperacillin and 0.5 g tazobactam.
- Piperacillin: An antipseudomonal penicillin with extended activity against Gram-negative anaerobes, streptococcal and enterococcal spp. It is preferred to ticarcillin for many Gram-negative infections. Because of this distinct characteristic, piperacillin is one of the more popular antibiotics to incorporate in antibiotic "beads" to treat acute and chronic orthopedic infections.

Macrolides
ERYTHROMYCIN
- Suspensions for oral administration:
  - The crushing of the enteric-coated tablets (e.g., stearate) is unlikely to be a problem if the patient is eating or is being treated with a histamine$_2$ (H$_2$) antagonist or proton pump blocker. Low gastric pH (<4.0), as reported among anorexic horses, can inactivate erythromycin in the crushed tablets.
- Products:
  - Erythromycin stearate phosphate (a poultry product) and estolate are reported to provide higher plasma concentrations of the active drug (at least in adults) than does erythromycin base or ethylsuccinate. All have been used with clinical success in foals and none is shown to have a higher incidence of diarrhea than others.
- Mix erythromycin lactobionate for intravenous infusion (mostly for ileus treatment), 1 g/450-kg adult, in *buffered* intravenous fluid.
- *Use oral erythromycin cautiously in the care of patients older than 5 months* because of increased risk of drug-induced clostridial colitis.
- May alter temperature homeostasis in foals, causing hyperthermia and respiratory distress during hot weather periods.
- Aminoglycosides may be antagonistic. If Gram-negative coverage is needed during erythromycin therapy, ceftiofur may be used.
- May increase serum theophylline level to toxic concentration when used concurrently.
- As with most orally administered antibiotics bioavailability is increased if the drug is given before feeding.

AZITHROMYCIN
- An azalide antimicrobial similar to macrolides
- Bioavailability (33%-53%) much better than erythromycin
- Plasma half-life ($t_{1/2}$) (10 hours) much greater than of erythromycin
- Larger apparent volume of distribution (V_d) and better phagocytic cell uptake (pulmonary macrophage) than of erythromycin
- Postantibiotic effect (PAE) against some organisms
- Tablet formulation equally absorbed in fasting as opposed to fed state in foals
- 10 mg/kg PO once a day for minimum of 5 days then every other day
- May be combined with rifampin

TRIMETHOPRIM-SULFONAMIDE
- Differences between trimethoprim (TMP)-sulfadiazine and TMP-sulfamethoxazole:
  - Sulfadiazine has a more favorable pharmacokinetic profile, but there is little difference in clinical success between the two products.
- Enteral absorption:
  - Paste and commercially prepared oral suspensions often are better absorbed than are suspensions of crushed tablets with little difference in clinical success or incidence of adverse reaction (diarrhea).
- Best absorbed when administered without feed.
- Toxicity:
  - The incidence of diarrhea after oral administration is very low. Diarrhea seems to be more common among postoperative patients that have had dramatic reductions in feed or have been treated with other antimicrobials before the TMP-sulfonamide and in those housed in referral hospitals. If diarrhea is an adverse effect of TMP-sulfonamide treatment, it usually occurs 2-6 days after treatment is started.
- Safety in treatment of pregnant mares: Unknown; however, decreases folate levels and rarely causes congenital anomaly.
- May falsely elevate serum creatinine concentration when administered to individuals with renal dysfunction.
- Frequency of treatment: Generally recommended to administer q12h for bacterial diseases.

TRIBRISSEN INJECTABLE 48% AQUEOUS SUSPENSION
- Each milliliter contains 80 mg trimethoprim and 400 mg sulfadiazine.
- Not for use in horses intended for food.
- Indicated for susceptible infections in horses, including acute strangles, acute urogenital infections, respiratory infections, and wounds or abscesses.
- Should not be used in patients showing marked liver dysfunction, blood dyscrasias, or those with a history of sulfonamide sensitivity.
- Transient pruritus has been found in a few individuals within the first 24 hours after administration.
- Swelling, pain, and tissue damage have been occasionally observed with subcutaneous, intramuscular, or extravasated administration.
- Rare shocklike convulsions and collapse have occurred within seconds of administration in some patients.
- Do *not* administer after detomidine hydrochloride (Dormosedan)!

PHARMACOLOGY

PYRIMETHAMINE

- Best administered without food or trimethoprim; has been used successfully in the management of equine protozoal myelitis with sulfa drugs. If TMP-sulfonamide and pyrimethamine are administered together, commercial source of folic acid supplementation is not routinely indicated; however, green forage is recommended.
- May rarely cause congenital anomalies in foals whose dams have been treated during pregnancy.
- May occasionally cause anemia and leukopenia, however clinical importance not proved.
- Feeding green forage recommended with the long term treatment.

OXYTETRACYCLINE, TETRACYCLINE, DOXYCYCLINE

- Administration:
  - ▫ Oxytetracycline administered intravenously can be diluted with any intravenous fluid except sodium bicarbonate or fluids containing calcium.
  - ▫ Administer slowly intravenously. Nonfatal collapse or hemolysis rarely occurs.
  - ▫ *Do not administer intramuscularly or subcutaneously.*
  - ▫ Orally administered tetracycline has not been shown to be well absorbed in horses.
  - ▫ When administered to volume depleted, hypotensive horses or horses with preexisting renal dysfunction, these drugs may cause acute renal failure.
  - ▫ When these drugs are administered at high dosage for contracted tendons in foals, renal failure may occur in a low percentage of cases, especially if the foal is not nursing adequately!
  - ▫ *Do not administer doxycycline intravenously!*
  - ▫ Doxycycline, 10.0 mg/kg PO q12h is frequently used in the horse but bioavailability is very low!
  - ▫ Doxycycline does not appear to have the nephrotoxic properties of oxytetracycline, is absorbed orally in horses, and rarely causes gastrointestinal (GI) side effects.
  - ▫ Doxycycline does not accumulate in patients with renal dysfunction.
  - ▫ Both doxycycline and tetracycline have antiinflammatory properties.

METRONIDAZOLE

- Anorexia directly associated with treatment is unusual in the horse but does occur; can be administered per rectum.
- Excellent distribution properties (e.g., peritoneum).
- Safety in pregnant mares has not been demonstrated, however this drug is frequently used to treat pregnant mares without known adverse effects.
- Neurologic signs have been reported when 25 mg/kg q6-8h is exceeded.
- Dosage interval should be prolonged in the treatment of patients with liver failure or in foals <1 week of age.

AMINOGLYCOSIDES

- Incompatibility:
  - ▫ Do not mix in the same solution or syringe with β-lactam drugs.
  - ▫ More effective when used in an alkaline pH.
  - ▫ Generally better to administer in one daily dose (q24h), although more frequent administration may be needed in the care of some adults and foals.

- Indications:
  - □ Life-threatening Gram-negative aerobic infection that cannot be managed with safer antibiotics.
  - □ Synergistic when administered with β-lactam drugs. Do not combine in the same syringe.
  - □ Ineffective for managing anaerobic infections (add metronidazole) and most intracellular bacteria.
- Contraindications:
  - □ Do not administer to dehydrated patients, premature foals, or hypokalemic patients without fluid support.
  - □ Do not administer to adults or foals with neuromuscular weaknesses (e.g., botulism).
- Drug monitoring:
  - □ Peak concentration of gentamicin 30-60 minutes after administration should be 40 µg/ml or greater in the management of severe Gram-negative infections; that of amikacin should be 60 µg/ml or greater. Trough levels of both drugs should be <2 µg/ml.
  - □ Foals may need a higher initial (loading) dosage.
- Can be used for nebulization after a bronchodilator is administered.

ENROFLOXACIN
- Contraindications and indications:
  - □ Because of the potential for cartilage damage in the young horse, it is best not to use enrofloxacin to treat individuals younger than 18 months unless there are no other logical antimicrobial alternatives
  - □ When administered orally, enrofloxacin should not be mixed with molasses (use corn syrup, e.g., Karo syrup, instead).
- Has been used safely to treat pregnant mares, but safety has not been documented.
- Enrofloxacin is preferred over ciprofloxacin in the treatment of horses because of better absorption.
- Fluoroquinolones are not effective against anaerobic bacteria!
  - □ Excellent distribution properties.
  - □ Bovine-approved injectable product can be used either intravenously or orally in the treatment of horses.
  - □ Increases the risk of theophylline toxicity.

CHLORAMPHENICOL
- Pharmacokinetics:
  - □ Protect from sunlight. Excessive cold may cause precipitation, for which warming and shaking are recommended.
  - □ Chloramphenicol is poorly absorbed when administered orally to horses and has a very short $t_{1/2}$ when administered intravenously. Therefore there are only a few indications for intravenous administration of chloramphenicol to horses. It is used orally for long-term management of aerobic and anaerobic infections.
- Adverse effects: None reported in the horse, but there is some risk (1 in 40,000) to humans handling the drug. Chloramphenicol is prohibited in Europe.
- A paste preparation can be purchased from several veterinary-compounding pharmacies in the United States.
- **Do not use florfenicol in the treatment of horses.**

PHARMACOLOGY

RIFAMPIN
- Adverse effects:
  - May cause urine discoloration, which is not clinically important
  - May increase rate of elimination of theophylline and diazepam
  - May cause diarrhea in adults

POLYMYXIN B
- Indications: May be of benefit in the management of endotoxemia.
- Warnings: Should be used only during endotoxemia and in the treatment of patients with normal renal function and after urination is observed. Concurrent or sequential use of other potentially nephrotoxic agents should be avoided. These include bacitracin, streptomycin, kanamycin, gentamicin, amikacin, cephaloridine, tetracycline, paromomycin, vancomycin, viomycin, and colistin.
- The neurotoxcity from polymyxin B can result in respiratory paralysis, especially if the drug is given soon after anesthesia or muscle relaxants.

SPECTINOMYCIN HYDROCHLORIDE
- The sterile solution for injection in poultry has been successfully used to treat horses, however clinical indications are limited. Dosage: 22 mg/kg IV q8h

VANCOMYCIN
- Primary indication is life-threatening staphylococcal and group D streptococcal (*Enterococcus* sp.) infection resistant to the more commonly used antistaphylo-coccal/antistreptococcal agents.
- May be used for management of colitis caused by *Clostridium difficile*.
- Clinical use should be restricted to bacterial infections resistant to all other tested antibiotics.

AMPHOTERICIN B
- Administer in D_5W!
- Amphotericin has potent nephrotoxic properties and should not be administered to dehydrated or azotemic patients.
- Bolus fluid therapy (adults) with 5 L 0.9% saline solution once a day may protect against nephrotoxicity.
- The proper dosage for horses is not known. One recommendation is 0.3 mg/kg IV on day 1, 0.45 mg/kg IV on day 2, and 0.6 mg/kg IV every other day.
- Amphotericin should be mixed in 1 L of D_5W to reduce the incidence of phlebitis.

ITRACONAZOLE
- Preparation for oral administration:
  - Empty capsules in 95% ethanol (24 capsules/4-5 ml ethanol). Let stand 3-4 minutes, then grind to paste and allow to dry.
  - Can be mixed with syrup and refrigerated for 35 days
  - Absorption is better than with other antifungal drugs.
  - Nonsteroidal antiinflammatory drugs (NSAIDs) administered concurrently with itraconazole may increase free itraconazole.

KETOCONAZOLE
- Absorption: *Very poor* after oral administration to horses. Mixing the drug with an acidic fluid (e.g., orange juice) or withholding feed improves absorption.

- Has antiinflammatory and antipyretic effects and slows the progression of several nonseptic inflammatory diseases (e.g., progressive pulmonary fibrosis).

ANTIHISTAMINES
Diphenhydramine Hydrochloride, Doxylamine Succinate, Hydroxyzine Hydrochloride, Tripelennamine, Pyrilamine Maleate
- Administer slowly intravenously. Most of these agents can be administered intramuscularly or subcutaneously.
- For an overdose causing hyperexcitability or a seizure, *do not* use barbiturates or diazepam. Chloral hydrate is recommended.
- Increases the effect of epinephrine.

SHORT-ACTING ANESTHETICS, TRANQUILIZERS, NARCOTICS, SEDATIVES, AND ANALGESICS
Diazepam
- Administration: Do not draw into plastic syringes except immediately before administration; adsorbs to plastic.
- Interactions: When used to treat foals receiving erythromycin, the effect can be prolonged.
- Do not use if the patient has hepatic encephalopathy.

Butorphanol Tartrate
- Compatibility: Can be combined in the same syringe with acepromazine or xylazine.
- Contraindications: Do not use in the management of head trauma because CSF pressure may be increased if respiratory rate and/or effort are decreased.
- When administered before tranquilization, may produce severe head shaking. No treatment is required, and the antagonist naloxone is not indicated.
- Controlled Schedule IV drug!
- Should not be used concurrently with fentanyl patches!
- May be used as a continuous rate infusion (CRI) starting at the dosage of 13 µg/kg/hr to control pain; however butorphanol may decrease intestinal motility.

Narcotic Agonists and Analgesics (Morphine, Meperidine, Oxymorphone, and Fentanyl)
- These drugs produce analgesia, sedation, respiratory depression, and decreased intestinal motility.
- Morphine, 0.1 mg/kg (preservative free) plus xylazine, 0.17 mg/kg, or detomidine, 0.06 mg/kg, is frequently used as epidural analgesia.
  □ Morphine has no effect on motor neurons and does not cause ataxia, which occurs with both xylazine and detomidine.
  □ Morphine has maximal effect approximately 2-6 hours after administration, and the effect may last 8-16 hours.
  □ Epidural morphine may provide analgesia up to the thorax.
- Administration: When these drugs are administered systemically before tranquilization, excitement can occur!
- Fentanyl patches can be used as a potent analgesic in the treatment of individuals that cannot receive NSAIDs or can be used in addition to NSAIDs.

PHARMACOLOGY

□ Therapeutic effect may not occur for 4-6 hours, maximum effect in 8 hours and quickly declines after 20 hours.

□ Apply to inside of clipped and/or shaved forelimb and/or withers with a dry bandage for the best skin to patch contact. This improves the absorption of the drug through the skin.

□ Dosage for horses is not published; some clinicians use 2-3× 100 μg/h patch every 48-72 hours for adults and 1× 100 μg/h for foals.

Acepromazine

- Incompatibility: May be mixed in same syringe with xylazine but not diazepam
- Contraindications: *Do not* use in the management of hypotensive shock or hypovolemia. Use barbiturates or chloral hydrate rather than acepromazine to treat patients with tetanus because of the effect of acepromazine on the extrapyramidal system.
- Do not administer to individuals with a history of seizures.
- Do not use to treat intact stallions unless absolutely necessary! If used to treat a stallion for laminitis, use a lower dose (10 mg/450 kg) and do not allow the stallion exposure to other horses, especially mares, or excessive movement, such as trailering, until tranquilization is no longer apparent.
- Management of acepromazine-induced hypotension: Administer hypertonic saline solution, ephedrine, phenylephrine, or norepinephrine.
- Management of *paraphimosis*: See p. 472.

Xylazine

- Compatibility: May be mixed in the same syringe with acepromazine or butorphanol and combined with acepromazine if *both* are administered at a lower than normal dosage.
- Contraindications:
  □ Do not use to treat patients with severe upper airway obstruction; can be used if the patient has a lower airway disorder (e.g., chronic obstructive pulmonary disease [COPD]) when tranquilization is needed.
  □ Xylazine has been used in pregnant mares without causing abortion.

CAUTION: Some breeds, such as draft breeds, are more susceptible to sedative effects.

□ Collapse may occur among some draft horses and immature equines.

CAUTION: Intestinal motility is inhibited, especially with repeated use.

- Hyperglycemia, caused by decreased insulin, and increased urine production occur with α_2 agonist administration.

Detomidine

- Indications: α_2-adrenergic agonist provides superficial and visceral analgesia.
- Contraindications: Previously existing atrioventricular or sinoatrial heart block, coronary disease, cerebrovascular disease, or head trauma.
- **Intravenous potentiated sulfonamides should not be used in anesthetized or sedated individuals because potentially fatal dysrhythmias can occur in this situation.**
- Be careful administering detomidine to patients with endotoxic or traumatic shock, advanced liver or kidney disease, or stress (i.e., extreme heat, cold, fatigue, high altitude).

- Adverse reactions: Occasional anaphylactic-type reactions have been reported. Urticaria, skin plaques, dyspnea, edema of the upper airways, trembling, recumbency, and death all have been reported.
- Avoid use of epinephrine because epinephrine can potentiate the effects of α_2-agonists.
- Side effects: Bradycardia is common. Piloerection, sweating, salivation, slight muscle tremors, and partial atrioventricular or sinoatrial heart block may occur. Incoordination may happen within the first few minutes after injection and increased urination 45-60 minutes after injection.

Guaifenesin (GG)
- Preparation and storage:
  □ Precipitation generally occurs when temperature is less than 22.2°C (72°F).
  □ Prepare as a 10% solution in sterile water or D_5W; may be stored at room temperature for 1 week. A 5% solution causes less endothelial irritation than does a 10% solution.
- Compatibility: Can be combined with ketamine, xylazine, barbiturates.

Ketamine Hydrochloride
- Compatibility:
  □ Can be mixed with xylazine in the same syringe, but induction of anesthesia is best achieved with tranquilization before administration of ketamine.
  □ May precipitate when mixed with barbiturates or diazepam.
  □ Can be mixed in polyionic fluids with GG and xylazine.

> **NOTE:** Do not use ketamine hydrochloride in the management of head trauma or deep corneal wounds because CSF pressure and intraocular pressure increase after administration.

Barbiturates
- Compatibility: May be mixed in polyionic intravenous fluid solutions
- Contraindications:
  □ Severe respiratory depression at high doses
  □ Perivascular injection results in severe inflammation (see p. 688)
  □ Depresses fetal respiration
- Indications for pentobarbital, phenobarbital:
  □ Head trauma (may need to assist ventilation to maintain normal to slightly low $PaCO_2$, which decreases cerebral vascular pressure)
  □ Most seizures
  □ Tetanus
  □ Has been used to stimulate bilirubin metabolism in neonatal foals

Chloral Hydrate
- Activity: Hypnotic-sedative, no analgesic properties
- Advantages:
  □ Inexpensive
  □ Minimal cardiopulmonary and GI side effects unless used at higher dosage
- Administration
  □ Use after tranquilization with acepromazine; an analgesic (meperidine or morphine) is preferred
  □ Administer 12% solution IV at approximately 22 mg/kg
  □ Titrate to effect 30-60 minutes after first dose

- □ Duration up to 12 hours
- □ Can be administered orally at the same dosage

| **CAUTION:** Do not administer perivascularly!

- Indications:
  - □ Medical colic with severe intractable pain that cannot be controlled with NSAIDs or a tranquilizer-narcotic combination and when these drugs are contraindicated or are needed frequently. In some cases of severe ileus and gas distention, neostigmine is administered while the patient is sedated with chloral hydrate.

Yohimbine

- α_2-Adrenergic antagonist that may be used to reverse the effects of xylazine or detomidine
- 0.075 mg/kg IV as needed
- May increase intestinal motility

Tolazoline Hydrochloride

- Reversal agent for xylazine and detomidine
- Decreases peripheral vascular resistance and blood pressure
- Recommended dosage on insert: 2-4 mg/kg administered *slowly* IV or IM. Recommend using the lower dosage
- Arrhythmias and sudden death have been reported

DRUGS USED TO MANAGE GASTROINTESTINAL EMERGENCIES

Antiulcer Treatment

RANITIDINE

- Administration: Do not give orally within 2 hours of administering sucralfate.

FAMOTIDINE

- Administration: As for ranitidine.
- Storage: Refrigerate the injectable form; it is stable at room temperature for at least 48 hours.

CIMETIDINE

- Administration: As for ranitidine.
- Storage: Do not refrigerate.
- Drug interactions: May prolong serum $t_{1/2}$ of drugs requiring hepatic metabolism (e.g., diazepam).

OMEPRAZOLE (GASTROGARD)

- Peak effect on gastric pH may not occur for 3-4 days, but clinical effect may be noticeable sooner.
- Pharmacokinetics in young foals not published; omeprazole is used in neonatal foals.
- Inhibits diazepam metabolism.

SUCRALFATE
- Administration: Administer *2 hours apart from other oral medication* because it can decrease absorption of orally administered drugs.

MISOPROSTOL
- Possible contraindications: Do not administer to pregnant mares or to individuals with COPD.
- Do not dispense without warning: ***Not to be handled by pregnant women!***
- Used in prophylaxis or management of NSAID GI toxicity.
- Higher dosages can cause diarrhea; may be of benefit in the management of cecal or colonic impaction.

METOCLOPRAMIDE
- Incompatibility: Do not mix with calcium gluconate or erythromycin in the same intravenous solution.
- Protect from prolonged exposure to light.
- Central nervous system (CNS) effects may be enhanced by some sedatives, tranquilizers, and narcotics. Diazepam has been used to help control CNS side effects.

BETHANECHOL
- Preparation of injectable solution from powder (Sigma). Commercially available parenteral product is preferred, but is expensive:
  - Powder is soluble in water (sterile).
  - Can be autoclaved without loss of potency.
  - Administer through 0.2-U filter.
  - Can be administered intravenously or subcutaneously.

DIOCTYL SODIUM SULFOSUCCINATE (DSS)
- Theoretically, DSS and mineral oil should not be administered together because DSS damages epithelial cells and may increase intestinal absorption of mineral oil. These two drugs are commonly administered in combination without reported clinical problems. *Do not use in foals.*

BISMUTH SUBSALICYLATE
- Manure turns black after administration, but this effect is of no clinical concern.
- Sufficient salicylate may be absorbed so that metabolism of salicylic acid may affect platelet function; therefore aspirin therapy to alter platelet function may not be needed.

NEOSTIGMINE
- Contraindications:
  - *Do not* use to treat patients with intestinal displacement.
  - *Do not* use to treat patients with severe COPD.
- Indications:
  - In foals or adults, ileus and severe large-intestinal *tympany* after GI obstruction has been ruled out (e.g., with radiographs).

PHARMACOLOGY

  □ Gravel obstruction of the rectum in adults.
  □ Atropine toxicity.
- Always use neostigmine cautiously; analgesics may be needed.

NONSTEROIDAL ANTIINFLAMMATORY DRUGS

Aspirin
- Contraindications: Do not administer to patients with known bleeding disorders.
- Indication: Administer 60-90 grains/450-kg adult (10-20 mg/kg) every 2 or 3 days PO or rectally to inhibit platelet function.
- Platelet function is suppressed in normal horses; in vitro aggregation is not suppressed after in vitro endotoxin stimulation.

Flunixin Meglumine
- Administration: Irritating when administered perivascularly. **Occasionally associated with clostridial myositis after intramuscular or perivascular injection.**
- Indications, possible contraindications:
  □ Preferred NSAID (0.25-0.3 mg/kg) to manage cardiopulmonary effects of endotoxemia.
  □ Do not use to treat foals with gastric ulceration or dehydration.
  □ Has minimal effect on platelet function.
  □ Use with caution to treat foals with diarrhea or dehydration; duodenal ulceration can result!

Phenylbutazone
- Administration: Irritating when administered perivascularly; do not administer intramuscularly.
- Use lower dosage recommendations to treat ponies.
- Indications, possible contraindications:
  □ Preferred NSAID by many clinicians to manage musculoskeletal and gastrointestinal disorders.
  □ Avoid using in the management of ulcerative colitis, gastric ulceration, or acute renal failure or in the care of dehydrated patients.
  □ Minimal effect on platelet function.
  □ May help to normalize intestinal motility in endotoxemia.

Carprofen
- Although this effect is not documented, carprofen may have more selective cyclooxygenase-2 (COX-2) inhibition than do approved equine NSAIDs.
- Hepatic disease has not been reported in horses in association with treatment.

Ketoprofen
- Reported to have lower incidence of adverse effects (e.g., GI ulceration) than does phenylbutazone.
- Use: Reported to inhibit prostanoids and leukotrienes, however superiority in the management of endotoxemia has not been demonstrated.
- Significance of L-arginine component not proved.

Meclofenamic Acid
- Use: Compared with other NSAIDs, infrequently used in practice
- May affect platelet function
- Adverse effects rarely reported

Dipyrone
- Indications: Generally believed to be the safest NSAID and is predominantly used in the management of hyperthermia and mild colic. Has not been associated with gastric ulcers in foals.
- Available only through compounding pharmacies.

Etodolac
- Has been evaluated for use in horses.
- In some species may have some preference for COX-2 inhibition; not proved in the horse.

➤ Additional Cautions on the Use of All NSAIDs
- All NSAIDs are highly protein-bound and can displace other drugs from protein-binding sites. This effect:
  - Increases free drug levels of the displaced drugs.
  - Enhances and speeds the therapeutic effect and toxicity of the displaced drug.
  - Speeds elimination of displaced drugs.
- Use with caution in the treatment of individuals with COPD, because inhibition of prostaglandin E can exacerbate airway function.
- All of the NSAIDs currently approved for use in the treatment of horses inhibit both COX-1 and COX-2 enzymes and should be used in the lowest dosage possible for horses with intestinal mucosal disease because all can inhibit normal regeneration of the intestinal mucosa.

DRUGS USED IN THE EMERGENCY MANAGEMENT OF RESPIRATORY DISORDERS
Bronchodilators
ATROPINE
- Administration:

CAUTION: Use only at low dosage for bronchodilator effect, 7-10 mg/450-kg adult IV, IM, or SQ q12-24h for 1 day only.

- Incompatibility: Do not mix with sodium bicarbonate
- Contraindications:
  - Severe tachycardia
  - Ileus
  - When combined with epinephrine, dobutamine or dopamine can increase risk of arrhythmia

CLENBUTEROL HYDROCHLORIDE
- Indication: β_2-adrenergic agonist, bronchodilator with minimal cardiac side effects. Antagonized by β-adrenergic blockers.

PHARMACOLOGY

- Used to manage airway obstruction such as that which occurs with COPD in horses.
- Loading dosage not required or recommended.
- Exists as a palatable syrup.
- Not intended for treatment of horses used for human consumption.
- Stability: Stable at room temperature.
- Contraindications:
  - Antagonizes the effects of prostaglandin-$F_{2\alpha}$ and oxytocin. Should not be used to treat pregnant mares "near term" unless delayed labor is the intention.
  - Can produce tachycardia as well as other cardiac changes including but not limited to altered heart rate, blood pressure changes, and electrocardiographic changes.
  - Do not use to treat individuals with suspected cardiovascular impairment.
- Impairment of reproductive performance in breeding stallions and mares has not been found.
- Adverse reactions: Mild sweating, muscle tremors, restlessness, urticaria, and tachycardia observed in some patients in the first few days of treatment. May increase serum creatine kinase levels. Ataxia observed in 1.3% of 239 horses in clinical trials.
- Dosing schedule as per package insert (Boehringer Ingelheim Vetmedica, Inc. St. Joseph, MO 64506; (800) 325-9167).
  - Initial dosage: 0.5 ml/100 lb (0.8 µg/kg) for 3 days (6 treatments). If no improvement, administer 1.0 ml/100 lb (1.6 µg/kg) for 3 days (6 treatments). If no improvement, administer 1.5 ml/100 lb (2.4 µg/kg) for 3 days (6 treatments). If no improvement, administer 2 ml/100 lb (3.2 µg/kg) for 3 days (6 treatments). If no improvement, patient is not responsive to clenbuterol, and treatment should be discontinued.
  - Recommended duration of treatment at effective dose is 30 days. At the end of this 30-day treatment period, drug should be withdrawn to assess for recurrence of signs. If signs return, the 30-day regimen may be repeated. If treatment is repeated, the stepwise dosage schedule should be used.

ALBUTEROL
- Contraindications:
  - Do not use to treat hypokalemic patients.
  - May delay labor in pregnant mares at term or uterine involution during the postpartum period.
  - Erratically absorbed when administered orally.
  - Useful for nebulization or metered-dose inhalation (approved for use in the horse).

AMINOPHYLLINE
- Drug interaction: Used with **caution** in foals treated with erythromycin because hepatic metabolism of theophylline (cytochrome P-450 system) can be delayed, causing toxicity (CNS signs). Rifampin can increase the rate of elimination.
- Administration: If administered intravenously, aminophylline can be mixed in most intravenous fluid solutions.

NOTE: Therapeutic index (10 µg/ml) to toxic (20 µg/ml) range is very narrow in horses.

- Has some beneficial effects in addition to bronchodilation, such as delaying diaphragmatic fatigue and immune modulation (antiinflammatory effects).

GLYCOPYRROLATE
- Administration: Has a pH of 2 to 3; do not mix in a solution with alkaline drugs or fluids.

DOXAPRAM HYDROCHLORIDE
- Compatibility: Do not mix with alkaline solutions (e.g., sodium bicarbonate or aminophylline).
- Use: Controversial. Main indication is primary apnea, and most cases of apnea are believed secondary to asphyxia or drug overdosage. Regardless, doxapram has been reported to be successful in the treatment of many apneic foals when used very early. Doxapram can be used for apnea when mechanical ventilation is impractical, but it should *not* be used if mechanical ventilation is available and should be supplemented with oxygen if feasible, because as the respiratory rate and depth of breathing increase, oxygen demand increases.
- Can be administered by injection in the umbilical vessels or jugular vein, for example, or can be placed on the tongue.

INHALATION DRUG THERAPY
- Aerosol metered-dose canisters
  - Beclomethasone, 500-1200 µg/450-kg adult q12h
  - Ipratropium, 720-1000 µg/450 kg q8-12h
  - Fluticasone, 1000 µg/450 kg q12h
  - Cromolyn, 200 mg/450 kg q12h
  - Albuterol, 720 µg/450 kg q6h
  - Clenbuterol, 200 µg/450 kg q8h
  - All are relatively safe when administered by aerosolization

Nebulization
- Brochodilators
  - Albuterol, 0.5% solution (5 mg/ml), 0.25-0.50 ml for foal and 1-2 ml for an adult
- Antibiotics
  - Amikacin, 250 mg or more depending on size of patient
  - Gentamicin, 100 mg or more

  Administration without a bronchodilator can cause respiratory distress
  Systemic absorption occurs and must be considered as a potential nephrotoxin, especially if nephrotoxic drugs are given systemically

- Mucolytic
  - Acetylcysteine, 10% solution, 2.5-5.0 ml
- Surfactant
  - Can be nebulized but ideally is administered through a nasotracheal tube
  - 100 mg/kg divided into four lung quadrants by turning and rolling the foal; lower doses can be used

Do not use antibiotics, mucolytics, or steroids in nebulizer without bronchodilators.

CORTICOSTEROIDS

- Administered intravenously, corticosteroids are best given as a bolus rather than mixed in intravenous solutions.
- Can cause hepatic lipidosis and elevation in serum γ-glutamyl transferase concentration when used for prolonged periods.
- Can cause late-term abortion in mares when administered in very high dosages (e.g., dexamethasone, 0.2 mg/kg for 3 consecutive days).
- If a corticosteroid is used to manage CNS inflammation or septic shock (empirical) a rapid-acting water-soluble agent (e.g., dexamethasone sodium phosphate or prednisolone sodium succinate or acetate) should be used.

Dexamethasone

- Store only at room temperature.
- Administration: Intravenous or intramuscular in emergency situations because oral bioavailability is variable.
- Indications: Commonly used to manage:
  - Acute, noncardiogenic edema.
  - Nonseptic respiratory disease.
  - Severe COPD.
  - Interstitial pneumonia.
  - Cerebrospinal trauma and inflammation: Efficacy not demonstrated!
  - Shock: Efficacy not demonstrated!

NOTE: Dexamethasone has been occasionally reported to cause laminitis. Use this drug with caution to treat patients with laminitis. It is frequently used in the dexamethasone suppression test without adverse effects.

Prednisone, Prednisolone

- Metabolism: Prednisone is converted to the active drug prednisolone by the liver. In horses prednisone is either poorly absorbed or is poorly converted to prednisolone.

NOTE: Do not use prednisone to treat individuals with severe hepatic dysfunction. Because of the poor bioavailability of prednisone, it is rarely administered orally to horses.

Methylprednisolone Sodium Succinate (Solu-Medrol)

- This is not Solu-Delta Cortef; however it is a methyl derivative reported in some studies to be effective in the management of acute CNS injury.
- Dosage is 5.4 mg/kg per hour immediately before expected CNS trauma (e.g., manipulation of cervical compressive myelopathy) or immediately (within 30 minutes) after CNS trauma. It is very expensive!

Triamcinolone

- Adverse effects: For unknown reasons, use of triamcinolone is reported to be associated with a higher incidence of laminitis than is use of other corticosteroids!

Pentoxifylline

- Can make red blood cells more deformable, decrease blood viscosity, and inhibit some inflammatory cytokines.

- Can be administered orally or can be dissolved, filtered, and administered intravenously.

Allopurinol
- A xanthine oxidase inhibitor used in early therapy for neonatal maladjustment syndrome with the goal of preventing oxidative damage in the brain.
- Research results indicate this drug would be of little or no benefit in the management of large-colon reperfusion injury.

INTRAVENOUS FLUIDS (ADJUNCTS)
Calcium Salts
- Compatibility: Calcium gluconate and calcium chloride are compatible with most fluids and drugs, *except* tetracyclines, intravenous lipids, and sodium bicarbonate.
- Adverse effects: Calcium gluconate is considered less irritating and safer than is calcium chloride.
- Contraindications: There is some evidence that the use of calcium is contraindicated in resuscitation therapy because it may enhance cellular death.
- **Subcutaneous, intramuscular, or perivascular administration causes a severe local injection site reaction.**

Dimethyl Sulfoxide (DMSO)
- Storage: Airtight container away from light.
- Incompatibility: If DMSO is mixed with water, heat is produced, which can cause local irritation or blistering when this agent is applied to wet skin that is bandaged tightly or covered with plastic.
- *Always* dilute to a concentration less than 20% for parenteral administration.
- Most commonly diluted with 0.9% saline solution.
- Hemolysis and hemoglobinuria occur in some adults even with proper dilution; these effects usually are of no concern.

NOTE: Use only medical-grade DMSO.

- Frequently administered through a nasogastric tube, and adverse effects have not been proved.

Magnesium Sulfate
- Can be given intravenously or orally.
- May have some effect on inactivating N-methyl-D-aspartate receptors in the brain and therefore decreasing brain injury caused by hypoxia and ischemia. Administer magnesium sulfate ($MgSO_4$), 50 mg/kg per hour IV for 1 hour then continue with 25 mg/kg per hour for 24-48 hours.
- Can be administered *slowly* IV as a 10% $MgSO_4$ solution, 100 g/L water, to individuals with severe hypomagnesemia.
- Can be mixed with calcium borogluconate for the management of hypomagnesemia.
- Use caution in administration of magnesium, either intravenously or orally, to patients with decreased renal function and/or severe hypotension.

Hyperimmune Serum
- Administer slowly intravenously.

PHARMACOLOGY

- Adverse effects, probably resulting from endotoxin in the product, have been reported.

Equine Plasma
- Administration: Administer at a moderately fast rate, 20-40 ml/kg per hour, and monitor closely for signs of adverse reaction (trembling, rapid respiration). *Adverse reactions are rare.*
- Pretreatment with antihistamine may prevent adverse reactions and maintain albumin in the intravascular space for a longer time, but this step generally is not performed.
- Indications:
  - Ideal fluid for most emergency and life-threatening conditions. Hetastarch and crystalloids (isotonic or hypertonic) can be used while plasma is thawing.
  - Shock.
  - Hypoalbuminemia, edema.
  - Synergistic with polyionic crystalloids.
- Heparin, 40-100 mg/kg body weight as total initial dose, can be mixed in plasma before administration to activate antithrombin III.
- Both normal plasma and hyperimmune plasma (high antibody against endotoxin or *Rhodococcus equi*) are available.

Hetastarch
- Colloidal solution frequently used in combination with crystalloids as a plasma volume expander in the management of shock and reperfusion type injuries.
- Do not use to manage hemorrhagic shock or in the presence of prolonged coagulation time; otherwise very safe for horses.
- Colloidal property approximately 30 mm (plasma approximately 20 mm).
- Frequently used with crystalloids (isotonic or hypertonic) as initial therapy for inflammatory shock (SIRS) while plasma is being thawed.
- Dosage: There is no correct dosage, because any quantity can be beneficial; 5-10 ml/kg is frequently used.
- Beneficial effects expected for 24-36 hours.

Phosphorus
- Available in most bovine milk fever preparations; Fleet enema mixed in crystalloids is an alternative.

Hypertonic Saline Solution
- Frequently used for severe hypovolemia and hypotension.
- Has beneficial effects of rapid and dramatic intravascular expansion with only a small administration volume, 4-8 ml/kg.
- Added advantage of:
  - Decrease in pulmonary arterial pressure, which inhibits pulmonary edema formation.
  - Rapid diuresis.
- Do not use to treat chronically dehydrated patients, because intracellular water is severely depleted in these patients.
- Additional polyionic crystalloids recommended simultaneously or within 1.5 hours after administration of hypertonic saline solution to prevent "rebound" intravascular volume depletion.

- Do not use, or use only as last resort, to treat individuals with uncontrolled bleeding.
- Use carefully to treat foals because hypernatremia can become severe in some cases.

Sodium Bicarbonate
- Can be administered as a hypertonic (e.g., 5%-8.4%) solution to patients with severe metabolic acidosis (pH <7.1) and intravascular volume depletion.
- For severe metabolic acidosis without intravascular volume depletion, best administered as an isotonic solution, 1.25% (100-g sodium bicarbonate in 8 L of sterile water).
- Do not use in the following situations:
  □ When hypokalemia is present.
  □ In respiratory acidosis.
  □ In head trauma.
- Controversial for use in resuscitation.

Dextrose
- Frequently added to crystalloids for IV fluid treatment of foals (solution generally 5%-10% dextrose).
- Do *not* use as sole source of fluid replacement in dehydrated patients.
- Avoid excessive administration and prolonged or severe hyperglycemia.
- Not recommended for use in resuscitation unless hypoglycemia is present.

Oxyglobin (Polymerized Bovine Hemoglobin)
- Ideal treatment for acute life-threatening anemia when whole-blood transfusion is not readily available. This product should be viewed as a temporary treatment to gain time for whole-blood transfusion.
- Cross-matching not required.
- Readily available, no refrigeration, shelf-life 2 years.
- Clinical effect lasts approximately 24 hours.
- No toxicity demonstrated in foals, although this agent is both a potent colloid and a nitric oxide scavenger, which can increase blood pressure through increases in intravascular volume and vasopressor effects, respectively. Use oxyglobin with caution in the management of uncontrolled hemorrhage (uterine artery rupture) and pulmonary hypertension (hypoxic, respiratory distress in foals).

CARDIAC DRUGS
β_1-Agonist
DOBUTAMINE
- Stability: Use diluted solutions within 24 hours.
- Compatible with most intravenous fluid solutions except lidocaine, aminophylline, furosemide, and sodium bicarbonate and is compatible with most other β- and α-agonists in the same solution. Do not mix with other drugs, including calcium chloride or gluconate, heparin, furosemide, or digoxin.
- Indications: To improve cardiac output when fluid therapy is unsuccessful or cannot be used. Synergistic when administered with nitroprusside or other vasodilators to improve peripheral circulation.

PHARMACOLOGY

- Solution preparation:
  - 1 vial (250 mg) in 1000 ml = 250 μg/ml.
  - Minidrip set = 60 drops (1 ml).
  - Normal drip set = 10 drops/1 ml (Baxter), 15 drops/1 ml (Abbott).

CAUTION is needed for calculating the dosage rate (generally 2-10 μg/kg per minute) because of the potency of dobutamine. Monitor for arrhythmias and discontinue administration if necessary.

- Dobutamine is the preferred drug for improving cardiac output (mostly through increased heart rate) in hypotensive patients that have not responded adequately to volume replacement.

β_1- and β_2-Agonist
ISOPROTERENOL
- Compatible with most fluids, however not with sodium bicarbonate, lidocaine, aminophylline, and furosemide
- Indications: Because of many adverse effects on the heart and blood pressure, rarely indicated except for increasing ventricular rate

β_1- and α_1-Agonist
DOPAMINE
- Solution stability: Use diluted solutions within 24 hours.
- Compatible with most other β- and α-agonists and with mannitol.
- Incompatibility: Furosemide, sodium bicarbonate, lidocaine, and potassium penicillin. More likely than dobutamine to be compatible with other drugs.
- Preparation of solution:
  - Add 5-ml vial (80 mg/ml) to 1 L of 0.9% saline solution or D_5W for 400 μg/ml.
  - Minidrop set = 60 drops (1 ml).
  - Normal drop set = 10 drops (1 ml).
- Pharmacologic properties and indications:
  - At lower dosage, 1-5 μg/kg per minute, dopamine may act primarily at renal dopaminergic receptors (use in renal failure with normal cardiac output).
  - At medium dose, 5-10 μg/kg per minute, dopamine stimulates β_1-adrenergic receptors (use in renal failure without normal cardiac output or non-cardiogenic shock with normal or high-normal central venous pressure).
  - At higher dosages, >10 μg/kg per minute, dopamine stimulates α effects and increases vascular tone (increased blood pressure with possible decrease in renal, splenic, **intestinal,** and coronary blood flow).
  - Use in the management of severe hypotension that is unresponsive to fluid therapy.
  - Use with caution. If heart rate increases 50% above normal, arrhythmias develop, and hypertension can occur. Discontinue administration.

β_1-, β_2-, and α_1-Agonist
EPINEPHRINE
- Incompatible with sodium bicarbonate, furosemide, lidocaine, hypertonic saline solution, and aminophylline.

NOTE: Does not have to be diluted in the treatment of adults when administered through the jugular vein.

▷ ▪ Indications:
  - □ Anaphylaxis: Drug of choice (antihistamines may enhance the effect of epinephrine).
  - □ Cardiac resuscitation: Drug of choice.
▪ Routes of administration:
  - □ Intravenous: Immediate effect—0.01-0.05 mg/kg (1 ml of 1:1000/50 kg) administered every 3-5 min.
  - □ Intratracheal: Effect within 5 minutes; larger dosage (2×-10×) may be needed.
  - □ Intramuscular: Effect within 5-10 minutes.
  - □ Subcutaneous: Effect within 10 minutes.
  - □ Intracardiac (injection above left lateral thoracic vein on left chest): *Rarely indicated.* Effect is immediate.
▪ Contraindications:
  - □ Shock with causes other than anaphylaxis. May increase oxygen demand and undesirable peripheral perfusion associated with β- and α-responses.
  - □ Do not inject undiluted into a small vessel.

α_1-*Adrenergics*

NOREPINEPHRINE
▪ Used to increase urine output in inflammatory shock (SIRS) when fluids and inotropic agents have failed.
▪ Has some β_1-agonist effect.
▪ Dosage 0.5-1.5 µg/kg per minute on the basis of blood pressure and urine output response
▪ May be administered in conjunction with dobutamine.
▪ Do not use with sodium bicarbonate, lidocaine, furosemide, or aminophylline.

PHENYLEPHRINE
▪ Compatible with all common intravenous preparations. Do not use with lidocaine.
▪ Indications:
  - □ Splenic contraction (3 µg/kg per minute) to correct left colon displacement.
  - □ To increase blood pressure during general anesthesia when dopamine or dobutamine may not be desirable owing to their arrhythmogenic properties and *after* intravenous fluids have been unsuccessful.
  - □ Topically as a hemostatic agent and to reduce nasal pharyngeal edema.

PHENYLPROPANOLAMINE HYDROCHLORIDE
▪ Indications: Used commonly in the treatment of patients to increase urethral sphincter tone (0.5-2.0 mg/kg PO q12h).
▪ Adverse effects: Restlessness, sweating, tachycardia.

PHENOXYBENZAMINE
▪ An α-**antagonist**
▪ May be used to relax urethral tone in herpes myelitis

VASOPRESSIN (ADH)
▪ Used in poorly responsive severe shock or CPR to increase blood pressure.
▪ May lead to a larger redirection of blood flow to the brain compared to epinephrine.

PHARMACOLOGY

- May inhibit or reverse the pathologic vasodilator changes occurring in shock.
- Should not be used when renal failure is present or a clinical concern.
- Dose for resuscitation 0.4-0.8 units/kg IV.

VASODILATOR DRUGS

Nitric Oxide Gas

- Inhaled nitric oxide gas may be "piggy backed" into the oxygen line in a 1:5-1:9 ratio for pulmonary hypertension.
- Should have minimal effect on systemic blood pressure at this dosage.

Nitroglycerin (Ointment)

- Primarily indicated for hypertension (e.g., laminitis, obesity syndrome, some cases of renal failure, pheochromocytoma).
- Efficacy in laminitis unproved.
- At low dosages, has primary vasodilator effect on venules but at higher dosages also relaxes arterioles.
- Wear gloves when applying.
- Do not use to treat hypotensive patients!
- Tolerance occurs, however proper interval therapy is unknown (e.g., 3 days on, 3 days off).
- Also may be used for pulmonary arterial hypertension.
- Part of treatment for heart failure to decrease resistance.

Isoxsuprine

- Administered orally does **not** increase digital blood flow
- Bioavailability very low after oral administration

Hydralazine

- Compatible with most isotonic intravenous fluid solutions and dobutamine.
- Indications:
  - In heart failure, to decrease afterload and improve cardiac output. Primary effect is to decrease arteriolar smooth-muscle contractions and arteriolar resistance to blood flow (see p. 173).
- Monitor heart rate carefully.

Enalapril (Angiotensin-Converting Enzyme Inhibitor)

- Compatibility: Most intravenous isotonic fluids; stable in solution for 24 hours
- Indications: Same as for hydralazine

Acepromazine

- See p. 658.

Phenoxybenzamine

- See p. 671.

Magnesium Sulfate

- See p. 667.

ANTIARRHYTHMIC DRUGS

Lidocaine

- Compatible with most intravenous solutions
- Incompatible with dopamine, epinephrine, dobutamine, isoproterenol, norepinephrine, ampicillin, and cefazolin
- Indications:
  - Antiarrhythmic (see p. 156)
  - Enhances intestinal motility (see p. 223)
  - Analgesic effect, either during anesthesia or in the awake horse
  - May also have some benefit in the management of endotoxic shock by decreasing neutrophil adherence
- Adverse effects (see Table 34–6)

CAUTION: For intravenous administration, make certain the lidocaine product does *not* contain epinephrine.

Quinidine

- Drug interactions:
  - Increases digoxin levels
  - Sodium bicarbonate decreases excretion
- Indications (see p. 143)
- Adverse effects (see Box 34–1 and Table 34–6)
  - Potentiated with hypokalemia or dehydration

Propranolol (β-Blocker)

- Administration: Do not combine with sodium bicarbonate
- Indications (see Table 34–5)
- Adverse effects (see Table 34–6)
  - Do not use in the treatment of patients with COPD

Phenytoin

- Administration: If solution for intravenous use is needed, it is available commercially or can be prepared, filtered, and administered with sodium bicarbonate
- Indications:
  - Digitalis-induced ventricular arrhythmias
  - Anticonvulsive therapy: Generally administered orally
  - Myopathy: Generally administered orally

Magnesium Sulfate

- Calcium channel blocker
- Use to treat ventricular tachycardia (see p. 159)
  - 4 mg/kg bolus q2min up to 50 mg/kg total dosage
- Has vasodilatory properties: Do not use in hypotensive conditions.
- Used to protect against reperfusion injury: 0.2-0.5 g/kg continually IV q24h

Bretylium Tosylate

- Use for ventricular arrhythmias unresponsive to lidocaine.
- Can cause severe hypotension!

PHARMACOLOGY

Positive Inotropic Drugs for the Management of Heart Failure
DIGOXIN (FOR INJECTION)
- Compatible with most intravenous solutions of near-normal pH. Incompatible with dobutamine.
- Orally administered digoxin is best used as follow-up treatment after intravenous digoxin or in a nonemergency situation.
- Indications: Heart failure (*except ionophore toxicity*) and supraventricular tachycardia (see pp. 153, 172-174 and Table 34–4).
- Contraindications: Do not use in the presence of ionophore toxicity.
- Adverse effects (see Table 34–6).
- Drug interactions:
  - Diazepam, tetracycline, quinidine, and erythromycin can increase the serum concentration of digoxin.
  - Hypokalemia (e.g., furosemide [Lasix] administration) can increase toxicity.

DIGITOXIN
- Indications, adverse effects, and drug interactions same as for digoxin.
- Digitoxin may be used instead of digoxin in the presence of renal insufficiency because digitoxin is metabolized by the liver.

DIURETICS
Furosemide
- Storage: A precipitate occurs with refrigeration, but the drug resolubilizes after warming without loss of potency
- May turn brown when exposed to air; however, it is usable if not past expiration date
- Compatible with all intravenous fluids. Incompatible with dobutamine, epinephrine, and aminoglycosides
- Indications:
  - Congestive heart failure
  - Pulmonary edema
  - Edema, especially noninflammatory
  - Oliguric renal failure when used with dopamine/dobutamine or mannitol
  - Inflammatory and septic shock: Controversial because it decreases cardiac output
- Contraindications:
  - Hypokalemia
  - Dehydration
  - May enhance digitalis, aminophylline, and aminoglycoside toxicity

Acetazolamide
- Compatible with all intravenous fluid solutions
- Oral administration is most common
- Indication: Hyperkalemia
- May increase gastric pH

Trichlormethiazide-Dexamethasone
- Indication: Use orally for nonseptic inflammatory edema (e.g., vasculitis)

Mannitol
- Precipitation occurs if mannitol is cooled or mixed with high-chloride–containing fluids
- Indications:
  - Cerebral edema, CNS ischemia, hypoxemia
  - Renal failure: Controversial, not anuric
  - To decrease ocular pressure
- Contraindications:
  - Progressive cerebral hemorrhage
  - Anuric renal failure

DRUGS SPECIFICALLY FOR MUSCLE DISORDERS
Methocarbamol
- Administration: Drug should be precipitate-free for intravenous injection. Do not administer by the subcutaneous route; perivascular administration is irritating.
- Sedation and ataxia may occur.

Dantrolene Sodium
- Storage: Use reconstituted product for injection within 6 hours and protect from light.
- Do not mix with saline solution or dextrose.

Phenytoin
- See p. 673.

NEUROMUSCULAR BLOCKING AGENTS
Succinylcholine
- Administration: Incompatible with sodium bicarbonate.
  - Do *not* use to treat Quarter Horses with genetic defect for hyperkalemia.
  - If succinylcholine is used for cesarean section, mechanical ventilation may be needed for the foal.
  - Do *not* use for debilitated, exhausted, or excited individuals recently treated with an organophosphate.
- Dosages higher than 0.088 mg/kg cause respiratory paralysis.
- Does not provide analgesia!
- Indications:
  - For muscle relaxation during surgery with mechanical ventilation and when atracurium is not available.
  - For muscle relaxation to remove physically entrapped horse when general anesthesia is not indicated or is unavailable.
  - Do not use if active bleeding is occurring.
  - In combination with euthanasia solution to prevent agonal movement (gasping).

Atracurium
- Neuromuscular blocking drug, preferred for horses because of minimal cardiovascular side effects

PHARMACOLOGY

- Onset of action is slower than that of succinylcholine
- Indications:
  - Muscle relaxation during surgery with mechanical ventilation
  - Muscle relaxation in foals receiving mechanical ventilation
  - Can be reversed with neostigmine, 0.06 mg/kg IV, after atropine, 0.02 mg/kg

MISCELLANEOUS DRUGS

Aminocaproic Acid
- Administration: Dilute in intravenous fluids
- Frequently used for uncontrolled bleeding when surgery is not an option

Cyproheptadine
- Safety: Reproductive safety has not been demonstrated, however this agent has been used frequently in pregnant mares without reported adverse effects
- Frequently used for management of pituitary adenoma (efficacy questionable)
- Used to control photophobic head shaking

Heparin Sodium
- Administration: Do not mix in solutions containing aminoglycosides.
- Can be mixed with fresh frozen plasma (40-100 U/kg body weight) before administration of plasma to activate antithrombin III activity as part of shock therapy.
- Compatible with total parenteral nutrition solutions.
- Contraindications: Do not administer intramuscularly.

➤ | **NOTE:** Blood gas values may be erroneous if heparin is more than 10% of the sample.

- Monitor the coagulation panel if heparin is used to manage hyperlipemic syndrome.

Insulin (Regular)
- Administration: Adheres to bottles, bags, and tubing unless "rinsed" first with other fluids
- Compatible with total parenteral nutrition, dextrose, potassium chloride, and other intravenous fluids (*except sodium bicarbonate*); however, bag should be mixed intermittently
- Indications:
  - Hyperlipemia: Controversial but may lower blood glucose concentration
  - Septic and inflammatory shock (used with glucose, potassium chloride, and magnesium); controversial
- Contraindications: Hypoglycemia and hypokalemia

Naloxone
- Administration: Do not mix in fluids with an alkaline pH.

Vasopressin
- Administration: Dilute in saline solution or D_5W and administer slowly in aqueous suspension only (see p. 671).

Oxytocin
- Administration: Dosage >20 IU/450-kg mare may cause "colicky" signs.

Domperidone
- Dopamine agonist
- Available from compounding pharmacies

Prostaglandins
FLUPROSTENOL SODIUM
DINOPROST TROMETHAMINE
- Contraindications: Do not use to treat individuals with COPD.

▶ **CAUTION:** Abortifacient for both humans and horses!

MISOPROSTOL
- See p. 661.

Progesterones
- Altrenogest: Synthetic progestational agent. Used orally, 0.044 mg/kg, with the goal of supporting pregnancy in mares experiencing endotoxemia, colic, systemic illness, or placentitis. If treatment is to be discontinued, gradual reduction over 2 weeks is recommended by some clinicians.
- Progesterone in oil for intramuscular injection used for purposes outlined previously and when oral route is not an option. Dosage: 0.3-0.6 mg/kg IM once a day. Product is available only through veterinary compounding pharmacies.

▶ CONSIDERATIONS FOR DRUG THERAPY IN THE NEONATAL FOAL
- Renal excretion of most drugs is approximately equal to that of adults.
- Premature foals may need prolonged treatment intervals if drug is excreted predominantly by the kidneys, particularly drugs with potential toxicity (e.g., aminoglycosides).
  - Trough and peak (30-60 min) concentrations ideally should be determined.
- Hepatic metabolism is slower in foals than in adults. The time of delayed metabolism varies owing to drug-induced enhanced activity. Sulfonamides, phenobarbital, trimethoprim, NSAIDs, diazepam, metronidazole, and theophylline may require extended dosing intervals and, in the case of inhalant anesthesia, lower concentrations. This has not been documented to be a clinically important concern.
- The albumin concentration in young foals is approximately that of adults. Protein binding is not very different between age groups. If hypoalbuminemia, as from enteritis, is present, highly protein-bound drugs such as diazepam, sulfas, and NSAIDs may have an enhanced effect. This effect may be partially offset by more rapid elimination.
- Extracellular fluid volume in neonatal foals is nearly double that of adults. The results are decreased blood concentration and prolonged excretion of many drugs. In the management of life-threatening infection, it may be advisable to administer a larger loading dosage (approximately 30% larger than an adult dose) and use prolonged treatment intervals to compensate for delayed metabolism or elimination. For example: amikacin, 25 mg/kg loading dose.

PHARMACOLOGY

- Oral absorption of many drugs may be more variable (usually increased absorption) in foals than in weanlings, yearlings, or adults.

DRUG DOSING ADJUSTMENTS IN RENAL FAILURE

- Discontinue all nephrotoxic drugs if possible.
- If it is absolutely necessary to administer potentially nephrotoxic drugs during renal failure, the interval of the treatments should be prolonged in accordance with the estimated decline in glomerular filtration rate (GFR). For example, occasionally it is necessary to continue aminoglycosides, tetracycline, polymyxin, sulfonamides, or NSAIDs despite an abnormally low GFR. A Thoroughbred mare with a creatinine concentration of 2.2-2.4 mg/dl conceivably has only 50% normal GFR. Therefore if any of the above treatments are required, the treatment interval should be doubled. Intravenous fluids also should be provided. There are more elaborate methods of estimating GFR (e.g., radionuclide studies), but serum creatinine concentration generally provides a reasonable estimate in a euvolemic (normal water content) patient. Most light-breed horses and foals have serum creatinine concentrations between 0.9 and 1.4 mg/dl. Quarter Horses may have a normal value as high as 2.1 mg/dl. The value in some foals born of mares with placentitis may be very high for the first 3 days of life without any abnormality in GFR.
- Increasing the interval of administration generally is preferred to decreasing dosage, although either method may be used.
- Measurement of peak and trough levels is ideal if assays are available.
- For drugs that are not nephrotoxic but eliminated almost entirely by the kidney (e.g. digoxin), similar adjustments should be made if there is concern about toxic effects. Many drugs (e.g., penicillins, doxycycline, cephalosporins, lidocaine, and barbiturates) do not require interval or dosage adjustments.

DRUG DOSING ADJUSTMENT IN LIVER FAILURE

- Prolongation of interval of treatment should be considered for potentially toxic drugs excreted predominantly by the liver (e.g., lidocaine, and metronidazole).
- Foals younger than 2 weeks *may* also have decreased hepatic clearance of these and other drugs such as diazepam, barbiturates, and aminophylline.

Information for the previous section is summarized from personal experience, various publications, and specifically Plumb DC: Veterinary drug handbook, ed 3, Ames, Iowa, 1999, Iowa State University Press. Plumb's handbook is an excellent pharmacology reference for equine clinicians.

ADVERSE DRUG REACTIONS

Thomas J. Divers

IMPORTANT ADVERSE DRUG REFERENCE INFORMATION

Drug Interaction
(888) FDAVETS

Director of Center for Veterinary Medicine
(301) 827-3800

United States Department of Agriculture
Veterinary Biologics and Diagnostics Hotline
(800) 752-6255 weekdays 8:00 A.M. to 4:30 P.M. CT
(message service after hours)
www.aphis.usda.gov/vs/cvb/ic/adverseeventreport.htm

National Animal Poison Control Center Hotline
(888) 426-4435

Veterinary Practitioners' Reporting Program
(800) 487-7776

FDA Internet Home Page
www.cvm.fda.gov

INTRACAROTID INJECTIONS

Many of the immediate adverse reactions to parenterally administered xylazine, detomidine, phenylbutazone, and trimethoprim-sulfadiazine are probably the result of inadvertent intracarotid injections.

Water-Soluble Intracarotid Drugs

These include acepromazine, detomidine, some barbiturates, and xylazine.

CLINICAL SIGNS
- Immediate *hyperexcitability* and possibly *collapse.*
- Seizure or coma may follow.

TREATMENT
- Usually can be successfully managed by sedation with pentobarbital or phenobarbital, 5-12 mg/kg IV (or to effect) q12h or as needed.
- Alternatively, administer chloral hydrate intravenously to effect as a relatively safe sedative.
- Administer antiinflammatory, edema-reducing drugs (e.g., DMSO), 1 g/kg, or dexamethasone, 0.5 mg/kg.
- Some patients may remain recumbent for several hours or days before standing.
- Manage wounds and corneal trauma that may occur as a result of the seizure.
- Cortical blindness occurs in some cases.
  - Include antiedema therapy:
    - DMSO, 1 mg/kg IV diluted in polyionic crystalloid fluid.
    - Dexamethasone, 0.2 mg/kg IV.
    - Mannitol (20%), 0.25-2.0 g/kg slowly IV.

Oil-Based Intracarotid Drugs

These include propylene glycol, trimethoprim-sulfadiazine, diazepam, procaine penicillin, and phenylbutazone.

CLINICAL SIGNS
- Seizure, collapse, and rapid death.

- Contralateral cortical blindness is a frequent finding among patients that survive.
- Cerebral hemorrhage often is present.

TREATMENT
- If the patient does not die immediately, administer treatment as for water-soluble drugs.

FLUNIXIN MEGLUMINE
- Intracarotid injection does not produce signs as severe as those of some of the drugs listed earlier. May produce neurologic signs such as ataxia and hysteria, hyperventilation, and muscle weakness. These signs are transient, according to the package insert, and require no antidote.

NOTE: When a 20-gauge needle is used to penetrate the carotid artery, blood may not spurt from needle hub.

Not all reactions to the drugs mentioned are the result of inadvertent intracarotid injection. For example, procaine penicillin can cause procaine reactions when the drug is inadvertently administered in a small vessel. This is more common among individuals receiving long-term injections in the same muscle mass. Similarly, acute tachypnea may follow xylazine or detomidine injections. This reaction usually is not fatal, however in a rare case may cause fatal pulmonary edema. Injectable trimethoprim-sulfadiazine can cause fatal reactions when detomidine is administered intravenously along with intravenous trimethoprim-sulfadiazine (Table 52–1).

Air Emboli
Catheters become disconnected frequently in equine practice, and in the majority of cases there is no problem with air emboli. If the horse keeps its head high, there is greater risk for air aspiration than when the head is lowered when bleeding from a disconnected intravenous catheter. If the air remains on the venous side, which is the usual case, clinical signs are those of poor perfusion and hypoxemia, elevated heart and respiratory rate, discolored mucous membranes, trembling, weakness, and disorientation. A bubbling or swishing sound may be heard at cardiac auscultation, and an ultrasound examination reveals air in the right side of the heart. Treatment includes intranasal oxygen and flunixin meglumine. If the problem is serious, place a long catheter through the jugular vein into the right atrium and remove the air. If the problem is severe enough to cause arrest, perform cardiac massage. In the rare instance, the air may pass to the arterial side, in which case neurologic signs predominate (e.g., seizure). Therapy for arterial air emboli includes seizure management: Pentobarbital, 5-12 mg/kg IV, oxygen, mannitol, fluids to decrease viscosity, aspirin, and pentoxifylline.

ACUTE ANAPHYLAXIS, POSSIBLE WITH ANY DRUG
Anaphylactic reactions are most frequent with intravenous administration of vaccines, occasionally penicillin, *selenium*, phytonadione (vitamin K), and other vitamins and minerals. In most cases, this is not a result of previous sensitization and antigen-antibody reaction but is an immediate "triggering" of the complement-kinin system caused by some part of the drug.

TABLE 52–1. Specific Acute Drug Reactions and Recommended Treatments

Drug	Clinical Signs and Overdose Information	Treatment
Acepromazine	Weakness, sweating, pale membranes, death, low PCV (chronic), penile paralysis	4 ml/kg hypertonic saline solution IV for hypotension (for paraphimosis, see p. 472)
Albuterol	Tremors, tachycardia, CNS excitement, some of which may be caused by hypokalemia	Usually requires no treatment, however, check serum K^+; if hypokalemia present, administer supplemental K^+
Altrenogest, oral	Colic, sweating rarely reported. Avoid human skin exposure.	Symptomatic
Aminoglycoside antibiotics	A single dose even 10× normal dosage is unlikely to cause clinical problems. Treatment of a dehydrated patient with aminoglycosides is the most common predisposing factor for aminoglycoside toxicity.	IV fluid therapy (see urinary chapter); monitoring serum creatinine values and urine production is advisable for prevention.
	Weakness due to neuromuscular blockade occurs rarely, unless other neuromuscular blocking drugs are administered or a neuromuscular disease (e.g., *botulism*) is present	If it occurs, neuromuscular blockage can be reversed with neostigmine, 0.01 mg/kg SQ, or slowly administered calcium IV mixed in polyionic fluids
Aminophylline (theophylline)	Seizures, tachydysrhythmia	If possible, discontinue drugs that reduce clearance: H_2 blockers, enrofloxacin, erythromycin. Administer phenobarbital to control seizures and enhance clearance. Keep serum concentration <15 µg/ml
Amitraz	Accidental exposure	See p. 692
Amphotericin B	Rarely recommended in treatment of horses, but can cause renal failure unless sodium diuresis is administered during treatment	See p. 531
Anthelmintics	Colic, diarrhea	Supportive; in most cases do not treat with atropine unless an organophosphate is used *and other clinical signs of organophosphate toxicity are present* (miosis, salivation)!
Atropine	Colic, abdominal distention	Analgesics plus neostigmine, 0.01-0.02 mg/kg SQ q2h or cecal trocarization
Barbiturates	Respiratory depression, hypothermia; irritating when administered perivascularly	Assisted respiration
Bethanechol	Rarely produces adverse effects other than salivation	None
Butorphanol	Head tremors, excitement, ataxia, death (rare). Most often occurs when used without tranquilizers	Xylazine

Continued…

PHARMACOLOGY

TABLE 52–1. Specific Acute Drug Reactions and Recommended Treatments *Continued*

Drug	Clinical Signs and Overdose Information	Treatment
Clenbuterol (see Albuterol)		
Detomidine	Do not administer with IV trimethoprim-sulfamethoxazole or sulfadiazine; sweating, cardiovascular and respiratory depression, collapse	Yohimbine, 0.07-0.1 mg/kg, or tolazoline, 0.5-1 mg/kg IV
Diazepam	Ataxia; coma with massive overdosage	None for ataxia; flumazenil, 0.01 mg/kg slowly, for coma
Dichlorvos	Colic or signs of organo-phosphate toxicity (salivation, miosis, diarrhea); rarely neuro-muscular weakness	NSAID for colic. Atropine only if certain organophosphate toxicity has occurred
Digoxin	See pp. 172-174	See pp. 172-174
Dimethyl sulfoxide (DMSO)	Hemolysis; do not use in concentrations greater than 10% dextrose	No treatment required unless severe. Transfusion
Dinoprost tromethamine (prostaglandin $F_{2\alpha}$)	Colic, sweating	Usually none required
Dobutamine	Heart rate increases more than 30%-50%, arrhythmias	Usually none required; decrease rate of administration or stop infusion
Dopamine	Tachycardia, very irritating if perivascular, decreased GI perfusion	Usually none required; decrease rate of administration
Doxapram HCl	Seizures	Pentobarbital to effect, intranasal oxygen
Doxycycline	Collapse, death, supraven-tricular tachycardia, hyper-tension when administered IV	*Do not use IV*
Embutramide, mebezonium, tetracaine	CNS signs, hyperactivity	Sedation rarely needed
Epinephrine	Collapse	Usually none; monitor cardiac rhythm and blood pressure. A β-blocker proponent should be used only if hypertension is demonstrated
Epogen (recombinant human erythropoietin)	Nonregenerative anemia (possibly life-threatening) may develop in horses receiving one or usually more injections of this product. Diagnosis is by history, presence of non-regenerative anemia, or low or absent levels of erythropoietin (EPO Trac RIA, Incstar) 1 week or more after the last injection	Treatment is blood transfusion. Steroids are used but of unknown efficacy. Recovery can occur in many cases
Fentanyl	No adverse effect reported in horses, but could cause respiratory and CNS depression	Naloxone

TABLE 52–1. Specific Acute Drug Reactions and Recommended Treatments *Continued*

Drug	Clinical Signs and Overdose Information	Treatment
Flunixin meglumine	Injection site swelling most common. Collapse if administered into carotid artery	If swelling occurs, monitor closely for sepsis
Fluphenazine decanoate (Prolixin decanoate), a phenothiazine derivative that blocks dopamine receptors	Bizarre behavior, restlessness (refractory to treatment with xylazine), recumbency, seizure	Phenobarbital, 12 mg/kg, administered in 1 L over 20 minutes rather than by bolus; antihistamines (e.g., diphenhydramine). Supportive therapy, hypnotic therapy. Chloral hydrate to effect IV may be used in place of barbiturates
Fluprostenol sodium	Sweating, colic	Treatment generally not needed
Glycopyrrolate	Tenesmus, small-colon impaction, possible cardiovascular effects	Analgesics, oral and IV fluids for impaction
Guaifenesin	Toxic at high dosage (3× normal) causes hypotension	IV fluids
Halothane	Respiratory or cardiac depression, arrhythmia	Stop anesthesia; CPR if arrest occurs
Heparin	Anemia	Discontinue treatment; PCV should return to pretreatment values within 2-4 d
Hyaluronate sodium	Swollen joints, lameness. See *Polysulfated glycosaminoglycan*	NSAIDs, joint lavage, hydrotherapy, antibiotics (especially if swelling does not occur for several hours)
Imipramine	Tricyclic overdosage causes CNS signs and hypotension	Diazepam or phenobarbital for CNS signs; fluids with NaHCO$_3$ for hypotension
Insulin	Overdosage can lead to hypoglycemia	Check glucose and K and administer 20%-50% dextrose with KCl if needed. Save blood sample if malicious administration suspected.
Iron	In newborn foals, produces acute hepatic failure and death when administered PO before colostrum. Can cause acute collapse followed by hepatic or renal disease in some patients when administered IV	Fluids
Isoflurane	Respiratory or cardiac depression	CPR if arrest occurs, O$_2$ therapy, stop anesthesia
Isoxsuprine	When administered IV, can cause hyperexcitability and hypotension	Diazepam and IV fluids
Ivermectin (oral)	Rare severe systemic reaction, ventral abdominal swelling caused by death of *Onchocerca* microfilaria not unusual. Injection of ivermectin (SQ or IM) can result in severe local swelling	For *Onchocerca* reaction, symptomatic usually. If severe, steroids Supportive therapy for uncommon CNS signs in neonatal foals.

Continued...

TABLE 52–1. Specific Acute Drug Reactions and Recommended Treatments *Continued*

Drug	Clinical Signs and Overdose Information	Treatment
Ketamine (see p. 659)	Respiratory depression	Mechanical or physical ventilation
Ketoprofen	Injection site reactions; collapse and death with intracarotid administration	None
Lidocaine (see p. 673). *Do not use lidocaine with epinephrine IV.*	CNS signs, hypotension	Diazepam, hypertonic saline solution for hypotension
Lincomycin	*Contraindicated* in horses; severe colitis	IV fluids; metronidazole, 25 mg/kg PO q12h
Magnesium toxicity	Rare, can produce weakness and respiratory distress when administered to oliguric patients	IV fluids slowly with calcium borogluconate
Mannitol	Electrolyte imbalances, pulmonary edema if patient is anuric	Stop treatment if urination is inadequate.
Meperidine HCl	Overdosage may produce respiratory depression and hypotension. Excitement may occur when used without tranquilization!	Naloxone, 0.01 mg/kg IV, repeated if necessary, and IV fluids
Methocarbamol	Sedation and ataxia	Supportive
Metoclopramide HCl	Bizarre behavior, head tremors, ataxia	Diphenhydramine and *phenobarbital. Do not use tranquilizers.* Chloral hydrate can be administered to effect as a sedative
Misoprostol	High dosages can cause diarrhea and colic. Abortion in pregnant animals	Stop treatment or reduce dosage if diarrhea occurs, especially in foals.
Monensin (oral)	Increased heart rate, diarrhea, recumbency, death	Supportive (see pp. 183, 722)
Morphine sulfate, oxymorphone, and pentazocine	After IV administration, hyper-excitability, ataxia may occur when pretreatment with tranquilizers has not been administered. Large dosages may depress respiration.	Naloxone, 0.01 mg/kg IV, repeated if necessary. Efficacy of naloxone in treating drugs (pentazocine, butorphanol) with both opiate agonist and antagonist properties is unknown; therefore, use it cautiously.
Moxidectin	A leading cause of serious adverse reaction in foals <4 months of age! Coma, death, hypothermia, bradycardia, blindness. Identical signs reported in a premature foal treated with ivermectin.	With supportive treatment some recover.
Neostigmine	Colic	Analgesics and fluids
Nitric oxide (inhaled)	Has little effect on systemic blood pressure. High levels (>40 ppm) can cause methemoglobinemia	Methylene blue for confirmed methemoglobinemia

TABLE 52–1. Specific Acute Drug Reactions and Recommended Treatments *Continued*

Drug	Clinical Signs and Overdose Information	Treatment
Nitroglycerin ointment	If used for laminitis in a hypotensive patient, hypotension can worsen.	IV fluids; remove ointment. *Avoid human contact.*
Organophosphate anthelmintics, e.g., trichlorfon	Rarely causes signs, loose feces, diarrhea, increased salivation, sweating, colic, ataxia, death	Supportive treatment, fluids and analgesics. If classic signs (salivation, miosis) of organophosphate poisoning are present and overdosing is known to have occurred, administer atropine, 0.22 mg/kg. *Do not use atropine unless certain of organophosphate toxicity.*
Oxytetracycline	Rapid IV infusion can cause collapse and hemolysis. Large dosages (3 g) administered to foals only to treat contracted/deformed tendons rarely results in renal failure. Do not use >15 mg/kg per day for prolonged periods.	Treatment usually not required. IV fluid diuresis (see p. 531)
Oxytocin	Colic	Treatment usually not required
Penicillin	Procaine penicillin reactions are more common in patients receiving long term injections in the same muscle mass. **Heating procaine penicillin increases procaine toxicity.** Rarely, immune-mediated anaphylaxis or hemolytic anemia. IV penicillin salts may cause salivation, "smacking" lips, head movement. (No treatment required.)	Prevent injury to the individual by removing dangerous objects from the area. Humans should leave the stall to prevent bodily harm unless the patient is persistently circling, in which case an experienced person may walk *carefully* with the horse. Diazepam has no effect after excitability has occurred For anaphylaxis, see p. 680. For hemolytic anemia, see p. 326
Phenobarbital	Sedation, ataxia, coma, respiratory depression	Activated charcoal PO decreases serum levels, fluids
Phenoxybenzamine	May cause hypotension when administered IV (little or no indication for IV use in horse)	Hypertonic saline solution IV, If Na fluid loading not indicated, administer phenylephrine. *Epinephrine contraindicated with any α-adrenergic-blocking agent adverse reaction.*
Phenylbutazone	Gross overdosing can cause GI ulceration, colic, diarrhea, hemorrhage, and ARF with hematuria. Perivascular injection can cause necrosis.	Misoprostol, omeprazole, sucralfate, and fluids
Phenylpropanolamine	Relatively safe in horses; gross overdosing can cause CNS signs and cardiovascular collapse.	IV fluids and oral charcoal and $MgSO_4$ if treatment within last hour
Phenytoin	Ataxia, depression, weakness, recumbency	Treatment usually not required however may administer IV fluids

Continued...

PHARMACOLOGY

TABLE 52–1. Specific Acute Drug Reactions and Recommended Treatments *Continued*

Drug	Clinical Signs and Overdose Information	Treatment
Phytonadione (vitamin K)	Immediate death when given IV; anaphylaxis?	Do not administer IV
Piperazine	Gross overdosing has occurred in horses and caused paralysis, salivation, and CNS signs. As with any anthelmintic effective against *Parascaris equorum*, it can cause colic if large numbers of the worms are killed.	IV fluids and oral charcoal and $MgSO_4$ for overdosage
Plasma, whole blood	Tremors, pyrexia, agitation, tachypnea, tachycardia, piloerection	If hemolysis occurs, stop. Slow plasma, blood infusion and administer antihistamine if other reactions
Polysulfated glycosaminoglycan	When administered intra-articularly, may cause subacute (within hours) swelling and pain. This usually is a nonseptic inflammatory response. Sepsis is always a concern and should be ruled out with arthrocentesis and cytology if pain or lameness does not occur for 12-24 h or more	Phenylbutazone systemically and cold hydrotherapy. Joint lavage if swelling is severe or sepsis is suspected. If sepsis is suspected, therapy should be directed against the most common organism, *Staphylococcus aureus*
Procainamide	Rarely used in horses; however, when used can cause hypotension	IV hypertonic saline solution
Promazine	See Acepromazine	Fluids or pressor drugs for hypotension
Propantheline bromide	GI ileus, colic	Dipyrone or low-dose flunixin meglumine, 0.3 mg/kg IV; cecal trocarization if needed; neostigmine, 0.01-0.02 mg/kg SQ; IV fluids
Propranolol	Rarely used in horses; however, can cause severe bradycardia and collapse	Atropine, 0.07 mg/kg IV, fluids
Pergolide	Overdosage can cause CNS signs similar to those of metoclopramide	Sedation (barbiturates) and fluid therapy
Quinidine	Tachycardia, sweating, colic (ileus), collapse, hypotension, ataxia (usually mild), mild nasal stridor, ileus, and colic	Digoxin, 1 mg/450-kg IV adult, fluids for hypotension. HCO_3 IV to increase excretion, and KCl
Selenium	Collapse occurs occasionally with IV injections, death, colic, ataxia	Supportive; **do not administer IV**
Sodium bicarbonate	Gross overdosage either IV or PO can cause alkalosis and synchronous diaphragmatic flutter.	0.9% NaCl with KCl and calcium borogluconate
Succinylcholine chloride	Respiratory paralysis	Mechanical ventilation
Terbutaline	Excitement, tachycardia, sweating, tremors	IV fluids containing potassium

TABLE 52–1. Specific Acute Drug Reactions and Recommended Treatments *Continued*

Drug	Clinical Signs and Overdose Information	Treatment
Tetracycline	Acute renal failure, in dehydrated or hypotensive individuals. Rarely causes ARF in foals. Occasional collapse or hemolysis when administered undiluted	Fluids for ARF (see p. 531)
Tolazoline	Cardiovascular collapse when administered in high dosages to some horses	Use with caution, lowest dosage possible, administer slowly.
Trimethoprim-sulfamethoxazole or sulfadiazine	Oral, rarely diarrhea; IV, rarely collapse. Fatal if administered by intracarotid route	Diarrhea (see p. 252). Do not administer IV with detomidine
Vasopressin	If administered IV, can cause CNS signs	Treatment usually not required
Vincristine	Rarely causes acute neutropenia, thrombophlebitis	Bactericidal antibiotics, hot pack area
Warfarin	See p. 726	Charcoal and MgSO$_4$ PO, vitamin K
Xylazine	Hyperventilation, death from pulmonary edema or rare occasion (when preexisting respiratory disease is present). Intracarotid administration (see p. 079) Some horses (e.g., draft breeds, Warmbloods, foals) can become recumbent with recommended dosage.	Do not use with upper respiratory obstruction. Treat with yohimbine, 0.075 mg/kg IV, or preferably tolazoline, 2.2 mg/kg IV. Use diazepam rather than xylazine when possible in foals <1 week of age. Treatment usually not required; however, if patient is severely hypotensive, administer IV fluids

PCV, Packed cell volume; *CNS,* central nervous system; *NSAID,* nonsteroidal antiinflammatory drug; *GI,* gastrointestinal; *CPR,* cardiopulmonary resuscitation; *ARF,* acute renal failure.
Note: For any adverse drug reaction, read the package insert.

Mild Forms

- Mild forms of anaphylaxis cause urticaria and minor increases in respiratory rate. May be simply treated with antihistamines:
  □ Doxylamine succinate, 0.5 mg/kg

  or

  □ Pyrilamine maleate, 1.0 mg/kg *slowly* IV, IM, or SQ

  or

  □ Tripelennamine, 1.1 mg/kg with close monitoring

NOTE: Administer all antihistamines slowly intravenously because excitement and hypotension are occasional adverse effects. Alternatively, but not simultaneously, administer epinephrine intramuscularly, 5-8 ml/450-kg adult, because when antihistamines and epinephrine are used, antihistamines potentiate the effect of epinephrine on vascular resistance.

Severe Forms

- See pp. 308 and 502.
- Epinephrine, 3-7 ml (1:1000 undiluted) slowly IV to a 450-kg adult. May be administered intramuscularly in less severe cases at the same dosage or 2 times this dosage intramuscularly for severe anaphylaxis (intratracheal route, 5× IV dosage, may be used when intravenous access is not possible or limited).
- Provide patent airway if needed by means of intubation. This is imperative when laryngeal edema becomes severe. It is also of some benefit in managing pulmonary edema when the upper airway is edematous and compromised. Stridor may not appear until 80% or more of the upper airway is obstructed.
- Furosemide, 1 mg/kg IV.
- Use plasma or hetastarch as an oncotic volume expander if pulmonary edema is believed to be progressive. If other fluids are needed for hypotension, administer hypertonic saline solution, 4 ml/kg.
- Corticosteroids: Although of no demonstrated benefit, dexamethasone, 0.2-0.5 mg/kg, frequently is administered to prevent delayed edema formation.
- Intranasal oxygen.

SPECIAL CONSIDERATIONS

Perivascular Injections

- Perivascular injections with irritating drugs are common.
- The most irritating drugs are those with high or low pH.
- Clinical signs include pain, swelling, cellulitis, and vessel necrosis. Vessel necrosis may occur several days after the perivascular injection and can be fatal.
- Recommendations:
  - Stop the infusion.
  - Infiltrate the area with 10 ml saline solution mixed with 1 ml procaine penicillin.
  - Apply heat to the area.
  - If a large volume of irritating drug is administered, ventral drainage and flushing may be indicated.

Drug Overdose

What to do if an *overdose* of a drug has occurred:

- Keep records and provide proper communication.
- Review clinical and physiologic effects of the overdose.
- Provide specific treatment if indicated.
- General treatment for most overdoses includes:
  - Intravenous fluids.
  - Activated charcoal, 0.5 kg/450-kg adult PO.

NOTE: Even when the overdose has been administered parenterally, the oral charcoal may act as a "sink" and "pull" some of the drug into the GI tract for excretion.

  - If overdose was administered orally, give $MgSO_4$, 0.5 kg/450-kg adult PO, in addition to fluids and charcoal.

Broken Jugular Catheters

Although alarming, breaking off a jugular catheter in an adult often is not a life-threatening occurrence. The catheter usually passes through the right side of the heart and lodges in the pulmonary circulation, where it is walled off and causes no clinical problems. Perform an ultrasound examination to confirm passage of the catheter into the lungs. In foals, the catheter often is too large to pass out of the right side of the heart and must be removed. For a foal or the rare adult in which the catheter is lodged in the heart, consult a vascular surgeon regarding the technique of retrieval of the catheter. Location of the broken end is important because some catheters lodge at the thoracic inlet and can be removed surgically.

Acute Drug Reactions
See Table 52–1.

REFERENCES

Gabel AA, Koestner A: The effects of intracarotid artery injection of drugs in domestic animals, *J Am Vet Med Assoc* 142:1397-1403, 1993.
Hausner EA: Toxicology—what every veterinarian needs to know, *Clinical Techniques in Equine Practice* 2:51-115.
Kauffman VG et al: Extrapyramidal side effects caused by fluphenazine decanoate in a horse, *J Am Vet Med Assoc* 195:1128-1130, 1989.
Plumb DC: *Veterinary drug handbook,* ed 3, Ames, Iowa, 1999, Iowa State University Press.
Riond JL et al: Cardiovascular effects and fatalities associated with intravenous administration of doxycycline to horses and ponies, *Equine Vet J* 24:41-45, 1992.

53 | Toxicology and Sudden Death
Robert H. Poppenga and Thomas J. Divers

■ TOXICOLOGY

A poisoning should be suspected if:

- Many horses are sick with no known exposure to infectious disease
- The affected individual has been exposed recently to a new environment
- There has been a recent change in feed
- There are unusual weather conditions
- The horse has limited feed or pasture
- An uncommon clinical condition exists
- An unexplained death has occurred

If toxicosis is suspected, a complete history is essential, as are a complete physical examination, laboratory testing, and a detective-like inspection of the premises. If unexplained deaths occur, perform a complete postmortem examination in all suspect cases, including thorough gross inspection of the entire body and all gastrointestinal (GI) contents.

The plant distribution maps accompanying the figures of plants in this chapter should be used as guides only. Plant distribution is not static. Some plants such as *Quercus* spp. (oaks) have many species, which are widely and variably distributed. Other plants such as *Taxus* spp. (yews), which are ornamental, also are widely distributed. Maps for these genera are not provided.

Collect specimens from all major organs and tissues, fix them in formalin, and submit them for histopathologic examination. Ancillary tests may include serologic testing, microbiologic culturing of suspect tissue or lesions, and virus isolation.

For toxicologic testing, the most important specimens to collect are liver, kidney, whole EDTA blood (10 ml), serum (10 ml), stomach and intestinal contents (500 g of each), urine (50 ml), half of the brain (right or left side), representative feed samples (1-2 kg of complete feed and each feed component), water (1 L), and any suspect plant or toxic substances in the environment.

For plant identification, submit the entire plant, including the roots. Wrap the roots in moist newspaper or towels. Place the plant in a plastic bag and keep it refrigerated before and during shipment.

Clearly label samples and package individually in sealable plastic bags or clean plastic containers. Tissues can be frozen, and whole blood should be refrigerated. Dry feed samples can be placed in a labeled paper bag. Double-bag samples and package them in an insulated container to avoid breakage or leakage and deliver the samples to the laboratory by overnight or second-day delivery service.

A letter of transmittal should accompany the specimens to the laboratory with specific identification of the affected horses and a list of all samples submitted. Include pertinent facts concerning background, history, clinical signs, gross postmortem findings, and an explanation of any treatments given.

► Despite the availability of broad-based analytical screens, *no toxicologic screen can be used to test for all poisons*, and a complete and accurate history helps the toxicologist test for the most likely toxicants.

Clinicians should strive to be as complete as possible in their examinations, to document their findings, and to keep an open mind.

Additional help in the diagnosis and management of suspected poisoning can be obtained by calling the National Animal Poison Control Center hotlines:

- **(800) 426-4435.** The fee is $45 per case unless a product is covered by a sponsoring company. Credit cards are accepted. Follow-up calls as necessary, treatment protocols, and literature citations are included when indicated.
- **(900) 680-0000.** The fee is $45 per case. Follow-up calls are included as necessary.

Use regional laboratories for diagnostic testing when possible because the regional laboratory is more likely to have information on common toxicants in the area. Box 53–1 contains a list of these laboratories.

Veterinary diagnostic laboratories are accredited by the American Association of Veterinary Laboratory Diagnosticians; website: www.aavld.org. This site links to the websites of the laboratories listed in Box 53–1, from which information on available toxicologic testing, test costs, appropriate samples for each test, and shipping instructions can be obtained. Keep in mind that testing may be available for specific toxicants that are not listed in laboratories' user guides. It is always worth a call to the laboratory to ask about what additional testing is available.

GENERAL DECONTAMINATION PROCEDURES

Decontamination after ingestion of a toxicant consists of three steps:

- Removal of material from the stomach
- Administration of activated charcoal (AC) to adsorb toxicant present in the GI tract
- Administration of a cathartic to hasten elimination of contents from the GI tract

BOX 53-1. Regional Diagnostic Testing Laboratories

**California Animal Health
and Food Safety Laboratory System**
School of Veterinary Medicine at UC Davis
West Health Science Drive
Davis, CA 95617
(530) 752-8700

**Veterinary Diagnostic and
Investigational Laboratory**
University of Georgia
PO Box 1389
Tifton, GA 31793
(912) 386-3340

**Laboratories of Veterinary
Diagnostic Medicine**
College of Veterinary Medicine
University of Illinois
2001 S. Lincoln Avenue
Urbana, IL 61801
(217) 333-1620

Animal Disease Diagnostic Laboratory
School of Veterinary Medicine
at Purdue University
West Lafayette, IN 47907
(765) 494-7448

Veterinary Diagnostic Laboratory
College of Veterinary Medicine
Iowa State University
Ames, IA 50010
(515) 294-1950

Veterinary Diagnostic Laboratory
Kansas State University
Manhattan, KS 66506
(913) 532-4605

Veterinary Diagnostic and Research Center
Murray State University
PO Box 2000 North Drive
Hopkinsville, KY 42240
(270) 886-3959

Animal Health Diagnostic Laboratory
Michigan State University
PO Box 30076
Lansing, MI 48909-7576
(517) 353-0635

Veterinary Diagnostic Medicine
University of Minnesota
1943 Carter Avenue
St. Paul, MN 55101
(612) 624-8707

**Veterinary Medical Diagnostic
Laboratory**
University of Missouri
PO Box 6023
Columbia, MO 65205
(573) 882-6811

Lincoln Diagnostic Laboratory
Fair Street, E. Campus Loop
University of Nebraska
Lincoln, NE 68583
(402) 472-1434

Veterinary Diagnostic Laboratory
College of Veterinary Medicine at
Cornell University
Upper Tower Road
Ithaca, NY 14853
(607) 253-3900

**Animal Disease Diagnostic
Laboratory**
College of Veterinary Medicine
Oklahoma State University
Stillwater, OK 74078
(405) 744-6623

PADLS-NBC Toxicology
University of Pennsylvania
382 West Street Road
Kennett Square, PA 19348
(610) 444-5800 ext. 2217
Fax: (610) 444-4617

**Veterinary Medical Diagnostic
Laboratory**
Texas A & M University
PO Box 3200
Amarillo, TX 79106
(806) 353-7478

**Texas Veterinary Medical
Diagnostic Laboratory**
Drawer 3040
College Station, TX 77841-3040
(979) 845-3414

**Poisonous Plants Research
Laboratory**
Utah State University
1150 East 1400 North
Logan, UT 84341
(435) 752-2941

TOXICOLOGY

Continued...

BOX 53-1. Regional Diagnostic Testing Laboratories *Continued*

Animal Disease Diagnostic Laboratory
Washington State University
PO Box 2037, College Station
Pullman, WA 99165
(509) 335-9696

Wyoming State Veterinary Laboratory
1174 Snowy Range Road
Laramie, WY 82070
(307) 742-6638

In horses, removal of material from the stomach is difficult because of the inability to administer an emetic and the time and effort required to perform gastric lavage. In most suspected intoxications resulting from ingestion of a toxicant, the best approach to decontamination is administration of an adsorbent such as AC with or without a cathartic as soon as possible after the ingestion. AC is administered as an aqueous slurry through a stomach tube at a dosage range of 1-5 g/kg body weight (~1 g of AC per 5 ml of water). Commonly used cathartics include sodium sulfate (Glauber's salts), magnesium sulfate (Epsom salts), and sorbitol. Sodium or magnesium sulfate can be administered at 250-500 mg/kg body weight mixed in the AC slurry. Sorbitol (70%), also mixed in the AC slurry, can be administered at 3-ml/kg body weight. There is little need to administer a cathartic if significant diarrhea is already present.

Mineral oil often is given after suspected exposure to a toxicant. This practice should be discouraged because there is *no* evidence that mineral oil is an effective adsorbent for most toxicants. It has a laxative, not a cathartic, effect. Mineral oil should not be administered with AC because of a possible diminution of the adsorptive capacity of the administered AC.

Dermal or ocular exposure to a toxicant necessitates thorough bathing with soap (a dish soap such as Dawn is recommended) or copious irrigation with tap water or normal saline solution, respectively. Always observe appropriate precautions during decontamination procedures to avoid self-exposure or exposure of others to the toxicant.

➤ There are relatively few antidotes for the toxicants most likely to poison horses. However, early and appropriate decontamination and vigorous symptomatic and supportive care often result in recovery.

COMMON TOXINS PREDOMINANTLY AFFECTING THE GASTROINTESTINAL TRACT

Amitraz

A formamide insecticide available in the United States as an acaricide dip or spray for cattle and hogs and used in the management of canine demodectic mange. ➤ Horses are very sensitive to this drug; *it should not be used on horses.*

Mechanism of Toxic Action

- α_2-adrenergic agonist activity

Clinical Signs

- Impaction, colic, depression, incoordination
- All occur within 24 hours of exposure

Treatment

- If dermal exposure, soap and water bath
- If oral exposure, AC, 1-5 g/kg PO
- Yohimbine is an α_2-adrenergic antagonist (appropriate dosage for reversal not determined, however 0.075 mg/kg IV is recommended for reversal of effects of xylazine).
- Intravenous fluids
- Flunixin meglumine, 1 mg/kg q24h

Atropine Toxicosis

Most commonly occurs when atropine has been administered (often incorrectly) for suspected organophosphate (OP) poisoning. Plants such as jimsonweed *(Datura stramonium)* (see Color Plate 23), nightshades *(Solanum nigra, S. dulcamara, S. eleagnifolium)*, and belladonna *(Atropa belladonna)* contain related tropane alkaloids. Foliage of potatoes and tomatoes contains tropane and steroidal glycoalkaloids and can be toxic.

Mechanism of Toxic Action

- Competitive inhibition of acetylcholine at postganglionic parasympathetic neuroeffector sites
- High dosages can block nicotinic receptors at autonomic ganglia and neuromuscular junctions

Clinical Signs

- Bloat, colic, dry membranes, and dilated pupils (anticholinergic toxidrome)
- Steroidal glycoalkaloids cause gastroenteritis

Treatment

- After plant ingestion, AC, 1-5 g/kg PO
- Flunixin meglumine, 1.0 mg/kg IV
- Neostigmine, 0.01 mg/kg SQ, repeated as needed (Use should probably be reserved for horses exhibiting extreme agitation or likely to injure themselves.)

Black Locust *(Robinia pseudoacacia)* (Fig. 53-1 and Color Plate 24)

Ingestion of young sprouts, bark, or pruned or fresh leaves can cause illness. Potential toxicity of other *Robinia* species is not clear.

Mechanism of Toxic Action

One hypothesized toxic principle, robin, is a toxalbumin that inhibits protein synthesis. However, a number of bioactive constituents have been isolated; their role in disease pathogenesis is not known with certainty.

Clinical Signs

- Anorexia, diarrhea (may be bloody), colic, depression, weakness, irregular pulse
- Rarely fatal, laminitis can be a severe sequela

Treatment

- AC, 1-5 g/kg PO, intravenous fluids, and nutritional support

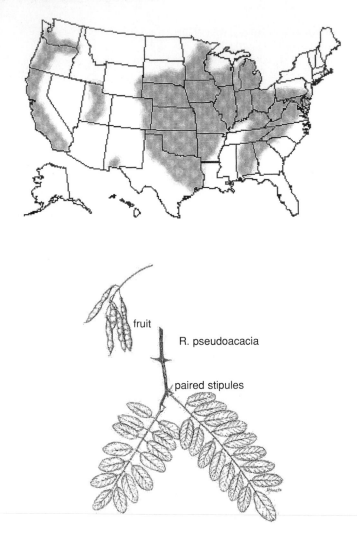

FIGURE 53-1. Distribution and drawing of *Robinia pseudoacacia* (black locust).

Blister Beetle (Cantharidin)

Toxicosis is caused by ingestion of the blister beetle (*Epicauta* spp., see p. 258), which can be found in alfalfa that has been simultaneously cut and crimped. Blister beetles usually are found in the plains states and the midwest and occasionally are found in other parts of the country.

Mechanism of Toxic Action
- Vesicant and irritant
- Inhibition of phosphatase 2A

- Cause of hypocalcemia is unknown

Clinical Signs
- Mucous membrane irritation, including oral cavity, GI tract, and urinary tract
- Colic, hypocalcemia with synchronous diaphragmatic flutter, frequent urination, shock, and death
- Cardiac damage is possible.
- Neurologic signs only in a few cases
- Sudden death

Diagnosis
- Compatible clinical signs, postmortem lesions (erythema and occasionally erosions of GI mucosa)
- Identification of blister beetles in hay or GI contents
- Submit GI contents and urine for analysis for cantharidin. The following laboratories commonly perform this test:

  Texas Veterinary Medical Diagnostic Laboratory; (979) 845-3414
  Michigan State University Diagnostic Laboratory; (517) 353-0635
  University of California at Davis Diagnostic Laboratory; (530) 752-8700
  Animal Disease Diagnostic Laboratory, Oklahoma State University; (405) 744-6623

Treatment
- Remove suspect feed, administer AC, 1-5 g/kg, or mineral oil (1 gal/adult), because this is a lipid soluble toxin.
- Administer intravenous fluid therapy.
- Monitor serum calcium concentration.
- Provide supportive care!
- Mucosal ulcerations may develop.
- There is no known antidote.

Prognosis
- Guarded
- Poor with neurologic signs

Buckeye *(Aesculus glabra)* (Fig. 53–2)
The most common species of *Aesculus*. Found in moist, well-drained soils of woods and thickets in the midwestern United States. Toxic effects believed to be caused by a number of saponins.

Buttercups (*Ranunculus* spp.)
Genus comprises several hundred species. Widely distributed. Plentiful in many pastures. Horses almost never eat the plant in a pasture setting, and drying renders the plant nontoxic. Toxic principle is ranunculin, which releases protoanemonin when damaged. Cyanogenic glycosides are present in some species.

Mechanism of Toxic Action
- Protoanemonin is a potent vesicant.

TOXICOLOGY

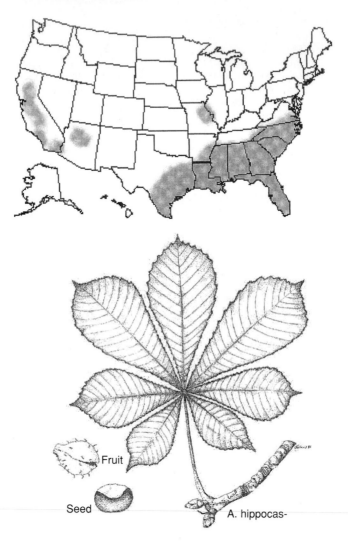

FIGURE 53-2. Distribution of *Aesculus glabra* (buckeye) and drawing of *A. hippocastanum* (horse chestnut).

Clinical Signs

- Irritated oral mucous membranes, colic, anorexia, diarrhea, muscle tremors that may proceed to excitement and convulsions
- Contact with crushed plant can cause skin irritation

Treatment

- AC, 1-5 g/kg PO
- Symptomatic and supportive care

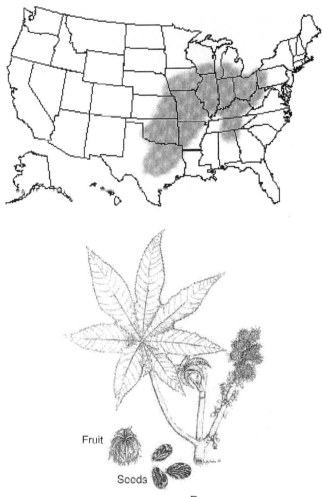

Fruit

Seeds

R. commu-

FIGURE 53-3. Distribution and drawing of *Ricinus communis* (castor bean).

Castor Bean *(Ricinus communis)* (Fig. 53–3)

Numerous cultivars are planted as ornamentals. Typically overwinters only in southernmost regions of the United States. Plants are grown commercially in California and Florida for castor oil. Seeds and foliage are poisonous. Ingested seeds that remain intact in the GI tract are not toxic. Contains the alkaloid ricinine and the glycoprotein ricin.

Mechanism of Toxic Action

- Ricinine can cause seizures through γ-aminobutyric acid type A ($GABA_A$) antagonism; there is a possible neuromuscular effect.
- Ricin inhibits protein synthesis and, secondarily, DNA and RNA synthesis, impairs sugar absorption, and is an irritant.

Clinical Signs

- Colic, profuse and watery diarrhea, fever, incoordination, depression, sweating, terminal convulsions, death
- Signs may be delayed 12 hours or more after ingestion

Diagnosis

- Identification of seeds in GI contents, evidence of consumption, and compatible clinical signs

Treatment

- AC, 1-5 g/kg PO
- Sedation if needed (xylazine, 0.4 mg/kg), fluids (hypertonic saline solution), followed by polyionic isotonic fluids
- Flunixin meglumine, 1.0 mg/kg IV

Horse Chestnut *(Aesculus hippocastanum)* (see Fig. 53–2)

Garden and park tree in North America.

Mechanism of Toxic Action

- Uncertain. Experimentally studied saponins are neurotoxic at low dosages and hemolytic at higher dosages. Also have hypoglycemic effect.

Clinical Signs

- Ingestion can cause colic, inflamed mucous membranes, hyperesthesia, and ataxia followed by muscle tremors, paresis, dyspnea, convulsions, and death.
- Mortality infrequent.

Treatment

- AC, 1-5 g/kg PO
- Analgesics (parenteral), supportive fluids (intravenous), and symptomatic treatment

Oak (*Quercus* spp.) (see Color Plate 25)

Oaks compose a variety of native and introduced species that are widely distributed in the United States. Species range in size from shrubs 2-3 feet (60-90 cm) in height to large trees. All species should be considered toxic. Toxic principles are polyphenolic complexes called tannins, which are categorized as either condensed or hydrolyzable. Hydrolyzable tannins such as gallotannins are responsible for clinical effects. Oak rarely causes poisoning in horses as opposed to cattle, although poorly fed horses may eat leaves, acorns, or oak buds. Relatively large amounts of the plant have to be ingested before clinical signs occur.

Mechanism of Toxic Action
- Tannins interact with and denature protein.
- Phenolic metabolites are likely responsible for liver and renal damage.

Clinical Signs
- Anorexia, colic, sometimes bloody diarrhea, tenesmus, depression followed by frequent urination and constipation.
- Dependent edema may develop.

Treatment
- Fluids, nutritional and other supportive care.
- Evaluate for possible kidney damage.

Organophosphate and Carbamate Insecticides

Poisoning with these compounds usually causes clinical signs of nervous and GI dysfunction. The most likely source of the poisoning is inappropriate or accidental oral or topical administration of an insecticide or anthelmintic containing OPs or carbamates. Clinical signs for both insecticides are similar.

Mechanism of Toxic Action
- Inhibition of acetylcholinesterase enzyme resulting in excessive cholinergic stimulation

Clinical Signs
- Colic, hypersalivation, sweating, diarrhea, muscle tremors, miosis, weakness, dyspnea, convulsions
- OPs and carbamates increase the peristaltic activity of the intestines and cause bradycardia

Diagnosis
- History of exposure and compatible clinical signs.
- Exposure confirmed by measurement of whole-blood cholinesterase activity or plasma pseudocholinesterase activity. If significant OP or carbamate exposure has occurred, the cholinesterase or pseudocholinesterase activity is much lower (<25%) than the normal value for the referring laboratory. If submitting samples to a laboratory for humans, submit a control (unexposed) equine sample. A postmortem sample of brain or retina shows decreased cholinesterase activity in OP or carbamate exposure.
- If submittal to the laboratory is delayed all samples of carbamate insecticides can exhibit a "regeneration" of active cholinesterase, resulting in a normal value.
- Submit GI contents and liver for detection of a specific OP or carbamate insecticide. Representative feed samples should be obtained and tested if the suspected source is feed. Concentrations of OPs and carbamates can be very high in feed and GI content samples. These insecticides can penetrate plastic. Therefore make sure that sample cross-contamination does not occur.

Treatment
- Atropine, 0.01-0.05 mg/kg IV and 0.05 mg/kg SQ as needed (up to four times daily) to control clinical signs of OP and carbamate poisoning.

- There should be obvious improvement in the muscarinic effects (salivation, miosis, and sweating) soon after treatment begins.
- Glycopyrrolate use may be associated with fewer adverse effects than atropine has. Not approved for use in horses. Titrate dosage to effect.
- Pralidoxime hydrochloride (2-PAM) is specific for OPs and does not help in carbamate poisoning. Administer 20 mg/kg IV q4-6h, if needed.
- If exposure is believed due to a cholinesterase inhibitor but it is unknown whether OPs or carbamates are involved, administer 2-PAM if available.
- Pass a stomach tube to remove any gastric reflux fluid.
- Administer AC, 1-5 g/kg PO, along with supportive care such as replacement fluids.
- ► Accurate diagnosis of OP or carbamate poisoning in horses is imperative because of the possible adverse effects of atropine administration. High-dosage atropine used in OP or carbamate poisoning therapy should never be administered without clear historical, clinical, and preferably laboratory evidence that OP or carbamate poisoning is responsible for the clinical signs!
- Transient abdominal pain following oral administration of OP anthelmintics is not uncommon; however, it is unusual that atropine treatment is required.

Red Clover *(Trifolium pratense)*

Under certain environmental conditions a fungus, *Rhizoctonia leguminicola*, can grow on the clover and produce a mycotoxin, slaframine, which increases saliva production and causes *slobbering*. The fungus is seen as blackish-brown spots on the clover. More commonly affects horses grazing pastures containing some red clover or, less commonly, when red clover is in the hay. The same fungus may produce clinical signs in horses when grown on other legumes, for example, white clover *(Trifolium repens)*, alsike clover *(Trifolium hybridum)*, or alfalfa *(Medicago sativa)*.

Fungus persists in vegetative tissue and seeds; therefore once a pasture is infested, slobbers can be a recurring problem, especially when weather is cool and moist.

Mechanism of Toxic Effect
- Cholinergic agonism

Clinical Signs
- Excess salivation. Duration can be several hours for mild cases or continuous.
- In severe cases, diarrhea and anorexia occur.

Treatment
- Remove affected individual from the pasture.
- Provide water and salt.
- Detoxification of contaminated hay is not possible.

Tobacco (*Nicotiana* spp.)

Toxic principles are nicotine and other alkaloids, such as anabasine. Tobacco plants (commercial, wild, and ornamental) are extremely unpalatable; therefore, poisoning is unusual. Poisoning may occur if horses are housed where tobacco is stored or where wild tobacco plants grow and there is little else to eat. Alkaloids are teratogenic.

Mechanism of Toxic Action
- Nicotine causes initial stimulation with subsequent depolarizing blockade of nicotinic receptors in sympathetic and parasympathetic ganglia, neuromuscular endplates, and the central nervous system.

Clinical Signs
- Initial excitement, colic, diarrhea, incoordination, muscle tremors, excess salivation followed by muscle weakness, recumbency, stupor
- Death from respiratory paralysis
- Survival beyond 12 hours is a good prognostic sign

Treatment
- AC, 1-5 g/kg PO
- Fluids and symptomatic treatment

Miscellaneous Toxic Plants

Those predominantly affecting the GI tract include:

- *Delphinium* spp. (larkspur)
- Rotten potatoes
- *Berteroa incana* (see p. 721), which produces fever, limb edema, diarrhea, mainly in northeastern and north central United States and Canada

Other Gastrointestinal Poisonings
Salt Poisoning
- Can cause diarrhea, colic, and neurologic signs when salt-deprived horses are fed salt and do not have adequate water available

DIAGNOSIS
- Elevated serum or cerebrospinal fluid concentration of sodium

TREATMENT
- Fluid therapy, 2.5% dextrose/0.45% saline solution, polyionic crystalloid; DMSO, 1 g/kg IV
- Do not use 5% dextrose!

Arsenic and Mercury
- Can produce sudden death with severe GI erosions

CLINICAL SIGNS
- Salivation
- Diarrhea
- Depression

DIAGNOSIS
- History plus examination of GI contents, liver, and kidney for arsenic or mercury concentration.
- Clinical signs plus hepatic and kidney arsenic concentrations >10 ppm are compatible with arsenic intoxication.

TOXICOLOGY

TREATMENT

- Dimercaprol, 3-5 mg/kg IM q8h on day 1 and 1 mg/kg IM q6h on days 2 and 3.
- Succimer is a newer, orally administered chelator that is effective for chelation of lead, arsenic, and mercury. There is little information on its use in horses, but it has been shown safe in other species for management of lead intoxication. Recommended dosage is 10 mg/kg PO q8h for 5-10 days. Measurement of blood concentration should be repeated several days after cessation of chelation therapy.

TOXINS PREDOMINANTLY AFFECTING THE NERVOUS SYSTEM

Ammonia Intoxication

This disorder should be strongly considered when horses have signs of acute encephalopathy, severe acidosis, normal liver enzyme values, and hyperglycemia. Supportive treatment can result in complete recovery. Colic and diarrhea also may be present. It may also exist with liver failure.

Australian Dandelion *(Hypochoeris radicata)* (Fig. 53–4)

This plant causes outbreaks of stringhalt and roaring in horses in Australia. Similar outbreaks of unknown etiology are reported in the western, southeastern and mid-Atlantic United States. The toxins have not been identified. Stringhalt also is associated with acute injury to the rear legs and hypocalcemia.

Mechanism of Toxic Action

- Unknown.

Treatment

- For severely affected individuals, phenytoin, 7.5 mg/kg PO q12h, may eliminate clinical signs.
- Acupuncture.

Avocado *(Persea americana)*

Found mainly in Florida and California. Only the Guatemalan type and its hybrids are known to be toxic. Toxic principle is believed to be persin. All parts of the tree are believed toxic, especially the leaves. Poisoning most commonly occurs when affected horses have access to pruned branches, which remain toxic when dried.

Mechanism of Toxic Action

- Unknown, although administration of persin experimentally has caused mammary gland and myocardial necrosis.

Clinical Signs

- Noninfectious mastitis, depression, mild tremors, and colic.
- Higher, repeated dosages are associated with cardiomyopathy.
- Edema of the head and neck
- Death is unusual.

Treatment

- Symptomatic and supportive care.
- Mastitis subsides within 1 week; however, no additional milk is produced during the lactation.

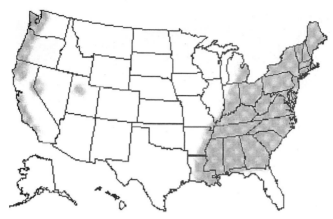

FIGURE 53-4. Distribution of *Hypochoeris radicata* (Australian dandelion).

Botulism (see p. 400)

Caused by *Clostridium botulinum*, this is mainly a clinical problem among foals 2-8 weeks of age; however, it can affect adults. In Kentucky, Pennsylvania, Maryland, New Jersey, and Virginia, it is usually caused by *C. botulinum* toxin type B. There are eight toxin types with variable regional distribution. Types A and C occur sporadically. In adults, botulism is most often a result of ingestion of preformed toxin in vegetative matter. In foals, it is a toxic-infectious process caused by ingestion of *C. botulinum* type B spores. Wound botulism occurs among horses but is uncommon.

Mechanism of Toxic Action
- Inhibition of the release of acetylcholine causing presynaptic blockade of nerve impulses

Clinical Signs
- Dysphagia, trembling; mydriasis (type C); weak tail, tongue, and eyelid tone; recumbency

Diagnosis
- Although it is difficult to isolate the toxin, submit samples of serum, gastric and intestinal contents, feces, and suspect feed. A laboratory for testing is at the University of Pennsylvania, New Bolton Center; (610) 444-5800 ext. 2244.
- In foals, culture of *Clostridium* type B from the feces is strongly supportive of the diagnosis in the presence of dysphagia and weakness.

Treatment
- Antiserum (see p. 402)
- Supportive care

Bracken Fern *(Pteridium aquilinum)* (Fig. 53–5 and Color Plate 26)

Although frequently listed in textbooks, this poisoning is uncommon among horses because a large quantity of the unpalatable plant must be consumed. Toxic principle is a type I thiaminase.

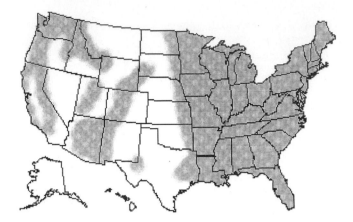

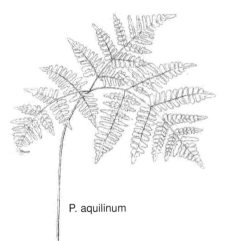

P. aquilinum

FIGURE 53–5. Distribution and drawing of *Pteridium aquilinum* (bracken fern).

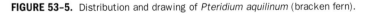

Mechanism of Toxic Action
- Competitive type inhibition of thiamine cofactor activity

Clinical Signs
- Unthriftiness, lethargy, ataxia, blindness, recumbency, and convulsions.
- Polioencephalomalacia can be found on postmortem examination.

Treatment
- Thiamine hydrochloride, 5 mg/kg slowly IV or IM q6h for 5 days.
- Response to early treatment is dramatic.

Fumonisin Mycotoxins

Fumonisins are mycotoxins produced by *Fusarium* spp. of fungus, are mainly found on corn, and can be present in high concentration in corn screenings. Fumonisins cause equine leukoencephalomalacia (ELEM, or moldy corn poisoning). Several fumonisins have been isolated; fumonisin B_1 is the most toxic.

Mechanism of Toxic Action

- Fumonisins inhibit sphingosine and sphinganine N-acetyltransferases, which are important for sphingolipid synthesis. Sphingolipids are important for normal cell structure, cell-cell communication, cell–extracellular matrix interactions, modulation of receptor kinases, and signal transduction.
- Sphinganine accumulation is cytotoxic, inhibits protein kinase C and other signal transduction pathways, and increases intracellular calcium concentration.

Clinical Signs

- Occur after the affected individuals eat the feed for several days
- Anorexia, ataxia, blindness, head pressing, occasionally icterus, and death

Diagnosis (see p. 411)

- Detection of fumonisins in suspect feed.
- The maximum recommended concentration of fumonisins in horse feed is 5 ppm.
- Malacia of the white matter of the cerebral cortex and in some cases hepatosis with elevation of serum hepatic enzymes.
- The contaminated corn usually appears normal on inspection.
- Many diagnostic laboratories test for fumonisins.

Treatment

- Supportive. Affected individuals infrequently completely recover.
- Do not feed corn screenings to horses.

Horsetail (*Equisetum hyemale* and *E. arvense*)

Rarely reported as a toxicosis in horses and can occur if little else is available to eat. Toxic principle is a thiaminase, similar to bracken fern (not known whether a type 1 or type 2 thiaminase).

Mechanism of Toxic Action, Clinical Signs, and Treatment

- See Bracken Fern, p. 703.

Insulin

Hypoglycemic shock has been reported in horses inappropriately treated with insulin.

Diagnosis

- High-pressure liquid chromatography (HPLC) is used to identify the source of insulin in the serum; performed by drug-testing centers.

TOXICOLOGY

Treatment

- Continuous 5%-10% dextrose administration, polyionic crystalloids with 40 mEq/L potassium chloride, and dexamethasone, 0.2 mg/kg IV initially followed by a decreasing dose for 2-3 additional days.

Prognosis

- Poor

Lead

Lead poisoning is rare but can be caused by ingestion of lead paint, old batteries, or lead weights.

Mechanism of Toxic Action

- Interferes with a variety of enzymes, especially those with a sulfhydryl group.
- Replaces zinc as an enzyme cofactor.
- Inhibits several enzymes necessary for heme synthesis: Aminolevulinic acid (ALA) synthetase, coproporphyrinogenase, and heme synthetase.

Acute Signs

- Weakness, ataxia, depression, and convulsions.
- Laryngeal paresis, especially with exercise or excitement, may be present with chronic lead poisoning.

Diagnosis

- Whole-blood lead concentration greater than 0.6 ppm (or greater than 0.3 ppm with compatible clinical signs).
- Liver or kidney, 5-10 ppm (wet weight) or greater. To approximate a liver or kidney dry weight value from a wet weight value, multiple the wet weight value by 3.3. Alternatively, if a wet weight value is desired from a dry weight determination, divide the dry weight value by 3.3. This assumes tissue moisture content of approximately 70%.

Treatment

- Calcium EDTA, 75 mg/kg per day slowly IV, divided q12h. Treat for 2 or 3 days and then stop for 2 or 3 days and repeat if needed.
- Succimer is a newer, orally administered chelator that is effective for chelation of lead, arsenic, and mercury. There is little information on its use in horses, but it has been shown safe in other species for management of lead intoxication. Recommended dosage is 10 mg/kg PO q8h for 5-10 days. Measurement of blood concentrations should be repeated several days after cessation of chelation therapy.
- Thiamine, 5 mg/kg IV or IM.
- Magnesium or sodium sulfate, 1 g/kg PO, helps remove lead from GI tract.
- Maintain adequate hydration of affected patient during treatment period.

Locoweeds (Certain *Astragalus* spp. and *Oxytropis* spp.) (Figs. 53–6 and 53–7 and Color Plate 27)

Grow in central and western range lands of North America. A large amount of the plant must be ingested (30% of body weight over 6-7 weeks). Toxic principle is

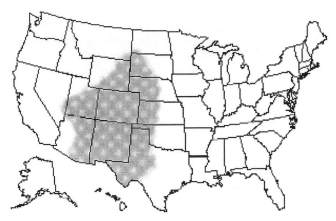

FIGURE 53-6. Distribution of *Astragalus mollissimus* (locoweed).

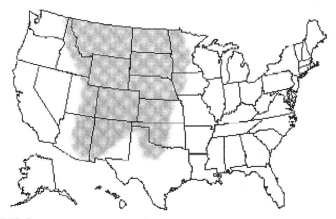

FIGURE 53 7. Distribution of *Oxytropis lambertii* (locoweed).

TOXICOLOGY

swainsonine. Horses eat the plant even though other forage is available and can become habituated to the plant.

Mechanism of Toxic Action
- Inhibition of α-mannosidase with subsequent intracellular accumulation of oligosaccharides and glycoproteins in lysosomes. Central nervous system, lymphoid tissue, endocrine tissues, and liver contain lysosomal vacuoles.

Clinical Signs
- Depression, ataxia, dysphagia, hyperexcitability, apparent blindness, stringhalt-like gaits, paraplegia, and death.

Diagnosis

- Swainsonine can be measured in serum samples. Contact the U.S. Department of Agriculture Poisonous Plant Research Laboratory in Logan, UT; (435) 752-2941.
- Histologic changes in affected tissues are highly suggestive.

Treatment

- None demonstrated to be effective; reserpine, 3.0 mg/450 kg IM or 1.25 mg/450 kg PO for 6 days, has been reported to eliminate the clinical signs.
- Horses should not be kept in areas where locoweeds grow.
- Recovery may occur in mild cases, but affected individuals should never be used for riding or work.

Marijuana, Hemp *(Cannabis sativa)*

Tall annual herb of the hemp family. Occasionally fed to horses. Active ingredients are δ-tetrahydrocannabinol and related resinoids.

Clinical Signs

- Excitement, incoordination, sweating, salivation, and subsequent weakness and depression.

Treatment

- AC, 1-5 g/kg PO, if ingestion within previous 2 hours.
- Symptomatic and supportive care.

Ryegrass *(Lolium perenne)*

A common pasture grass of the southeastern United States and West Coast that can be parasitized by an endophytic fungus called *Neotyphodium lolii*. Ryegrass staggers is caused by toxic alkaloids, especially lolitrem B, produced by the fungus. Ryegrass staggers is a sporadic disease that occurs during years that are apparently conducive to the fungal growth. May rarely be seen with other grasses (e.g., Bermuda grass and dallisgrass).

Mechanism of Toxic Action

- Inhibition of GABA receptor function

Clinical Signs

- If at rest and left undisturbed, affected individuals can appear normal.
- If disturbed or forced to move: Stiffness, tremors, weakness, incoordination.
- Death usually is accidental (e.g., falling into water and drowning).

Treatment

- Remove from pasture; recovery generally occurs rapidly.

Selenium Toxicosis

Acute form from inappropriate selenium injections (see Table 52–1) or feeding toxic amounts. Errors in feed formulation can occur but rarely cause problems. Toxicity reported in horses administered 3.3 mg/kg PO (smaller amounts can be toxic).

Mechanism of Toxic Action
- Oxidative stress.
- Displacement of sulfur in sulfur-containing amino acids.

Clinical Signs
- Acute form can exhibit excess salivation, tremors, ataxia, apparent blindness, respiratory distress, diarrhea, inability to stand, and death.
- Chronic form can exhibit hair or hoof abnormalities, coronary band separation, and joint stiffness.
- If poisoning is suspected, measure selenium concentrations in the blood and liver samples.

Treatment
- Symptomatic and supportive care.
- Acetylcysteine, beginning at 140 mg/kg IV then 70 mg/kg IV q6h, is suggested for acute poisoning.

Sudan Grass (*Sorghum vulgare* Var. *Sudanese*) (see Color Plate 28)

In addition to the risk of acute cyanide poisoning, grazing on Sudan grass for several weeks can cause equine cystitis and ataxia syndrome. It has occurred in the central and southern Great Plains of North America in pastures almost exclusively composed of sorghum species. Problems do not occur from eating dry, well-cured hay. Cyanide and nitriles are hypothesized to cause the cystitis and ataxia, although neither has been shown to reproduce the disease.

Mechanism of Toxic Action
- Unknown.

Clinical Signs
- Ataxia of the rear limbs, a hopping gait, dribbling of urine (the bladder is enlarged).
- Abortion at any time during gestation, dystocia due to deformed fetus, deformed or weak newborn
- Acute poisoning (cyanide) frequently causes death.

Diagnosis
- Clinical signs, exposure, cyanide levels in gastric contents or forage.

Treatment
- Remove from pasture and manage any bladder infection with antibiotics.
- Full recovery is unusual.
- Use sodium thiosulfate, 30-40 mg/kg IV q12h, to manage acute poisoning due to cyanide.

White Snakeroot (*Eupatorium rugosum*) (Fig. 53–8 and Color Plate 29)

Toxic principle is unknown (older texts list tremetol), is cumulative, and can be passed in the milk. Grows in shady areas and is a problem in late summer and fall; remains toxic after frost or when dried.

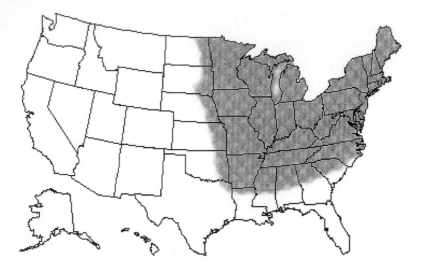

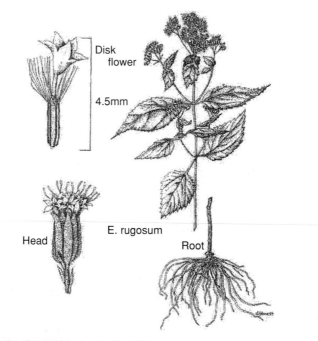

FIGURE 53-8. Distribution and drawing of *Eupatorium rugosum* (white snakeroot).

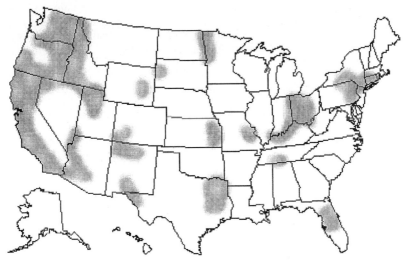

FIGURE 53-9. Distribution of *Centaurea solstitialis* (yellow star thistle).

Mechanism of Toxic Action

- Not certain; metabolic alterations secondary to tricarboxylic acid cycle impairment and decreased utilization of glucose.

Clinical Signs

- Weakness, depression, trembling, sweating, salivation, and recumbency.
- Arrhythmias, jugular vein distention and pulsation, cardiac damage and dependent edema are possible.
- Increases in serum values of lactate dehydrogenase and creatine kinase.

Treatment

- Symptomatic and supportive care.
- Remove from source.
- May have long-term cardiac compromise.

Yellow Star Thistle *(Centaurea solstitialis)* (Fig. 53–9 and Color Plate 30)

Grows predominantly in the western United States. **Russian knapweed** (*Centaurea repens*) causes identical signs and is considered more toxic. Numerous sesquiterpene lactones are present and are believed to be involved in disease pathogenesis.

Mechanism of Toxic Action

- Lesions restricted to the globus pallidus and substantia nigra.
- Several of the lactones have been found cytotoxic to neurons in vitro.

Clinical Signs

- Begin suddenly after chronic ingestion of the plant.

TOXICOLOGY

- Affected individuals can prehend food with their incisors but cannot move the food back into the mouth. They have difficulty in drinking water and may immerse the head deep into the water to swallow. The lips may be retracted from hypertonic facial muscles, and the tongue may protrude.
- Depression, ataxia, circling, and starvation.
- May have secondary aspiration pneumonia.
- Nigropallidal encephalomalacia is found at necropsy.
- Oxidative stress may play a role in the toxicity.

Treatment
- No specific treatment; vitamin E should be administered. Affected individuals do not recover but if not severely diseased may learn to accommodate.

TOXINS PREDOMINANTLY AFFECTING THE LIVER
Aflatoxicosis

Aflatoxins B_1, B_2, G_1, and G_2 are produced in *Aspergillus flavus* and *A. parasiticus*, which grow on corn, peanuts, cottonseed, and other small grains in warm, wet conditions. Aflatoxins have been reported to cause acute hepatic failure (neurologic signs and icterus) in horses; it is apparently rare.

Mechanism of Toxic Action
- Aflatoxins and their liver metabolites react with enzymes, RNA, and DNA within the hepatocytes, and the result is acute or chronic liver dysfunction.

Diagnosis
- Evidence of exposure (have feed tested for mycotoxins), clinical signs, laboratory findings of liver disease and failure.
- Many laboratories can test for aflatoxin metabolites in urine (submit 1 L) or liver.

Treatment
- Remove from suspect feed
- General therapy for hepatic failure (see p. 315)
- L-Methionine, 25 mg/kg PO
- Vitamin E, 6000-10,000 units q24h PO, in adult

Alsike Clover *(Trifolium hybridum)*

A pasture legume found mostly in Canada and the northeastern United States. A cluster of cases may occur among horses grazing alsike clover grown on clay soil during certain years, probably owing to wet weather conditions. Alsike must be predominant feed for several days to several weeks to cause subacute intoxication. Longer-term ingestion is reported to be associated with liver damage and hepatogenous photosensitization. The toxic principle has not been identified; it may be a plant toxin or a mycotoxin.

Mechanism of Toxic Action
- Subacute intoxication: Uncertain, but toxin may be a primary photosensitizer
- Chronic intoxication: Uncertain, but toxin may be a hepatotoxin causing hepatogenous photosensitization

Clinical Signs
- Photosensitivity (erythema, swelling, edema and sloughing of skin in lightly or nonpigmented areas, icterus)

Treatment
- Remove alsike from diet.
- Protect from direct sunlight.
- General therapy for photosensitization and liver failure.

Prognosis
- Good if identified early in the syndrome before significant liver damage has occurred

Iron Toxicosis

May occur in horses given one large dose (overuse of a hematinic, oral or injectable) or be caused by long-term accumulation (hemochromatosis). Foals receiving even small-dosage iron supplements before nursing may experience fatal hepatopathy.

Mechanism of Toxic Action
- Oxidative cell damage

Clinical Signs
- In acute exposure, colic signs predominate.
- Clinical signs of liver failure generally do not occur unless more than 60%-75% of hepatic function is lost.

Diagnosis
- Signs of liver failure, laboratory findings of liver disease (increased serum value of γ-glutamyl transferase [GGT]), and failure (increased serum concentration of conjugated bilirubin)
- Liver iron concentration >300 ppm (most horses with iron toxicosis have values threefold or more above the upper normal range). The concentration of iron in the liver can be abnormally high without liver disease (hemosiderosis), as in vitamin E deficiency.
- Serum value of iron is frequently normal in chronic hemochromatosis and may be increased with acute toxicosis.
- Elevation of serum and liver concentrations of iron is *not* specific for iron toxicosis and is found in a variety of liver disorders. Correlation with laboratory and histopathologic lesions is necessary.

Treatment
- Supportive for hepatic failure
- After oral exposure, magnesium hydroxide (milk of magnesia) to precipitate iron in the GI tract
- Vitamin C, 0.5 g/kg PO, and desferrioxamine, 10 mg/kg IM or slowly IV twice, 2 hours apart
- If urine is reddish-gold, additional treatment may be needed to hasten excretion in acute cases

TOXICOLOGY

Klein grass and Fall Panicum (*Panicum* spp.)

Klein grass poisoning is primarily a problem in Texas and the southwestern United States, whereas fall panicum occasionally is a problem in the mid-Atlantic states. Liver damage is associated with the presence of saponins such as diosgenin; hepatogenous photosensitization results.

Mechanism of Toxic Action

- Possible reaction of saponins with calcium results in precipitation of insoluble calcium salts in bile ducts.

Clinical Signs

- Chronic poor appetite and weight loss
- Depression, icterus, photosensitization, and more rarely neurologic signs of hepatic encephalopathy

Treatment

- General therapy for hepatic failure (see p. 325)

Prognosis

- Guarded if signs of hepatic failure are present

Pyrrolizidine Alkaloids

Contained in the following plants: *Senecio* spp. (ragwort, groundsel; Fig. 53–10 and Color Plate 31), *Crotalaria* spp. (rattlebox; Fig. 53–11 and Color Plate 32), *Amsinckia* spp. (fiddleneck), *Echium vulgare* (viper's bugloss), *Heliotropium*

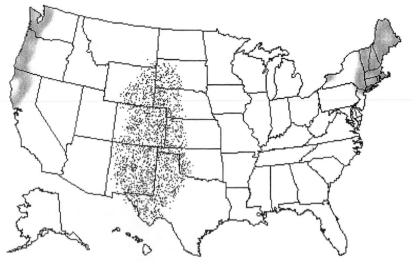

FIGURE 53-10. Distribution of *Senecio jacobea* (ragwort) (solid) and *S. riddellii* (stippled).

europaeum (heliotrope), *Cynoglossum officinale* (hound's tongue; Fig. 53–12 and Color Plate 33), and others. Toxicity from pyrrolizidine alkaloid–containing plants is a clinical problem mostly in the western United States, although some areas of eastern Canada and the United States have reported cases. Toxicity occurs from chronic ingestion of the plants, mostly in spring-cut alfalfa hay. Pyrrolizidine

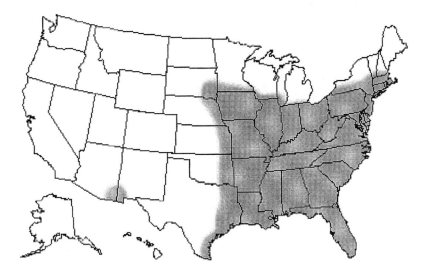

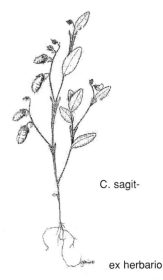

C. sagit-

ex herbario

FIGURE 53-11. Distribution and drawing of *Crotalaria sagittalis* (rattlebox).

TOXICOLOGY

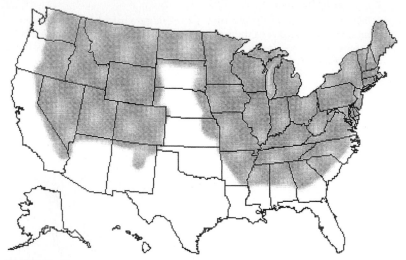

FIGURE 53-12. Distribution of *Cynoglossum officinale* (hound's tongue).

alkaloids produce a chronic hepatic disease, and the onset is often acute several weeks after ingestion.

Mechanism of Toxic Action
- Pyrrolizidine alkaloid liver metabolites interact with cellular constituents and cause a decrease of DNA-mediated RNA and protein synthesis.
- Hepatocyte degeneration, necrosis, and impairment of cell division result in megalocytosis.

Clinical Signs
- Head pressing, circling, blindness, ataxia, icterus, photosensitization, and weight loss.

Diagnosis
- May be difficult because exposure may have occurred long before the onset of clinical signs.
- Inspection of the hay.
- Liver biopsy with characteristic findings of megalocytosis, centrilobular necrosis, portal fibrosis, and biliary hyperplasis.
- Suspect feed can be analyzed for alkaloids (Poisonous Plant Research Laboratory, Logan, UT 84341 or California Animal Health and Food Safety Laboratory, Davis, CA 95617).
- See p. 317 for additional information on diagnosis, including the use of GGT measurement in detecting subclinical cases.

Treatment
- Supportive for hepatic failure (see p. 325; most affected individuals have signs of liver failure and die within days to several months after exposure.

Sensitive Fern *(Onoclea sensibilis)*

Found throughout eastern North America in open woods and meadows. Poisoning is rare because quantities must be ingested over long periods.

Clinical Signs

- Incoordination, anorexia, hyperesthesia
- Affected individuals have liver disease (fatty degeneration) and cerebral edema with neuronal degeneration.

Blue-Green Algae

See p. 729.

TOXINS PREDOMINANTLY AFFECTING THE SKIN

Lower Limb Dermatitis

Acutely developing dermatitis of one or more lower limbs on a horse is common under certain conditions, usually owing to excessive moisture (from wash racks or wet pasture). It appears more noticeably on white legs. The limb is swollen, has many scabs, and is painful. **Rule out** *Dermatophilus* infection!

Treatment

- Systemic glucocorticoids (e.g., prednisolone), 0.5-1.0 mg/kg PO q24h.
- Clean the leg and apply chlorhexidine cream.

Snow-on-the-Mountain *(Euphorbia marginata)*

This and other *Euphorbia* spp. are in the spurge family. Spurges contain an irritant milky sap that causes *contact irritation* of the skin, mouth, and GI tract.

Treatment

- Wash skin with water; apply topical steroid or antihistamine emollients.
- Administer demulcents or mineral oil orally.
- If severe clinical signs are present: Steroids, antihistamines, and analgesics.

Stinging Nettle *(Urtica dioica* and Others)

Plants have stinging hairs containing formic acid, histamine, serotonin, and other constituents that cause local irritation. Affected individuals have been reported to exhibit ataxia, distress, and muscle weakness for several hours after extensive contact with nettle; the mechanism is unknown.

Treatment

- Steroids, antihistamines, analgesics, local cleansing of affected area, and topical emollients as needed.

St. John's Wort *(Hypericum perforatum)* (Fig. 53–13 and Color Plate 34)

Found throughout the United States along roadsides and in abandoned fields and open woods. Toxic principle is hypericin, a pigment that directly reacts with light

TOXICOLOGY

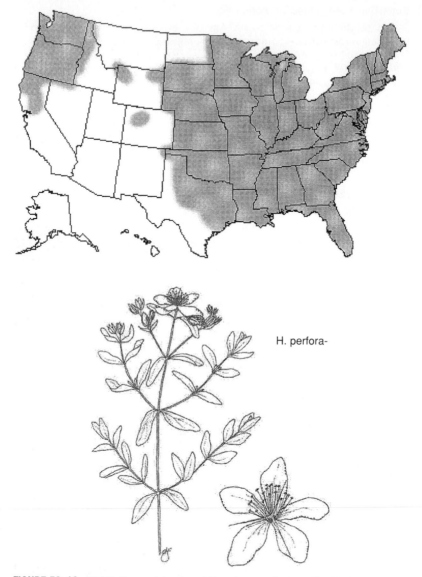

H. perfora-

FIGURE 53–13. Distribution and drawing of *Hypericum perforatum* (St. John's wort).

to cause primary photosensitization, often within 24 hours after ingestion. Buckwheat *(Fagopyrum esculentum)* also causes primary photosensitivity; however, exposure is unusual. Both plants remain toxic when dried.

Mechanism of Toxic Action

- Photodynamic agent (hypericin) activated by long ultraviolet light to a reactive compound. Interaction of reactive compound with cellular constituents.

Clinical Signs
- Dermatitis, pruritus, and ulceration, all of which are more severe in nonpigmented areas of the skin and areas of the body with more exposure to sunlight.
- Lacrimation, conjunctival erythema, corneal ulceration, and anorexia due to irritation around the mouth also may occur.

Treatment
- Remove the affected individuals from plant exposure and sunlight.
- Topical treatment of the dermatitis (e.g., silver sulfadiazine cream), antihistamines, or systemic glucocorticoids if pruritus is severe.
- Ophthalmic antibiotics as needed.
- Oral antibiotics (e.g., trimethoprim-sulfamethoxazole) in cases of severe dermatitis.

PHOTOSENSITIZATION (SECONDARY)
In *primary photosensitization* (e.g., St. John's wort), there is no biochemical evidence of liver disease. *Secondary photosensitization* involves failure of the liver to excrete a normal metabolite of chlorophyll, phylloerythrin, and subsequent accumulation of this substance. Phylloerythrin is a photodynamic agent that becomes reactive after activation by ultraviolet light. The differential diagnosis of secondary or hepatogenous photosensitivity includes hepatic failure (use biochemical tests, GGT, bilirubin) and other plants such as alsike clover, panicum, and pyrrolizidine alkaloid–containing plants. Prognosis for horses with secondary photosensitization is worse than for primary photosensitization because of the severe liver disease.

TOXINS PREDOMINANTLY AFFECTING THE MUSCULOSKELETAL SYSTEM
Black Walnut *(Juglans nigra)* (see Color Plate 35)
Walnut and related hickories are important trees of the eastern deciduous forests. Problems arise after horses are bedded on wood shavings containing black walnut. The toxic principle of black walnut shavings is unknown.

Mechanism of Toxic Action
- Unknown, but toxin may enhance the vasoconstrictive actions of hormones such as epinephrine.

Clinical Signs
- Laminitis often occurs within 12-24 hours of bedding on fresh black walnut shavings. As little as 5% black walnut shavings in the bedding can cause clinical disease.
- There may be marked edema of all four limbs and mild pyrexia.
- Laminitis with edema of all four limbs affecting more than one horse on a farm should arouse suspicion of black walnut shaving toxicity.

Diagnosis
- Rule out other causes of laminitis.
- Black walnut can be identified in shavings by diagnostic laboratories or wood technologists.

Treatment

- Remove from the shavings.
- Wash legs with mild soap and administer hydrotherapy.
- Treat for laminitis, for example, analgesics such as phenylbutazone, 4.0 mg/kg IV; flunixin meglumine, 1.0 mg/kg IV; or ketoprofen, 2.2 mg/kg IV (see p. 368).
- Apply frog pads or place in sand bedding.
- Apply support wraps.
- Pentoxifylline, 8.4 mg/kg q12h, and aspirin, 60-90 grains (10-20 mg/kg) PO every other day for a 450-kg adult.
- 2% Nitroglycerine cream (wear gloves) placed around the palmar/plantar digital arteries and covered with a light bandage.

Prognosis

- Generally better than for other causes of laminitis.

Day-Blooming Jessamine *(Cestrum diurnum)*

Toxic principle is cholecalciferol glycoside, which causes hypervitaminosis D_3 (hypercalcemia). Found in southeastern United States, Texas, California, and Hawaii.

Mechanism of Toxic Action

- Excessive vitamin D_3 causes increased absorption of calcium from the GI tract and renal tubules and increased osteoclastic activity, which results in hypercalcemia.
- Hypercalcemia leads to dystrophic tissue calcification.

Clinical Signs

- Lameness, loss of weight, stiffness, and reluctance to move.
- Acute poisoning does not occur; however, chronic ingestion can cause calcification of tendons, ligaments, arteries, and kidneys.
- Serum calcium concentration is elevated.

Treatment

- Remove from source.
- Normal saline solution and furosemide diuresis with glucocorticoid administration may decrease calcium concentration.
- Symptomatic and supportive care.
- Evaluate kidney function.

Fescue Foot in Foals

Arterial constriction in a limb is a rare occurrence in otherwise healthy foals grazing on fescue pasture. Most reported cases occurred during one summer; this finding suggests unusual environmental conditions are needed. Ergotism produced from the growth of *Claviceps purpurea* on grains has a similar presentation.

Treatment

- None.
- Nitroglycerin cream can be applied over affected arteries.

Hoary Alyssum *(Berteroa incana)* (Fig. 53–14 and Color Plate 36)

A plant in the mustard family found throughout the midwest and northeastern United States. Often grows in older alfalfa fields where considerable winterkill occurs; remains toxic and palatable in dried hay.

Mechanism of Toxic Action

- Unknown.

Clinical Signs

- Acute onset of limb edema, along with lethargy, fever, and sometimes diarrhea.
- Joint stiffness, laminitis, and hematuria may develop.
- Death is unusual.
- Clinical signs develop 18-36 hours after ingestion.

Treatment

- Symptomatic and supportive care.
- When plant is removed from diet, remission of signs generally occurs within 2-4 days.

TOXINS PREDOMINANTLY AFFECTING THE CARDIOVASCULAR SYSTEM

Foxglove *(Digitalis purpurea)*, Milkweed *(Ascleplas* spp.), Yellow Oleander *(Thevetia peruviana)*, Dogbanes *(Apocynum* spp.), Lily-of-the-Valley *(Convallaria majalis)*

These are all potentially toxic plants that contain cardiac glycosides. Poisoning of horses by these plants is uncommon but can occur if the plants are mixed in hay and the affected individuals have little else to eat.

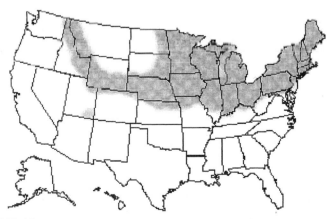

FIGURE 53–14. Distribution of *Berteroa incana* (hoary alyssum).

Mechanism of Toxic Action

- Inhibition of Na^+-K^+-ATPase with subsequent alteration of Na^+, K^+ flux across membranes. Increase in intracellular Ca^{2+} level results in alterations of cardiac conduction.

Clinical Signs and Treatment

- See Oleander.

Ionophore Antibiotic Poisoning

Ionophore antibiotics are used in cattle and poultry feed to improve feed efficiency and as coccidiostats. They are capable of carrying ions across biologic membranes. Common ionophores include monensin (Rumensin, Coban), lasalocid (Bovatec, Avatec), narasin (Monteban), laidlomycin (Cattlyst), and salinomycin (Sacox, Bio-Cox). Horses are extremely susceptible to ionophore antibiotics; the minimal lethal dosage of monensin may be as low as 1 mg/kg body weight.

Mechanism of Toxic Action

- Mediate an electrically neutral exchange of cations for protons across cell membranes
- Influx of calcium into cells.
- Disruption of electrochemical gradients across mitochondrial membranes leading to loss of cellular energy production.

Clinical Signs

- Vary depending on the amount ingested and ionophore involved: Anorexia, colic, diarrhea, depression, sweating, labored breathing, prostration, and death
- Hyperventilation, jugular pulsation, tachycardia, and bright-red mucous membranes are found with cardiac failure (especially monensin).
- Sudden death has been reported, presumably from cardiac failure (especially with monensin).
- Recumbency occurs in some cases without signs of heart failure (especially with lasalocid). The cause of the recumbency has not been found.
- Stranguria (straining) and excess urination (polyuria) are reported in some horses.

Diagnosis

- Send the suspect feed or GI (stomach and colon) contents to a laboratory. Most diagnostic laboratories can test for ionophores.
- Serum concentration of muscle enzymes generally is increased.
- Histologic evidence of cardiac muscle lesions.

Treatment

- Remove the suspect feed.
- Administer AC.
- Administer intravenous polyionic fluids.
- Administer vitamin E and intramuscular selenium injection.
- Provide other supportive care.
- Do not administer digoxin!

Japanese Yew *(Taxus cuspidata)* (see Color Plate 37)

A common ornamental shrub throughout the United States; the toxic principles are taxine alkaloids, especially taxine B. Horses are most commonly exposed to yew plants when they are allowed to graze around show barns, offices, or homes or when clippings from the bushes are thrown into the pasture. Ingestion of as little as 1.0 kg of Japanese yew can kill a 450-kg adult. The English yew *(Taxus baccata)* also is toxic.

Mechanism of Toxic Action

- In vitro, taxines decrease cardiac contractility, maximal rate of depolarization, and coronary blood flow.
- In vivo, taxines slow atrial and ventricular rates with ventricles stopping in diastole.

Clinical Signs

- Ataxia, muscle trembling, and collapse occur. The heart rate is abnormally low.
- Sudden death, within 1-5 hours of ingestion, can occur. If the individual survives, mild colic and diarrhea develop.

Diagnosis

- Compatible history and clinical signs.
- Identification of needle fragments in the stomach contents and possible isolation of alkaloids.

Treatment

- If ingestion is suspected and no clinical signs are exhibited, administer AC and place the patient in a quiet area.
- Administering any treatment *after clinical signs* are manifested can lead to excitement-induced death.

Oleander *(Nerium oleander)* (Fig. 53–15 and Color Plate 38)

Introduced into the United States and grows mostly in the southern states from California to Florida. Can be a potted houseplant in northern climates. Affected individuals become exposed from browsing on plants around buildings or eating dried leaves in the hay. All parts of the plant are toxic, and as little as 1 ounce (28 g) of leaves can be lethal to a 450-kg adult. Toxic principles are steroidal glycosidic cardenolides, which remain when the plant is dried.

Mechanism of Toxic Action

- See Foxglove.

Clinical Signs

- Colic, muscle tremors, hemorrhagic diarrhea, recumbency, arrhythmias, weak pulse, and signs of cardiac failure.
- Onset of clinical signs may be delayed several hours after ingestion.
- Signs may persist for 1-2 days after last ingestion.

Diagnosis

- Evidence of consumption, compatible clinical signs.

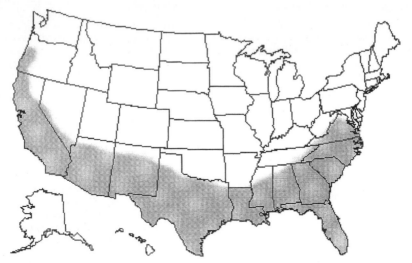

FIGURE 53–15. Distribution of *Nerium oleander*.

- Identification of leaf fragments in the stomach or GI contents. Some laboratories (California Animal Health and Food Safety Laboratory, Davis, CA 95617) test for cardiac glycosides in the stomach contents.
- Histologic evidence of cardiac necrosis.

Treatment
- AC orally.
- Magnesium sulfate by mouth.
- Supportive care and confinement in a quiet area.
- Evaluate cardiac irregularities and treat with appropriate antiarrhythmic drugs; if arrhythmia is life-threatening, see p. 134.

TOXINS PREDOMINANTLY CAUSING HEMOLYSIS OR BLEEDING
Moldy Yellow Sweet Clover *(Melilotus officinalis)*, Moldy White Sweet Clover *(M. alba)*

Grown as forage crops, especially in northwestern United States and western Canada. Only when moldy are these plants toxic. The mold converts normal plant constituents to dicoumarol, an anticoagulant. Occurrence is rare among horses, because horses are less likely than cattle to be chronically fed or ingest the moldy sweet clover hay.

Mechanism of Toxic Action
- Interference with normal vitamin K_1 function with resultant decline in vitamin K_1–dependent clotting factors.

Clinical Signs
- Bleeding abnormalities, as seen in anticoagulant rodenticide poisoning.

Diagnosis
- History and clinical signs.
- Prolonged prothrombin time or other abnormalities in coagulation profile.
- Liver function is otherwise normal.

Treatment
- Remove from suspect hay.
- See Anticoagulant Rodenticide.

Red Maple *(Acer rubrum)* (Fig. 53–16 and Color Plate 39)

A common tree throughout eastern North America, also known as the swamp maple. Red maple poisoning is the most common cause of hemolytic anemia among adult horses in the eastern United States. The poisoning most commonly follows a storm that causes limbs to fall into the pasture or occurs when cut trees are left lying in a pasture. Wilted leaves are the most toxic; toxicity slowly decreases as the leaves dry. Fresh leaves are apparently not toxic. The toxic principle is unknown. Although not well documented, other *Acer* spp. should be considered potentially toxic.

Mechanism of Toxic Action
- Oxidative damage to red blood cells.

Clinical Signs
- Depression, red urine, jaundice, ataxia, and sometimes sudden death.
- Hemolysis, Heinz body formation, and methemoglobinemia occur, although one may predominate. If hemolysis is the primary clinical finding of the disease, the course of the disease is 2-10 days. If methemoglobinemia predominates, then sudden death may occur.

Diagnosis
- History and clinical signs.
- Clinical pathologic examination reveals Coombs-negative hemolytic anemia with Heinz bodies and a variable degree of methemoglobinemia (8%-50%).

Treatment
- Blood transfusion if packed cell volume is less than 11% over 2 or more days or if it is less than 18% in 1 day (see p. 336)
- Large dosages of vitamin C (1 g/kg PO) may be of some benefit; however, the efficacy has not been demonstrated.
- Methylene blue, 8.8 mg/kg slowly IV, for individuals with methemoglobin over 20%, however, results may not be dramatic because of relatively low methemoglobin reductase activity in horses.
- Intravenous polyionic fluids are important to prevent hypovolemia, dilute red blood cell fragments that may trigger disseminated intravascular coagulation, and prevent tubular necrosis. Although the packed cell volume decreases with fluids, the number of red blood cells remains the same, and function may improve.

TOXICOLOGY

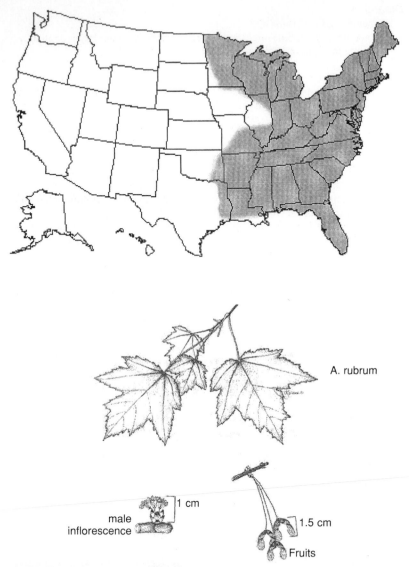

FIGURE 53-16. Distribution and drawing of *Acer rubrum* (red maple).

Anticoagulant Rodenticide Poisoning

This condition is caused by overzealous administration of warfarin in the management of navicular disease and by ingestion of anticoagulant rodenticides (e.g., warfarin, indanediones, brodifacoum). Newer anticoagulant rodenticides are 40-200 times as potent as warfarin and are much more commonly used.

Mechanism of Toxic Action
- Interference with normal vitamin K_1 function with resultant decline in vitamin K_1–dependent clotting factors.

Clinical Signs
- Excessive bleeding from wounds, failure of blood to clot. Often pale mucous membranes from intraabdominal bleeding. Hematoma may form or dyspnea may occur because of intrapleural bleeding.
- Clinical signs are delayed for 1-5 days after ingestion owing to persistence of functional clotting factors.

Diagnosis
- History and clinical signs.
- Prolonged prothrombin time or other abnormalities in coagulation profile (submit citrate sample with control).
- Detection of a specific anticoagulant rodenticide in serum, whole blood, or liver samples. Testing is widely available through diagnostic laboratories.
- Liver function is otherwise normal.

Treatment
- Administer vitamin K_1, 0.5-1 mg/kg SQ q4-6h for the first 24 hours. *Do not administer vitamin K_1 intravenously.*
- Follow with oral vitamin K_1, 5 mg/kg per day with food for an additional 7 days. With newer anticoagulants (indanediones, brodifacoum), vitamin K_1 is recommended for a minimum of 21 days.
- Administer fresh-frozen plasma to affected individuals with clinical bleeding.
- Avoid steroid use or other drugs that are highly protein bound, because they can exacerbate the anticoagulant effects.
- *Do not use vitamin K_3 in the treatment of horses.*

Wild Onions (*Allium* spp.), Domestic Onions (*A. cepa*)

Wild onions are found in moist areas of most states, and the feeding of cull onions is associated with clinical problems. Onions cause Heinz body hemolytic anemia in horses ingesting large quantities of the plant or bulbs. The toxic principle is *n*-propyl disulfide.

Mechanism of Toxic Action
- Oxidative damage to red blood cells; hemoglobin denaturation.

Clinical Signs
- Vary from a mild anemia to acute hemolytic anemia.
- Other signs as with red maple poisoning.
- Affected individuals often have a sulfur or onion odor to their breath.

Treatment
- Remove onions from diet.
- Symptomatic and supportive.
- Generally not life threatening; anemia is unusual.

TOXINS PREDOMINANTLY AFFECTING THE URINARY SYSTEM
Aminoglycosides

Toxicity especially common when used in dehydrated or hypotensive patients. See p. 530.

Mercury

Inorganic mercury may be ingested in toxic amounts when horses lick mercury poultices or blisters (mercuric iodide, mercuric oxide) applied to the legs. If mercury is ingested, severe tubular nephrosis and gastrointestinal ulceration occur.

Mechanism of Toxic Action
- Direct reaction of mercury with cellular constituents.

Clinical Signs
- Anorexia, weight loss, colic, stomatitis, and diarrhea.
- Progressive signs of renal failure, laboratory findings of azotemia.

Treatment
- Intravenous fluids (see treatment of renal failure, p. 531)
- Acute cases are managed with oral sodium thiosulfate, 30-500 mg/kg slowly IV, and dimercaprol BAL, 2.5 mg/kg IM q6h for 2 days and continued q12h for an additional 8 days.
- Succimer is a newer, orally administered chelator effective for chelation of lead, arsenic, and mercury. There is little information on its use in horses; however, it has been shown safe in other species for management of lead intoxication. Recommended dosage is 10 mg/kg PO q8h for 5-10 days. Measurement of blood concentration should be repeated several days after cessation of chelation therapy.
- Supportive care with GI protectant: Sucralfate, 4 g PO q6h.

Nonsteroidal Antiinflammatory Drugs

All nonsteroidal antiinflammatory drugs (NSAIDs) are potentially toxic. Toxicity generally is dosage and duration dependent. Mechanism of toxic action is probably related to inhibition of prostaglandin synthesis. Clinical signs include depression, bruxism, oral ulceration, polyuria and, less frequently, diarrhea. Therapy for intoxication is symptomatic and supportive.

Vitamin K$_3$ (Menadione)

Signs of depression and renal failure may occur in affected individuals 3-4 days after parenteral administration of vitamin K$_3$ (no longer commercially available).

Treatment
- Intravenous fluids (see treatment of renal failure, p. 531)

■ SUDDEN AND UNEXPECTED DEATH IN HORSES

SUDDEN DEATH WITHOUT CLINICAL SIGNS

Sudden death is one of the most frustrating emergency calls for clinicians. Rather than managing a medical emergency, it is the clinician's role to determine the cause of death. This becomes especially urgent when there is a chance of foul play, the affected individual is insured, or there is a possibility that other horses may be affected. A complete history is imperative, including:

- Use of the horse
- Management changes, including personnel, at the stable
- Changes
  - Feed
  - Pasture
  - Treatments
  - Ownership
  - Insurance
  - Weather

Perform a complete postmortem examination initially, looking for obvious causes of death: Hemorrhage, gastric rupture, or cardiac abnormalities, as discussed later. If the cause of death is not obvious, obtain samples of all appropriate tissues for histopathologic evaluation and toxicologic testing, as listed at the beginning of this chapter. If there is the suspicion of foul play, take photographs or video footage of the affected individual and surroundings. Label all samples, and document all reports regarding the case.

Cases of sudden, unexplained death of horses often involve litigation. It is critical to thoroughly document all investigative work. It is prudent to follow chain-of-custody procedures when submitting samples for analysis. Diagnostic laboratories often can advise practitioners about appropriate sample submission in such situations.

Sudden death is defined as death that occurs acutely without previous illness or illness of only a few minutes. The most common causes among horses are as follows.

TOXIC CAUSES OF SUDDEN DEATH (INGESTION)
Blue-Green Algae (*Microcyotis* spp. and others)

Rarely reported among horses but can cause sudden death, especially in the plains states in summer when horses drink from ponds in full bloom with algae. Algae often are concentrated at the side of the pond by the wind. Affected individuals may have sudden onset of gastroenteritis and hemorrhagic diarrhea; acute liver failure and seizures precede death.

Diagnosis

- Preserve algae bloom material with 10% formalin (9 parts water to 1 part 10% formalin) for testing for the pathogenic algae.
- Freeze fresh algae bloom material for toxin testing or mouse bioassay.

- Freeze samples of stomach and intestinal contents for toxin testing.
- Perform histopathologic examination of fixed liver.

Treatment
- For other exposed horses: AC
- Symptomatic and supportive care

Cyanide Poisoning

Has been reported as a cause of sudden death among horses ingesting wild cherry (*Prunus* spp.) leaves, saplings, or bark (Figs. 53–17 and 53–18 and Color Plate 40).

Diagnosis
- Cyanide in stomach contents or blood. Freeze stomach contents immediately in airtight container.

Treatment
- For known exposed horses on the farm: 16 mg/kg sodium nitrate (1%), followed by sodium thiosulfate, 30-40 mg/kg slowly IV.

Monensin Poisoning

See pp. 181 and 722

Oleander Poisoning

See p. 723

Red Maple

See p. 725. Sudden illness and rapid death may result from acute methemoglobinemia and for an unexplained reason. Occurs more commonly late in the leaf season. Death may precede jaundice; however, urine is dark black.

Taxus

See p. 723.

Diagnosis
- Plants found in stomach
- Detection of alkaloid in GI contents

CARDIAC DEFECTS AND EXERCISE-INDUCED DEATH

A variety of cardiac abnormalities have been blamed for sudden and unexpected death among horses either during or immediately after exercise:

- **Aortic valve thickening.**
- **Ruptured chordae tendineae:** More commonly results in acute respiratory distress and signs of heart failure.

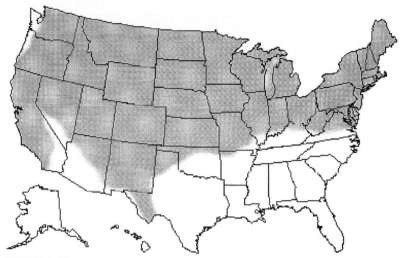

FIGURE 53-17. Distribution of *Prunus virginiana* (wild cherry).

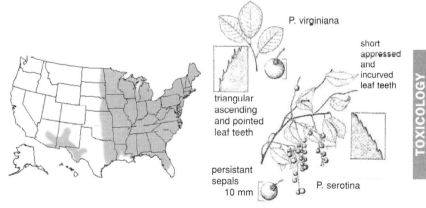

FIGURE 53-18. Distribution of *Prunus serotina* and drawings of *P. virginiana* and *P. serotina*.

- **Occlusion of the coronary artery;** rarely if ever documented in the horse.
- **Lacerated coronary artery** in foals, associated with fractured ribs.
- **Cardiac arrhythmias** and **myocarditis**, as in humans, result in unexplained and unexpected death associated with exercise.

- **White-muscle disease** in foals younger than 8 months should be considered in areas with severe selenium deficiency (e.g., Canada, northeastern United States, Ohio, and other areas). Measure liver and heart blood selenium concentrations. Also HYPP dominant in Quarter Horse foals.
- **Air emboli** are unlikely to cause problems in the horse unless large volumes are rapidly injected and/or the air enters the arterial circulation.
- **Electrolyte abnormalities** (hypocalcemia, hypercalcemia, hypokalemia, hyperkalemia) and cardiac arrhythmia are a common cause of sudden death and generally occur in horses with severe predisposing illness.

BLEEDING AS A CAUSE OF SUDDEN AND UNEXPECTED DEATH

- **Ruptured uterine artery** in mares: More common in older brood mares in late pregnancy or at foaling.
- **Lacerated iliac artery:** May or may not be associated with a fractured pelvis.
- **Ruptured kidney:** History of trauma or rib fracture in many cases.
- **Ruptured aorta:** Most common in middle-aged or older breeding stallions; frequently occurs immediately after breeding.
- **Ruptured spleen or liver:** In most cases associated with trauma.
- **Rupture of the internal carotid or maxillary artery** in association with guttural pouch mycosis: Massive external hemorrhage occurs.
- **Pulmonary hemorrhage** in a racehorse rarely causes sudden death.
- **Acute hemolytic anemia** rarely causes sudden death in horses without previous clinical signs. Sudden death rarely occurs among foals with neonatal isoerythrolysis.

NEUROLOGIC CAUSES OF SUDDEN DEATH

- **Trauma.**
  - Rearing and falling backward, fracturing the junction between the basisphenoid and basioccipital bones resulting in cerebral trauma, hemorrhage. Evidence of blood in the external ear canal or from the nostrils supports this premise.
  - Fractured cervical vertebrae.
  - Other traumatic events causing severe head injury (i.e., kicks).
- **Botulism** causes sudden death if a large amount of preformed toxin (e.g., as from silage) is ingested.
- **Accidental feeding of 4-aminopyridine** (a bird-repellent agent) produces severe neurologic signs or sudden death in horses fed 2-3 mg/kg. Diagnosis is by testing the suspect source such as feed and GI contents along with a history of exposure.
- **Heat stroke, hypothermia, and hypoglycemia** cause coma and sudden death.
- **OP poisoning** causes acute paralysis and death if horses are exposed to sufficient quantities of the toxin (seed corn) (see p. 699).

INTESTINAL CAUSES OF SUDDEN AND UNEXPECTED DEATH

Intestinal diseases rarely cause sudden death without evidence of illness (colic, diarrhea, toxemia) preceding the death. In some cases these signs may be brief:

- **Gastric rupture**, most commonly from tympany and from impaction in a few peracute cases or in foals with perforating ulcer. Duodenal perforations may occur in foals.
- **Colitis** rarely causes death from endotoxemia with only a brief clinical illness (e.g., <1 hour).
- **Ruptured cecum:** In most cases there is evidence of mild discomfort for hours or days preceding the death and in a few cases after foaling.
- **Rupture of the colon** rarely occurs without mechanical displacement.
- **Blister beetle poisoning** (see p. 694)
- **Volvulus of the small intestine:** Acute abdominal signs or evidence of colic usually precede death.

SEPTICEMIA, BACTEREMIA, AND ENDOTOXEMIA AS CAUSES OF SUDDEN DEATH

These conditions are more common among young foals than they are among adults. Among foals, death occasionally occurs within 1 hour of the clinical signs. In 8- to 42-day-old foals, Tyzzer's disease is a primary differential diagnosis. In a 2- to 4-day-old foal, *Actinobacillus* infection is a primary differential diagnosis.

RESPIRATORY CAUSES OF SUDDEN AND UNEXPECTED DEATH

- **Pneumothorax:** Most cases are associated with trauma, although some are idiopathic
- **Pulmonary hemorrhage:** Most common among racehorses during or immediately after a race. In most cases blood is seen at the nares or on the ground
- **Airway obstruction:** Acute laryngeal obstruction caused by edema, food bolus, paralysis, or spasms (postoperatively after removing an endotracheal tube) may result in sudden death. In rare instances, horses with hyperkalemic periodic paralysis die of laryngeal obstruction
- **Acute pulmonary edema:** The most common causes are:
  □ *Acute heart failure* (e.g., ionophores, ruptured chordae tendineae, acute myocarditis associated with a viral infection)
  □ *Anaphylaxis*
  □ *Endotoxemia*
  □ *Laryngeal obstruction*
  □ Hyperkalemic periodic paralysis in Quarter Horses

In most cases clinical signs are noticeable before death.

- **Smoke inhalation** (see p. 513)

OTHER CAUSES OF SUDDEN AND UNEXPECTED DEATH

- **Lightning strike or electrocution:** A history of a storm and evidence of exposed electrical wires support the diagnosis. A *select few* affected individuals may have linear burn marks on the body.
- **Gunshot wounds:** Look for penetrating wounds entering and exiting the body. The bullet is found in the body in some cases.
- **Black fly swarms** occasionally kill horses.
- **Drowning.**

TOXICOLOGY

ADVERSE DRUG REACTIONS

See Table 52–1.

CAUSES OF MALICIOUS OR CRIMINAL DEATH

- **Electrocution:** Examine the skin closely for injury from placement of needles or clamps used to electrocute the horse. The head (especially the lips), back, tail, and perineal area are the most common sites used for malicious electrocution.
- **Insulin injections:** Collect serum from the heart blood clot and determine insulin concentration and type with HPLC.
- **Potassium injection:** Examine the jugular veins closely for evidence of needle entrance.
- If **deliberate feeding of a poison** is suspected, collect the gastric contents, remaining feed and water, kidney, urine, liver, and fat, and test, at the minimum, for the following: Ionophores, arsenic, strychnine, chlorinated hydrocarbons, and OPs.

REFERENCES

Toxicosis

Brown C, Bertone J: *5 Minute veterinary consult: equine,* Philadelphia, 2001, Lippincott Williams & Wilkins.

Burrows GE, Tyrl RJ: *Toxic plants of North America,* Ames, Iowa, 2001, State University Press.

Galey FD: Toxicology. In Robinson NE, editor: *Current therapy in equine medicine IV,* Philadelphia, 1997, WB Saunders.

Galey FD: Disorders caused by toxicants. In Smith BP, editor: *Large animal internal medicine,* ed 3, St. Louis, 2002, Mosby.

Galey FD, editor: Toxicology. *Vet Clin North Am Equine Pract* 17(3), 2002.

Hall JO, Buck WB, Cote J: *Natural poisons in horses,* ed 2, Urbana, Ill, 1995, National Animal Poison Control Center, University of Illinois.

Hausner EA: Toxicology—what every veterinarian needs to know, *Clinical Techniques in Equine Practice* 2:51-115.

Knight AP: Plant poisoning of horses. In Lewis L, editor: *Equine clinical nutrition: feeding and care,* Media, Pa, 1995, Williams & Wilkins.

Knight AP, Walter RG: *A guide to plant poisoning of animals of North America,* Jackson, Wyo, 2001, Teton New Media.

Plant Identification

The following websites contain excellent photos that may be of assistance in identifying a plant. They also provide considerable plant toxicity data.

http://cal.nbc.upenn.edu/poison/
http://sis.agr.gc.ca/pls/pp/poison?p_x=px
http://www.ansci.cornell.edu/plants/index.html
http://vet.purdue.edu/depts/addl/toxic/cover1.htm
http://www.ces.ncsu.edu/depts/hort/consumer/poison/poison.htm
http://education.vetmed.vt.edu/Curriculum/VM8424/toxicplants/index.html
http://www.caf.wvu.edu/~forage/library/poisonous/index.htm

Acute and Unexpected Death

Brown CM et al: Sudden and unexplained death in adult horses, *Comp Cont Educ Pract Vet* 9:78-85, 1987.

Platt H: Sudden and unexplained deaths in horses: a review of 69 cases, *Br Vet J* 138:417-429, 1982.

Management of Special Problems

54 Disaster Medicine

Tomas Gimenez, Rebecca M. Gimenez, and Richard A. Mansmann

INDIVIDUAL SITUATIONS

Clinicians frequently equate emergencies with "disasters," or at a minimum, some complex emergencies are referred to as "disasters!" Emergencies are incidents that require immediate response, such as a trailer accident on a highway, but that do not exhaust the local resources. Although a disaster also can be an emergency, this term is more commonly used in the case of natural disasters, such as hurricanes or floods, in which the response to individual incidents within the disaster can take place from a few hours to a day to a week after the initial event. The difference between an emergency and a disaster is the number of persons involved:

- In an emergency, the clinician and staff work with the owner to help the patient.
- In a disaster, the veterinarian works with rescue personnel as a member of a team to safely assist the patient.

This is true of disasters involving small numbers of individuals and of disasters with large numbers of individuals.

Types of Emergencies/Disasters

- Road emergencies (trailer and van accidents, loose horses)
- Off-road emergencies (fall or entrapment)
- Competition emergencies
- Barn fires
- Natural disasters (hurricane, flood, tornado, wild fire, earthquake)
- Hazardous spills

Veterinarians are creative and independent. This creativity allows clinicians to help horses in difficult situations by being able to process many "helpful" suggestions. However, the independence frequently results in humane destruction of patients that could have been helped by a well-organized team. Emergency horse rescue performed in a way that is safe for both the rescuers and the patient requires training in technical rescue procedures for all emergency responders, *including the veterinarian.*

Preparation

Planning for disasters requires detailed protocols and training at several **levels.** *The basis of disaster medicine is sharpening standard emergency skills rehearsed in routine clinical emergencies.* Emergencies are more difficult to plan for, necessitating training and preparation in coordination with a team of rescuers. Written emergency protocols are mandatory, and "emergency kits" must be prepared for every imaginable scenario. For example, the horse:

- Is stuck in mud
- Has fallen into a ravine

- Has crawled into a culvert
- Is hanging from a railroad trestle

The emergency kit contains everything needed for a *specific emergency.* It is portable, clearly marked, and readily accessible. These kits can serve several functions in the routine practice:

- *Crash kit:* For chemical restraint, resuscitation, or euthanasia, with dosages of each drug listed. This kit is most valuable at the side of an anesthetized patient and in the management of adverse drug reactions (see Chapter 52).
- *Catheter kit:* Contains all the materials for placing an intravenous catheter and for fluid administration (several boxes of fluids readily available). The catheter kit saves valuable time in an emergency and facilitates routine catheter placement in nonemergency situations (see p. 11).
- *Respiratory kit:* Contains tracheotomy equipment and instruments and includes tubing for oxygen delivery, a humidifier, and a small oxygen tank (see p. 64).
- *Splint kit:* Contains precut polyvinyl chloride (PVC) pieces, tape, bandage material, hack saw, and cast material, all of which can be tailored to the specific type of limb problem (see p. 345).

These emergency kits can be kept in the ambulatory clinician's vehicle and stored as part of the hospital's inventory. Plastic inventory tags on each bag or kit facilitate any rescue operation.

Disaster Equipment

The most important universal principle to follow in any emergency or disaster is to use the simplest approach that results in a quick and safe rescue. *Training in the use of rescue equipment is beyond the scope of this book.* Veterinarians and other emergency responders should attend one of the equine technical emergency rescue courses available through regional or national (e.g., American Humane Association) organizations. Equipment used for equine emergencies and disasters can be classified into the categories in Box 54–1.

Some specialized large-animal rescue equipment is commercially available. Research on the use of these types of equipment is ongoing. Many items are simple to make or to convert from conventional or human rescue use. Larger and more expensive equipment needs for a community should be proposed and purchased by the community and used under the direction of a veterinarian skilled in large-animal rescue.

Personnel

- Disaster planning is positive and nonthreatening and brings together many different persons working as a team.
- Area veterinarians can exchange ideas on how to respond to various problems.
- Volunteer groups, such as volunteer fire companies and colic or foal teams in academic institutions, can be organized.
- Any volunteer group is a means to involve persons of various skills, including county and emergency professionals.
- Practice drills for various emergency situations train an emergency team that is interested and up to date on disaster medicine.

MANAGEMENT

BOX 54–1. Equipment for Equine Emergencies and Disasters

PERSONAL PROTECTIVE EQUIPMENT
- Gloves
- Boots
- Protective headwear (helmet or hard hat)
- Goggles
- Ear protection
- Protective clothing (durable, long sleeves and pants)
- Rappelling gear (harness, helmet, gloves)
- Water rescue gear (personal flotation device [PFD], dry suit, boots, and specialized helmet)

NOTE: Do not attempt to perform a rescue operation in either swift water or flood water without training.

CRITICAL EQUIPMENT
- Halters of different sizes (nylon, sturdy hardware)
- Lead ropes (10-ft [3 m] cotton, sturdy hardware and chain shank)
- Two 35-ft (10.7 m) sections of 0.5-inch (1.3 cm) kernmantle static rescue rope
- 20 ft (6 m) of 3-inch (7.6 cm) nylon web with a loop on each end (forward assist sling)
- Santa Barbara sling (Fig 54–1)
- 4-6 ft (1.2-1.8 m) of 5-inch-wide (12.7 cm) fire hose web with loops sewn on each end
- Spread bar
- Fleece-lined breast collar (sturdy hardware)
- One set of fleece-lined hobbles
- 1 gallon (3.8 L) of lubricant
- Six 6-ft (1.8 m) loops of 0.5-inch (1.3-cm) rescue rope with mariner's knots
- Protective gear for the horse's head
- 12 large steel carabiners
- One leg-handling cane
- Cotton horse earplugs
- Canvas tarp (minimum 8 ft × 8 ft [2.4 m × 2.4 m])
- Camera (loaded with film)

Important Equipment
- One containment portable fence (e.g., 5-ft × 110-ft [1.5 m × 33.5 m] Polygrid fence)
- One 4:1.5 rope anchor system (with 2 double pulleys and Prusik loops [Fig. 54–2])
- One 3:1 Z-rig rope anchor system (with two single pulleys and Prusik loops)
- 300 ft (91.4 m) of 0.5-inch (1.3-cm) rescue rope
- One human class III full body harness
- Two canvas tarps (at least 12 ft × 12 ft [3.7 m × 3.7 m])
- Blankets
- Cutting saws, axes, shovels
- Boat hook
- Documentation forms
- Portable screen (for competition or public rescues)
- Emergency lights and signs
- Large rubber mat, or Rescue glide set (Fig 54–3) with ratchet straps and hobbles

MECHANIZED EQUIPMENT
- Four-wheel drive truck with winch (minimum 8000 lb [3629 kg]), CB or 2-way radio, and public-address system
- Portable winch (minimum 3000 lb [1361 kg])

BOX 54-1. Equipment for Equine Emergencies and Disasters
Continued

- Wrecker, crane, or rough-terrain forklift (minimum 10-ft [3 m] boom clearance above ground)
- Equine "ambulance," such as a converted horse trailer (with intravenous fluid capability)
- Not critical but important when helicopter rescue is the only option: Anderson sling with cable, web connector, frame (Fig. 54-4)

NOTE: Helicopter rescue of horses is dangerous and should not be attempted without proper training in ground procedures for helicopter rescue.

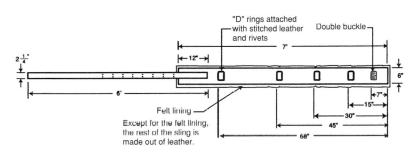

FIGURE 54-1. Santa Barbara sling.

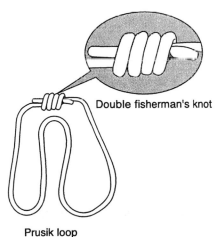

Double fisherman's knot

Prusik loop

FIGURE 54-2. Prusik loop.

MANAGEMENT

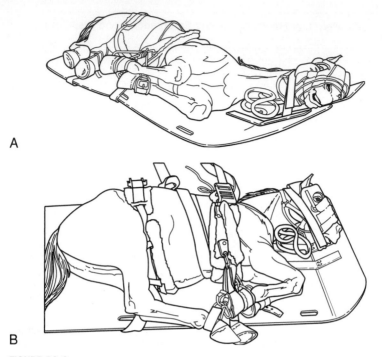

FIGURE 54–3. Rescue glide set. **A,** Side glide. **B,** Top glide.

Chronologic Walk-Through of a Disaster

Step at Which Decisions Must Be Made	Specific Considerations at Step
Assessment of the situation during initial contact	If humans are injured, need for emergency medical services (EMS); whether EMS has been called to the scene
	Physical access to patient; need for police escort
	Additional equipment needs
	Additional personnel needs
Development of a mental protocol on the way to the scene	**Restraint:**
	Calming techniques (massage, voice)
	Physical (earplugs, blindfold, twitch)
	Chemical (drugs and dosages)
	Physical examination:
	Procedures for special circumstances
	Scene security:
	"Onlooker" recruitment or dispersement
	Jobs to fill: Traffic control, animal handler
Arrival on the scene	Meeting with incident commander (chief emergency worker on scene)

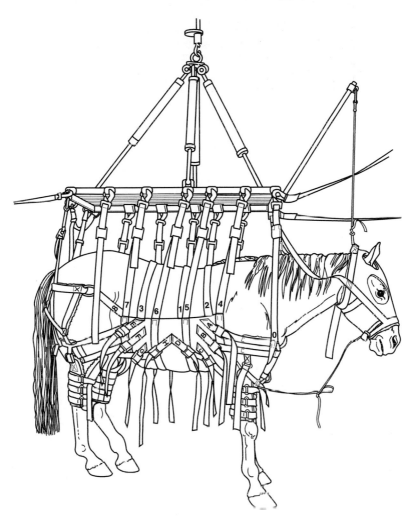

FIGURE 54-4. Anderson sling.

Assessment of overall situation: Whether the horse's rescue is a primary or a secondary concern (humans always are rescued first!)

Assessment of the patient's situation

Whether the horse is dead or alive
Attitude: Quiet, sulking, or depressed
Struggling: Coordinated or uncoordinated
Concept of self-preservation
Obvious medical problems (e.g., wounds, shock)
Less obvious problems (e.g., temperature, pulse,

MANAGEMENT

	respiration [TPR], neurologic and musculoskeletal status)
	Legal: Whether owner or authorized agent wants documentation (photographs, video, written account); notification of insurance company (for euthanasia cases)
Finalization of team plan	Specific equipment and personnel needed
	Notification of incident commander about rescue options
	Additional specialized equipment needed (e.g., jaws of life)
	Specific restraint (none, sedation, anesthesia, euthanasia); when in doubt, be conservative!
	Whether rescue workers understand their jobs (everyone should!)
	Safety first: Check and recheck; use a checklist
Rescue	Technical steps of rescue performed as prescribed
Aftermath of rescue	Examination, assessment
	Treatment of patient
Debriefing, review after rescue	Sharing of written information
	Thanking all participants
	Review of entire protocol, mental and written procedures
	Scheduling follow-up examinations

PRACTICE AND COMMUNITY INVOLVEMENT

Dealing with the effects of large-scale natural and manmade disasters involves more personnel and equipment than does an individual emergency. It requires knowledge of how the state's emergency preparedness and response divisions are organized and how individual veterinarians and volunteers should work within that system.

- Within the disaster are numerous emergencies. Training in large-animal rescue, organizing emergency kits (see Box 54–1), experience, and planning ready the clinician for specific situations within the disaster.
- Counterproductive thinking (e.g., *"These things happen in other places, not here!"*) is to be avoided.
- The goal of the veterinarian should be to facilitate the preparedness of horse owners *ahead* of time. There is no substitute for owners taking responsibility for their animals and facilities. Many owners never take into account how difficult it is to simply help their animals survive without electricity, communication, city water, and food.

A clinician involved in disaster planning should understand four specific points:

- The present level of interest and organizational skills of the equine community
- The office of emergency planning and community response and its relation to other emergency response groups (e.g., fire, police, emergency medical services [EMS], and hospitals)

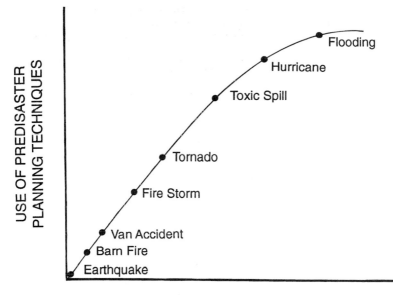

FIGURE 54-5. Disaster curve for intelligent planning.

- The veterinary skills available at the local, state, and national levels that can help in a disaster
- Learning the national, state, and local emergency preparedness and response systems that are in place

To accomplish disaster preparedness and response successfully, all four areas must be carefully assessed and the most common types of disasters that can occur in the community prioritized. Use the disaster curve (Fig. 54–5) to determine the time needed for specific catastrophes.

Involvement of the Horse Community

Veterinarians are ideal leaders in a community's animal disaster planning. Clinicians interested in disaster preparedness and response organize their practices or are involved in routine emergencies at all levels of disaster preparedness.

- Groups need 6-12 owners with basic skills to form an organization of other local owners.
- Close coordination with trained emergency rescue personnel (e.g., police, fire, EMS, animal control) in the early stages of development of an organization greatly stimulates rescue training and practice opportunities. Ask them to share their experiences with rescuing large animals. What worked? What did not? Once the emergency community knows you are interested, trained, and available, prepare to be used regularly.
- Disaster response can be a unifying experience for different horse groups.

MANAGEMENT

Involvement of the Local Office of Emergency Services

▶ *For success, a strong working relationship and trust must be developed between local volunteer groups of animal owners and the office of emergency planning for the community.*

- This is the most critical component for any animal group doing community emergency work.
- The issue of incorporating animals in disaster planning can be organized into local planning by representatives attending emergency service meetings.
- Owners and veterinarians must learn the protocols for emergency preparedness and response.
- Organizations such as humane societies and the American Red Cross are excellent resources for training and help.
- Large facilities such as racetracks, fairgrounds, and show facilities can develop shared needs in an emergency.
- Insurance for volunteers who work in a disaster may be available through county emergency services.

Available Emergency Services

- The American Veterinary Medical Association (AVMA) is heavily involved in veterinary disaster preparedness and response and has published an excellent guide.
- In cooperation with the United States Department of Public Health, the AVMA is helping to organize veterinary medical assistance teams (VMATs) that can be used in a national disaster.
- The VMAT system is an excellent model to integrate several county organizations and therefore act as a regional group.
- The American Academy of Veterinary Disaster Medicine has crossover with the human disaster-preparedness groups and significant organizational skills. For additional information, contact:

  Lyle Vogel, DVM, Secretary/Treasurer, AAVDM
  1931 N. Meacham Road, Suite 100
  Schaumburg, IL 60173

- Several state veterinary medical associations are involved in their states' emergency planning. Contact the association for specifics.
- The American Humane Association and the Humane Society of the United States are designated as the animal arm of the American Red Cross. The American Humane Association provides training in large-animal emergency rescue. For more information, see www.americanhumane.org.
- The Federal Emergency Management Agency (FEMA) has an educational campus:

  Emergency Management Institute
  16825 South Seton Avenue
  Emmitsburg, MD 21727

A complete definition of funding and roles of all animal-related organizations in various disasters is undetermined. It is the responsibility of every veterinarian, horse owner, and community to work within the framework of existing emergency planning to help reduce losses in disasters and identify the necessary funding and part played by everyone involved in emergency management.

- Several states have large-animal emergency rescue volunteer organizations. Contact the state emergency operations/preparedness division. Fire departments and fire academies in several states are training personnel in this aspect of rescue.
- A catalog of activities and several self-study and on-campus courses are available from this agency (see References).

REFERENCES

Rescue

FEMA: *Animals in disaster,* www.femagov/emi/train.htm. Emmitsburg, Md, 1999, Emergency Management Institute.

Fox J: *The horse/large animal extrication unit,* www.feltonfire.com/nmeq3b.html. Felton, Calif, 1998, Felton Fire District.

Heath SE: *Animal management in disasters,* St. Louis, 1999, Mosby.

Ray S: *Animal rescue in flood and swiftwater incidents,* Asheville, NC, 1999, CFS Press.

Sandberg R: *Helsinborg veterinary ambulance,* www.helsinborg.se/brand/engleska/vetrans.html. Helsinborg, Sweden, 1995, Helsinborg Animal Hospital.

Segerstrom J: *Technical animal rescue,* www.rescue3.com. Elk Grove, Calif, 1997, Rescue 3 International.

Product Manufacturers of Emergency Equipment

CUSTOM WEB SLINGS
New Haven Moving Equipment
2490 Verna Court
San Leandro, CA 94577-4223
(800) 624-7950; (510) 760-8901 (talk to Frank)
www.newhaven-usa.com

HORSE RESCUE GLIDE
(accessories must be purchased separately)
B & M Plastics
Greenville, SC
Ben McCracken
(864) 270-1344
ben@leaguemfg.com

RESCUE ROPE AND HARDWARE
CMC Rescue Equipment
P.O. Box 6870
Santa Barbara, CA 93160-6870
(800) 235-5741
www.cmcrescue.com

RESCUE ROPE AND HARDWARE
PMI-Petzl Distribution, Inc.
P.O.Box 803
LaFayette, GA 30728-0803
(800) 282-7673
www.pmi-petzl.com

MANAGEMENT

Rock-n-Rescue
P.O. Box 213
Valencia, PA, 16059-0213
(800) 346-7673
www.rocknrescue.com

PROTECTIVE CLOTHING
Cascade Fire Equipment
P.O. Box 4248
Medford, OR 97501
(800) 654-7049
www.cascadefire.com

PROTECTIVE CLOTHING AND RESCUE EQUIPMENT
Forestry Suppliers, Inc.
P.O. Box 8397
Jackson, MS 39284-8397
(800) 647-5368
www.forestry-suppliers.com

PUBLIC SAFETY CLOTHING AND EQUIPMENT
Galls
2680 Palumbo Drive
Lexington, KY 40509-1000
(800) 477-7766
www.galls.com

WATER RESCUE AND OTHER RESCUE EQUIPMENT
The Rescue Source
P.O. Box 519
Elk Grove, CA 95759
(800) 45-RESCUE
www.rescuesource.com

LARGE HOOKS, STEEL RODS, ETC
McMaster-Carr Industrial Supply Company
P.O. Box 740100
Atlanta, GA 30374-0100
(404) 346-7000
www.mcmaster.com

PORTABLE FENCE
Polygrid Ranch Fence
Jerry B. Leach Co.
P.O. Box 279
Cheraw, SC 29520-0279
(800) 845-9005
www.jerrybleach.com

BOAT HOOK
Westport Marina, Inc.
Part No. DAV4132
(877) 744-7786
www.shipstore.com

HELICOPTER SLING (ANDERSON SLING)
CDA Products
P.O. Box 53
Potter Valley, CA 95469
(707) 743-1300
Fax: (707) 743-2530

LIFTEX SLING
443 Ivyland Road
Warminster, PA, 18974
(800) 448-3079

ALUMINUM LEG SPLINT
Kimzey Veterinary Products
(888) 454-6039

SAM SPLINT
Southeastern Emergency Equipment
P.O. Box 1196
Wake Forest, NC 27588
(800) 334-6656
www.seequip.com

TACTICAL & SURVIVAL SPECIALTIES, INC.
P.O. Box 1890
Harrisonburg, VA 22801
(540) 434-8974
www.tacsurv.com

Basic for Client Distribution

Filkins ME, editor: *Veterinary medicine for back country horsemen,* P.O. Box 11095, Bakersfield, Calif 93389, 1994. Kern Sierra Unit of the Backcountry Horsemen of California. (P.O. Box 11095, Bakersfield, Calif 93389.)

Goodman J, Abronson S: Emergency-red alert! What do I do with my horse in fire, flood, and/or earthquake? Monte Nido, Calif, 1993, E.T.I. Corral 63. (543 Cold Canyon Road, Monte Nido, Calif 91302-2206.)

Hamilton JM, Scheve NK: Hawkins guide: equine emergencies on the road, Southern Pines, NC 28327, 1994, Bluegreen Publishing Co. (P.O. Box 1255, Southern Pines, NC 28327.)

Sakach E, editor: *Disaster relief: designing a disaster plan for your community,* Gaithersburg, Md, 1996, The Humane Society of the United States. (700 Professional Drive, Gaithersburg, Md 20879.)

Organizers

Catalog of Activities of the Emergency Management Institute, 16825 South Seton Avenue, Emmitsburg, Md 21727.

Dey S: *Equine trailer rescue* [film], Horse Park of New Jersey, P.O. Box 548, Allentown, NJ 08501.

Lundin CS, editor: *AVMA emergency preparedness and response guide,* Schaumburg, Ill, 1994, American Veterinary Medical Association. (1931 N. Meacham Road, Schaumburg, Ill 60173.)

Mansmann RA, and others: Disaster planning model for an equine assistance and evacuation team, *J Equine Vet Sci* 12:268-271, 1992.

Natural Hazards Observer [monthly newsletter]. Natural Hazards Research and Application Information Center, Institute of Behavioral Science #6, University of Colorado at Boulder, Campus Box 482, Boulder, Colo 80309-0482.

MANAGEMENT

Proceedings of the First International Conference on Equine Rescue, *J Equine Vet Sci* 13(5), 1993.

Proceedings of the Second International Conference on Equine Rescue, *J Equine Vet Sci* 15(4), 1995.

Medical Personnel

Auf der Heide E: *Disaster response: principles of preparation and coordination*, St. Louis, 1989, Mosby.

Bertone JJ, editor: Emergency treatment in the adult horse, *Vet Clin North Am Equine Pract* 10(3), 1994.

Duffy JC, editor: *Health and medical aspects of disaster preparedness*, New York, 1990, Plenum Publishing.

Prehospital and disaster medicine [human disaster medical journal], Jems Communications, PO Box 2789, Carlsbad, Calif 92018.

55 Acute Pain Management

Michael Tomasic

The presence and degree of pain are a useful diagnostic guide; however, persistence of long-term pain can be harmful to the equine patient.

Acute pain is an important biologic signal that is supposed to last a relatively short time. It is often associated with anxiety and with sympathetic nervous system hyperactivity:

- Tachycardia
- Increased blood pressure
- Increased respiratory rate
- Diaphoresis (sweating)
- Pupillary dilatation

After local injury, due to either trauma or disease, peripheral nociceptors are activated, and as a result of release of local mediators, some peripheral sensitization develops. Segmental and suprasegmental motor activity in response to noxious stimuli can result in muscle spasm, which can further increase pain. This "circle of pain" generally leads to marked increases in sympathetic activity and further sensitization of peripheral nociceptors. Persistent pain and limitation of movement may be associated with:

- Impairment of muscle metabolism
- Atrophy
- Delayed restoration of function

Increased sympathetic activity results in:

- Increased intestinal secretions
- Increased smooth muscle sphincter tone
- Decreased intestinal motility

Gastric stasis and paralytic ileus may occur. In addition, increased sympathetic activity as a result of pain can increase urinary sphincter tone and result in urinary retention. Sympathetic overactivity with increases in heart rate, peripheral resistance, and blood pressure result in increased cardiac work and myocardial oxygen consumption. Because heart rate is greatly increased, diastolic filling time is decreased and there may be reduced oxygen delivery to the myocardium. In the peripheral circulation, acute pain is associated with decreased limb blood flow. Severe postoperative pain and high levels of sympathetic activity may be associated with reduced arterial inflow and decreased venous emptying.

Surgery and other forms of injury generate a catabolic state through changes in endocrine hormonal control with increased secretion of catabolic hormones and decreased secretion or action of anabolic hormones. The results for the patient include:

- Pain
  - Nausea
  - Intestinal stasis

- Alteration in blood flow
  □ Coagulation
  □ Fibrinolysis
- Alteration in substrate metabolism
- Alteration in water and electrolyte handling
- Increased demands on the cardiovascular and respiratory systems

Specific effects of acute pain on the respiratory system include:

- Small tidal volumes
- High inspiratory and expiratory pressures
- Decreased functional residual capacity
- Decreased alveolar ventilation

These effects can progress to regional atelectasis, ventilation-perfusion mismatch, and impairment of pulmonary gas exchange. Infection can follow and lead to pneumonia.

The development of effective pain management requires not only a general understanding of the processes involved in the pain experience but also information regarding available analgesics, their mechanisms of action, and effective methods of application with regard to the pain type. This section briefly reviews the pain process and provides general guidelines for the use of available drugs for an acute pain management plan.

Three general neural regions are involved in the experience of pain:

- The brain
- The spinal cord
- The peripheral sensory receptors (so-called nociceptors) and associated nerve fibers

The complex processes occurring in the brain to integrate the physiologic signals emanating from the cord and the cognitive and experiential functions of the cortex are not well understood. The relation between experienced pain intensity and the peripheral stimulus that evokes it depends on several factors interacting in a complex manner to influence a response to a noxious stimuli:

- Age
- Breed
- Sex
- Instinctive behavior
- Socialization
- Training
- Disposition
- Stress level

Psychological factors are influenced by contextual cues that establish the significance of the stimulus and help determine an appropriate response. The alteration of neural, behavioral, and subjective pain responses by arousal, attention, and expectation result from the action of central nervous system networks that modulate the transmission of nociceptive messages.

NOTE: For each patient, the pain experienced as the result of a given noxious stimulus is unique.

Pharmacologic modulation of pain at the level of the **brain** *is aimed primarily at reducing the response to incoming nociceptive signals through depression of the response centers and by enhancing the activity in supraspinal inhibitory pathways.*

The **spinal cord** *is the intermediary processing center for information regarding pain generated at the periphery.* Nociceptive signaling from activated peripheral afferents is carried to the spinal cord, where it stimulates the release of fast-acting neurotransmitters and slower acting mediators from the afferent terminals in the dorsal horn. The spinal cord does not act as a simple conduit for nociceptive signaling to the brain. Rather, modulation is exerted through bidirectional control over dorsal horn nociceptive transmission neurons. Interaction of peripheral signaling, both noxious and innocuous, and supraspinal inhibitory signals within the dorsal horn creates a balance of neuroactive substances to modulate the flow of information to the brain. Simple spinal reflex response to noxious input from the injured area also may occur. These responses result in reflex muscle spasm in the immediate region of the injury and in adjacent muscle groups, often increasing the volume of nociceptive signaling to the dorsal horn. Continued neural activity from peripheral nociceptive fields can lead to sensitization of second-order and wide dynamic range neurons within the dorsal horn. This central sensitization is characterized by:

- Increased size and duration of response to a specific stimulus
- Reduced stimulus threshold for activation
- An apparent increase in the receptor field size

Analgesics that function at the spinal cord level may enhance supraspinal inhibition and reduce the activity of interneurons involved in nociceptive transmission. The overall effect is a reduction in the level of nociceptive signaling transmitted to the brain.

Acute pain has its beginning at the level of the peripheral receptors. Nociception involves the transduction of specific noxious signals and the generation of action potentials by the peripheral terminals of small-diameter sensory neurons. These action potentials are propagated to the spinal cord for further processing. Nociceptors are sensitive to specific types of stimuli.

- Thermal
- Mechanical
- Chemical
- Polymodal (responsive to all three modalities)

Through antidromic (conducting impulses opposite to normal) signaling, nociceptors may also be stimulated to release neuroactive substances. Thus they have a peripheral effector role in mediating responses associated with neurogenic inflammation and neuroimmune regulation. The action of nonneural and neural substances released at the site of injury or inflammation can result in (peripheral) sensitization of local nociceptors (lowered stimulus threshold for activation and increased response activity once threshold is reached). *Analgesic agents acting at the peripheral level effectively raise the threshold for nociceptor activation or reduce the signal-carrying capacity of the sensory neuroaxons.*

Immediate resolution of the inciting injury or disease process through medical or surgical management is the key to limiting the pain experienced by the patient. However, minimizing pain before and during the therapeutic processes and during

MANAGEMENT

the healing phase may reduce physiologic stress and actually speed healing. The ➤ **goal** in acute pain management is to break the circle of pain. It is accomplished primarily through the use of pharmaceutical agents that:

- Decrease the susceptability of the brain to recognize spinal transmissions as pain
  □ Local anesthetic agents
  □ Nonsteroidal antiinflammatory drugs (NSAIDs)
  □ Opioids
  □ Parasympathomimetics
  □ Sedatives
- Directly affect the activity of spinal neural pathways
  □ Local anesthetic agents
  □ NSAIDs
  □ Opioids
  □ Parasympathomimetics
- Interfere with or diminish nociceptive signaling from the periphery
  □ Local anesthetic agents
  □ NSAIDs
  □ Opioids

Environmental factors also likely play a role in the pain response.

| **NOTE:** Whenever possible, provide a well-ventilated, draft-free area without excessive visual or auditory stimuli.

Remember, the pain a patient experiences from a given noxious stimulus is unique. Therefore the therapeutic plan for pain management for each patient is ➤ unique. Whenever possible, combine drugs with different mechanisms of action (Table 55–1) and use drug combinations to modulate pain at the peripheral level, spinal cord, and brain simultaneously (Fig. 55–1).

Table 55–1 lists classes of drugs, mechanisms of action, and recommended dosages. Figure 55–2 depicts a simplified decision tree with drug class recommendations for the more common pain problems. Both serve as a guideline for developing an acute pain management plan in a clinical setting.

The modalities of alternative medical therapy, such as acupuncture, chiropractic manipulation, and massage therapy, can be successfully added to any pain management plan. The practitioner is encouraged to consult with professionals trained in these specialties for their application in pain management.

TABLE 55–1. Drug Actions and Dosages

Drug	Dosage	Approximate Dosage for 1000-lb (450-kg) Horse
LOCAL ANESTHETICS		
In addition to their recognized effect in decreasing neuronal excitability through inhibition of voltage-dependent sodium channels, evidence indicates local anesthetics have additional antinociceptive effects through blockade of cellular potassium currents, presynaptic muscarinic receptors, and dopamine receptors. Local anesthetics also are potent modulators of the inflammatory process; they must be used with caution in the care of patients with overwhelming bacterial or viral infections. Local anesthetic agents function at the peripheral, spinal cord, and brain levels.		
Regional anesthesia		
Bupivacaine (Marcaine)	0.25%-0.75% solution	
Lidocaine (Xylocaine)	0.5%-2% solution with	

TABLE 55–1. Drug Actions and Dosages *Continued*

Drug	Dosage	Approximate Dosage for 1000-lb (450-kg) Horse
	or without epinephrine	
Mepivacaine (Carbocaine)	1%-2% solution	
Procaine	1%-2% solution	
Ropivacaine (Naropin)	0.5%-0.75% solution	
Lidocaine* CRI	Loading dosage: 1-1.3 mg/kg IV (administer over 5-15 min); maintenance at 0.05 mg/kg per minute	50 g lidocaine in 1 L D$_5$W at 150 ml/h over 6.7 h

NONSTEROIDAL ANTIINFLAMMATORY DRUGS (NSAIDs)
A heterogeneous group of compounds that probably express their antiinflammatory and analgesic properties through the inhibition of cyclooxygenase-mediated prostaglandin synthesis and phospholipase A$_2$. NSAIDs function primarily at the peripheral and spinal cord levels.

Aspirin	5-20 mg/kg	1-2 240-grain (15.6-g) boluses PO q24h
Carprofen	0.7-1.4 mg/kg	3-5 100-mg caplets PO q24h
Flunixin meglumine	1.1 mg/kg IV or IM	1 ml/100 lb (45 kg)
Ketoprofen	2.2 mg/kg IV	1 ml/100 lb of 100 mg/ml solution
Meclofenamic acid	2-4 mg/kg	2 500-mg packets PO q24h
Naproxen	5 mg/kg IV	Followed by 4 g PO q12h (granules)
Phenylbutazone	2.2-4.4 mg/kg IV	1-2 g/1000 lb or 2-4 g PO q12h
DMSO	Apply DMSO gel (90%, medical grade) topically over affected area q8-12h, not to exceed 100 ml/d	

OPIOIDS
Block the transmission of noxious stimuli by mimicking the action of endogenous ligands for the opioid receptors within the spinal cord and activating receptors on peripheral sensory nerves. Through action on opioid receptors in the brain, supraspinal inhibitory systems are activated. *The use of pure opioid agonists in the care of horses can cause extreme agitation if sedatives are not administered beforehand.* Excitement can occur with the mixed agonist-antagonists when administered alone at high levels.

Buprenorphine[†]	0.001-0.003 mg/kg IV	1-3 0.3-mg ampules q6-8h
Butorphanol	0.01-0.1 mg/kg IV IM	0.5-5 ml of 10-mg/ml solution q3-6h
Butorphanol CRI[†]	Add 50 mg (5 ml of 10 mg/ml solution) to 5 L balanced salt solution (e.g., Normosol-R); administer at 1 L/h	
Fentanyl[†]	Regional nerve infiltration; apply as for local nerve block 2-3 ml per injection site every 3-4 days; may cause mild local pruritus	
	Transdermal patch application 100-µg/h patch, apply 1 each over regional nerve supply (as for local nerve block)	
	Alternatively, apply 3 patches over shaved area at withers (appears less effective)	
Meperidine[†]	2.2 mg/kg IM	10 ml of 50-mg/ml solution q1-6h
Morphine[†]	0.1-0.6 mg/kg IV or IM q8h	3-20 ml of 15-mg/ml solution
Intraarticular	5-10 mg per joint	5-10 ml of 1-mg/ml preservative-free solution
Epidural		

SEDATIVES
Whereas acepromazine has no primary analgesic properties, it is very useful in pain management protocols as an anxiolytic. Its action is thought to be inhibition of CNS dopamine transmission and inhibition of dopamine turnover. The centrally mediated

Continued...

TABLE 55–1. Drug Actions and Dosages *Continued*

Drug	Dosage	Approximate Dosage for 1000-lb (450-kg) Horse

analgesia and muscle relaxation of α_2-agonists are important in the short-term management of acute pain; however, the strong sedative action and short duration of analgesia render these agents impractical in the long term. The effects of α_2-agonists are believed to be mediated through inhibition of norepinephrine release by activation of the inhibitory presynaptic α_2-receptor. Both acepromazine and the α_2-agonists are effective in the control of opioid-mediated excitement in the horse.

Drug	Dosage	Approximate Dosage for 1000-lb (450-kg) Horse
Acepromazine	0.01-0.06 mg/kg IV or IM	0.5-3 mg of 10-mg/ml solution
α_2-Agonists[†]		
Detomidine	0.01-0.02 mg/kg IV or IM	0.5-1.0 ml of 10-mg/ml solution
Xylazine	0.3-1.0 mg/kg IV or IM	1.5-5 ml of 100-mg/ml solution

MISCELLANEOUS

Ketamine: An analgesic through its actions as a noncompetitive NMDA receptor antagonist working primarily at the brain and spinal cord levels, although there is some speculation about a peripheral effect as well. High dosages induce dissociative anesthesia, thereby limiting the usefulness of this agent in the long-term management of acute pain.

Drug	Dosage	Approximate Dosage for 1000-lb (450-kg) Horse
CRI[§]	0.01-0.02 mg/kg per minute	2-3.5 g ketamine in 1 L D_5W at 150 ml/h over 6.7 h

Methocarbamol: A centrally acting muscle relaxant and mild sedative with unknown mechanism of action. This agent does not directly affect the muscle fiber. Its use in acute pain management is limited to conditions in which muscle spasm contributes to the overall pain experience of the horse. Its CNS depressant effects are additive with those of other administered central depressants. Known or suspected renal abnormality is a contraindication to the use of injectable methocarbamol owing to the vehicle, polyethylene glycol 300.

Drug	Dosage	Approximate Dosage for 1000-lb (450-kg) Horse
Parenteral	5-20 mg/kg IV loading dose	25-100 ml of 100-mg/ml solution
Oral	10-40 mg/kg	7-25 750-mg tablets q12h

EPIDURAL MORPHINE PROTOCOL[#]

Drug	Dosage	Approximate Dosage for 1000-lb (450-kg) Horse
Morphine	0.1 mg/kg	50 ml of 1-mg/ml preservative-free solution
Bupivacaine	15 mg	3 ml of 0.5% solution
Neostigmine**	5 mg	5 ml of 1-mg/ml solution

For the initial injection, combine morphine, bupivacaine, and neostigmine in one syringe and administer slowly, 5-10 ml/min in caudal epidural space (Co3-2, Co2-1, or Co1-S5). Repeat bupivacaine and neostigmine, diluted to original volume (~50 ml) in 0.9% saline solution q8h. Repeat morphine q24h. Recommend placement of epidural catheter to facilitate repeated treatment (see Appendix for method of catheter placement).

CRI, Constant rate infusion; *CNS,* central nervous system; *NMDA,* N-methyl-D-aspartate.

*Muscle twitching and tremors, especially about the head and neck, are indicative of lidocaine overdose. Stop the infusion until toxic signs resolve, then resume at a reduced rate of administration (5%-20% reduction).

[†]Previous sedation with acepromazine or α_2-agonist necessary to reduce or eliminate opioid-induced excitement.

[†]Strong sedative effects and short duration of analgesia make long-term pain management with α_2 agonists impractical.

[§]Limit to maximum 12-hour continuous in 24-hour period to reduce risk of drug accumulation. Muscle tremors, clonic contractions, spastic movements, and ataxia are indicative of excessive ketamine levels; if these effects occur, discontinue infusion and administer diazepam, 10-20 mg IV.

[#]Morphine may also be combined with xylazine or detomidine for long (morphine) and short (α agonist) analgesic effects (see p. 125).

**Optional.

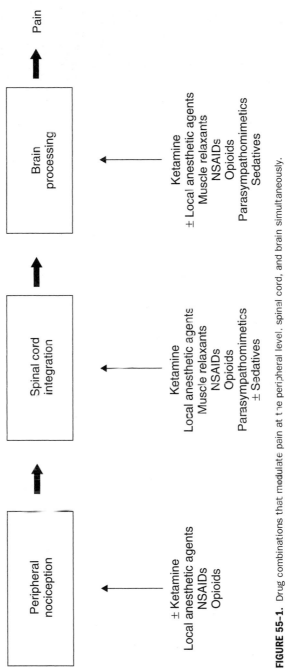

FIGURE 55-1. Drug combinations that modulate pain at the peripheral level, spinal cord, and brain simultaneously.

MANAGEMENT

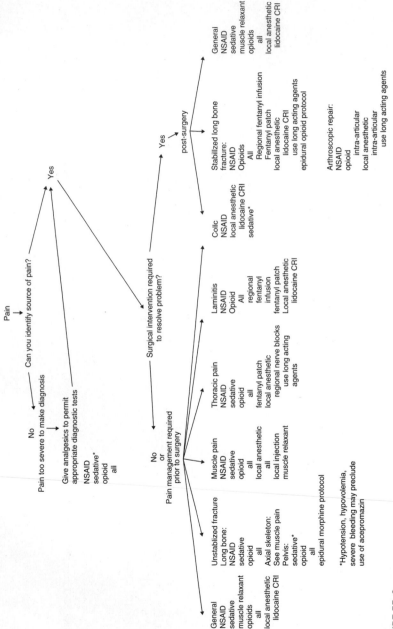

FIGURE 55-2

56 Anesthesia for Field Emergencies and Euthanasia

ANESTHESIA FOR FIELD EMERGENCIES
Ann Townsend and Robin D. Gleed

Emergencies requiring field anesthesia occur often and require the clinician to be familiar with current techniques. The focus of this section is on methods to provide short-term (<40 minutes) general anesthesia when analgesia, unconsciousness, and complete immobility are needed and inhalant anesthesia is not practical. Emergencies requiring only sedation and tranquilization are not discussed.

The goal of emergency anesthesia is usually one or more of the following:

- To enable immediate, definitive treatment to be administered on site (e.g., suture laceration, control of bleeding)
- To allow life-threatening conditions to be stabilized before and during transportation to a surgical facility (e.g., long-bone fractures)
- To prevent further injury to the patient and personnel while the patient is evaluated and plans are made for treatment

Normal risks associated with general anesthesia are amplified when anesthesia is administered in an emergency away from the hospital. Increased risk may be caused by:

- The compromised condition of the patient
- Unsatisfactory environment for administering anesthesia
- Minimal time for planning

Increased risk can be reduced by preparing standard emergency anesthetic protocols that are understood by everyone involved and by having all materials assembled for easy transportation. "Up front" investment in time and resources results in quality emergency care.

BASIC EMERGENCY ANESTHESIA KIT
Suggested Equipment

- Halter for restraining head during induction, made from webbing with 1-inch (2.5-cm) cotton rope braided to it (EquuSport, Monument, CO 80132; [719] 481-4200)
- Two 30-ft (9.1-m) × 1-in (2.5-cm) cotton ropes:
  □ Tail rope
  □ General
- Protective hood (A and A, Maryville, TN 37801; [865] 970-7400)
- Body sling (CDA Products, Potter Valley, CA 95461; [707] 431-1300)
- Endotracheal tubes with intact cuffs (Cook Veterinary Products, Bloomington, IN 47402; [800] 826-2380)
- Syringe, 60 ml (to inflate and deflate cuff)

MANAGEMENT

757

- Tracheotomy tubes, 8- to 26-mm inner diameter (ID) with functional cuffs (Bivona Veterinary Products, Gary, IN 46406; [800] 348-6064)
- Oxygen, medical grade, size E tanks with transport dolly
- Oxygen regulator (two-stage, downstream pressure set at 60 psi for use with the demand valve)
- Quick release adaptor for oxygen regulator
- Oxygen demand valve (Model-LSP, 160 L/min capacity, Chesapeake Breathing Services, Ephrata, PA 17522; [800] 732-0028)
- Oxygen hose, 20-40 ft (6.1-12.2 m)
- Adaptor (to connect demand valve to the endotracheal tubes larger than 22-mm ID)*
- Portable electrocardiographic (ECG) monitor (battery-operated, telemetry preferred)
- Cable hoist puller, come along (Mini Mule, Deuer, Dayton, OH 45439; [937] 298-6040)
- Hobbles
- Space blankets
- General surgical pack
- 2-inch-long (5-cm) polyvinyl chloride (PVC) pipe for mouth gag (wrapped with porous white tape)
- Cordless clippers (Lazor Clip, Kim Laube & Co., Oxnard, CA 93033; [800] 869-8225)
- Injection pole (Simmons heavy duty syringe pole, Zulu Arms Co., Omaha, NE, distributed by Fuhrman Diversified Inc., LaPorte, TX 77586; [281] 474-1388)
- Tackle box (containing needles, syringes, injection caps, over-the-needle catheters (22- to 10-gauge), 4 × 4 gauze, heparinized saline solution, and drugs (Tables 56–1 and 56–2). Advance labeling of essential syringes minimizes confusion during emergency anesthesia (Time Med Label Systems, Burr Ridge, IL 60527; [800] 323-4840)
- Oscillometric sphygmomanometer (GE Medical Systems; [800] 558-5120)
- Fluid Bag Compressor ("Infusable" Vital Signs, Inc., Totowa, NJ 07512; [800] 932-0760)†
- Extension cord, 100 ft (30.5 m)

ANALGESIC, ANESTHETIC, AND RESTRAINT DRUGS

See Table 56–1.

- Atracurium (Tracrium), 0.10-0.20 mg/kg IV, blocks neuromuscular transmission and causes apnea. *Equipment for controlling ventilation must be readily available when this drug is used.* Atracurium is a nondepolarizing neuromuscular blocking agent without anesthetic or analgesic properties and is used to enhance muscle relaxation. The palpebral reflex is diminished or absent, making depth of anesthesia difficult to assess. Consider judicious use in horses in which severe central nervous system (CNS) depression is part of the problem and, hence,

---

*This adaptor has to be machined to match the tapered connections on the demand valve and endotracheal tubes. Delrin, a plastic, is suitable because it can be turned easily, is biologically inert, and can be sterilized with steam or ethylene oxide.

†Three-liter pressure bag can accommodate a 5-L bag of intravenous fluid.

TABLE 56–1. Analgesic, Anesthetic, and Restraint Drugs for the Tackle Box

Agent	No. Vials or Bags	Volume and Concentration
Atracurium	3 vials	5 ml (10 mg/ml)
Butorphanol	1 vial	50 ml (10 mg/ml)
Detomidine	1 vial	20 ml (10 mg/ml)
Diazepam	3 vials	10 ml (5 mg/ml)
Edrophonium	6 vials	10 ml (10 mg/ml)
Guaifenesin	2 bags	1000 ml (50 mg/ml) (5% solution)
Ketamine	5 vials	10 ml (100 mg/ml)
Thiopental sodium	2 vials	5 g
Xylazine	1 vial	50 ml (100 mg/ml)
Euthanasia solution	1 vial	250 ml

TABLE 56–2. Resuscitation Drugs for the Tackle Box

Agent	No. Vials or Bags	Volume and Concentration
Atropine	1 vial	100 ml (0.5 mg/ml)
Dextran 70 in 0.9% saline solution	10 bags	500 ml
Dobutamine	1 vial	20 ml (12.5 mg/ml)
Doxapram	1 vial	20 ml (20 mg/ml)
Epinephrine	2 vials	30 ml (1 mg/ml)
Flunixin meglumine	1 vial	50 ml (50 mg/ml)
Hetastarch	10 bags	500 ml
7% hypertonic saline solution	6 vials	1000 ml
Lactated Ringer's solution (or other crystalloid electrolyte solution)	6 bags	5000 ml
Lidocaine	1 vial	100 ml (20 mg/ml)
Prednisolone sodium succinate	3 vials	10 ml (20 mg/vial)
Tolazoline HCl	1 vial	100 ml (100 mg/ml)

large dosages of centrally active anesthetics are contraindicated. Duration of action of the initial dosage (0.20 mg/kg) is approximately 20 minutes. Subsequent dosages are 0.05-0.10 mg/kg. Dehydration, hypothermia, and some antibiotics (e.g., aminoglycosides, gentamicin) prolong the effects of atracurium. Reverse the effects of atracurium with edrophonium. Unlike succinylcholine, atracurium is reversible, does not cause muscle injury, and does not exacerbate hyperkalemia.

- Butorphanol (Torbugesic), 0.01-0.04 mg/kg IV, is an opioid that produces unreliable sedation when used alone. It has opioid agonist and antagonist properties. It can produce excitement or dysphoria when it is the only agent used in some individuals. It potentiates the analgesic effects of α_2-agonist drugs and can be used in conjunction with xylazine to produce analgesia and chemical restraint (butorphanol, 0.01-0.02 mg/kg, plus xylazine, <0.6 mg/kg IV).
- Detomidine (Dormosedan), 0.005-0.02 mg/kg IV, 0.02-0.04 mg/kg IM, is an α_2-agonist that produces reliable sedation and analgesia. It has a long duration of action (up to 2 hours). Because of its profound cardiovascular depressant effects, use detomidine carefully in the care of patients with cardiovascular

MANAGEMENT

➤ compromise. *Draft breeds* are more susceptible to its effects than are other horses. Conversely, mules may need larger doses. Donkeys may assume sternal recumbency.

- Diazepam (Valium), 0.1-0.2 mg/kg IV, is a sedative frequently administered to promote muscle relaxation with drugs such as ketamine. It can produce excitement in adults when used on its own. In foals up to 4 weeks of age, diazepam has sedative effects and can be used as a preanesthetic. Its primary use is to manage seizures.

- Edrophonium (Enlon), 0.5 mg/kg IV, is used for competitive reversal of nondepolarizing neuromuscular blockers (e.g., atracurium). It is preferred to neostigmine for this purpose because it produces less bradycardia and, therefore, does not necessitate atropine administration. Administer slowly (over >2 minutes) to avoid excitement and bradycardia.

- Euthanasia solution (e.g., Beuthanasia, >0.2 ml/kg IV). *Approved for humane destruction only!* Because this solution often produces transient motor activity and gasping, it is advisable to sedate the horse before administering it (e.g., with xylazine).

- Guaifenesin, 40-80 mg/kg IV to effect, is a centrally acting muscle relaxant used in conjunction with the anesthetic drugs ketamine and thiopental to induce and maintain anesthesia. It has no analgesic or anesthetic properties. *Overdosage causes apnea.* Guaifenesin usually is administered as a 5% solution. Precipitates during storage; therefore make solutions fresh. Peak effect is reached 10 minutes after administration.

➤ | **NOTE:** Mules and donkeys may be more sensitive to guaifenesin than are horses.

- Ketamine (Ketaset, Ketaject), 2.2 mg/kg IV, is a dissociative anesthetic that may be preferred to a barbiturate because of its relatively benign effects on the cardiovascular system. It increases heart rate and overrides the bradycardia caused by xylazine and detomidine tranquilization. *Ketamine causes increased cerebral and ocular pressure and may be contraindicated when cerebral and intraocular pressures are a primary concern.* May cause excitement and even seizure-like activity if administered without preexisting CNS depression; hence precede administration with a sedative (e.g., xylazine).

- Romifidine, 40-100 μg/kg IV, is an α_2-agonist used in Europe. It has preanesthetic and tranquilizing effects similar to those of other α_2-agonists. Romifidine can be combined with diazepam and ketamine for short-duration intravenous anesthesia. The sedation and analgesia achieved with romifidine are not as great as those achieved with detomidine.

- Thiopental sodium (Pentothal), 4-10 mg/kg IV alone, or 3-4 mg/kg IV, with 5% guaifenesin. An ultrashort-acting barbiturate used for rapid induction of anes-
➤ thesia after bolus administration. Transient apnea often occurs. *Use with caution in emergency situations because thiopental sodium depresses ventilation, cardiac output, and systemic blood pressure.* It also can be used at 3-4 mg/kg, either mixed with guaifenesin or as a bolus after pretreatment with guaifenesin.

- Xylazine (Rompun), 0.2-1.1 mg/kg IV, is an α_2-agonist that produces reliable sedation and analgesia. It also causes bradycardia and reduces cardiac output. Use xylazine with caution in the treatment of patients with cardiovascular compromise. To some extent, the adverse effects of xylazine on the cardiovascular
➤ system are ameliorated by ketamine. *Draft breeds are more sensitive to xylazine than are other horses.* Mules may need higher dosages than do either donkeys or horses.

RESUSCITATION DRUGS AND SUPPORT DRUGS

See Table 56–2.

- Atipamezole (Antisedan), 0.05-0.2 mg/kg IV, is a synthetic α_2-adrenergic antagonist. As for all α_2-antagonists, administer atipamezole slowly and monitor the effect carefully. This drug can produce excitement and reverse analgesic effects and sedation. It is advisable to administer one-half the calculated dosage initially.
- Atropine, 0.01-0.02 mg/kg IV, is used to manage sinus bradycardia. It can produce ileus at higher dosages.
- Dextran 70 (Gentran 70) in 0.9% saline solution, 5-10 ml/kg per hour, is a colloidal solution used as a blood volume expander. Indicated for hypovolemia and when total plasma protein level is decreased.

> **CAUTION:** During the first minutes of infusion, observe for signs of an adverse reaction (e.g., tachycardia, tachypnea, etc.) due to antigenic properties of dextran 70.

- Dobutamine (Dobutrex), 0.001-0.008 mg/kg per minute (1-8 µg/kg/min) IV, is a β_1-agonist that increases mean cardiac output and arterial blood pressure. It has a short half-life and is best used in an infusion (50 mg in 500 ml of 0.9% saline solution equals 0.01% solution or 0.1 mg/ml or 100 µg/ml). Overdosage produces tachycardia, tachydysrhythmia, and hypertension. In hypovolemic patients, do not use dobutamine as a substitute for blood volume replacement. It produces severe sinus tachycardia when used with atropine.
- Doxapram (Dopram), 0.2 mg/kg IV, is a respiratory stimulant that is contraindicated if severe hypoxia has already occurred. In an emergency, resuscitation by positive-pressure ventilation with 100% oxygen is the preferred management of apnea.
- Epinephrine (Adrenalin), 0.02 mg/kg by the jugular vein or intratracheal route and repeated as necessary, is the drug of choice for cardiopulmonary resuscitation. It is a mixed α- and β-sympathomimetic agent that produces peripheral vasoconstriction and cardiac stimulation. Through the jugular vein, inject this agent in conjunction with fluid therapy to ensure that the drug is flushed centrally.
- Flunixin meglumine (Banamine), 0.25-1.0 mg/kg IV, is a nonsteroidal antiinflammatory drug (NSAID) used to manage endotoxic shock.
- Hetastarch (Hespan), 10-20 ml/kg per hour, is a colloid solution that has a higher molecular weight and less antigenic properties than those of dextran.
- 7% hypertonic saline solution, 4 ml/kg per 5 minutes (*3 L maximum dose to a 450-kg adult*), is used principally as a blood volume expander to manage shock. It causes hypernatremia. It is contraindicated in cardiogenic shock. The mechanism of action is to shift intracellular and interstitial water into the intravascular space. Therefore, hypertonic saline solution is viewed as emergency treatment only; administer in conjunction with conventional replacement fluids.
- Lactated Ringer's solution (and other "balanced" electrolyte solutions), 10-40 ml/kg per hour, is an isotonic crystalloid solution used to correct hypovolemia, dehydration, shock, and acidosis. It can be used with colloidal or hypertonic saline solutions.
- Lidocaine, 0.5 mg/kg IV, is used to manage ventricular tachydysrhythmias. These are relatively uncommon in horses, but prompt treatment may be critical when they are present in anesthetized horses.

MANAGEMENT

- Prednisolone sodium succinate (Solu-Delta Cortef), 2-5 mg/kg, is used to stabilize cell membranes during shock and after resuscitation.
- Yohimbine (Yobine), 0.1 mg/kg IV, is used to reverse the effects of α_2-agonists, xylazine, and detomidine. Yohimbine can cause excitement and cardiac arrhythmias; minimize this effect by administering one-half the calculated dosage slowly. Administer the second half of the dosage only if necessary. Use when early termination of an α_2-agonist is desirable or to manage inadvertent α_2-agonist overdosage. Repeated dosage may be needed.

GENERAL ANESTHETIC CONSIDERATIONS
Depth of Anesthesia

Distressed horses in emergency situations are likely to have different sensitivity to anesthetics compared with nondistressed horses. Therefore depth of anesthesia should be monitored closely by trained personnel.

Pain and distress increase sympathetic tone and circulating catecholamine levels. These increases can cause a hyperdynamic cardiovascular state characterized by increased cardiac output. *Drug requirements may markedly increase under these circumstances, but use caution to prevent an overdosage when catecholamine levels decline. In hypovolemic horses, the reduced volume of distribution of injected drugs can increase susceptibility.* Exhaustion also can complicate an emergency, because it is often associated with muscle damage, dehydration, electrolyte imbalance, and decreased circulating levels of catecholamines.

Monitoring

A pulse oximeter (9847V, Nonin Medical, Inc., Minneapolis, MN 55447; [763] 553-9948) shows continuous evidence of a pulse and is used to measure oxygen saturation. Heska, Corp., 1613 Prospect Parkway, Fort Collins, CO 80525, makes a pulse oximeter that may prove useful in equine practice.

Portable oscillometric sphygmomanometers (Dinamap Critikon Veterinary Blood Pressure Monitor 8300, Tampa, FL 33634; [813] 887-2000) assists the anesthetist by warning of hypotension. Systemic arterial hypotension indicates cardiovascular collapse due to a primary problem or anesthetic overdosage.

"Bedside" units (e.g., i-STAT Portable Clinical Analyzer, Heska; [800] GO HESKA; www.heska.com) can be used to measure various blood values, including acid-base status and blood gas values.

A portable ECG monitor is used to detect dysrhythmias and to monitor response to treatment. A telemetry unit (recorder and Holter monitor, Hewlett Packard, Andover, MA 01810; [800] 752-0900) is particularly useful.

Systemic arterial hypotension indicates the presence of cardiovascular collapse due to a primary problem or anesthetic overdosage. Modern portable oscillometric sphygmomanometers assist the anesthetist by warning of hypotension.

An accurate anesthetic record is the best defense against claims of negligence. The best way to ensure safe anesthesia and an accurate record is to designate someone to be personally responsible for anesthesia and supportive care.

Respiratory Support

Orotracheal intubation is the best method to ensure airway patency and is mandatory if ventilation is controlled. A demand valve attached to a two-stage regulator valve and type E oxygen cylinder is suitable for controlling ventilation with oxygen. Demand valves allow spontaneous ventilation to be supplemented with oxygen. For larger horses, the regulator may have to be adjusted to 60 psi to maintain sufficiently high inspiratory flow. E cylinders contain approximately 660 gaseous liters; therefore 3 or 4 cylinders may be needed to ventilate a 450-kg adult for 30 minutes. A 30-ft (9.1-m) length of hose allows isolation of the compressed gas cylinder from the patient. A dolly also helps secure the cylinder.

Cardiovascular Support

A 14-gauge (or larger), 5.5-inch (14-cm) over-the-needle catheter should be secured (with cyanoacrylate glue [Superglue] or suture [2-0 Ethilon]) in a peripheral vein; the jugular vein is preferred. If the patient is hypovolemic, administer balanced electrolyte solution at a rate of 10-20 ml/kg IV. Use 7% hypertonic saline solution at a rate of 4-6 ml/kg if hypovolemia is severe. A 450-kg adult should receive no more than 3 L of 7% hypertonic saline solution. Hetastarch (2-10 mg/kg) can be used with other crystalloids to manage hypovolemia.

Dobutamine in conjunction with fluid therapy should be used only with adequate preload.

Increasing the heart rate in a less than full ventricle increases the cardiac oxygen requirements and may be detrimental to the patient.

Positioning and Padding

Pad pressure points (shoulder, hips) and large muscle groups during anesthesia. Protect the eyes, especially when moving the patient.

Ileus

Horses that need emergency anesthesia may have a full gastrointestinal (GI) tract. The reduction in GI motility caused by anesthetic drugs can predispose these patients to ileus and colic. A full GI tract can complicate ventilation and result in hypoxemia during anesthesia. Many anesthetic and tranquilizing drugs decrease intestinal motility; therefore consider the risk of postanesthesia colic. Minimize positional changes while the patient is recumbent to decrease the risk of torsion.

Hyperkalemic Periodic Paralysis

Hyperkalemic periodic paralysis (HYPP) is a genetic disorder among Quarter Horses. Stress is a primary factor in the disease. In the emergency setting and with anesthesia, it is important to recognize and manage HYPP immediately (see p. 425).

Hypothermia

Hypothermia usually is a problem only among foals. However, monitor body temperature in all emergencies when shock and environmental temperature extremes are possible.

Euthanasia

Humane or economic considerations may necessitate destruction of the patient. Anesthesia (see Protocol 1, p. 765) makes euthanasia easier to accomplish and more humane.

MANAGEMENT

SPECIFIC CASES

In most cases necessitating emergency anesthesia, consider sedation or tranquilization and local anesthesia initially. Reserve general anesthesia for patients that need complete immobilization. Minimizing general anesthesia time decreases the incidence of complications.

Severe Lacerations

- It is often difficult to determine the volume of blood lost after a laceration. Presume tachycardia (heart rate >50 beats/min) to be secondary to hypovolemia until proved otherwise, and treat by blood volume replacement with crystalloid or colloidal solutions. Heart rate increases and blood pressure drops when 25% or more of the blood volume is lost.
- When possible, control severe bleeding before anesthesia.
- Cardiodepressant effects of α_2-agonists and barbiturates are dangerous in hypovolemic patients. Diazepam, 0.1 mg/kg IV, and ketamine, 2 mg/kg IV (see Protocol 4, p. 767) are preferred for induction because they cause minimal depression of the cardiovascular system.

Fractures

- It often is necessary to stabilize fractures before transport to a surgical facility.
- Considerations are the same as those for severe lacerations.
- Ameliorate anxiety associated with pain with butorphanol.
- When hypovolemia is not evident, use α_2-agonists for analgesia.
- Higher than normal dosages may be required in excitable horses.

Seizures

- Treat a patient with seizures by administering diazepam, 0.1-0.2 mg/kg IV.
- If anesthesia is needed for immediate transport and diagnostic tests, a thiopental bolus or thiopental with 5% guaifenesin (Protocol 2, see p. 765) is the protocol of choice.
- Avoid ketamine because it produces seizure-like activity of the CNS and increases intracranial pressure.

Dystocia

- General anesthesia can produce enough vaginal and uterine relaxation to facilitate manipulation of malpresented foals.
- Elevating the caudal end of the anesthetized mare allows abdominal viscera to move cranially and improves the ease of fetal manipulation. Do not maintain this Trendelenburg (head down) position for long periods because it is associated with reduced ventilation and cardiac output. Controlling ventilation with a demand valve minimizes ventilatory compromise.
- Protocol 1 (see p. 765) is satisfactory for these situations, followed by maintenance with a "triple drip."
- General anesthesia for field cesarean section rarely results in a live foal and places the mare at increased risk; extensive manipulation per vagina increases the risk of complications during cesarean section.

Colic

- Horses with colic are frequently unresponsive to analgesics and are unmanageable to the point at which they injure themselves and are dangerous to transport.

Injectable anesthesia may be needed before definitive treatment or transport to a surgical facility.
- Intravenous fluids and other supportive treatment usually are needed in these situations.
- Diazepam with ketamine combination is a suitable induction technique.
- Abdominal distention may necessitate controlled ventilation.
- Correct nephrosplenic entrapment in the field by "rolling" the patient from right to left lateral recumbency under general anesthesia. Protocol 1 (see below) usually is used for this purpose. Appropriate medical therapy is important in conjunction with "rolling," if phenylephrine and exercise do not correct the problem.

Extrication, Entrapment
- Horses may need to be anesthetized for safe removal from dangerous situations.
- Often impossible to assess accurately the physiologic status.
- Sometimes difficult or unsafe to get close to the patient. Use of a pole syringe may allow intramuscular administration of drugs.
- Skills and equipment needed for safe removal of horses are important in disasters such as hurricanes, floods, and trailer accidents (see p. 736).

Cardiopulmonary Resuscitation
- Emergency field anesthesia can result in respiratory and cardiac arrest from hypovolemia, upper airway obstruction, pneumothorax, hypokalemia, and so on.
- Careful continuous monitoring and early intervention are the keys to success in cardiopulmonary resuscitation (CPR). Figure 56–1 is a guide for patient evaluation.
- Box 56–1 is a guide for CPR.

SELECTED PROTOCOLS FOR EMERGENCY ANESTHESIA
Protocol 1
- *Premedication:* Xylazine, 0.3-0.6 mg/kg IV, and butorphanol, 0.01-0.02 mg/kg IV. Wait 3-5 minutes for peak effect.
- *Induction:* Ketamine, 2.2 mg/kg IV, with diazepam, 0.05-0.10 mg/kg IV.
- *Maintenance:* "Triple drip," 1 L 5% guaifenesin, 1-2 g ketamine, and 250-500 mg xylazine in solution. Titrate carefully to approximately 1-2 ml/kg per hour to produce the desired level of anesthesia. (With a standard 10 drops/ml administration set, this equates to 1-2 drops per second for a 450-kg adult.).

Protocol 2

CAUTION: This protocol is not recommended in cases of hypovolemia and shock.

- *Premedication:* Xylazine, 0.2-0.4 mg/kg IV; wait 3-5 minutes for peak sedation.
- *Induction:* 5% guaifenesin in 1 L 5% dextrose or sterile water until patient becomes ataxic (after approximately 0.6-1.0 ml/kg IV), then a bolus of thiopental, 3-4 mg/kg IV.
- *Maintenance:* 2 g thiopental in 1 L of 5% guaifenesin titrated to approximately 1-1.8 ml/kg per hour.

MANAGEMENT

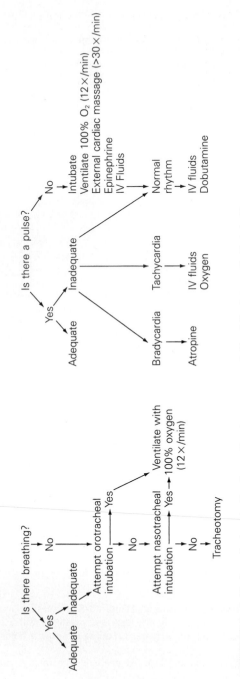

FIGURE 56–1. Guide for patient evaluation for cardiopulmonary resuscitation following anesthetic induction.

BOX 56-1. Cardiopulmonary Resuscitation

Verify Arrest, Discontinue Anesthetics, Note Time of Arrest
A. Airway: Pass orotracheal or nasotracheal tube
B. Breathing: Start positive-pressure ventilation with 100% oxygen
C. Circulation: Establish external cardiac massage 30/min by knee drops on chest
Epinephrine: 0.02 mg/kg IV, intracardiac or intratracheal
Administer fluids (lactated Ringer's solution, physiologic saline solution) at shock dosage so heart has something to pump (40 ml/kg). A capnograph can be used to monitor results of resuscitative efforts.

Protocol 3 *(For Foals ≤4 Weeks of Age)*

- *Premedication:* Diazepam, 0.1 mg/kg IV, wait for peak sedation to take effect. The foal may lie down.
- *Induction:* Ketamine, 2.2 mg/kg IV.
- *Maintenance:* Modified "triple drip," 1 L 5% guaifenesin with 125-250 mg of xylazine and 1 g of ketamine titrated to approximately 0.5-1.0 ml/kg per hour.

Protocol 4

CAUTION: In healthy individuals, induction can cause excitement. This protocol is indicated *only* in cases of severe hypovolemic, endotoxic shock or CNS depression.

- *Premedication:* None
- *Induction:* Diazepam, 0.1-0.2 mg/kg IV, followed immediately by ketamine, 2.2 mg/kg IV
- *Maintenance:* See Protocol 1. Manage shock with large-volume fluid therapy

■ EUTHANASIA

Thomas J. Divers

Properly performed euthanasia is important to ensure humane destruction of terminally ill or distressed horses and is particularly important when viewed by the client. Before administering any euthanasia solution:

- Properly identify the patient being euthanized and *recheck* that this is the correct horse and owner/insurance company consent is verified.
- Consider the location, distracting noise, surface, surrounding objects, condition of the jugular veins, placement of the needle or catheter, location of burial, condition of the halter, and shank and holder.

PERFORMING EUTHANASIA WITHOUT TRANQUILIZATION

Insert a 12-gauge, 2-inch (5-cm), nondisposable needle or 14-gauge, 5.25-inch (13.3-cm) intravenous catheter in the jugular vein. Prepare two 60-ml syringes of euthanasia solution, one syringe containing 40 mg of succinylcholine. After aspiration, to ensure that the needle is properly positioned in the vein, *rapidly* inject

MANAGEMENT

the syringe of succinylcholine and 50 ml of the euthanasia solution into the jugular vein. Immediately attach the second syringe (60 ml) to the needle and administer quickly. The individual usually falls within 30 seconds after injection of the two doses.

PERFORMING EUTHANASIA WITH TRANQUILIZATION

To ensure a tranquil state during administration of the euthanasia solution, heavily sedate the patient with detomidine, 0.01-0.02 mg/kg IV, or xylazine, 0.5-1.0 mg/kg IV. Once sedation is established, administer the solutions, as described in the preceding paragraph, through a 12-gauge needle or a 14-gauge, 5.25-inch (13.3-cm) catheter properly placed in the jugular vein. Tranquilized horses are slower to collapse than non-tranquilized individuals.

NERVOUS OR NEEDLE-SHY PATIENT

Heavily sedate the individual with detomidine, 10 mg IV or 40 mg IM (use an injection pole if necessary). Place a 14-gauge, 3.5- or 5.25-inch (8.9- or 13.3-cm) catheter in the jugular vein, and administer euthanasia-succinylcholine solution rapidly.

EUTHANASIA UNDER ANESTHESIA

This procedure can be performed with administration of euthanasia solution.

EUTHANASIA OF PATIENTS WITH THROMBOSED JUGULAR VEINS

Place a 14- or 16-gauge, 3.5-inch (8.9-cm) catheter in the lateral thoracic vein. Tranquilize the patient and administer the euthanasia-succinylcholine solution. If the lateral thoracic vein cannot be catheterized, use detomidine, 20 mg IV, injected into the cephalic vein, or 40 mg IM. Once the patient is sedated, intracardiac administration of euthanasia solution and succinylcholine can be performed with an 18-gauge, 3.5- to 6-inch (8.9- to 15.2-cm) needle and 30-60 ml syringe.

57 Nutritional Guidelines for the Injured Horse

Jonathan M. Naylor

The only true nutritional emergency is hypoglycemia, and this is discussed on Chapter 47 p. 541.

Food deprivation often is required before surgery to allow the gastrointestinal tract to empty. Approximately 80% of intestinal fill is lost in the first 24 hours when food is withheld. If more complete intestinal evacuation is required, the recommendation is 24-hour food deprivation in combination with use of a laxative such as mineral oil. This method leads to rapid emptying with minimal loss of body condition and immune function, which occurs with prolonged fasting.

Equine clinicians generally choose diets for their patients as part of the therapeutic regimen. This is an important decision made early in the patient care cycle. Different feeding regimens are presented in this section. Some clinicians feed only complete feeds or alfalfa hay cubes as the standard hospital diet. These feeds are convenient but often lead to stall chewing because of boredom. The absence of long-stem fiber may increase the incidence of colic.

Most sick horses can be fed a diet of a high-quality grass hay or a grass–alfalfa hay mixture, either free choice or at a minimum of 1.5% of body weight with a salt block and free-choice water.

CAUTION: Some horses are not used to automatic waterers, so watch them closely for the first 24 hours to be sure they are drinking.

Hay usually is supplemented with approximately 1 kg of whole oats twice a day. Feeding oats helps maintain acclimation to grain and therefore makes it easier to return the horse to a high-grain diet after recovery. Whole oats are palatable and unlikely to cause digestive problems because the thick fibrous capsule is intact. If the patient is thin, the usual remedy is to feed more grain and avoid poor-quality hay.

The general rule for changing grain is to increase it slowly by no more than 0.5 kg/d.

Specific disease problems may necessitate the modified approaches in Table 57–1. In addition to changes in nutritional requirements dictated by disease, normal physiologic changes can increase nutrient needs. The two most important are heavy lactation and growth. Growing or lactating horses usually need high-quality hay, grain, and a mineral supplement (Table 57–2). Alfalfa hay and alfalfa–grass hay mixtures are particularly suited for growing or lactating horses because alfalfa has a high protein and calcium content.

Nursing foals have special requirements; if the mare is present, the foal can be encouraged to nurse, or the mare can be milked out and the foal fed by hand.

NOTE: A general guideline is that the foal should receive 12% or more of body weight as mare's milk, according to the schedules in Table 57–3.

Healthy, hand-fed foals may drink no more than 12% of body weight as milk. It has been suggested that this is the most a foal's stomach can accommodate on a

TABLE 57–1. Dietary Guidelines for Specific Disease Conditions

Disease	Nutritional Objectives	Dietary Recommendations
Cervical vertebral malformation (wobbler)	Maintenance of steady growth without periods of excessive rapid growth	Balanced diet including adequate copper so that nutritional objectives are met
Choke (esophageal obstruction)	Soft diet to prevent further obstruction at site of spasm or stricture	After relief of choke, feed soft, short particle size feeds (e.g., soak complete feed pellets to make a soft mash, fresh tender grass). Continue until esophageal ulceration and inflammation have resolved
Diarrhea		
No weight loss	Increased water and electrolyte absorption	Good quality hay: fiber may bind water, loose salt
Weight loss	Reduced maldigestion	Grain, small amounts frequently. Watch for signs of worsening of diarrhea. Loose salt in small amounts
Colic after surgical or medical treatment	General objective: minimization of catabolic state	If no gastrointestinal reflux, feed small quantities of high-quality grass hay or grass to promote intestinal contractions. Gradually increase amounts
Extensive small-intestinal resection	Increased soluble fiber, decreased bulk	Ground alfalfa pellets, restricted amounts of grain. Vitamin B supplementation
Enterolithiasis	Decreased large-intestinal pH, calcium, magnesium, phosphorus	Grass hay, grain (up to 50% of diet)
Large-colon surgery	Decreased postoperative diarrhea	Initially feed grass or grass hay, avoid alfalfa hay
Extensive large-colon resection	Increased water, carbohydrates, protein, minerals, especially phosphorus	Initially, grass hay. Long term most horses do best on alfalfa hay or alfalfa cubes; can add small amounts of grain as energy and phosphorus supplement
Chronic obstructive pulmonary disease (heaves)	Avoidance of fungi associated with hay and bedding	Keep outside if possible; if not, house in well-ventilated, clean stall at end of barn. Feed alfalfa cubes from feeder on ground. Complete pelleted feeds can be fed but the fiber length is shorter. Use shredded paper or wood shavings for bedding
Geriatric (older than 20 y)	Increased protein, phosphorus; decreased fiber; calcium to phosphorus ratio, 1:1 to 3:1	High-quality grass hay and grain, pelleted feeds (12%-14% CP). Supplement with linseed or soybean meal (200-400 g), B vitamins. Ascorbic acid (10 g), phosphate (5 g). Can feed mashes or slurries if necessary (dental problems)
Hepatic encephalopathy	Reduced protein, increased branched-chain amino acids, simple sugars, B vitamins	Mature grass hay (8% CP); corn grain, milo, soaked beet pulp

TABLE 57–1. Dietary Guidelines for Specific Disease Conditions
Continued

Disease	Nutritional Objectives	Dietary Recommendations
Hyperkalemic periodic paralysis (HYPP)	Decreased serum potassium	Avoid lush green feeds, lush hay made from young grass or molasses. Feed late-cut grass hays, sugar beet pulp, grain; supplement with sodium bicarbonate 15-30 g/d (500-kg horse). Proprietary low potassium HYPP feeds available made from alfalfa hay (provides protein, minerals) and sugar beet pulp (low potassium)
Renal disease with azotemia	Increased water, salt; reduced protein, calcium	Loose salt. Grass hay (8% CP). Feed grain (oats, corn) as necessary to maintain condition or reduce hypercalcemia
Rectal or vaginal surgery	Low bulk, laxative diet	Green grass. Finely ground pelleted feed (alfalfa pellets or complete feed)

CP, Crude protein.

TABLE 57–2. Nutritional Guidelines for Pregnant, Lactating, and Growing Horses

Condition	Hay (% of Body Weight)	Grain (% of Body Weight)
Mares, late gestation	1.0-1.5	0.5 1.0
Mares, early lactation	1.0-2.0	1.0-2.0
Mares, late lactation	1.0-2.0	0.5-1.5
Nursing foal, 3-6 mo	0	1.0-2.0
Weanling foal, 6-12 mo	0.5-1.0	1.5-3.0
Weanling foal, 12-18 mo	1.0-1.5	1.5-3.0
Long yearling, 18-24 mo	1.0-1.5	1.0-1.5
Two-year-olds	1.0-1.5	1.0-1.5

In general, try to feed good-quality hay and restrict grain to the lower end of the recommended ranges. Alfalfa or grass alfalfa mix hays are preferred because they are good sources of calcium and protein needed to support growth and lactation. Feed a mineral block containing appropriate amounts of trace minerals (especially copper) and calcium and phosphorus if needed. Mineral blocks should contain salt to promote and control intake. Only feed one type of block; horses can eat plain salt blocks and ignore the trace mineral fortified block.

hand-feeding regimen. However, foals nursing from mares ingest small amounts at frequent intervals and drink more (22%-25%).

➤ *During the first few days of life, a foal should be fed at least every 2 hours. The intervals can be slowly increased between feedings over 10 days. If the foal is sick and has to be tube fed, it is important to check for reflux through the tube before each feeding.*

The presence of reflux suggests the presence of ileus and is a reason for discontinuing or decreasing the amount of milk fed. Indwelling 12F, enteral feeding

TABLE 57–3. Feeding Regimen for a Foal Fed Milk Replacer as a 14.3% wt/wt Solution (125 g Powder in 750 ml Water)

Days of age	2-3	4	5	6	7	8	9	10	11	12	13	14	15+
Volume (ml)	250	375	500	625	750	1000	1125	1250	1376	1500	1625	1750	2625
Feedings per day	12	8	8	8	8	6	6	6	6	6	6	6	4
Total daily intake (L)	3	3	4	5	6	6	6.75	7.5	8.26	9	9.75	10.5	10.5

Adapted from Cymbaluk NF, et al: Importance of milk replacer and composition in rearing orphan foals, *Can Vet J* 34:479-486, 1993.

tubes* used in humans have been used successfully to feed foals. These are generally placed with the tip in the distal esophagus with a plastic collar taped to the halter to reduce the risk of dislodgment. These tubes can be connected to fluid delivery sets,† and the liquid meal slowly delivered over 1 hour.

If a lactating mare is not available, the foal can be fed a commercial foal milk replacer, which contains only milk proteins (casein, whey) as the protein source. These are believed closer in composition to mare's milk and are used more extensively in the care of foals than are human enteral preparations. Some foals are raised on goat's milk; however, 2% fat in cow's milk is closer in composition to mare's milk. Care of sick foals frequently necessitates that the amounts recommended on the package be divided into several smaller meals.

Once a foal is healthy, it can be fostered onto a nursemare or trained to drink from a bucket. Milk can be prepared several times a day and left for the foal to drink. Weighing the quantity of powder added to water is a good practice because variation in the amount of powder scooped into a cup can result in overconcentrated solutions. Mare's milk is approximately 12% dry matter, whereas foal milk replacers are slightly more concentrated at 14% dry matter. The slight increase in concentration over mare's milk helps compensate for the reduced-volume intake of hand-fed foals.

With good management and early provision of high-quality hay and creep feed, foals can be weaned at 7 weeks of age. Socialization is important, so access to equine role models (an old, quiet pony) should be provided as early as possible. Fostering onto a mare usually is accomplished by:

- Rubbing the dead foal's placenta or skin onto the foal to be fostered
- Placing Vicks VapoRub ointment on the mare's nostrils
- Tranquilizing and hobbling or twitching as needed
- Assisting the foal to nurse
- Transferring a blanket from the orphaned foal to the orphan foal

Some mares may require as long as a week or more of continuous observation and restraint.

Some sick adult patients are unable or unwilling to eat normal diets and require tube feeding with liquid diets or slurries. The three basic types of diet used are:

- **Soaked pelleted feeds** made from finely ground ingredients. The liquid gruel is administered through a large-bore stomach tube. Typically, approximately 500 g of pellets, 50 ml of vegetable oil, and 3 L of water are mixed together. A blender helps to grind the ingredients. Initially, a 500-kg horse receives approximately 4-8 3-L meals a day. Over a week the volume fed can be increased to 6-8 L per meal and the number of feedings gradually reduced to 4 per day. A wide-bore tube and large funnel or high-capacity hand pump, such as a marine bilge pump, helps the gruel flow through the tube. This approach is inexpensive; however, it can be difficult to get sufficient gruel through the tube to meet daily requirements.
- **Defined diet** with a mixture of electrolytes, glucose, and casein (Table 57–4). It is important to add some alfalfa meal because the addition of a fiber source can

---

*Flexiflo Enteral Feeding Tube. Ross Products Division of Abbott Laboratories, Columbus, OH 43215-1724.

†Flexitainer-500, Ross Products Division of Abbott Laboratories.

MANAGEMENT

TABLE 57–4. Alfalfa, Casein, Dextrose Slurry

INDIVIDUAL FEEDING (4 FEEDINGS PER DAY)	
Alfalfa meal	500 g
Casein*	225 g
Dextrose*	225 g
Electrolyte mixture (see below)	58 g
Water	5.25 L
ELECTROLYTE MIXTURE (1-DAY SUPPLY)	
Sodium chloride (NaCl)	10 g
Sodium bicarbonate (NaHCO$_3$)	15 g
Potassium chloride (KCl)	75 g
Potassium phosphate (dibasic anhydrous) (K$_2$HPO$_4$)	60 g
Calcium chloride (CaCl$_2$ 2H$_2$O)	45 g
Magnesium oxide (MgO)	25 g
Total	230 g

Adapted from data in Naylor JM, Freeman DE, Kronfeld DS: Alimentation of hypophagic horses, *Compend Contin Educ Pract Vet* 6:S93-100, 1984.
Initially feed only 100-g amounts of dextrose and casein in the slurry. Slowly increase the amounts to the levels in the table over 5-7 days. Casein (Sigma Chemical Co., St. Louis, MO 63178; [800] 325-3010) or dehydrated cottage cheese; 82% crude protein with less than 2% lactose.

reduce the incidence of diet-induced diarrhea. Although the ingredients are inexpensive, weighing the components is time-consuming.

- **Commercial enteral diet.** Human enteral diets are expensive, and horses fed solely on these diets often have diarrhea (Table 57–5). Mature horses have been satisfactorily maintained with Osmolite HN administered at a total daily caloric intake of 155 × (body weight in kilograms) × 0.75 or approximately 15 Mcal for a 500-kg horse. The solution comes at an energy density of 1 Mcal/L, so the total volume fed is approximately 16 L for a 500-kg horse and is divided among three feedings. Additional water usually is added to each feeding to provide a total daily water intake of 45 ml/kg. Giving each meal over a 30-minute period by gradual infusion from a container or adding a fiber source, such as ground alfalfa meal (1 kg per feeding) is likely to reduce the risk of digestive upset. The diet should be introduced at 25% of caloric needs on day 1, 50% of caloric needs on day 2, 75% on day 3, and 100% of maintenance requirements thereafter.

NOTE: Whichever approach is chosen, it is important to begin the diet gradually and monitor the patient's hydration, electrolyte balance, and gastrointestinal function carefully.

Tube feeding can be highly successful when lack of food intake is caused by a temporary functional or painful problem affecting the mouth or pharynx. Individuals with these types of conditions can be satisfactorily maintained for several weeks with a liquid diet. When anorexia is secondary to systemic disease, some degree of weight loss can be tolerated. Forced feeding becomes more important with chronic inappetence (>3 days) and poor body condition.

Deliberate underfeeding often is practiced in veterinary medicine to empty or rest the intestine (e.g., before surgery or after major abdominal surgery). Because prolonged fasting predisposes horses to diarrhea and gastric ulcers, which can be severe in some cases, *it is better to allow patients with digestive tract problems access to small amounts of food when possible rather than to err on the side of complete food restrictions.*

TABLE 57-5. Commercial Preparations of Hyperalimentation and Enteral Diets

Manufacturer	Address	Telephone	Toll-Free Telephone	Fax	E-Mail	Product
Abbott Laboratories	1401 Sheridan Road, North Chicago, IL 60064	(847) 937-3183	(800) 323-9597	(847) 938-0659	www.abbott.com	Aminosyn,* Liposyn*
Baxter Healthcare Corporation	One Baxter Parkway, Deerfield, IL 60015	(847) 948-2000	(888) 229-0001 customer service	(888) 228-0020	www.Baxter.com	Clinimix 5/25*

*Hyperalimentation.

58 Emergency Diseases Seen in Europe

Tim Mair

GRASS SICKNESS

A dysautonomia of Equidae (horses, ponies, donkeys, and exotic Equidae) with damage to neurons of the autonomic, enteric, and somatic nervous systems. The disease occurs throughout the United Kingdom and many northern European countries, including Norway, Sweden, Denmark, France, Switzerland, and Germany. Mal seco (dry sickness) is a similar condition that occurs in the Patagonia region of Argentina and in Chile and the Falkland Islands.

The acute and subacute forms of the disease are fatal; however, a proportion of horses with the chronic form may survive. The cause of grass sickness remains unknown, although a natural neurotoxin is probably involved.

Signalment and Epidemiology
- All ages can be affected, but the highest incidence occurs among 2- to 7-year-olds.
- Usually affects only individuals in good bodily condition.
- In the northern hemisphere, the highest incidence occurs in the spring and summer (April-July). In the southern hemisphere, the highest incidence occurs in October-February.
- Affects grazing horses only.
- Disease often recurs on certain premises or pastures.
- Recent movement to a new pasture or new premises is a predisposing factor.
- Cool (7°C-10°C [46°F-50°F]), dry weather tends to occur in the 10-14 days preceding outbreaks.

Subdivisions of the Disease
- Acute
- Subacute
- Chronic

Clinical Signs
ACUTE
- Depression and somnolence
- Inappetence
- Colic
- Tachycardia (heart rate up to 100 beats/min)
- May be pyrexic (up to 40°C [104°F])
- May have bilateral ptosis
- Muscle fasciculations of the triceps and quadriceps muscle groups
- Sweating, generalized or localized to the flank, neck, and shoulder regions
- Dysphagia
- Dribbling of saliva

- Dehydration
- Small-intestinal distention
- Gastric reflux with malodorous green or brown fluid
- Reduced or absent bowel sounds
- Abdominal distention
- Most patients die or require humane destruction within 2 days

SUBACUTE
The clinical signs are similar to but less severe than those of acute cases.

- Dysphagia
- Persistent tachycardia
- Patchy sweating on flanks, neck, shoulder
- Muscle tremors (triceps and quadriceps)
- Weight loss and development of marked "tucked-up" abdomen
- Ptosis
- Nasogastric reflux and episodes of colic possible
- Most patients die or require humane destruction within 7 days

CHRONIC
The clinical signs in the chronic form are insidious in onset

- Severe weight loss with the development of a "tucked-up" abdomen
- Base narrow stance and adoption of an "elephant on a tub" posture
- Weakness and toe dragging
- Ptosis
- Persistent tachycardia (up to 60 beats/min)
- Muscle tremors
- Patchy sweating
- Mild colic
- Mild dysphagia and accumulation of food in the mouth
- Rhinitis sicca with accumulation of dry mucoid discharge around the nares and the presence of a distinctive "snuffling" sound during breathing

Diagnosis
Signalment, clinical signs, and results of rectal examination allow a tentative diagnosis. Confirmation of grass sickness can be made only by demonstrating histopathologic lesions in the autonomic or enteric ganglia at postmortem examination or by ileal biopsy at laparotomy.

- Exploratory laparotomy and ileal biopsy may be needed to differentiate acute grass sickness from surgical diseases causing small-intestinal obstruction.
- Phenylephrine eye drops cause a greater increase in the size of the palpebral fissure (as measured by the change in the angle of the eyelashes with the head observed from a frontal view) than occurs in normal horses.
- Endoscopic examination of the distal esophagus of patients with acute or subacute grass sickness may reveal longitudinal linear ulceration of the mucosa.
- Contrast esophagography (barium swallow) may show abnormal esophageal motility.

MANAGEMENT

Treatment

Acute and subacute grass sickness should be managed with humane destruction. Individuals with mild chronic disease may survive after prolonged treatment and nursing care.

CRITERIA FOR SELECTION OF CHRONIC CASES
- Some ability to swallow
- Some appetite present
- Some intestinal motility present
- Heart rate less than 60 beats/min

MANAGEMENT OF SELECTED CHRONIC CASES
- General nursing care with frequent human contact, frequent grooming, and regular hand walking and grazing
- Palatable high-energy, high-protein feeds offered 4-5 times a day
- Cisapride, 0.5-0.8 mg/kg PO 3 times a day for 7 days
- Flunixin meglumine, 0.5-1.1 mg/kg IV, or phenylbutazone, 2.2-4.4 mg/kg, may be administered as necessary to control abdominal pain
- Diazepam, 0.05 mg/kg IV every 2 hours, can be administered as an appetite stimulant

AFRICAN HORSE SICKNESS

African horse sickness is an arthropod-borne viral disease. Although the disease is normally restricted to tropical and subtropical Africa south of the Sahara, it regularly spreads southward to South Africa and northward to other parts of the African continent. Occasionally it has spread to Asia (as far as Pakistan and India) and to southern Europe (Portugal and Spain).

Signalment
- The horse is the most susceptible host.
- Mules and European donkeys are susceptible, but less so than horses.
- African donkeys are generally resistant.

Clinical Signs

Four forms of the disease are recognized:

- Pulmonary
- Mixed
- Cardiac
- Horse sickness fever

The pulmonary form is peracute or acute and is usually rapidly fatal. The cardiac form usually is subacute and has an incubation period of up to 3 weeks. The mixed disease is a combination of pulmonary and cardiac forms. Horse sickness fever is a mild condition caused by less virulent trains of the virus and is characterized by pyrexia and edema of the supraorbital fossae.

PULMONARY FORM
- May result in "sudden death"
- Depression and fever (39°C-41°C [102°F-106°F])

- Respiratory distress
- Paroxysmal coughing
- Head and neck extended
- Sweating
- Recumbency
- Frothy nasal discharge (terminally)

CARDIAC FORM
- Fever
- Edema of the head, neck, chest, and supraorbital fossae
- Conjunctival congestion
- Petechial hemorrhage on mucous membranes
- Colic

Diagnosis
- Virus isolation from blood or tissues (spleen, lung, liver, heart, lymph nodes)
- Serology: Agar gel immunodiffusion (AGID), enzyme-linked immunosorbent assay (ELISA), complement fixation (CF) test, or virus neutralization tests

Treatment
- Symptomatic treatment only

Prognosis
- The mortality among susceptible horses is 80%-90%.

ATYPICAL MYOGLOBINURIA
Reported in the United Kingdom, continental Europe, and Australia. Occurs typically in horses and ponies on pasture. Affected individuals usually are on a low plane of nutrition and are either not being exercised or are only minimally exercised. Adverse climatic conditions (heavy rain and gales) often occur before an outbreak. One or more individuals in a group may be affected.

Signalment
- Any age, however most common among young horses (<6 years)

Clinical Signs
- May be found dead or recumbent
- Less severely affected individuals may have a sudden onset of stiffness, which may progress over several hours to recumbency.
- Usually no signs of pain or distress
- Appetite and thirst normal, even in recumbent individuals
- Temperature, heart rate, and respiratory rate are normal.
- Dark brown or red urine

Diagnosis
- Epidemiologic characteristics and clinical signs
- Marked elevations of creatine kinase (CK) and aspartate aminotransferase (AST) values
- Urine contains myoglobin.

MANAGEMENT

- Some patients have elevations of sorbitol dehydrogenase and γ-glutamyl transferase.
- Some patients have hypocalcemia, especially in terminal stages.

Treatment

- Symptomatic treatment of recumbent patient and to limit further muscle damage
- Correction of any fluid-electrolyte imbalances
- Monitoring urea and creatinine values to assess renal function
- Prednisolone, 0.5-1 mg/kg PO q24h, may help in some cases

Prognosis

- Mortality is high, up to 100% in some outbreaks.
- Recumbent individuals have a poor prognosis.
- Horses that are stiff but remain standing after 2-3 days have a good prognosis.
- Prognosis and clinical features show poor correlation with degree of elevation of CK and AST.

PLANT TOXINS (see Chapter 53)
Deadly Nightshade (*Atropa belladonna*)

Deadly nightshade contains atropine, which is a muscarinic antagonist of acetylcholine.

Clinical Signs

- Mydriasis and impaired vision
- Anorexia
- Hyperexcitability
- Shivering and muscle spasms
- Ataxia
- Polyuria, occasionally with hematuria
- Convulsions

Diagnosis

- History and clinical signs
- Identification of plant fragments in stomach and intestinal tract

Treatment

- Neostigmine, 0.005-0.01 mg/kg IM or SQ
- Activated charcoal by mouth
- Supportive care

Hemlock (*Conium maculatum*)

Hemlock is widely distributed in the United Kingdom. It contains the alkaloid coniine. Only fresh plant material is toxic because drying inactivates the alkaloid.

Clinical Signs

- Pupillary dilatation
- Weakness

- Ataxia
- Bradycardia followed by tachycardia
- Bradypnea with increased respiratory effort
- Death due to respiratory arrest

Diagnosis
- Compatible history and clinical signs
- Identification of plant fragments in the stomach or intestinal contents

Treatment
- Activated charcoal by mouth
- Supportive care

Rhododendron (*Rhodendron ponticum*)
Rhododendron is a widely distributed naturalized species in the United Kingdom and is poisonous because of its content of the polyol andromedotoxin. Poisoning usually occurs in winter when snow interferes with grazing or in summer when pastures are scorched by drought.

Clinical Signs
- Hypersalivation (ptyalism/sialorrhea)
- Retching and repeated ineffective attempts to vomit
- Colic
- Diarrhea
- Excitement
- Depression
- Cardiovascular collapse
- Ataxia
- Death after several days due to respiratory depression and failure

Diagnosis
- Compatible history and clinical signs
- Identification of plant fragments in the stomach or intestinal contents

Treatment
- Activated charcoal by mouth
- Supportive care

Water Dropwort (*Oenanthe* spp), Water Hemlock (*Cicuta virosa*)
These plants are toxic because of their content of resinous toxins oenanthetoxin and cicutoxin. The roots are particularly toxic and are usually eaten when they are dug up during ditching operations and left on the banks.

Clinical Signs
- Hypersalivation
- Abdominal pain
- Pupillary dilatation
- Muscle spasms

MANAGEMENT

- Seizures
- Death often occurs within a few minutes of the onset of clinical signs due to respiratory failure.

Diagnosis

- Compatible history and clinical signs
- Identification of plant fragments in the stomach or intestinal contents

Treatment

- Activated charcoal by mouth
- Supportive care
- In most cases death occurs before treatment can be initiated.

REFERENCES

Grass Sickness

Hahn CN, Mayhew IG: Phenylephrine eyedrops as a diagnostic test in equine grass sickness, *Vet Rec* 147:603-606, 2000.

Hunter LC, Miller JK, Poxton IR: The association of Clostridium botulinum type C with equine grass sickness: a toxicoinfection? *Equine Vet J* 31:492-499, 1999.

Milne E, Wallis N: Nursing the chronic grass sickness patient, *Equine Vet Ed* 6:217-219, 1994.

Scholes SFE et al: Diagnosis of grass sickness by ileal biopsy, *Vet Rec* 133:7-10, 1993.

African Horse Sickness

Mellor P: African horse sickness (AHS), *Equine Vet Ed* 6:200-202, 1994.

Rodriguez M, Hooghus H, Castono M: Current status of the diagnosis and control of African horse sickness, *Vet Rec* 24:189-198, 1993.

Atypical Myoglobinuria

Whitwell KE, Harris P, Farrington PG: Atypical myoglobinuria: an acute myopathy in grazing horses, *Equine Vet J* 20:357-363, 1988.

Equine Emergency Drugs: Approximate Dosages

Drug Name, Trade Name,* Conversion Factor	Indication	Dosage	Route	1000-lb (450-kg) Dose	Precautions and Comments
Acepromazine, 10 mg/ml	Restraint, sedation, preanesthetic, peripheral vasodilator	0.02-0.05 mg/kg q8h	IV, IM	0.9-2.25 ml	Produces hypotension
Acetazolamide, 250 mg/tab[†]	Diuretic, glaucoma, HYPP prophylaxis, hyperkalemia	2-4 mg/kg q6h	PO	3.6-7.2 tabs	
Acetylcysteine, *Mucomyst,* 10% or 20% solution	Mucolytic, anticollagenase	140 mg/kg	PO	315 ml	ARDS, oxidative disorders
N-Acetyl-L-cysteine (powdered)	Meconium impaction	Add 8 g powder and 1.5 tbsp (22.5 g) sodium bicarbonate (baking soda) to 200 ml water; infuse 120-180 ml	Nebulization, IT	120-180 ml	ARDS or tenacious exudate in airways
			Per rectum		
Acetylsalicylic acid, aspirin, (240 gr) bolus[†]	Antithrombotic	15-20 mg/kg q48h	PO	½ boluses	May not inhibit platelet activity in endotoxemia
Acyclovir, *Zovirax*	Acute herpes infection	10-20 mg/kg q12h	PO, IV		Oral bioavailability unknown
Albuterol, *Proventil,* 90 µg/puff 0.5% for nebulization	Bronchospasm	720 µg/kg q3-4h for adult	Inhaler	8 puffs	Do not use in hypokalemic patients
			Nebulization		Dilute with sterile saline
Altrenogest, *Regumate,* 2.2 mg/ml	Pregnancy maintenance, estrus suppression	0.044-0.088 mg/kg q24h	PO	9-18 ml	For pregnant mares experiencing toxemia or indications of premature delivery
Amikacin, *Amiglyde,* 250 mg/ml	Antibiotic	15-25 mg/kg q24h	IV, IM	27-45 ml	Preferred over gentamicin in foals

Continued

EQUINE EMERGENCY DRUGS: APPROXIMATE DOSAGES—*cont'd.*

Drug Name, Trade Name,* Conversion Factor	Indication	Dosage	Route	1000-lb (450-kg) Dose	Precautions and Comments
Aminocaproic acid, *Amicar,* 250 mg/ml	Hemorrhage	10-20 mg/kg	IV diluted in 1-3 L 0.9% saline solution and administered slowly	18-36 ml	Used for uncontrollable bleeding when surgery not an option
Aminophylline, *Corophyllin, Palaron,* 200 mg/tab,† 25 mg/ml	Bronchodilator, diminishes diaphragmatic fatigue, muscle fatigue, respiratory stimulant, antiinflammatory	4-10 mg/kg q8-12h	PO	9-22 tabs	May improve glomerular filtration rate; rarely recommended as a bronchodilator
Ampicillin sodium, *Amp-Equine,* 1 and 3 g/vial (40 mg/ml)†	Antibiotic	2-5 mg/kg q8-12h 5 mg/kg q8-12h 15-20 mg/kg q8h	IV Nebulization IV	36-126 ml 168-225 ml	More concentrated solutions may be used.
Ampicillin trihydrate, *Poly-Flex,* 10 and 20 g/vial (40 mg/ml)	Antibiotic	11-22 mg/kg q8-12h	IV, IM	123-247 ml	More concentrated solutions may be used.
Antacids, *Maalox, Di-Gel*	Esophagitis, gastric hyperacidity, peptic ulcer, gastritis	30-100 ml q3-4h for foal	PO	30-100 ml **(foals)**	Buffers acid for a brief period
Atracurium, 10 mg/ml	Neuromuscular blocker	0.1-0.2 mg/kg	IV	4.5-9.0 ml	Paralytic agent
Atropine, 15 mg/ml	Bradyarrhythmias	0.005-0.01 mg/kg for sinus bradycardia	IV	0.15-0.3 ml	Tachycardia, arrhythmia, ileus, mydriasis may occur; do not use with inotropes

EQUINE EMERGENCY DRUGS: APPROXIMATE DOSAGES—cont'd.

Drug Name, Trade Name,* Conversion Factor	Indication	Dosage	Route	1000-lb (450-kg) Dose	Precautions and Comments
	Bronchodilator	0.014-0.02 mg/kg for bronchodilatation	IV, IM	0.6 ml	Repeat in 5 min if indicated
	Organophosphate toxicity	0.15 mg/kg	IV, IM, SQ		Administer only for organophosphate toxicity and observe for signs of ileus
Azithromycin, Zithromax, 100 mg/tab, 250 mg/tab	Antibiotic	10 mg/kg q24h for 5 days, then every other day	IV, IM, SQ PO		Can be combined with rifampin
Beclomethasone, Beclovent, Vanceril, 42 µg/puff	Antiinflammatory	1-2 µg/kg q12-24h	Inhaler	10-20 puffs	
Benztropine mesylate, Cogentin, 1 mg/tab	Anticholinergic	8 mg/450 kg	PO	8 tabs	
Bethanechol, Urecholine, 5 mg/ml 5 mg/tab†	Bladder atony	0.03-0.04 mg/kg q6-8h	SQ, IV		Can be formulated for IV or SQ use
Beuthanasia solution, 290 mg/ml pentobarbital	Euthanasia	0.22 mg/kg q6-8h 10-15 ml/100 lb (45 kg)	PO IV	20 tabs 100-150 ml	Poorly absorbed Has been approved for **euthanasia only;** emergency seizure control: 5-10 ml/500 kg IV
Bismuth subsalicylate, Pepto-Bismol, 262 mg/15 ml	Antidiarrheal	4.5 ml/kg q4-12h	PO	2000 ml	

Continued

EQUINE EMERGENCY DRUGS: APPROXIMATE DOSAGES—*cont'd.*

Drug Name, Trade Name,* Conversion Factor	Indication	Dosage	Route	1000-lb (450-kg) Dose	Precautions and Comments
Bovine hemoglobin	Transfusion	5-20 ml/kg	IV slowly	2.250-9.000 ml	Used to manage life-threatening anemia when an equine donor transfusion is unavailable
Bretylium, *Tosylate* 50 mg/ml	Ventricular fibrillation	5-10 mg/kg (every 10 min)	IV	45-90 ml	Do not exceed 30-35 mg/kg total dose
Butorphanol tartrate, *Torbugesic,* 10 mg/ml	Analgesic, sedation, preanesthetic, antitussive	0.01-0.1 mg/kg	IV, IM	0.45-4.5 ml	Ataxia and head tremors when used without tranquilization
Ca-EDTA, *Meta-Dote,* 50 mg/ml	Lead toxicity	75 mg/kg per day divided q12h	IV slowly	675 ml	
Caffeine, *NoDoz*[†] Vivarin 200 mg/tab	Respiratory stimulant	10 mg/kg loading dose, then 2.5-3 mg/kg, q24h maintenance dose	PO or per rectum		Toxic level >40 µg/L
Calcium borogluconate (23%), 230 mg/ml (20.7 mg Ca, 1.08 mEq/ml)	Hypocalcemia, hyperkalemia	150-250 mg/kg	IV slowly	112.5-450 ml	Can be mixed with most crystalloids. Monitor cardiac rate and rhythm
Calcium chloride, 100 mg/ml	Cardiac resuscitation	5-7 mg/kg	IV	22.5-31.5 ml	
Carprofen, *Rimadyl,* 100 mg/tab[†]	Analgesic, antiinflammatory	1.4 mg/kg q24h	PO	6.3 tabs	
Cefazolin[†]	Antibiotic	11-22 mg/kg q6-8h	IV		First-generation cephalosporin
Cefoperazone, *Cefobid,* 1 g/vial (40 mg/ml)[†]	Antibiotic	30 mg/kg q8h	IV	37 ml for **50 kg**	Third-generation cephalosporin

Drug Name, Trade Name,* Conversion Factor	Indication	Dosage	Route	1000-lb (450-kg) Dose	Precautions and Comments
Cefotaxime, *Claforan,* 500 mg (20 mg/ml)†	Antibiotic	40-50 mg/kg q6-8h	IV	125 ml for **50 kg**	Third-generation cephalosporin
Ceftazidime, *Fortaz,* 1 g/vial (40 mg/ml)	Antibiotic	20-40 mg/kg q8-12h	IV, IM	38 ml for **50 kg**	Third-generation cephalosporin
Ceftiofur, *Naxcel,* 50 mg/ml, 4 g/vial†	Antibiotic	1-5 mg/kg q6-12h	IV, IM	9-45 ml	Dose varies with severity of disease; third-generation cephalosporin
Cephapirin, *Cefadyl,* 500 mg (20 mg/ml)†	Antibiotic	20-30 mg/kg q4-8h	IM, IV	62 ml/**50 kg**	Reports of diarrhea, anaphylaxis; first-generation cephalosporin
Charcoal, *ToxiBan*† or chemical grade	Gastrointestinal adsorbent	0.5-1 g/kg	PO		
Chloral hydrate, *Chloropent*	Restraint, sedation, preanesthetic	22 mg/kg (moderate sedation) 30-60 mg/kg (profound sedation)	IV 12% solution by slow infusion		Perivascular administration causes phlebitis
Chloramphenicol, 500 mg tabs†	Antibiotic	44 mg/kg q8h	PO	40 tabs q8h	Compounded paste may decrease human contact during treatment; illegal in some countries.
Cimetidine, *Tagamet,* 150 mg/ml, 800 mg/tab	Gastroduodenal ulceration	6.6 mg/kg q6-8h	IV	198 ml	
Clarithromycin	Antibiotic	16-25 mg/kg q8h 7.5 mg/kg q12h	PO PO	9-14 tabs 4-5 tabs (250 mg/tab)/ 150 kg foal	Diarrhea may occur more commonly than with Azithromycin, *Biaxin*
Clavulanic acid-ticarcillin, *Timentin* 3.1 and 31 g vial	Antibiotic	100 mg/kg loading dose, then 50 mg/kg q6h	IV		
Clenbuterol, *Ventipulmin,* 72.5 µg/ml Inhaler†	Bronchodilator	0.8-3.2 µg/kg q12h 0.5 µg/kg q8h	IV, PO Nebulization	5-20 ml	Tachycardia and restlessness may occur at higher doses

Continued

EQUINE EMERGENCY DRUGS: APPROXIMATE DOSAGES—cont'd.

Drug Name, Trade Name, * Conversion Factor	Indication	Dosage	Route	1000-lb (450-kg) Dose	Precautions and Comments
Colchicine, 0.6 mg tabs	Hepatic fibrosis	0.03 mg/kg q24h	PO	22 tabs	
Colony-stimulating factor, *Neupogen,* 300 μg/ml	Life-threatening leukopenia	5 μg/kg q24h	IV slowly over 30 min	1 ml/50 kg	
Cromolyn sodium, *Intal Nasalcrom,* 100 mg/ml	Chronic obstructive pulmonary disease	0.2-0.5 mg/kg	Nebulization	0.9-2.25 ml	
Cyproheptadine, *Periactin,* 4 mg/tab	Pituitary, hyperplasia	0.25-0.5 mg/kg q12h	PO	28-56 tabs	Efficacy unproven
Dantrolene, *Dantrium,* 100 mg capsules	Rhabdomyolysis, muscle relaxation	2.5-5 mg/kg q12-24h	PO	11-22 capsules	May cause sedation at higher doses
Desferrioxamine, 500 mg (20 mg/ml)	Iron toxicity	10 mg/kg	IM, IV slowly	225 ml	
Detomidine hydrochloride, *Dormosedan,* 10 mg/ml	Sedation, analgesia	5-40 μg/kg	IV, IM	0.23-1.8 ml	Higher dosage for IM only; breed variation in dosage; 6 μg/kg for epidural use, may have some effect when given orally
Dexamethasone, *Azium,*† 2 mg/ml	Antiinflammatory	0.02-0.05 mg/kg q24h	IV, IM, PO	4.5-11 ml	Prolonged treatment may cause laminitis; prolonged high dose may cause abortion
Azium SP, 4 mg/ml (equivalent to 3 mg dexamethasone)	Antiedema	0.5 mg/kg q6-24h	IV	75 ml	
Dexamethasone-trichlormethiazide, *Naquasone*	Inflammatory edema	5 mg/200 mg boluses q24h	PO		

EQUINE EMERGENCY DRUGS: APPROXIMATE DOSAGES—cont'd.

Drug Name, Trade Name,* Conversion Factor	Indication	Dosage	Route	1000-lb (450-kg) Dose	Precautions and Comments
Dextrose	Hypoglycemia, hyperkalemia	5% or 10% solution at 4-8 mg/kg per minute; 0.5 ml/kg	IV	225 ml	May cause rebound hypoglycemia
Diazepam, *Valium,* 5 mg/ml	Sedation, anticonvulsant, preanesthetic	0.05-0.44 mg/kg for adult; 0.1-0.2 mg/kg for foal	IV	4.5-39.6 ml 1-2 ml foal	Respiratory depression may occur at higher doses; may precipitate in PVC lines
Digoxin, *Lanoxin,* 0.1 mg/ml	Cardiac failure, supraventricular arrhythmias	0.0022-0.0075 mg/kg q12h	IV	10-33 ml	Depression, anorexia, colic may occur; lower dose most commonly used
0.5-mg tab		0.011-0.0175 mg/kg q12h	PO	10 tabs	For longer-term use
Dimercaprol, 100 mg/ml	Arsenic, lead toxicity	2.5-5 mg/kg	IM	11.25-22.5 ml	
Dimethyl sulfoxide 90% (DMSO), *Domoso solution*	Antiedema	10%-20% solution at 0.5-1.0 g/kg q12-24h	IV in 0.9% saline solution or D_5W	500 ml	Antiedema
	Antiinflammatory	10%-20% solution at 100 mg/kg q8h	IV in 0.9% saline solution or D_5W		Postoperative treatment, antiinflammatory
Dinoprost tromethamine, *Lutalyse,* 5 mg/ml	Abortion	0.011-0.022 mg/kg	IM	0.9-1.98 ml (1-2 ml)	Early and midgestation; abortifacient

Continued

EQUINE EMERGENCY DRUGS: APPROXIMATE DOSAGES—cont'd.

Drug Name, Trade Name,* Conversion Factor	Indication	Dosage	Route	1000-lb (450-kg) Dose	Precautions and Comments
Dioctyl sodium sulfosuccinate, 100 mg/ml	Emollient laxative	10-20 mg/kg; up to 2 doses, 48 h apart	PO	45-90 ml	May cause mild abdominal pain and diarrhea
Diphenhydramine hydrochloride, *Benadryl,* 10 mg/ml	Antihistamine, antipyretic, analgesic	0.5-2 mg/kg	IV, IM	22.5-90 ml	May enhance or inhibit the effects of epinephrine
Dipyrone, *Novin, Metamizole*	Antiinflammatory analgesic	10-22 mg/kg	IV, IM		Compounded only in United States
Dobutamine, *Dobutrex,* 12.5 mg/ml	Cardiac failure, hypotension, AV block	1-20 µg/kg per minute	IV after dilution to 500 µg/ml		Do not use with magnesium; see Chapter 52 for incompatibilities and dilution
Domperidone (approval pending)	Agalactia, fescue toxicity	1.1 mg/kg q12h	PO		May enhance GI motility
Dopamine, *Intropin,* 40 mg/ml	Oliguric renal failure, cardiac failure, AV block	1-20 µg/kg per minute	IV		See Chapter 52
Doxapram, *Dopram,* 20 mg/ml	Respiratory stimulant	0.2 mg/kg	IV	4.5 ml	
Doxycycline, 100 mg/tab[†]	Antibiotic	5-10 mg/kg q12h	PO	22-45 tabs	Do not give IV, poorly absorbed orally
Doxylamine succinate, 11.36 mg/ml	Antihistamine	0.5 mg/kg q6-12h	IV slowly, IM, SQ	20 ml	May enhance or inhibit the effects of epinephrine
Edrophonium, *Tensilon,* 10 mg/ml	Supraventricular arrhythmia, reversal of atracurium	0.5-1 mg/kg	IV	22-45 ml	Antagonist for atracurium
Enalapril, *Enacard,* 20 mg/tab[†]	Vasodilator	0.25-0.5 mg/kg q12-24h	PO	5.6-11 tabs	Bioavailability unproven in horses

EQUINE EMERGENCY DRUGS: APPROXIMATE DOSAGES—cont'd.

Drug Name, Trade Name,* Conversion Factor	Indication	Dosage	Route	1000-lb (450-kg) Dose	Precautions and Comments
Enrofloxacin, *Baytril*, 100 mg/ml	Antibiotic	3.3 mg/kg q12h, 7.5 mg/kg q24h	PO	15-33 ml	Safety not demonstrated in foals
Epinephrine, *Adrenaline chloride*, 1:1000 (1 mg/ml)	Anaphylaxis, asystole, glaucoma, resuscitation, bradycardia	5-7.5 mg/kg q12-24h 0.01-0.02 mg/kg anaphylaxis	IV IV, IM	22.5-33.7 ml 4.5-9 ml	
		0.1-0.2 mg/kg anaphylaxis	IT		
		0.03-0.05 mg/kg to asystole	IV		
		0.3-0.5 mg/kg to asystole	IT		
Equine plasma	Sepsis, shock, hypogamma-globulinemia, hemorrhage, decreased oncotic pressure	1 or more liters	IV		Can generally be administered rapidly
Erythromycin lactobionate[†]	GI ileus	1-2.5 mg/kg as 1-h infusion q6h	IV	4.5-11 ml[†]	To improve intestinal motility; observe for colic, diarrhea, intussusception
Erythromycin estolate[†]	GI ileus	25-30 mg/kg q8-12h	PO		One of the preferred products for oral use in horses
Famotidine, *Pepcid AC* 20 mg/tab	GI ulceration	0.23-0.5 mg/kg q8-12h	IV		Minimal pharmacokinetic data available
		4 mg/kg q8h	PO	10 tabs **(foal)**	
Febantel (FBT), 93 mg/ml	Anthelmintic	6 mg/kg	PO	29 ml	
Fenbendazole (FBZ), *Panacur*, 100 mg/ml	Anthelmintic	5-10 mg/kg	PO	22.5-45 ml	

Continued

791

EQUINE EMERGENCY DRUGS: APPROXIMATE DOSAGES—cont'd.

Drug Name, Trade Name, * Conversion Factor	Indication	Dosage	Route	1000-lb (450-kg) Dose	Precautions and Comments
Fentanyl, *Duragesic,* 50- or 100-μg/hr patches	Analgesia		Dermal	2-3 × 100 μg/hr patches	Change every third day; do not use with butorphanol, decreases intestinal motility
Fluconazole, *Diflucan,* 200 mg/tab	Antifungal	4 mg/lb (45 kg) loading dose; 2 mg/lb maintenance q24h	PO	9 tabs; 4.5 tabs	
Flumazenil, *Romazicon,* 0.1 mg/ml	Benzodiazepine (Valium) antagonist, uncontrolled hepatic coma	0.011-0.022 mg/kg	IV slowly	50 ml	Expensive treatment with questionable benefit for hepatic encephalopathy
Flunixin meglumine, *Banamine,* 50 mg/ml	Endotoxemia	0.25 mg/kg q8h	IV	2.3 ml	
	Analgesia, antiinflammatory, antipyretic	0.25-1.1 mg/kg	IV, IM	2.3-9.9 ml	IM injections infrequently associated with Clostridial myositis
Fluprostenol sodium, *Equimate,* 50 μg/ml	Abortion	2.2 μg/kg	IM	20 ml	Induce parturition
Fluticasone, *Flovent*	Heaves	1 mg/450 kg q12-24h	Inhaler		
Furosemide, *Lasix,* 50 mg/ml	Diuretic	1-2 mg/kg for acute edema; 0.25-1 mg/kg q12-24h (maintenance); 0.25-0.5 mg/kg every 30-60 min during dopamine infusion or begin continuous infusion	SQ, IM, IV, PO	9 ml	Protect solution from light

EQUINE EMERGENCY DRUGS: APPROXIMATE DOSAGES—cont'd.

Drug Name, Trade Name,* Conversion Factor	Indication	Dosage	Route	1000-lb (450-kg) Dose	Precautions and Comments
Gentamicin, *Gentocin,* 100 mg/ml	Antibiotic	(0.25-2 mg/kg per hour) for oliguric acute renal failure 6.6 mg/kg	IV	30 ml	Nephrotoxic; use cautiously and only in well-hydrated foals and adults
Glycopyrrolate, *Robinul-V,* 0.2 mg/ml	Vagally induced bradyarrhythmias	0.005-0.01 mg/kg	IV	11-22.5 ml	Tachycardia, arrhythmia, ileus, mydriasis
Guaifenesin, *Gecolate,†* 50 mg/ml	Bronchodilator Muscle relaxant, preanesthetic, expectorant	0.005 mg/kg q8-12h 40-80 mg/kg	IV, IM, SQ IV as 5% solution	360-720 ml	
Haloperidol decanoate HCG, *Haldol,* 50 mg/ml	Long-acting tranquilizer Induction of ovulation	0.01 mg/kg	IM IM		Adverse effects occur; may cause sedation for 5-7 d; do not give IV
Heparin, 1000 IU/ml	Persistent ovarian follicles Anticoagulant, hyperlipidemia, prevention of abdominal adhesions	1000-5000 U 40-100 IU/kg q6h	SQ, IM, IV IV, SQ, mixed in equine plasma for SIRS	18-45 ml	Monitor for RBC agglutination and decreasing hematocrit
Hetastarch, *Hespan,* 60 mg/ml	Shock	10-20 ml/kg per hour	IV	4500-9000 ml	Do not use with hemorrhage
Hydralazine, *Apresoline,* 50 mg/tab†	Congestive heart failure	0.5-1.5 mg/kg q12h	PO	4.5-13.5 tabs	Arterial dilatation

Continued

DRUG DOSAGES

EQUINE EMERGENCY DRUGS: APPROXIMATE DOSAGES—*cont'd.*

Drug Name, Trade Name,* Conversion Factor	Indication	Dosage	Route	1000-lb (450-kg) Dose	Precautions and Comments
Hydrochlorothiazide, *Hydrozide,* 25 mg/ml	Diuretic	0.56 mg/kg q24h	PO	10 ml	
Hydroxyzine hydrochloride, *Atarax,* 100 mg tabs[†] 25 mg/ml	Antihistamine	1-1.5 mg/kg q8-12h	PO	5 tabs	
		0.5-1 mg/kg q12h	IM	9-18 ml	May have unpredictable results when used with epinephrine
Hyperimmune plasma, 2-4/450 kg	Endotoxemia	2-4 L/450 kg	IV	2-4 L	
Imidocarb, *Imizol,* 120 mg/ml	Babesiosis	2.2-4 mg/kg	IM	8-15 ml	
Imipenem, *Primaxin IV,* 250 mg (10 mg/ml)	Antibiotic	15 mg/kg q6-8h	IV in fluids	75 ml/kg	
Imipramine, *Tofranil,* 50 mg tabs	Narcolepsy, cataplexy	1.5 mg/kg q8-12h	PO	13 tabs	IV preparation also available
Insulin, protamine Zn	Hyperglycemia	0.4 IU/kg q24h	IM, SQ	180 IU	Available in Europe
Insulin, regular, *Humulin,* 100 IU/ml	Hyperglycemia	0.1 IU/kg PRN	IM, IV	0.45 ml	
	Hyperkalemia	0.1-1 IU/kg	IM, IV	0.45-4.5 ml	Should be used as a last resort for hyperkalemia
Insulin, ultralente,[†] 100 IU/ml	Hyperlipidemia	0.4 IU/kg q24h	IV, IM	1.8 ml	Dose and duration of treatment variable
Ipratropium bromide, *Atrovent,* 18 μg/puff	Bronchodilator	0.5-3 μg/kg q8h	Nebulization, inhaler	12.5-75 puffs	Can be used in addition to β_2 agonist

EQUINE EMERGENCY DRUGS: APPROXIMATE DOSAGES—*cont'd.*

Drug Name, Trade Name,* Conversion Factor	Indication	Dosage	Route	1000-lb (450-kg) Dose	Precautions and Comments
Isoflupredone acetate, *Predef 2x*	Heaves	0.02 mg/kg q24h	IM		Decrease dose and prolong interval after 3-5 d; no hypokalemia reported in horses
Isoproterenol, *Isuprel,* 0.2 mg/ml	Bronchodilator, resuscitation	0.05-0.2 µg/kg per minute	IV		Rarely used
Itraconazole, *Sporanox,* 100 mg/tab	Antifungal	2.6 mg/kg q12h	PO	9.7 caps	
Ivermectin, *Eqvalan,* 10 mg/ml	Anthelmintic	200 µg/kg	PO	9 ml	
Kaolin, 4-8 ml/kg	GI adsorbent	4-8 ml/kg q12h	PO	1800-3600 ml	
Ketamine, 100 mg/ml	Anesthesia	1-2 mg/kg for adult; 1 mg/kg for foal	IV	4.5-10 ml	
Ketoconazole, *Nizoral,* 200-mg tabs	Inflammatory respiratory disease, antifungal	3-10 mg/kg q24h	PO	11 tabs	Absorption may be improved by fasting; do not use with proton pump or H_2 blockers
Ketoprofen, *Ketofen,* 100 mg/ml	Analgesia, antiinflammatory, antipyretic	1.1-2.2 mg/kg	IV	5-10 ml	
Lactulose, 666 mg/ml	Liver failure	0.2 ml/kg q6-8h	PO	60-120 ml	May cause diarrhea
Lidocaine without epinephrine, 20 mg/ml	Ventricular tachyarrhythmias	0.25 mg/kg (bolus)	IV slowly	6 ml	For ventricular arrhythmias, excitement, seizures
	Systemic analgesia, antiinflammatory, gastrointestinal ileus	1.3 mg/kg, followed by 0.05 mg/kg per minute	IV slowly	30 ml slow bolus	Ataxia may occur if drug is delivered too fast; do not exceed 3 mg/kg total dose

Continued

EQUINE EMERGENCY DRUGS: APPROXIMATE DOSAGES—*cont'd.*

Drug Name, Trade Name,* Conversion Factor	Indication	Dosage	Route	1000-lb (450-kg) Dose	Precautions and Comments
Loperamide, *Imodium,* 2 mg/tab	Antidiarrheal	4-16 mg/foal; then increase by 2-mg increments every 2-3 doses q6h	PO	20-80 tabs	Enhances toxin absorption in cases of acute, infectious enteritis
Magnesium oxide	Hypertension	3-5 g/500 kg	PO		
Magnesium sulfate 50%,† 500 mg/ml, 4 mEq/ml	Ventricular tachyarrhythmia	1-2.5 g/450 kg per minute	IV	2-5 ml	Do not exceed 25 g IV total dose
	Hypomagnesemia, reperfusion injury	50-100 mg/kg q24h	IV		
	Malignant hyperthermia	6 mg/kg	IV		
Magnesium sulfate, Epsom salts	Laxative	0.2-1 g/kg diluted in warm water q24h	PO	450 g	Do not use longer than 3 d to avoid enteritis and magnesium toxicity
Mannitol, 20% 200 mg/ml	Cerebral edema	20% solution at 0.25-2 g/kg over 15-40 min	IV	560-4500 ml	May exacerbate cerebral hemorrhage
Mebendazole (MBZ), *Vermox,* 100 mg/tab	Anthelmintic	8.8 mg/kg	PO	40 tabs	
Meperidine hydrochloride, *Demerol,* 50 mg/ml	Analgesia, sedation	1.1-2.2 mg/kg	IV, IM	10-20 ml	IV administration may cause severe hypotension and excitement
L-Methionine, 500 mg tabs	Laminitis	25 mg/kg	PO	22 tabs	
Methocarbamol, *Robaxin-V, Robaxin,* 500 mg/tab, 100 mg/ml	Muscle relaxant	40-60 mg/kg q24h
10-50 mg/kg	PO
IV	36-54 tabs
45-112 ml	

EQUINE EMERGENCY DRUGS: APPROXIMATE DOSAGES—cont'd.

Drug Name, Trade Name,* Conversion Factor	Indication	Dosage	Route	1000-lb (450-kg) Dose	Precautions and Comments
Methylene blue, 10 mg/ml	Nitrate/nitrite and cyanide toxicities	5-8.8 mg/kg	IV slowly	225-400 ml	
Methylprednisolone sodium succinate, *Solu-Medrol*	Acute CNS trauma	30 mg/kg over 15 min	IV		Do not use unless trauma occurred within 4 hrs
Metoclopramide, *Reglan,* 5 mg/ml	GI ileus	0.25-0.5 mg/kg q4-8h as a continuous infusion	IV	22.5-45 ml	May produce CNS excitement
1 mg/ml oral solution		0.6 mg/kg q4-6h	PO	270 ml	
Metronidazole, *Flagyl,* 500 mg tabs†	Antibiotic, antiprotozoal	15-25 mg/kg q6-8h	PO, suppository	13-22 tabs	Suppository bioavailability is 50% of that of orally administered drug
Milk of magnesia	Laxative	6-8 L/500 kg	PO		
Milrinone, *Primacor,* 1 mg/ml	Cardiotonic	10 µg/kg per minute	IV	4.5 ml	
Mineral oil, 6-8 L/450 kg	GI laxative	0.5-1 mg/kg q12h	PO		
		2-4 L/450 kg	PO	2-4 L	
		4.5-9 ml/kg	PO through NG tube		
Misoprostol, *Cytotec,* 200 µg/tab†	Prevention of NSAID GI ulceration	2.5-5 µg/kg q12h	PO	5-11 tabs	Do not use in pregnant horses, and **do not allow pregnant women to handle**
Morphine sulfate, 50 mg/ml†	Analgesic	0.3-0.66 mg/kg	IV	2.7-6 ml	Use only with xylazine (0.66-1.1 mg/kg IV) or detomidine to avoid CNS excitement

Continued

DRUG DOSAGES

797

EQUINE EMERGENCY DRUGS: APPROXIMATE DOSAGES—cont'd.

Drug Name, Trade Name,* Conversion Factor	Indication	Dosage	Route	1000-lb (450-kg) Dose	Precautions and Comments
1 mg/ml preservative-free	Epidural analgesic	0.1 mg/kg q24h	Epidural		Use preservative-free solution for epidural (this can be compounded at a higher concentration per milliliter)
Moxidectin, *Quest,* 20 mg/ml	Anthelmintic	0.4-0.5 mg/kg	PO	9-11.25 ml	***Do not use in foals younger than 4 mo***
Naloxone, 0.4 mg/ml	Opioid antagonist, hemorrhage	0.01-0.02 mg/kg	IV	11.25-22.5 ml	
Neomycin, *Biosol,* 50 mg/ml†	Antibiotic for decreasing enteric ammonia production	8-20 mg/kg q8h	PO	72 ml	Prolonged administration (3-4 doses) or higher doses may cause diarrhea
Neostigmine, *Prostigmin,* 2 mg/ml	GI ileus	0.005-0.01 mg/kg	SQ, IM	1-2.25 ml	Higher doses may cause increased abdominal pain
Nitric oxide	Pulmonary hypertension	20-80 ppm, 1:5 to 1:9 ratio with oxygen	Inhalation		
Nitroglycerine cream, *Nitro-Bid*	Laminitis	15 mg over each digital artery (1-inch [2.5-cm] strip) q24h	Topical		Do not exceed 60 mg/d; use gloves
Norepinephrine, 1 mg/ml	Refractory hypertension and anuria	0.05-1 µg/kg per minute	IV		Do not exceed 10 µg/kg per minute
Omeprazole, *Gastrogard,* 2.28 g/tube	GI ulceration	1-4 mg/kg q24h	PO	0.2-0.8 tube	May require 2-3 d to effectively increase pH
Oxfendazole (OFZ), *Benzelmin,* 90.6 mg/ml†	Anthelmintic	10 mg/kg	PO	50 ml	

EQUINE EMERGENCY DRUGS: APPROXIMATE DOSAGES—cont'd.

Drug Name, Trade Name,* Conversion Factor	Indication	Dosage	Route	1000-lb (450-kg) Dose	Precautions and Comments
Oxibendazole (OBZ), *Anthelcide,* 100 mg/ml†	Anthelmintic	10-15 mg/kg	PO	45-67.5 ml	
Oxytocin, 20 IU/ml	Milk letdown, retained fetal membranes, induction of parturition	2.5-20 units/450 kg	IV, IM, SQ	0.25-1 ml	Higher doses produce pain
Paromomycin, *Humatin,* 250 mg/tab	Antiprotozoal	100 mg/kg q24h × 5 d	PO	20 tabs/50 kg	Efficacy unproven in foals; for *Cryptosporidia*
Pectin-kaolin, 4-8 ml/kg	GI adsorbent	4-8 ml/kg q12h	PO	1800-3600 ml	
Penicillin, Na+ or K+, 20,000 IU/ml†	Antibiotic	22,000-44,000 IU/kg q4-6h	IV, IM	22.5-66 ml	Higher dosages may be used for clostridial cellulitis
Penicillin, procaine, 300,000 IU/ml	Antibiotic	15,000-44,000 IU/kg q12h	IM		
Pentazocine, *Talwin,* 30 mg/ml	Analgesia	0.3-0.6 mg/kg	PO, IV	4.5-9 ml	
Pentobarbital, 64.8 mg/ml	Anesthesia, euthanasia anticonvulsant	3-10 mg/kg	IV	20-70 ml	To effect for sedation or seizure control
Pentoxifylline, *Trental,* 400 mg/tab	Endotoxemia, laminitis	8.4 mg/kg q8-12h	PO, IV	9 tabs	Can be prepared for IV use through 0.5-µg filter
Pergolide, *Permax,* 0.25 mg/tab†	Pituitary pars intermedia hyperplasia	0.0017-0.01 mg/kg q24h	PO	3-18 tabs	Higher concentration tablets may be more convenient.
Perphenazine *Trilafon*	Fescue toxicity	0.3-0.5 mg/kg q8h	PO		

Continued

EQUINE EMERGENCY DRUGS: APPROXIMATE DOSAGES—*cont'd.*

Drug Name, Trade Name,* Conversion Factor	Indication	Dosage	Route	1000-lb (450-kg) Dose	Precautions and Comments
Phenobarbital, 130 mg/ml	Anticonvulsant, dopamine antagonist	2-10 mg/kg q8-12h	PO	6.9-34.6 ml	Respiratory depression, hypotension; monitor serum levels (10-40 µg/ml) IV for seizure control
Phenoxybenzamine, *Dibenzyline,* 10 mg/cap	Laminitis, diarrhea, decreased urethral sphincter tone	5-15 mg/kg 0.4 mg/kg q6h	IV PO	18 caps	
Phenylbutazone, 200 mg/ml	Antiinflammatory, analgesic, antipyretic	2.2-4.4 mg/kg q12h	PO, IV	5-10 ml	
Phenylephrine hydrochloride, *Neo-Synephrine,* 10 mg/ml	Nephrosplenic entrapment, occasionally used for hypotension	3 µg/kg per minute for 15 min	IV	2 ml diluted in 1L NaCl over 15 min	Contracts spleen, increases vascular resistance, reflex bradycardia; perivascular injections may cause necrosis
	Nasal, pharyngeal hemorrhage and edema	10 mg diluted to 10 ml for nasal spray	Intranasal		
Phenylpropanolamine, *Prion,* 25, 50 & 75 mg/tabs†	Bladder atony, urethral sphincter hypotonus	0.5-2 mg/kg q12h	PO		
Phenytoin, *Dilantin,* 500 mg/ml†	Anticonvulsant, digoxin, toxicity, supraventricular, tachyarrhythmias	5-10 mg/kg (first 12h)	IV		Sedation, drowsiness, lip and facial twitching, gait deficits
100 mg cap†	Stringhalt, chronic intermittent exertional rhabdomyolysis prophylaxis	7.5 mg/kg q12h	PO	33 caps	Erratic absorption may cause weakness
Piperazine (PPZ)	Anthelmintic	110 mg/kg	PO		
Polymyxin B, 500,000 U/vial	Antibiotic, endotoxemia	6000 U/kg q12h	IV slowly diluted	2.7 million units	For endotoxemia

EQUINE EMERGENCY DRUGS: APPROXIMATE DOSAGES—*cont'd.*

Drug Name, Trade Name, * Conversion Factor	Indication	Dosage	Route	1000-lb (450-kg) Dose	Precautions and Comments
Ponazuril, *Marquis*	Antiprotozoal (for EPM)	5 mg/kg q24h	PO		
Potassium chloride (KCl), 2 mEq/ml	Hypokalemia	1 mEq/kg	IC	225 ml	For ventricular fibrillation only if electrical defibrillation not available
Pralidoxime (2-PAM), 300 mg/ml†	Organophosphate toxicity	0.5 mEq/kg/h 0.1 g/kg 20 mg/kg q4-6h	IV PO IV	30 ml	
Prednisolone, *Delta-Cortef,* 20 mg/tab†	Antiinflammatory	0.4-1.6 mg/kg q24h	PO	9-36 tabs	Antiinflammatory
Prednisolone sodium succinate, *Solu-Delta Cortef,* 125 mg/ml, 20 mg/ml	Inflammatory shock	2-5 mg/kg	IV	45-112 ml	
	Shock, cerebral edema	10 mg/kg q6h	V	36 ml	Use only for CNS trauma within past hour
Procainamide, *Pronestyl,* 100 mg/ml, 500 mg/cap	Supraventricular tachyarrhythmia	1 mg/kg per minute	IV	4.5 ml	Do not exceed 20 mg/kg IV total dose
Progesterone (in oil) compounded	Suppression of estrus, maintenance of pregnancy	25-35 mg/kg q8h	PO		GI, neurologic signs are similar to those of quinidine
		0.8 mg/kg q24h	IM		For pregnant mares experiencing endotoxemia or premature separation of placenta; compounded product for injection

Continued

EQUINE EMERGENCY DRUGS: APPROXIMATE DOSAGES—*cont'd.*

Drug Name, Trade Name,* Conversion Factor	Indication	Dosage	Route	1000-lb (450-kg) Dose	Precautions and Comments
Propafenone, *Rythmol*	Supraventricular and ventricular tachyarrhythmias	0.5-1 mg/kg in 5% dextrose (slowly to effect over 5-8 min)	IV		GI, neurologic signs similar to those with quinidine; bronchospasm
Propofol, 10 mg/ml	Anesthesia	2 mg/kg q8h	PO		
		4 mg/kg	IV after tranquilization	180 ml	
Propranolol, *Inderal,* 1 mg/ml	Ventricular tachycardia	0.03 mg/kg	IV	13.5 ml	Lethargy, worsening of COPD
		0.38-0.78 mg/kg q8h	PO		
Psyllium hydrophilic mucilloid, *Metamucil,* 400 g/kg†	Bulk laxative, sand colic	400 g/450 kg q6-13h	PO	400 g	
Pyrantel (PRT), 50 mg/ml	Anthelmintic	6.6 mg/kg	PO	60 ml	
Pyrimethamine, *Daraprim,* 25 mg/tab	Antiprotozoal (for EPM)	1-2 mg/kg q24h	PO	18 tabs	
Quinidine gluconate, 80 mg/ml	Atrial fibrillation, supraventricular and ventricular tachyarrhythmias	0.5-2.2 mg/kg (bolus every 10 min to effect)	IV	2.8-12.3 ml	Do not exceed 12 mg/kg IV total dose; depression, paraphimosis, urticaria, wheals, nasal mucosal swelling, laminitis, neurologic, GI effects

EQUINE EMERGENCY DRUGS: APPROXIMATE DOSAGES—cont'd.

Drug Name, Trade Name,* Conversion Factor	Indication	Dosage	Route	1000-lb (450-kg) Dose	Precautions and Comments
Quinidine sulfate, *Quinidex,* 300 mg/tab†	Atrial fibrillation	22 mg/kg q2h until converted, toxic, or plasma quinidine concentration >4 µg/ml; continue q6h until converted or toxic signs begin	NG tube	33 tabs	Do not exceed 6 doses q2h; depression, paraphimosis, urticaria, wheals, nasal mucosal swelling, laminitis, neurologic, GI effects
Ranitidine, *Zantac,* 300 mg/tab 25 mg/ml	Gastroduodenal ulceration	6.6 mg/kg q8h	PO	10 tabs	
Rifampin, *Rifadin,* 150 mg/tab	Antibiotic	1.5 mg/kg q8h 5-10 mg/kg q12h	IV PO	27 ml 15-30 tabs	
Saline solution, hypertonic 5% or 7%, 4 ml/kg		4 ml/kg	IV	1800 ml	Immediate management of life-threatening hypotension or cerebral trauma
Salmeterol, *Serevent,* 21 µg/puff	Bronchodilator	0.5 µg/kg q6-12h	Inhaler	10 puffs	
Selenium–vitamin E, *E-Se,* 2.5 mg Se and 68 U vitamin E per milliliter	Selenium and vitamin E deficiency	1 ml/100 lb (45 kg)	**IM only**	10 ml	IV administration can cause death
Sodium bicarbonate, 1 mEq/ml 8.4%	Metabolic acidosis; hyperkalemia	Variable up to 150 g PO	IV, PO		Do not use if patient has respiratory acidosis; see Chapter 52 for incompatibilities
Sodium nitrite 1%, 10 mg/ml	Cyanide toxicity	16 mg/kg	IV	720 ml	
Sodium thiosulfate, 300 mg/ml	Cyanide and arsenic toxicity	30-500 mg/kg	IV slowly	45-750 ml	

Continued

EQUINE EMERGENCY DRUGS: APPROXIMATE DOSAGES—cont'd.

Drug Name, Trade Name, * Conversion Factor	Indication	Dosage	Route	1000-lb (450-kg) Dose	Precautions and Comments
Succinylcholine, 20 mg/ml†	Muscle relaxation	0.1 mg/kg	IV	2.4 ml	Often used at time of euthanasia
Sucralfate, oral *Carafate,* 1 g/tab	GI ulceration	1 g/50-100 kg q6-8h	PO		Do not give within 1-2 h of other medication
Tetracycline, *Oxytetracycline,* 100 mg/ml, 200 mg/ml (L.A. 200)	Antibiotic	6.6 mg/kg q12h	IV slowly	30 ml (100 mg/ml) or 15 ml (200 mg/ml)	May cause renal failure in dehydrated horses
	Contracted tendons in foals	30-60 mg/kg 1-3 treatments EOD	IV		
Thiabendazole (TBZ)	Antifungal	50-100 mg/kg	PO		
Thiamine, 200 mg/ml	Thiamine deficiency, lead poisoning, CNS injury	1-10 mg/kg	IV, IM	2.25-22.5 ml	
Thiopental sodium, 20 mg/ml	General anesthesia	3-10 mg/kg	IV	67.5-225 ml	
Ticarcillin-clavulanate, *Timentin* 3.1 and 31 g/vial	Antibiotic	50 mg/kg q6h	IV		Higher loading dose may be used in foals (100 mg/kg)
Tolazoline, *Tolazine,* 100 mg/ml	α_2-Antagonist	0.5-1 mg/kg	IV slowly	4.5 ml	Occasional serious reactions; rapid administration of labeled dose may cause cardiac arrhythmias and death
Torbugesic, 10 mg/ml	See **Butorphanol**	0.01 mg/kg	IV	0.45 ml	

EQUINE EMERGENCY DRUGS: APPROXIMATE DOSAGES—cont'd.

Drug Name, Trade Name,* Conversion Factor	Indication	Dosage	Route	1000-lb (450-kg) Dose	Precautions and Comments
Trimethoprim-sulfadiazine,† *Tribrissen,* 960 mg (1:5) tablets,† 480 mg/ml (1:5)†	Antibiotic	20-30 mg/kg q12h	PO, IV		Do not use if patient has ileus; do not give IV after detomidine!
Tripelennamine HCl, *Re-Covr,*† 20 mg/ml	Antihistamine	1 mg/kg q6-12h	IM	22 ml	Do not give IV
Vancomycin, *Vancocin,* 500 mg/ml	Antibiotic	4.3-7.5 mg/kg q8h	IV slowly diluted	3.87-6.75 ml	
Verapamil, 2.5 mg/ml	Supraventricular tachyarrhythmia	0.025-0.05 mg/kg every 30 min	IV	4.5-9 ml	Do not exceed 0.2 mg/kg IV total dose
Vitamin C, 1 g/tab	Antioxidant	0.5-1 g/kg q24h	PO	225-450 tabs	
Vitamin E, *Aquasol E,* 1000 U/tab†	Vitamin E deficiency, equine motor neuron disease, equine degenerative myeloencephalopathy prophylaxis and treatment	2,000-10,000 IU q24h	PO	2-10 tabs	
Vital E-300, 300 U/ml	Acute neurologic injury	2000 IU/adult (once)	IM	7 ml	After initial treatment, switch to oral administration if possible
Vitamin K₁, phytonadione, *Veda-K1,* 10 mg/ml	Rodenticide (warfarin) toxicity	0.5-2 mg/kg	SQ, IM	22.5-90 ml	Do not administer IV!

Continued

EQUINE EMERGENCY DRUGS: APPROXIMATE DOSAGES—cont'd.

Drug Name, Trade Name,* Conversion Factor	Indication	Dosage	Route	1000-lb (450-kg) Dose	Precautions and Comments
Xylazine hydrochloride, *Rompun, Sedazine,* 100 mg/ml	Restraint, sedation, preanesthetic, analgesia	0.2-1.1 mg/kg q8-12h	IV slowly, IM	1-5 ml	May cause tachypnea when given to a febrile patient
Yohimbine, *Yocon,* 5 mg/ml	α_2-Antagonist	0.7 mg/kg 0.1 mg/kg	Epidural IV slowly	9 ml	

IV, Intravenous; *IM,* intramuscular; *HYPP,* hyperkalemic periodic paralysis; *PO,* by mouth; *ARDS,* acute respiratory distress syndrome; *IT,* intratracheal; *SQ,* subcutaneous; *PVC,* polyvinyl chloride; *AV,* atrioventricular; *RBC,* red blood cell; *PRN,* as necessary; *NG,* nasogastric; *NSAID,* nonsteroidal antiinflammatory drug; *GI,* gastrointestinal; *CNS,* central nervous system; *EPM,* equine protozoal myelitis; *COPD,* chronic obstructive pulmonary disease; *EOD,* every other day.
*Italics indicate trade name.
†Other products and concentrations are available.

P A R T

6

Appendices

Reference Values

REFERENCE VALUES FOR NORMAL BLOOD CHEMISTRY

Test	Normal Value
Acetylcholinesterase	450-790 IU/L
Adrenocorticotrophic hormone (ACTH)	8-35 pg/ml, horses
	8-20 pg/ml, ponies
Alanine aminotransferase* (ALT)	3-23 IU/L (14 ± 11)
Albumin	2.9-3.8 g/dl
	29-38 g/L
Alkaline phosphatase* (ALP)	138-251 IU/L
Ammonia (on ice) plasma	7.63-63.4 μmol/L (35.8 ± 17.0)
	13-108 μg/dl
Amylase	75-150 IU/L
Anion gap	10 mEq/L
Arginase	0-14 IU/L (11 ± 18)
Aspartate aminotransferase* (AST)	226-336 IU/L (296 ± 70)
Bicarbonate	20-28 mmol/L
Bile acids (total)	5-15 μmol/L; values in newborn foals unknown
	Up to 20 μmol/L in anorexia
Bilirubin (conjugated)*	0-6.48 mmol/L (1.71)
	0-0.4 mg/dl (0.1)
Bilirubin (total)*	7.1-34.2 mmol/L (17.1)
	1-2 mg/dl (1.5)
Bilirubin (unconjugated)*	3.42-34.2 mmol/L (17.1)
	0.2-2 mg/L (1.0); a few normal horses much higher
Butyrylcholinesterase	2000-3100 IU/L
Calcium*	2.8-3.4 mmol/L (3.10 ± 0.14); ionized 1.0-1.3 mmol/L
	11.2-13.6 mg/dl (12.4 ± 0.58)
Carbon dioxide, P_{CO_2} (venous and arterial)	38-46 mm Hg (42.4 ± 2)
Carbon dioxide, total*	24-32 mmol/L (28)
β-Carotene	150-397 μg/dl
Chloride*	99-109 mmol or mEq/L (104 ± 2.6)
Cholesterol (ester)	(81.1) mg/dl
Cholesterol (free)	(0.41) mmol/L
	15.7 mg/dl
Cholesterol (total)*	1.94-3.89 mmol/L (2.88 ± 0.47)
	75-150 mg/dl (111 ± 18)
Cortisol	36-81 nmol/L
Creatine kinase	2.4-23.4 IU/L (12.9 ± 5.2)
Creatine phosphokinase	119-287 IU/L
Creatinine*	106-168 μmol/L
	0.9-1.9 mg/dl; Quarter horses and newborn foals may be higher

REF VALUES

REFERENCE VALUES FOR NORMAL BLOOD CHEMISTRY *Continued*

Test	Normal Value
Fibrinogen*	2.94-11.8 µmol/L (7.65 ± 2.35)
	1-4 g/L (2.6 ± 0.8)
	100-400 mg/dl (260 ± 80)
Glucose*	4.1-6.4 mmol/L (5.30 ± 0.47)
	75-115 mg/dl (95.6 ± 8.5)
Glutamate dehydrogenase	0-11.8 IU/L (5.6 ± 4.2)
γ-Glutamyl transferase (GGT)	4-44 IU/L
Globulin, α_1*	7-17 g/L
Globulin, α_2*	7-17 g/L
Globulin, β*	8-16 g/L
Globulin, γ*	9-15 g/L
Hemoglobin*	110-190 g/L (144 ± 17)
Icterus index	5-20 IU
Insulin	10-30 µIU/mL (fasting level)
Iodine	394-946 nmol/L
	5-12 µg/dl
Iodine, protein bound	1.5-3.5 µg/dl
Iron	13.1-25.1 µmol/L (19.9 ± 1.97)
	73-140 µg/dl
Iron-binding capacity, total*	(59.1 ± 5.71) µmol/L
	270-390 µg/dl (330 ± 32)
Iron-binding capacity, unbound*	35.8-46.9 µmol/L (39.0 ± 3.78)
	200-262 µg/dl 218 ± 21
Isocitrate dehydrogenase	4.8-18 IU/L (10 ± 3.3)
Ketones, acetoacetate	(0.029 ± 0.003) mmol/L
Ketones, β-hydroxybutyric acid	(0.06 ± 0.006) mmol/L
	(0.67 ± 0.06) mg/dl
Lactate	1.11-1.78 mmol/L
	10-16 mg/dl
Lactate dehydrogenase (LDH)	162-412 IU/L (252 ± 63)
LDH-1	6.3%-18.5% (11.5 ± 4)
LDH-2	8.4%-20.5% (14.8 ± 3.2)
LDH-3	41%-65.9% (50.2 ± 7.2)
LDH-4	9.5%-20.9% (16.2 ± 3.8)
LDH-5	1.7%-16.5% (7.3 ± 4)
Lead	0.24-1.21 µmol/L
	5-25 µg/dl
Magnesium*	0.9-1.15 mmol/L, ionized 0.4-0.55
	2.2-2.8 mg/dl (2.5 ± 0.31)
Ornithine carbamoyltransferase (OCT)	(3.3 ± 4.2) IU/L
Osmolality	270-300 mOsm/kg
pH (venous and arterial)	7.32-7.44 (7.38 ± 0.03)
Phosphorus	3.1-5.6 mg/dl
Potassium	2.4-4.7 mmol or mEq/L (3.51 ± 0.57)
Protein (total)*	52-79 g/L (63.5 ± 5.9)
Albumin*	26-37 g/L (30.9 ± 2.8)
Globulins (total)*	26.2-40.4 g/L (33.3 ± 7.1)
α_1*	0.6-7 g/L (1.9 ± 2.6)
α_2*	3.1-13.1 g/L (6.5 ± 1.3)
β_1*	4-15.8 g/L (9.2 ± 3)
β_2*	2.9-8.9 g/L (5.7 ± 1.1)
γ*	5.5-19 g/L (10 ± 1.4)
Albumin/globulin ratio*	0.62-1.46 (0.96 ± 0.17)

Continued

REFERENCE VALUES FOR NORMAL BLOOD CHEMISTRY *Continued*

Test	Normal Value
Selenium	15-25 mg/dl
Sodium*	132-146 mmol or mEq/L (139 ± 3.5)
Sorbitol dehydrogenase* (SDH)	1.9-5.8 IU/L (3.5 ± 1.3)
Thyroxine (T_4)	11.6-36 mmol/L (0.024 ± 0.004)
	0.9-2.8 µg/dl (1.55 ± 0.27)
Triiodothyronine (T_3)	0.7-2.2 ng/mL
Urate	53.5-65.4 mmol/L
	0-1 mg/dl
Urea	3.57-8.57 mmol/L
Urea nitrogen*	10-24 mg/dl
Vitamin A	20-175 µg/dl (100)
Vitamin E (α-tocopherol)	>1.5 µg/mL

Data from Kaneko JJ et al: *Clinical biochemistry of domestic animals,* ed 5, San Diego, 1997, Academic Press.
Some values are affected by hemolysis.
Numbers in parentheses are mean value or mean ± SD.
Venous values normally only slightly higher than arterial.
*The values for these parameters are given for foals at various ages in subsequent tables.

REFERENCE VALUES FOR NORMAL URINE CHEMISTRY

	Adult	Foal
Allantoin, mg/kg per day	5-15	
Hydrogen ion, pH	7-8	5.5-8
Total nitrogen, mg/kg per day	100-600	
Specific gravity	1.020-1.050	1.001-1.027
Uric acid, mg/kg per day	1-2	
Urine volume, ml/kg per day	3-18	
Creatinine, mg/dl	156-232.5	26.5 ± 13.7
Osmolality, mOsm/kg	727-1456	101.7 ± 24
Alkaline phosphatase, IU/L	10.2 ± 4	2.4 ± 2
γ-Glutamyl transferase, IU/L	3.3-40.7	2.4 ± 2
Protein	Neg. to 30	Neg. to 30
Glucose	Neg.	Neg.
Crystal calcium carbonate	None	None
Casts	Neg.	Neg.
Hemoprotein	Neg. to +2	Neg. to +2
Bacteria	Neg.	Neg.
Epithelial cells	Squamous or caudate	Squamous or caudate
Red blood cells	Neg.	Neg.
White blood cells	3 per high power field	3 per high power field
Mucus	Neg. to abundant	Neg. to abundant

Data from Kaneko JJ et al: *Clinical biochemistry of domestic animals,* ed 5, San Diego, 1997, Academic Press.
Protein: Creatinine ratio <1.

REFERENCE VALUES FOR PLEURAL FLUID

Measurement	Observed Range	Comments
Red blood cell count, ×10⁹/L	22-540	<370 in 94% of horses
Total nucleated cell count, ×10⁹/L	0.8-12.1	<8 in 94% of horses
Differential cell count, ×10⁹/L		
Neutrophils	0.5-10.3	0.5-7.1 in 94% of horses
	32%-91%	
Lymphocytes	0 0.7	0%-10% in 94% of horses
	0%-22%	
Large mononuclear cells	0.1 2.6	
	5%-66%	
Eosinophils	0-0.2	No eosinophils found in 89% of horses, 0%-1% in 94% of horses
	0%-9%	
Specific gravity	1.008-4.7	<2.5 (25 g/L) in 83% of horses
Total protein, g/L	2-47	<34 in 94% of horses

BIOCHEMISTRY REFERENCE VALUES FOR PERITONEAL FLUID

	Blood	Peritoneal Fluid
Albumin, g/dl	1.7-3.9	0.3-1
Albumin, g/L	17-39	3-10
Globulin, g/dl	3.9-4.6	0.7-1.4
Globulin, g/L	39-46	7-14
Total protein, g/dl	4.7-8.9	0.1-2.8
Total protein, g/L	47 89	1-28
Amylase, IU/L (37°C)	14-35	0-14
Alkaline phosphatase IU/L	28-543	0-161
Aspartate aminotransferase, IU/L	133-459	25-213
Total bilirubin, mg/dl	0-5.3	0-1.2
Total bilirubin, μmol/L	0-90	0 20
Creatinine, mg/dl	1.5-1.8	1.8-2.7
Creatinine, μmol/L	130 160	160-240
γ-Glutamyl transferase, IU/L (37°C)	9-29	0-6
Glucose, mg/dl	45-167	74-203
Glucose, mmol/L	2.5-9.3	4.1-11.3
Inorganic phosphorus, mg/dl	0.6-6.8	1.2-7.4
Inorganic phosphorus, mmol/L	0.2-2.2	0.4-1.2
Lactate, mg/dl	6.3-15.3	3.6-10.8
Lactate, mmol/L	0.7-1.7	0.4-1.2
Lactate dehydrogenase, IU/L	151-590	0-355
Lipase, IU/L (37°C)	23-87	0-36
Urea (BUN), mg/dl	8.1-24.9	10.9-23.2
Urea (BUN), mmol/L	2.9-8.9	3.9-8.3

BUN, Blood urea nitrogen.

NORMAL HEMATOLOGIC VALUES

Hemoglobin concentration, g/dl	11-19
Packed cell volume	32%-53%
Red blood cells, ×10^9/µl	6.8-12.9
Mean corpuscular volume, fl	37-58.5
Mean corpuscular hemoglobin, pg	12.3-19.9
Mean corpuscular hemoglobin concentration, g/dl	31-38.6
Platelets, K/µl/10^3/µl	1-6
White blood cells, ×10^3/µl	5.4-14.3
Neutrophils, mature, ×10^3/µl	2.3-8.6 (22%-72%)
Neutrophils, band, /µl	0-100 (0%-8%)
Lymphocytes, ×10^3/µl	1.5-7.7 (17%-68%)
Neutrophil/lymphocyte ratio	0.8-2.8
Monocytes, /µl	0-1000 (0%-14%)
Eosinophils, /µl	0-1000 (0%-10%)
Basophils, /µl	0-290 (0%-4%)
Platelet count, ×10^3/µl	100-600
Plasma proteins, g/dl	5.8-8.7
Fibrinogen, mg/dl	100-400
Red blood cell diameter, µm	5-6

Data from Feldman BV, Zinkl JG, Jain NC: *Schalm's veterinary hematology,* ed 5, Philadelphia, 2000, Lippincott Williams & Wilkins.

CAUSE OF ALTERED LEUKOCYTE COUNTS

Condition	Etiology
NEUTROPHILIA	
Physiologic	Fear, excitement, brief but strenuous exercise
Corticosteroid-associated	Drugs, severe stress
Inflammation	Various causes
Infection	Bacterial, viral, fungal
Granulocytic leukemia	Very rare
NEUTROPENIA	
Defective neutrophil production in bone marrow	Drugs, bacterial bone marrow necrosis, myelophthisis, myelofibrosis, osteopetrosis, disseminated granulomatous inflammation, neoplasia, hereditary (Standardberds)
Excessive tissue demand for neutrophils (margination)	Septicemia/endotoxemia (salmonellosis, foal septicemia), severe bacterial infection, blister beetle toxicosis, cecal perforation, colic, chronic enteritis, monocytic ehrlichiosis (Potomac horse fever), phenylbutazone toxicity, immune-mediated neutropenia
LYMPHOCYTOSIS	
Physiologic	Especially high-strung light breeds
Chronic infection	Bacterial, viral
Postvaccination	
Lymphosarcoma/lymphocytic leukemia	Unusual to rare

CAUSE OF ALTERED LEUKOCYTE COUNTS *Continued*

Condition	Etiology
LYMPHOPENIA	
Corticosteroid-associated	Drugs, severe stress
Acute infection	Bacterial, viral
Combined immunodeficiency	Especially Arabian horses
MONOCYTOSIS	
Suppuration, tissue necrosis	
Hemolysis, hemorrhage	
Potomac horse fever	
Pyogranulomatous inflammation	
Nonhematopoietic neoplasia	
Monocytic/myelomonocytic leukemia	Very rare

From Cowell RL, Tyler RD: *Cytology and hematology of the horse,* ed 2, St Louis, 2002, Mosby.

REFERENCE VALUES FOR CELLULAR COMPOSITION OF BONE MARROW

Cell Type	Range (%)	Mean (%)
Myeloblasts	0-5	1
Promyelocytes	0.5-3.5	1.7
Neutrophilic myelocytes	1-7.5	3.2
Eosinophilic myelocytes	0-0.3	0.05
Neutrophilic metamyelocytes	1.1-15	5.6
Eosinophilic metamyelocytes	0-0.3	0.1
Basophilic metamyelocytes	0-0.3	0.08
Band neutrophils	6-26.5	15.7
Neutrophils	3 16.5	8.4
Eosinophils	0-5	1.8
Basophils	0-1.0	0.3
Total myeloid cells	26.5-45	35.7
Rubriblasts	0-2	0.7
Prorubricytes	1 0.5	3.6
Rubricytes	14.5-44	28.2
Metarubricytes	14 36	23.2
Total erythroid cells	47 69	58
Monocytes	0-1	0.2
Lymphocytes	1.5-8.5	3.8
Plasma cells	0 0.2	0.6
Megakaryocytes	0-1.0	0.3
Mitotic figures	0-3.5	8
Myeloid-erythroid ratio	0.48-0.91:1	0.71:1

Data from Feldman BV, Zinkl JG, Jain NC: *Schalm's veterinary hematology,* ed 5, Philadelphia, 2000, Lippincott Williams & Wilkins.

SERUM ELECTROLYTE CONCENTRATIONS IN FOALS (MEAN ± 2 SD)

Age	Na⁺ (mEq/L)	K⁺ (mEq/L)	Cl⁻ (mEq/L)	CO_2 (mEq/L)	HPO_{4-} (mg/dl)	Ca^{2+} (mg/dl)	Mg^{2+} (mg/dl)	Anion Gap (mEq/L)
HOURS								
<12	148 ± 15	4.4 ± 1	105 ± 12	25 ± 5	4.7 ± 1.6	12.8 ± 2	1.5 ± 0.8	21 ± 12
DAYS								
1	141 ± 18	4.6 ± 1	102 ± 12	27 ± 6	5.6 ± 1.8	11.7 ± 2	2.4 ± 1.8	16 ± 8
3	142 ± 19	4.8 ± 1.4	101 ± 11	28 ± 12	6.4 ± 2.6	12.1 ± 4.4	2.1 ± 0.9	23 ± 4
5							2.2 ± 2	
7	142 ± 12	4.8 ± 1.0	102 ± 8	28 ± 4	7.4 ± 2	12.5 ± 1.2	2 ± 0.6	17 ± 8
14	143 ± 8	4.6 ± 0.8	103 ± 6	26 ± 7	7.8 ± 1.8	12.4 ± 1.2	2.1 ± 1.1	18 ± 6
21	144 ± 8	4.6 ± 1.0	104 ± 11	27 ± 6	7.6 ± 0.8	12.3 ± 1	2.3 ± 3	18 ± 8
28	145 ± 9	4.6 ± 0.8	103 ± 6	27 ± 5	7.1 ± 2.2	12.2 ± 1.2	2 ± 1	19 ± 6
MONTHS								
2	148 ± 12	4.8 ± 1	105 ± 12	27 ± 5	7.4 ± 1.4	12.3 ± 0.6	2 ± 0.8	21 ± 10
3	148 ± 8	4.6 ± 1.2	106 ± 4	27 ± 3	7.3 ± 1	12.2 ± 1	2.2 ± 0.6	20 ± 8
4	147 ± 12	4.8 ± 1	105 ± 11	27 ± 4	6.7 ± 1.8	12.3 ± 1.6	2.4 ± 0.7	21 ± 8
5	145 ± 12	4.5 ± 1.4	107 ± 7	27.5 ± 5	6.3 ± 1.6	11.8 ± 1.4	2.4 ± 0.6	16 ± 10
6	143 ± 10	4.2 ± 1.4	105 ± 7	26 ± 4	6.2 ± 1.4	11.8 ± 1.6	2.4 ± 0.7	17 ± 8
9	143 ± 5	3.7 ± 1	102 ± 6	28 ± 4	6 ± 1.4	12 ± 1.2	2.3 ± 0.4	16 ± 8
12	146 ± 12	3.8 ± 1.6	104 ± 5	29 ± 2	6.0 ± 0.8	12.7 ± 1.4		17 ± 12
ADULTS	139 ± 8	4.2 ± 1	101 ± 6	26 ± 4	4.5 ± 1.4	12.0 ± 1.2	2.2 ± 0.6	18 ± 8

From Koterba AM, Drummond WH, Koseh PC: *Equine clinical neonatology*, Philadelphia, 1990, Lea & Febiger.

SERUM IRON AND RELATED PARAMETERS

Age	Iron (µg/dl)	UIBC (µg/dl)	TIBC (µg/dl)	Iron Saturation (%)	Ferritin (ng/ml)
HOURS					
<1	345-592	4-156	386-663	73-99	34-161
<12	262-488	10-133	339-535	69-98	
DAYS					
1	78-348	28-416	208-620	22-90	79-263
3	29-191	47-494	175-552	6-66	52-200
5	21-258	129-460	250-581	7-59	54-170
WEEKS					
1	30-273	35-503	222-619	10-72	57-173
2	22-215	168-643	337-706	4-52	21-136
3	46-241	228-669	408-745	7-46	27-117
MONTHS					
1	49-288	250-668	437-777	9-50	33-140
2	43-340	201-529	397-716	19-57	32-144
3	61-306	163-478	410-596	12-63	33-223
4	44-236	215-441	356-573	10-49	53-278
5	52-229	185-444	322-591	13-50	30 304
6	85-264	159-467	341-635	16-58	81-331
9	82-277	139-392	320-570	20-62	103-362
12	96-249	159-402	321-584	22 55	103-278
ADULT	74-209	177-379	305-542	21-48	58-365

From Koterba AM, Drummond WH, Koseh PC: *Equine clinical neonatology,* Philadelphia, 1990, Lea & Febiger.
UIBC, Unbound iron-binding capacity; *TIBC,* total iron-binding capacity.

NORMAL HEMATOLOGIC VALUES IN FOALS

Age	Total Plasma Protein (g/dl)	Fibrinogen (mg/dl)	Haptoglobin (mg/dl)	Icterus Index (units)	Platelets (× 10³/µl)
HOURS					
<1	4.4-5.9	100-500		20-100	
<12	5.1-7.6	100-350	8-120	15-50	105-446
DAYS					
1	5.2-8.0	100-400	0-136	10-75	129-409
3	5.3-7.9	150-500	8-162	10-50	105-353
5	5.4-7.6	100-500		15-50	
WEEKS					
1	5.2-7.5	150-450	0-143	5-25	111-387
2	5.2-7.2	150-600	0-202	5-25	133-457
3	5.2-6.8	150-600	11-184	5-20	134-442

Continued

REF VALUES

NORMAL HEMATOLOGIC VALUES IN FOALS *Continued*

Age	Total Plasma Protein (g/dl)	Fibrinogen (mg/dl)	Haptoglobin (mg/dl)	Icterus Index (units)	Platelets (× 10³/μl)
MONTHS					
1	5.1-7.1	200-700	0-214	5-20	136-468
2	5.2-6.8	150-650	15-214	5-25	152-456
3	5.5-7.1	100-800	23-187	5-25	200-376
4	5.9-7.5	250-800	53-182	5-20	140-388
5	6.1-7.3	300-800	32-198	5-20	132-376
6	5.9-7.1	200-550	0-125	5-20	128-368
9	5.6-6.8	200-550	16-127	5-20	105-337
12	5.4-7	200-550	0-179	5-20	120-316
ADULTS	6.2-8	100-600	19-177	5-20	100-350

From Koterba AM, Drummond WH, Koseh PC: *Equine clinical neonatology,* Philadelphia, 1990, Lea & Febiger.

RENAL FUNCTION

	2-4-Day-Old Foal	Adult
GFR (ml/kg per min)	2.3-2.8	1.5-2.2
ERPF (ml/kg per min)	15.2-18.2	12.1
FF (GFR/ERPF)	0.15	0.14-0.16

From Koterba AM, Drummond WH, Koseh PC: *Equine clinical neonatology,* Philadelphia, 1990, Lea & Febiger.
GFR, Glomerular filtration rate; *ERPF,* effective renal plasma flow; *FF,* filtration fraction.

SERUM ENZYME ACTIVITIES (RANGE, IU/L)

Age	ALP	GGT	SDH	AST*	ALT	CK*
HOURS						
<12	152-2835	13-39	0.2-4.8	97-315	0-47	65-380
DAYS						
1	861-2671	18-43	0.6-4.6	146-340	0-49	40-909
3	283-1462	9-40	0.6-3.7	80-580	0-52	21-97
5	156-1294	8-89	0.8-5.3			29-208
7	137-1169	14-164	0.8-8.2	237-620	4-50	52-143
14	182-859	16-169	0.6-4.3	240-540	1-9	46-208
21	146-752	16-132	1-8.4	226-540	0-45	44-210
28	210-866	17-99	1.2-5.9	252-440	5-47	81-585

SERUM ENZYME ACTIVITIES (RANGE, IU/L) *Continued*

Age	ALP	GGT	SDH	AST*	ALT	CK*
MONTHS						
2	201-747	8-38	1.1-4.6	282-484	7-57	50-170
3	206-458	0-27	1.1-3.9	282-480	8-65	57-204
4	124-222	0-27	1.5-4.4	280-520	8-65	60-266
5	105-239	0-30	1.3-4.8	225-420	0-65	60-125
6	155-226	0-26	0.3-3.3	300-620	7-20	97-396
9	158-232	0-26	0.3-3.3	246-728	4-27	97-396
ADULTS	64-214	5-28	0.5-3	149-267	4-10	69-272

From Koterba AM, Drummond WH, Koseh PC: *Equine clinical neonatology,* Philadelphia, 1990, Lea & Febiger.
ALP, Alkaline phosphatase; *GGT,* γ-glutamyl transferase; *SDH,* sorbitol dehydrogenase; *AST,* aspartate aminotransferase; *ALT,* alanine transaminase; *CK,* creatine kinase.
*Upper range may be considered abnormal.

LEUKOCYTE COUNTS (× 10^3/μl)

Age	Total Leukocytes	Neutrophils	Lymphocytes	Monocytes	Eosinophils	Basophils
HOURS						
<12	6.9-11.4	5.55-12.38	0.46-0.43	0.04-0.43	0	0-0.02
DAYS						
1	4.9-11.7	3.36-9.57	0.67-2.12	0.07-0.39	0-0.02	0-0.03
3	5.1-10.1	3.21-8.58	0.73-2.17	0.08-0.58	0-0.22	0-0.12
WEEKS						
1	6.3-13.6	4.35-10.55	1.43-2.28	0.03-0.54	0-0.09	0-0.18
2	5.2-11.9	3.99-9.08	1.32-3.12	0.07-0.58	0-0.10	0-0.1
3	5.4-12.4	3.16-8.94	1.47-3.26	0.06-0.69	0-0.16	0-0.09
MONTHS						
1	5.3-12.2	2.76-9.27	1.73-4.85	0.05-0.63	0-0.12	0-0.08
2	5.4-13.5	2.7-9.48	2.37-4.72	0.06-0.61	0-0.28	0-0.1
3	6.7-16.8	3.92-10.35	2.88-7.15	0.12-0.76	0-0.55	0-0.07
4	6.2-14.2	3.01-7.48	2.8-7.32	0.08-0.66	0-0.99	0-0.07
5	6.4-14.6	1.7-8.4	2.37-7.88	0.09-0.51	0-0.58	0-0.06
6	7.8-11.6	2.89-5.56	3.2-6.01	0.04-0.45	0-0.55	0-0.06
9	6.3-11.1	2.60-5.38	2.98-6.59	0.05-0.42	0-0.7	0-0.07
12	6.5-11.8	2.66-5.9	2.01-6.53	0.04-0.44	0-0.078	0-0.09
ADULTS	5.4-14.3	2.26-8.58	1.5-7.7	0-1	0-1	0-0.4

From Koterba AM, Drummond WH, Koseh PC: *Equine clinical neonatology,* Philadelphia, 1990, Lea & Febiger.

SERUM PROTEIN VALUES (g/dl)

Age	Total Protein*	Albumin	Total Globulin	Albumin:Globulin
HOURS				
<12	4-7.9	2.7-3.9	1.1-4.8	0.7-2.8
DAYS				
1	4.3-8.1	2.5-3.6	1.5-4.6	0.6-1.9
3	4.4-7.6	2.8-3.7	1.6-4.5	0.7-2.1
5				
7	4.4-6.8	2.7-3.4	2.7-3.4	0.7-1.8
14	4.8-6.7	2.6-3.3	2.6-3.3	0.7-1.7
21	4.7-6.5	2.6-3.2	2.6-3.2	0.8-1.8
28	5-6.7	2.7-3.4	2.7-3.4	0.8-1.5
MONTHS				
2	5.2-6.5	2.7-3.5	1.9-3.8	0.7-1.6
3	5.5-7.0	2.8-3.5	2.6-4.1	0.7-1.7
4	5.7-7.3	2.8-3.7	2.7-3.9	0.7-1.3
5	6-6.9	2.9-3.4	2.7-4	0.8-1.2
6	6-6.9	3-3.5	2.8-3.7	0.8-1.4
9	5.6-6.7	3-3.6	2.2-3.1	1-1.6
12	5.8-6.6	3.1-3.8	2.2-3.5	1-1.6
ADULTS	5.5-7.9	2.8-4.8	1.9-3.8	0.7-1.9

From Koterba AM, Drummond WH, Koseh PC: *Equine clinical neonatology,* Philadelphia, 1990, Lea & Febiger.
*Some values within these reported ranges may be considered abnormal.

ERYTHROCYTE VALUES

Age	PCV	Hb (g/dl)	RBC (x 10⁶/µl)	MCV (ff)	MCHC (g/dl)
HOURS					
<1*	40-52	13.4-19.9	9.3-12.9	37-45	33-39
<12†	37-49	12.6-17.4	9-12	36-45	32-40
DAYS					
1	32-46	12-16.6	8.2-11.0	36-46	32-40
3	30-46	11.5-16.7	7.8-11.4	35-44	34-40
5	30-44	11-16.6	7.2-11.6	35-45	34-40
WEEKS					
1	28-43	10.7-15.8	7.4-10.6	35-44	35-40
2	28-41	10.1-15.3	7.2-10.8	35-41	34-40
3	29-40	10.5-14.8	7.8-10.6	34-41	34-40

ERYTHROCYTE VALUES *Continued*

Age	PCV	Hb (g/dl)	RBC ($\times 10^6/\mu l$)	MCV (ff)	MCHC (g/dl)
MONTHS					
1	29-41	10.9-15.3	7.9-11.1	33-40	34-40
2	31-44	11.6-16	9.1-13.2	32-38	33-40
3	32-42	11.7-15.3	9.2-12.0	31-38	34-40
4	32-43	11.6-17.2	8.9-12.7	31-37	34-40
5	29-41	10.5-15.2	8.8-11.4	32-38	34-41
6	29-41	10.8-15.4	7.9-11.6	32-39	33-40
9	31-44	10.9-15.9	8-11.2	36-43	32-40
12	31-42	11-15.4	7.7-10.9	35-44	34-40
YEARS					
>4	31-47	11-18	5.9-9.9	41-51	33-41

From Koterba AM, Drummond WH, Koseh PC: *Equine clinical neonatology*, Philadelphia, 1990, Lea & Febiger.
PCV, Packed cell volume; *Hb,* hemoglobin; *RBC,* red blood cells; *MCV,* mean corpuscular volume; *ff,* free fraction; *MCHC,* mean corpuscular hemoglobin concentration.
*Before nursing.
†After nursing.

SERUM CHEMISTRY CONCENTRATIONIS: SMALL ORGANIC MOLECULES (RANGE, mg/dl)

Age	Glucose	BUN	Creatinine	TBR	CJBR	UNCJBR	Cholesterol	Triglycerides
HOURS								
<12	108-190	12-27	1.7-4.2	0.9-2.8	0.3-0.6	0.8-2.5	111-432	24-88
DAYS								
1	121-233	9-40	1.2-4.3	1.3-4.5	0.3-0.7	1-3.8	110-562	30-193
3	101-226	2-29	0.4-2.1	0.5-1.2	0.2-0.8	0.2-3.3	142-350	63-342
5				1.2-3.6	0.1-0.7	0.8-2.8	127-361	52-340
7	121-192	4-20	1-1.7	0.8-3	0.3-0.7	0.5-2.3	139-445	30-239
14	137-205	6-13	0.9-1.8	0.7-2.2	0.3-0.6	0.5-1.6	164-287	39-200
21	130-240	6-14	0.6-2	0.5-1.6	0.2-0.5	0.2-1.1	74-276	34-124
28	130-216	6-21	1.1-1.8	0.5-1.7	0.1-0.6	0.4-1.2	83-233	45-155
MONTHS								
2	119-204	6-11	1.1-1.2	0.5-2	0.2-0.5	0.3-1.5	98-242	10-148
3	88-179	7-20	0.7-2.2	0.4-2	0.1-0.7	0.4-1.4	110-226	28-151
4	113-196	9-25	1.3-2.1	0.3-1	0.1-0.6	0.2-0.4	91-207	14-148
5	95-210	11-33	1.2-2.1	0.3-1.8	0.1-0.7	0.1-1.1	51-137	14-57
6	110-210	15-30	1.2-2.1	0.3-1.3	0.1-0.7	0.1-0.6	83-173	35-76
9	104-207	16-26	1.1-2.2	0.3-1.1	0.1-0.7	0.2-0.6	11-187	38-86
12	105-165	15-24	1.3-2.1	0.4-1.4	0.1-1.0	0.2-0.6		
ADULTS	57-96	12-24	0.9-2	0.5-1.8	0.2-0.7*	0.3-1	58-109	6-44

From Koterba AM, Drummond WH, Koseh PC: *Equine clinical neonatology*, Philadelphia, 1990, Lea & Febiger.
BUN, Blood urea nitrogen; *TBR*, total bilirubin; *CJBR*, conjugated bilirubin, *UNCJBR*, unconjugated bilirubin.
*Higher than most texts report.

Worming Schedules

WORMING SCHEDULE

Class	Generic Name	Trade Name	Source	Route of Administration	Dosage
Avermectins	Ivermectin	Eqvalan	Merial	Liquid, paste	200 µg/kg
		Zimectrin	Farnam	Paste	
		Rotectin	TRC Animal Health	Paste	
	Moxidectin	Quest	Fort Dodge Animal Health	Paste	0.4 mg/kg; *do not use in young foals!*
Benzimidazoles	Fenbendazole (FBZ)	Panacur	Hoechst	Liquid, feed, paste	5-10 mg/kg
		Safeguard	Hoechst	Paste	
	Mebendazole (MBZ)	Telmin	Mallinckrodt	Tube, feed, paste	1 g/125 kg
	MBZ + TCF	Telmin B	Mallinckrodt	Liquid, feed, paste	
	Oxfendazole (OFZ)	Benzelmin	Syntex/Roche	Liquid, feed, paste	10 mg/kg
	OFZ + TCF	Benzelmin Plus	Syntex/Roche	Liquid, paste	
	Oxibendazole (OBZ)	Anthelcide EQ	Pfizer Animal Health	Liquid, feed, paste	10-15 mg/kg
		Equipar	Coopers	Liquid, paste	
	Thiabendazole (TBZ)	Equizole	Merial	Liquid	
	TBZ + PIP	Equizole-A	Merial	Liquid	
Phenylguanidines	Febantel (FBT)	Rintal	Bayer	Liquid, feed, paste	6 mg/kg
		Cutter horse dewormer	Cutter	Paste	
	FBT + TCF	Combotel	Bayer	Paste	
Organophosphates	Dichlorvos (DDVP)*	Equiguard	Squibb	Feed	20 mg/kg
	Trichlorfon (TCF)*	Combotel	Bayer	Liquid, paste	
Piperazines	Piperazine (PPZ)	Several	Several	Liquid	1 oz (30 ml)/45 kg
	PPZ + PTZ + TCF*	Dyrex TF	Ft. Dodge	Tube formula	
Pyrimidines	Pyrantel (PRT)	Strongid T	Pfizer	Liquid	6.6 mg/kg†
		Strongid paste	Pfizer	Paste	
		Strongid C	Pfizer	Feed	

WORMING

WORMING SCHEDULE—*cont'd.*

Class	Generic Name	Trade Name	Source	Route of Administration	Dosage
Other	Phenothiazine (PTZ)*	Several	Several	Feed	
	Carbon disulfide (CDS)*	Several	Several	Tube	
	Imidocarb*	Imizol	Coopers	Injection	

From Smith BP: *Large animal internal medicine,* ed 2, St. Louis, 1996, Mosby.

*No longer available in the United States.

†Double or triple dose used for tapeworms.

Praziquantel 0.5-1 mg/kg has been used and proved efficacious against Anoplocephala perfoliata in the horse but is currently not approved for use in the horse.

ANTHELMINTIC ACTIVITY ACCORDING TO CLASS OF DRUG

Class	Large Strongles[†]	Small Strongles[†]	Ascarids	Pinworms	Gasterophilus Organisms (Bots)
Avermectins*	X	X	X	X	X
Benzimidazoles	X	X	X	X	
Phenylguanidines	X	X	X	X	
Organophosphates					
Dichlorvos			X		X
Trichlorfon			X	X	X
Piperazines		X	X	X	
Pyrimidines	X	X	X	X	
Phenothiazines	X	X		X	
Carbon disulfide			X		X

From Smith BP: *Large animal internal medicine,* ed 3, St. Louis, 2002, Mosby.
*Also eliminates threadworms, cutaneous onchocerciasis, and summer sores.
[†]Efficacy variable depending on specific drug used, dose, and parasitic stage.

SAMPLE ANTHELMINTIC PROGRAMS FOR FOALS 8 WEEKS OR OLDER

Month	Program A	Program B
March/April	Anthelcide EQ	Equizole A
May/June	Eqvalan	Eqvalan
July/August	Rintal	Panacur
September/October	Strongid T paste	Strongid T paste
November/December	Eqvalan, Benzelmin Plus, or Telmin B	Eqvalan, Benzelmin Plus, or Telmin B

From Koterba AM, Drummond WH, Koseh PC: *Equine clinical neonatology,* Philadelphia, 1990, Lea & Febiger.

SAMPLE ANTHELMINTIC PROGRAMS FOR OLDER HORSES

Month	Program A	Program B	Program C
February	Equizole, Panacur, Telmin, or Rintal (alone or with piperazine or trichlorfon)	None	None
April	Eqvalan	Eqvalan	Eqvalan
June	Equiguard	Equizole A or Anthelcide EQ	None
August	Anthelcide EQ	Strongid T paste (double dose)	None
October	Strongid T paste (double dose)	None	None
December	Eqvalan, Equiguard, Telmin B, or Quest	Eqvalan, Equiguard, Dyrex TF, Telmin B, Combotel, or Quest	Eqvalan, Dyrex TF, Telmin B, Combotel, or Quest

From Smith BP: *Large animal internal medicine,* ed 3. St. Louis, 2002, Mosby.
Do not treat mares within 1 month of foaling.

Immunization Schedules

SUGGESTED IMMUNIZATION SCHEDULE FOR HORSES*

Disease	Etiologic Agent	Foals and Weanlings	Yearlings	Performance Horses	Pleasure Horses	Brood Mares	Comments
Anthrax	*Bacillus anthracis*	2 doses, 2-3 wk apart	Annual	Annual	Annual	Annual	Immunize 4 wks before potential exposure. Placing a horse in a dark stall for 10 days may be beneficial. Local reactions may occur. Do not administer antibiotics within 1 wk of immunization. **Not used in United States.**
Botulism	*Clostridium botulinum* type B toxin	3-dose series at 30-d intervals. Age at first injection dependent on local factors	Annual	Annual	Annual	Annual; 4 wk prepartum	Only in endemic areas or if travel to endemic area is planned.
Encephalomyelitis	EEE, WEE West Nile	First dose, 3-4 mo; second dose, 4-5 mo	Annual, in spring	Annual, in spring	Annual, in spring	Annual; 4-6 wk prepartum	In endemic areas, booster every 6 mo.
Encephalomyelitis	VEE	First dose 3-4 mo; second dose, 4-5 mo	Annual, in spring	Annual, in spring	Annual, in spring	Annual; 4-6 wk prepartum	Needed only when threat of an outbreak exists. This antigen is only available as a combination vaccine with EEE and WEE.

SUGGESTED IMMUNIZATION SCHEDULE FOR HORSES*—cont'd.

Disease	Etiologic Agent	Foals and Weanlings	Yearlings	Performance Horses	Pleasure Horses	Brood Mares	Comments
Equine influenza	Equine influenza A-equine-1 and A-equine-2	First dose, 3-6 mo; second dose, 4-7 mo; third dose, 5-8 mo. Repeat at 3-mo intervals	Every 3 mo	Every 3 mo	Annual with added boosters before likely exposure	At least biannual; with 1 booster 4-6 wk prepartum	A series of at least 3 doses is recommended for primary immunization of foals. Immunization response might not be seen in foals younger than 7 mo.
Equine viral arteritis	Equine arteritis virus					Annual; immunize mares to be bred to a positive stallion at least 3 wk before breeding. Pregnant mares should not be immunized the last 2 mo of gestation	Immunization of stallions at least 3 wk before breeding season is occasionally performed. Authorization by state veterinarian is required. Permit may be necessary. Regulations vary with state. Immunized horses may be ineligible for export because of seroconversion.

Continued

SUGGESTED IMMUNIZATION SCHEDULE FOR HORSES*—cont'd.

Disease	Etiologic Agent	Foals and Weanlings	Yearlings	Performance Horses	Pleasure Horses	Brood Mares	Comments
Potomac horse fever	*Neorickettsia risticii*	First dose, 3-4 mo; second dose, 4-5 mo	Biannual	Biannual	Biannual	Biannual with 1 dose 4-6 wk prepartum	Booster during May to June in endemic areas.
Rabies	Rabies virus	First dose, 3-6 mo; second dose, 6-7 mo	Annual	Annual	Annual	Annual; before breeding	Rabies immunization recommended in endemic areas.
Rhinopneumonitis	Equine herpesvirus type I (EHV-1) and type IV	First dose, 2-3 mo; second dose, 3-4 mo; third dose, 4-5 mo. Repeat at 3-mo intervals	Every 3 mo	Every 3 mo	Optional; biannual if deemed necessary	5th, 7th, 9th months of gestation (inactivated EHV-1 vaccine). Immunize mares before breeding and 4-6 wk prepartum	If primary series is started before 3 mo of age, a 3-dose primary series is preferred.
Strangles	*Streptococcus equi*	First dose, 8-12 wk; second dose, 11-15 wk; third dose, 14-18 wk	Biannual	Optional; biannual if risk is high	Optional; biannual if risk is high	Biannual, with 1 dose 4-6 wk prepartum	Vaccines containing M-protein extract may be less reactive than whole-cell vaccines. Can be used when endemic conditions exist or risk is high. Efficacy of

SUGGESTED IMMUNIZATION SCHEDULE FOR HORSES*—cont'd.

Disease	Etiologic Agent	Foals and Weanlings	Yearlings	Performance Horses	Pleasure Horses	Brood Mares	Comments
		(depending on product); fourth dose, weaning (6-8 mo)					vaccination with the intranasal vaccine in the face of an outbreak unproved but commonly used.
Tetanus	Clostridium tetani	First dose, before 3-4 mo; second dose, 4-5 mo	Annual	Annual	Annual	Annual; 4-6 wk prepartum	Booster at time of penetrating injury or surgery if last dose not administered within the last 6 mo.

Modified from Smith BP: *Large animal internal medicine*, ed 3, St. Louis, 2002, Mosby.

As with administration of all medications, read the label and product insert before administering any vaccine. Stallion schedules should be consistent with the immunization program of the adult population or the farm and modified according to risk.

EEE, Eastern equine encephalomyelitis virus; *WEE*, western equine encephalomyelitis virus; *VEE*, Venezuelan equine encephalomyelitis virus.

*Varies between regions and farms.

Product Manufacturers

PRODUCT MANUFACTURERS

Manufacturer	Address	Phone	Toll-Free Phone	Fax	Website	Products*
Abbott Laboratories	1401 Sheridan Road, North Chicago, IL 60064	(847) 937-6100	(800) 323-9100	(847) 938-0659	www.abbott.com	Extension set (7- or 30-in), Abbocath-T radiopaque FEP Teflon IV catheter (14 gauge, 2 in long)
Air Vet (Bivona)	5425 Raines Road, Suite 3, Memphis, TN 38115		(800) 343-6237		www.bivona.com	Silicone-cuffed endotracheal tubes (sizes 7, 9, 10, 12 mm, 55 cm long)
A.J. Buck and Son	See Buck					
Allegiance Health Care	100 Raritan Center Parkway Edison, NJ 08837		(800) 964-5227	(732) 417-4532	www.cardinal.com	Rayport muscle biopsy clamp
Allied Health	St. Louis, MO		(800) 444-3960			LSPO2 Regulator 270-020; LSP demand valve (with 6-ft [1.8-m] hose and female DISS fitting) 063-03
Arrow International, Inc.	P.O. Box 12888, 3000 Bernville Road, Reading, PA 19612	(610) 378-0131	(800) 523-8446	(800) 343-2935	www.arrowintl.com	Central venous catheter (16-gauge, 8-in)
Ayerst Laboratories	See Wyeth Pharmaceuticals					
Baker Cummins Dermatologicals	8800 N.W. 36th Street, Miami, FL 33178-2403	(305) 590-2200	(800) 347-4474			Baker's biopsy punch
C.R. Bard	8195 Industrial Boulevard, Covington, GA 30014	(770) 385-2300	(800) 526-4455	(770) 385-2310	www.crbard.com	Bard Monopty biopsy instrument
Bausch & Lomb Surgical	St. Louis, MO 63122				www.endoscopia.com	Dow-Corning Silastic tubing

Continued

831

PRODUCT MANUFACTURERS—cont'd.

Manufacturer	Address	Phone	Toll-Free Phone	Fax	Website	Products
Baxter Healthcare Corp.	One Baxter Parkway, Deerfield, IL 60015	(847) 948-2000	(800) 422-9837	(847) 948-3642	www.baxter.com	Jamshidi disposable bone marrow biopsy/ aspiration needle, Tru-Cut biopsy needle, 6 French Fogarty venous thrombectomy catheter
Baxter Healthcare Corp., Pharmaseal Division	1919-T South Butterfield Road, Mundelein, IL 60060 or Valencia CA 91355-8900			(201) 847-6475		Pharmaseal K75 3-way stopcock
Bayer Corporation, Agriculture Division, Animal Health	P.O. Box 390, Shawnee Mission, KS 66201		(800) 633-3796	(800) 344-4219	www.bayer.com	Pharmaceuticals
Becton-Dickinson	1 Becton Drive, Franklin Lakes, NJ 07417	(201) 847-6800			www.bd.com	Spinal needles; Culturette collection and transport system, Port-a Cul; Vacutainer needles, Vacutainer cuffs, Vacutainer blood tubes
Bivona	5700 West 23rd Avenue, Gary, IN 46406	(219) 989-9150	(800) 348-6064	(219) 898-7435	www.bivona.com	Cuffed silicon nasogastric tube, 7B 10-mm diameter, 55 cm long, uterine flush tubes
Boehringer Mannheim	St. Joseph, MO 64506		(800) 325-9176			Pharmaceuticals

PRODUCT MANUFACTURERS—cont'd.

Manufacturer	Address	Phone	Toll-Free Phone	Fax	Website	Products
Breathing Services	P.O. Box 817, 931 East Main Street, Ephrata, PA 17522	(800) 732-0028				Flowmeter/humidifier, Hudson model 5040 demand valve, adult human Ambu bag, PMR-2 manual resuscitator (self-inflating bag with accumulator)
A.J. Buck and Son	11407 Cronhill Drive, Owings Mills, MD 21117	(410) 531-1800	(800) 638-8672	(410) 581-1809	www.ajbuck.com	Jacobs chuck Pharmaceuticals
Burrow Medical, Inc.	824 Twelfth Avenue, Bethlehem, PA 18018	(800) 353-2439				Accu-Bloc Periflex, 18-gauge polyethylene epidural catheter
Butler Company	5000 Bradenton Avenue, Dublin, OH 43017-0753	(614) 751-9095		(614) 761-1045	www.wabutler.com	Ideal udder infusion cannula
CDA Products	P.O. Box 53. Potter Valley, CA 95461	(707) 431-1300		(707) 443-2530		Anderson sling
Cook Veterinary Products	P.O. Box 489, Bloomington, IN 47402	(812) 339-2235	(800) 457-4500	(800) 554-8335	www.cookgroup.com	Silicone cuffed endotracheal tubes (sizes 7, 9, 10, 12 mm, 55 cm long)
Critikon	5820 West Cypress, Suite B, Tampa, FL 35634	(813) 887-2000				Noninvasive blood pressure monitor
Datascope Corporation	580 Winters Avenue, Paramus, NJ 07632	(888) 949-9917	(800) 777-4222		www.datascope.com	Noninvasive blood pressure monitor, electrocardiogram
Davol Inc.	100 Sockanosset Crossroad, Cranston, RI 02920	(401) 463-7000		(401) 946-5379	www.davol.com	Intranasal oxygen tubing (16F Levin, 127-cm tubing)

Continued

PRODUCT MANUFACTURERS—cont'd.

Manufacturer	Address	Phone	Toll-free Phone	Fax	Website	Products
Deseret Medical	Becton-Dickinson and Co., Sandy, UT 84070					Intracath intravenous catheter placement unit
Edwards Lifesciences	1 Edward Way Irvine, CA 92614		(800) 424-3278			
Fort Dodge Animal Health	800 5th Street N.W., P.O. Box 518, Fort Dodge, IA 50501	(515) 955-4600		(515) 955-3730	www.fortdodge.com	Pharmaceuticals
Hartford Veterinary Supply	9100 Persimmon Tree Road, Potomac, MD 20854					Double-guarded uterine swab
Heska Corporation	1613 Prospect Parkway, Fort Collins, CO 80525	(970) 493-7272	(800) GO HESKA	(970) 472-1640	www.heska.com	NEEd PROduct
High Horse	Reno, NV 72851-1217					Velcro foam leg wraps, Velcro foam helmet
Howmedica	359 Veterans Boulevard, Rutherford, NJ 07070				www.howmedica.com	Surgical Simplex PMMA (polymethyl-methacrylate)
IMED Corporation	9775 Businesspark Avenue, San Diego, CA 92131-1192		(800) 854-2003			IV pumps (Gemini PC-1)
Immvac	6080 Bass Lane, Columbia, MO 65201	(573) 443-5363	(800) 944-7563	(573) 874-7108	www.immvac.com	Endoserum
IDEXX Blue Ridge Pharmaceutical	One IDEXX Drive, Westbrook, MA 04092	(207) 856-8601				Snap IgG Test
International Win, Ltd.	340 North Mill Road, Suite 6, Kennett Square, PA 19348-2853	(610) 444-0170	(800) 359-4946	(610) 444-0171	www.internationalwin.com	Large animal extension set (large-bore, 7 in), Stat large animal IV set (large-bore, 10 ft long)
J.A. Webster (see Webster)						

PRODUCT MANUFACTURERS—cont'd.

Manufacturer	Address	Phone	Toll-Free Phone	Fax	Website	Products
Johnson & Johnson Medical	Arlington, TX 76004-3-30				www.johnsonandjohnscn.com	Elasticon, K-Y lubricating jelly
Jorgensen Laboratories	1450 North Van Buren Avenue, Loveland CO. 80538	(970) 669-2500	(800) 525-5614	(970) 633-5042	www.jorvet.com	Jackson uterine biopsy forceps, tracheotomy tube (18- or 28-mm internal diameter), metal bitch urinary catheter
Karl Storz Veterinary Endoscopy-America	175 Cremona Drive, Goleta, CA 93117	(805) 967-7776	(800) 955-7832	(805) 685-2588	www.karlstorz.com	Flexible fiberoptic endoscopes: 11-mm outer diameter, 100 cm long; 12-mm outer diameter, 160 cm long; 8-mm outer diameter, 150 cm long
Laerdal Medical Corporation	P.O. Box 1037, Riverview, FL 33568-1037	(813) 677-3124		(813) 671-0772	www.laerdal.com	Laerdal silicone resuscitator (adult size, 1600 ml; with oxygen reservoir bag, 2600 ml), compact suction unit
Lake Immungenics	348 Beg Road, Ontario, NY 14519	(716) 265-1973	(800) 648-9990	(716) 265-2306	www.lakeimmunogenics.com	Plasma products
Mallinckrodt	675 McDonnell Boulevard, Hazelwood, MO 63042	(314) 654-2000	(888) 744-1414		www.mallinckrodt.com	Bubble jet humidifier
Merial Limited	3239 Satelite Boulevard, Duluth, GA 30096	(888) 637-4251	(800) MERIAL1		www.merial.com	Pharmaceuticals

Continued

835

PRODUCT MANUFACTURERS—cont'd.

Manufacturer	Address	Phone	Toll-Free Phone	Fax	Website	Products
Mg Biologics	1721 Y Ave, Ames, IA 50014	(515) 769-2340		(515) 769-2390		Equine plasma
Mila International	7604 Dixie Highway, Florence, KY 41042	(859) 371-1722	(888) MILA-INT	(859) 371-4792	www.milaint.com	Milacath polyurethane catheter (14- or 16-gauge, 8-in); single and double lumen styles available, endoscopic microbiology aspiration catheter, subpalpebral eye lavage kit
Mill-Rose Labs	7310 Corporate Boulevard, Mentor, OH 44060	(216) 255-7995	(800) 321-1380	(440) 255-5061	www.mrlabsinc.com	Darien microbiological aspiration catheter
Olympus America	2 Corporate Center Drive, Melville, NY 11747	(516) 844-5000	(800) 645-8160		www.olympusamerica.com	Flexible videoendoscopes: GIF 130 gastroscope (9.8-mm outer diameter, 200 or 300 cm long), SIF 100 (11.2-mm outer diameter, 300 cm long), CF 100 TL (12.9-mm outer diameter, 200 or 300 cm long)
Pall Biomedical Products Corporation	77 Crescent Beach Road, Glen Cove, NY 11542	(516) 759-1900	(800) 645-6578			HME filter (heat-moisture exchange filter)

PRODUCT MANUFACTURERS—cont'd.

Manufacturer	Address	Phone	Toll-Free Phone	Fax	Website	Products
Pfizer, North America Region, Animal Health Group	235 East 42nd Street New York, NY 10017	(610) 363-3100	(800) 733-5530	(888) 596-4469	www.pfizer.com/ah	Pharmaceuticals
Pharmacia Animal Health	7000 Portage Road, Kalamazoo, MI 49001	(616) 833-4000		(616) 833-4077	www. pnuanimalhealth. com	Pharmaceuticals
Physiocontrol Corporation (Medtronic) Puritan Bennett Corporation	P.O. Box 97006, Redmond, WA 98073-9706 See Mallinckrodt	(425) 867-4000	(800) 442-1142		www.medtronic physiocontrol.com	Defibrillator with ECG (Life Pak-10)
Roche Diagnostic Systems	P.O. Box 50457, Indianapolis, IN 46256	(317) 521-2000		(317) 521-2090	www.roche.com	Septi-Check, BB blood culture bottle; Dexatrometer (ACCU-CHEK III- Chemstrip bG)
Rusch Inc.	2450 Meadowbrook Parkway, Duluth, GA 30096	(770) 623-0816	(800) 553-5324	(770) 623-1829	www.ruschinc.com	Nasal catheter Levin tubes 235200-160; silicone-cuffed endotracheal tubes 7, 9, 10, 12 mm, 55 cm long
Safe and Warm	Boulder City, NV 89005		(800) 421-3237			Intratherm (warm IV fluid pouch); Safe and Warm reusable instant heat, 7 in, 9 in
Schein Pharmaceutical	100 Campus Drive, Florham Park, NJ 07932	(973) 593-5500	(800) 356-5790	(973) 593-5500	www.schein-rx.com	Progesterone injection USP

Continued

PRODUCT MANUFACTURERS—cont'd.

Manufacturer	Address	Phone	Toll-Free Phone	Fax	Website	Products
Schering-Plough Animal Health Corporation	1095 Morris Avenue, Union, NJ 07083	(908) 629-3490	(800) 648-2118	(908) 629-3306	www.sp-animalhealth.com	
Sherwood Medical	1915 Olive Street, St. Louis, MO 63103		(800) 428-4400			Monoject 60-ml syringe with catheter tip, polypropylene catheter, feline indwelling catheter (20 gauge)
StatPal II-PPG Industries	11077 Torrey Pines Road, La Jolla, CA 92037		(800) 369-3457			Blood gas analyzer
Synthes (USA)	P.O. Box 1766, 1690 Russell Road, Paoli, PA 19301-0800		(800) 523-0322		www.synthes.com	Steinmann pin (2.5, 3.2, 4.5, 6.34 mm)
Thomas Register of American Manufacturers	5 Penn Plaza, New York, NY 10001	(212) 290-7277	(800) 222-7900		www.thomasregister.com	Information on every manufacturer in the United States
Upjohn	See Pharmacia Animal Health					
Veterinary Dynamics	1535 Templeton Road, Templeton, CA 93465		(800) 654-9743	(805) 434-3840	www.thegrid.net/vdi/	Equine plasma
VWR Scientific	200 Center Square Road, Bridgeport, NJ 08014	(856) 467-2600	(800) 932-5000	(856) 467-5499	www.vwrsp.com	Oxygen line (clear vinyl tubing $\frac{3}{8}$-in ID, $\frac{1}{2}$-in OD, $\frac{1}{16}$-in thick
J.A. Webster	86 Leominster Road, Sterling, MA 01564	(978) 422-8211	(800) 225-7911	(978) 422-8959	www.jawebster.com	400-ml nylon dose syringe
Wedgewood Pharmacy	279-C Egg Harbor Road, Sewell, NJ 08080		(800) 331-8272	(800) 589-4250	www.wedgewoodpharmacy.com	Compounded prescription medications

PRODUCT MANUFACTURERS—cont'd.

Manufacturer	Address	Phone	Toll-Free Phone	Fax	Website	Products
Wyeth Pharmaceuticals	555 E. Lancaster Avenue, St. Davids, PA 19087	(610) 971-1200		(610) 688-9498	www.wyeth.com	Fluor-I-Strip (fluorescein sodium ophthalmic strip)

*Each company may make and/or distribute additional products. Those listed are ones used by at least one of the contributors to the manual.

Breed Chart

BREED CHART

Breed	Association	Address	Phone/Fax	Description
American Albino	International American Albino Association	Route 1, Box 20, Naper, NE 68755-2020	(402) 832-5560	Includes two colors: American White and American Cream. Both must have pink skin.
American Paint Horse	American Paint Horse Association	P.O. Box 961023, Fort Worth, TX 76161-0023	(817) 834-APHA; (Fax) (817) 834-3152	The American Paint Horse has a unique combination of white and any one of the colors of the equine rainbow.
Andalusian	International Andalusian Horse Association	1201 S. Main, #D-7, Boerne, TX 78006	(512) 249-4027	Of Spanish descent and usually white, gray, or bay. Stands approximately 15.2 hands.
Appaloosa	Appaloosa Horse Club	2720 W. Pullman Road, Moscow, ID 83843	(208) 882-5578; (Fax) (208) 882-8150	Noted for its spotted coat, the Appaloosa usually stands approximately 15.2 hands with a sparse mane and tail.
Arabian	International Arabian Horse Association	10805 E. Bethany Drive, Aurora, CC 80014	(303) 696-4500; (Fax) (303) 696-4599	Typical characteristics include a dished profile, prominent eyes, large nostrils, small, teacup muzzle, and a short, strong back.
Australian Stock Horse (Waler)	Australian Stock Horse Society	P.O. Box 288, 92 Kelly Street, Scone, NSW 2337, Australia	065/45-1122; (Fax) 065/45-2165	Developed from Thoroughbreds, Arabians, Welsh Ponies, and some Spanish stock, this breed is very versatile and used for a variety of disciplines.
Belgian	Belgian Draft Horse Corporation of America	P.O. Box 335, Wabash, IN 46992-0035	(219) 563-3205	Native to Belgium. A heavy, powerful, drafty breed. Usually stands between 16 and 17 hands.

Continued

BREED CHART—*cont'd.*

Breed	Association	Address	Phone/Fax	Description
Buckskin	American Buckskin Registry Association International Buckskin Horse Association	P.O. Box 3850, Redding, CA 96049-3850 P.O. Box 268, Shelby, IN 46377	(530) 223-1420; (Fax) (530) 223-1420 (219) 552-1013	A color designation for horses with tan or light brown coats.
Camargue	Association des Eleveurs de Chevaux de Race Camargue	Mas du Pont de Roustry, 13200 Arles, France	33 (0) 4 90 97 86 32; (Fax) 33 (0) 4 90 97 70 82	Hardy breed native to the marshy Camargue region of France. Stands between 13 and 14 hands.
Canadian Horse	Canadian Horse Breeders Association (Societe des Eleveurs de Chevaux Canadians)	200 Rang St-Joseph est, St-Alban, QC, G0A 3B0, Canada	(418) 268-3443; (Fax) (418) 268-3599	Rare breed. All-around riding and driving horse. Usually black, bay, or chestnut; 14-16 hands.
Carpathian Pony (Hucul)	Ministry of Agriculture of the Slovak Republic	Dobrovicova 12, 81266 Bratislava, Slovak Republic		Descended from Tarpan and Mongolian horses. Most common colors are bay, black, grullo, and chestnut.
Chincoteague Pony	National Chincoteague Pony Association	Gale Park Frederick, 2595 Jenson Road, Bellingham, WA 98226	(360) 671-8338	Small, hardy, and compact. These wild ponies live on the islands of Chincoteague and Assateague off the coast of Virginia and Maryland.
Cleveland Bay	Cleveland Bay Horse Society of North America	P.O. Box 221, South Windham, CT 06266		"The English Warmblood." This is the oldest established breed of English horse. Noted for intelligence, temperament, strength, stamina, and longevity.
Clydesdale	Clydesdale Breeders of the USA	17378 Kelly Road, Pecatonica, IL 61063	(815) 247-8780	A breed of heavy draft horse originating in Scotland. Most stand 16.2 to 18 hands and weigh 1600-1800 lb (726-816 kg).

BREED CHART—cont'd.

Breed	Association	Phone/Fax	Description
Comtois	Syndicat d'elevage du Cheval Comtois	33 (0) 3 81 52 46 97; (Fax) 33 (0) 3 81 41 01 00	Bred in the French province of Franche-Comte and the Jura Mountains. Heavy draft breed used for hauling wood.
Connemara Pony	American Connemara Pony Society	(540) 722-2277	Native of Ireland. Usually 13-14.2 hands; sturdy, general purpose riding pony.
Dartmoor Pony	American Dartmoor Pony Association		Sensible and surefooted, with a reputation as a naturally good jumper. Native to Britain. 12.2-hand height limit.
Donkey	American Donkey and Mule Society	(940) 382-6845; (Fax) (940) 484-8417	
Dutch Warmblood	North America Department, Royal Warmblood Studbook of the Netherlands	(541) 459-3232; (Fax) (541) 459-2967	
Exmoor Pony	American Exmoor Pony Registry	(919) 542-5704	An exceptionally tough, strong pony noted for its endurance. Highly intelligent and independent. The height limit is 12.2 hands for mares and 12.3 hands for stallions. No white markings permitted.
Fell Pony	Fell Pony Society	(Phone, Fax) 01768-891001	Large British pony bred in northern England and descended from the Frisians and the Galloway ponies. Generally stands 13-14 hands. Good riding and driving ponies.

Continued

843

BREED CHART—*cont'd.*

Breed	Association	Address	Phone/Fax	Description
Finnish Horse		Suomen Hippos, Tulkinkuja 3, SF-02600 Espoo, Finland	358 9 5 11 002 50	Only native Finnish breed. Used for riding, driving, and hauling heavy loads. Usually 14.2-15.3 hands. Many are chestnut, with flaxen mane and tail.
Frisian	Frisian Horse Association of North America	P.O. Box 11217, Lexington, KY 40574-1217		One of Europe's oldest breeds. Relatively small in stature, standing approximately 15 hands. The color is exclusively black with no white markings.
Genderland	KWPN (Royal Warmblood Studbook of the Netherlands)	Postbus 382, 3700 AJ, Zeist, Holland	31 30 693 4600; (Fax) 31 30 693 1455	Warmblood horse from Holland. Has been absorbed into the Dutch Warmblood breed.
Groningen	KWPN (Royal Warmblood Studbook of the Netherlands)	Postbus 382, 2700 AJ, Zeist, Holland	31 30 693 4600; (Fax) 31 30 693 1455	Bred in the Dutch province of Groningen. Heavy farm horse, draft type. Has been absorbed mostly into the Dutch Warmblood.
Hackney	NA/WPN (Dutch Warmblood Studbook of North America) American Hackney Horse Society	P.O. Box 828, Winchester, OR 97495 4059 Iron Works Road, Suite 1 Lexington, KY 40511-8462	(606) 255-8694	Originated in great Britain, a descendant of both Arabian and Thoroughbred lines. Usually used as a driving horse; average height approximately 15 hands.
Hanoverian	American Hanoverian Society	4059 Iron Works Road, Suite 1, Lexington, KY 40511-8462	(859) 255-4141; (Fax) (859)-255-8467	The foremost German Warmblood. Big and strong, usually between 16 and 17 hands. Primarily in demand as a dressage horse and in show jumping.

BREED CHART—cont'd.

Breed	Association	Address	Phone/Fax	Description
Highland Pony	Highland Pony Society	22 York Place, Perth, Scotland	(Phone, Fax) 01738-451861	Pony bred in the Scottish Highlands and used for riding and driving. Stands approximately 13-14.2 hands.
Holsteiner	American Holsteiner Horse Association	222 East Main Street, Suite 1, Georgetown, KY 4C324	(502) 863-4239	German Warmblood. Ideally suited as a sport horse in dressage, jumping, driving, and eventing. Usually between 16 and 17 hands.
Icelandic	United States Icelandic Horse Congress	38 Park Street, Montclair, N. 07042	(973) 783-3429	One of the toughest pony breeds. Noted for intelligence and homing instinct; between 12 and 13 hands.
Irish Draught Horse	Irish Draught Horse Society	Harkway Farm, 5480 Major Lane, Platteville, WI 53818	(Phone and Fax) (608) 348-2519	Rare draft breed of Ireland considered endangered. Between 15.1 and 16.3 hands.
Japanese Native Horses	Japanese Equine Affairs Association	1-2 Kanda Surugadai, Chiyoda-ku, Tokyo, Japan		All are technically ponies and are hardy survivors bred in the various local regions of Japan. Include the Masaki Horse, Tokara Horse, Hokkaido Washu Horse, Noma Horse, Kiso Horse, Tiashu Horse, and the Yunaguni Horse.
Lipizzan	United States Lipizzan Registry	707 13th Street SE, Suite 275, Salem, OR 97301	(503) 589-3172	Sturdy, intelligent, and docile. Born dark, black-brown, brown, or mousy gray; turn white between the ages of 6 and 10 years. A smallish horse, averaging 14.3 to 15.3 hands.
Lusitano	International Andalusian and Lusitano Horse Association	101 Carnoustie N, #20C, Shoal Creek, AL 35242	(205) 995-8900; (Fax) (205) 995-8960	Spanish breed used in modern Portugal as a bullfighter. Intelligent. Usually gray, bay, or chestnut.

Continued

BREED CHART—*cont'd.*

Breed	Association	Phone/Fax	Address	Description
Mangalarga Marchador	ABCCMM (Associacao Brasileira dos Cridores do Cavalo Mangalarga Marchador)		Rua Goitacazes 14, 13 Edificio Bom Destino, 30 000 Belo Horizonte, Minas Gerais, Brazil	Gaited Brazilian breed descended from Iberian stock. Noted as the National Horse of Brazil. Good endurance and temperament. Usually 15 hands
Marwari Horse	Marwari Horse Breeder's Association	(Fax) 635373	Umaid Bhawan Palace, Jodhpur, India (342006)	Native to India. Distinct inward curving of the tips and the ears. Usually 14-15.2 hands. Riding horse.
Miniature	American Miniature Horse Association	(817) 293-0041	5601 South Interstate 35 W, Alvarado, TX 76009	Small, sound, well-balanced horse; must measure not more than 34 in (86 cm) at the base of the last hair on the mane for Division A and not more than 38 in (97 cm) for division B.
	American Miniature Horse Registry	(309) 263-4132	6748 N. Frostwood Parkway, Peoria, IL 61615-2402	
Morab	International Morab Breeders Association (IMBA)	(414) 594-3667; (Fax) (414) 594-5136	S. 101 W. 34828 Highway 99, Eagle, WI 53119-1857	Combines the best genetic traits of its parents' breeds, the Arabian and Morgan horses.
Morgan	American Morgan Horse Association	(802) 985-4944; (Fax) (802) 985-8897	122 Bostwick Road, P.O. Box 960, Shelburne, VT 05482-0960	Stands up to 15.2 hands and makes an ideal all-around pleasure horse. Frequently shown both under saddle and in harness.
National Show Horse	National Show Horse Registry	(502) 266-5100; (Fax) (502) 266-5806	11700 Commonwealth Drive, Louisville, KY 40299	Cross between the American Saddlebred and Arabian. Exhibited in show classes throughout the United States.

BREED CHART—*cont'd.*

Breed	Association	Address	Phone/Fax	Description
Oldenburg	Oldenburg Registry North America	939 Merchandise Mart, Chicago, IL 60654	(312) 527-6544; (Fax) (312) 527-6573	This German-bred horse is one of the oldest Warmbloods. Standing 16.0 to 16.3 hands, the Oldenburg makes a fine sport horse, well suited for anything from dressage to show jumping.
Orlov	All-Russian Institute of Horsebreeding	Russia 391128 Ryazan, Rybnovsky Area, VNII konevodstva, G.A. Rozhdestvenskaya, G.V. Kalinkina		Russian light harness breed. Used for driving in the Russian troika. Generally gray, although black and bay are common.
	International Council on the Protection of the Orlov Trotter	Russia 125252 Moscow, Chapaezskii per. 5-1-101, A.P. Polzunova	(Phone and Fax) (095) 157-39 91	
Paint	American Paint Horse Association	P.O. Box 96102, Fort Worth, TX 76161-0023	(817) 439-4300	To register, must prove parentage from one of three approved registries: AQHA, TB, or APHA, as well as meet minimum color requirements.
Palomino	Palomino Horse Breeders of America	15253 E. Skelly Drive, Tulsa, OK 74116-2637	(918) 438-1234	A color registry. Horses stand between 14 and 17 hands and exhibit a coat color with variations from light to dark of a U.S. 24-karat gold coin. The skin usually is gray, black, brown, or motley, without underlying pink skin or spots except on the face and legs. The mane must be white. Three divisions include the Western Horse, Golden American Saddlebred, and pleasure type.

Continued

BREED CHART—*cont'd.*

Breed	Association	Address	Phone/Fax	Description
Paso Fino	Paso Fino Horse Association	101 N. Collins Street, Plant City, FL 33566	(813) 719-7777	Uniquely inherent lateral four-beat gait in which the horse's feet fall in a natural lateral pattern rather than the usual diagonal pattern. Size ranges from 13.2 to 15.2 hands.
Percheron	Percheron Horse Association of America	P.O. Box 141, Fredericktown, OH 43019	(614) 694-3602	A more high-strung horse than the other draft-type horses. Well-portioned gray or black heavy horse, standing between 15.2 and 17 hands.
Pinto	Pinto Horse Association of America	1900 Samuels Avenue, Fort Worth, TX 76102-1141	(817) 336-7842; (Fax) (817) 336-7416	Color registry. Pintos may be of any breed.
Pony of the Americas	Pony of the Americas Club	5240 Elmwood Avenue, Indianapolis, IN 46203-5990	(317) 788-0107	Cross between a Shetland stallion and an Appaloosa mare. The height must be between 11.2 and 13 hands. Useful child's pony with plenty of substance. Height must be between 11.2 and 13 hands.
Quarab	United Quarab Registry	31100 NE Fernwood Road, Newburg, OR 97132-7012	(503) 538-0351	
Quarter Horse	American Quarter Horse Association	P.O. Box 200, 1600 Quarter Horse Drive, Amarillo, TX 79168	(806) 376-4811	Used as an all-purpose riding and harness horse and raced over short distances. Exceptionally good mount for working cattle. Average height is 15.2 hands.
Rocky Mountain Horse	Rocky Mountain Horse Association	National Headquarters, 2805 Lancaster Road, Danville, KY 40422	(606) 238-7754	Medium sized (14-16 hands), gaited horse developed in eastern Kentucky and used as a pleasure mount.

BREED CHART—*cont'd.*

Breed	Association	Phone/Fax	Address	Description
Russian Heavy Draft			Russia 391128 Ryazan, Rybnovsky Area, VNII konevodstva, G.K. Konovalova	Short, muscular, powerful draft breed. Has had significant influence on improving Russian agricultural breeds.
Saddlebred	American Saddlebred Horse	(859) 259-2742; (Fax) (859) 257-1628	4093 Iron Works Parkway, Lexington, KY 40511-8462	Primarily bred for the show ring, where they compete in light harness, as a three-gaited saddler, or as a five-gaited saddler. Average height is 15 to 16 hands.
Selle Français	North American Selle Français Horse Association	(703) 662-2870	P.O. Box 646, Winchester, VA 22604-0646	Good-quality type of hunter horse standing between 15.2 and 16.3 hands. Chestnut is the predominant color, although any color is permissible.
Shetland Pony	American Shetland Pony Club	(309) 691-9661	81-B E Queenwood, Morton, IL 61550	Maximum height of 46 in (117 cm). These sturdy ponies have been in the United States for more than 100 years.
Shire	American Shire Horse Association	(970) 876-5980; (Fax) (970) 876-1977	P. O. Box 739, New Castle, CO 81647	One of the largest horses in the world. It stands up to 18 hands and may be bay, brown, black, or gray. An immensely strong but gentle, good-natured agricultural and draft worker.
Spanish Barb	Spanish Barb Breeders Association	(601) 372-8801	183 Springridge Road, Terry, MS 39170	

Continued

BREED CHART—*cont'd.*

Breed	Association	Address	Phone/Fax	Description
Spanish Mustang	Spanish Mustang Registry	HCR 3, Box 7670, Willcox, AZ 85643-9748	(520) 384-2886	Direct descendant of horses brought to North America from Spain. Different from the feral horses managed by the Bureau of Land Management. Favorite mounts of the Apaches. Stand 13.2-15 hands. Spanish-type appearance.
Spotted Saddle Horse	Spotted Saddle Horse Breeders and Exhibitors Association	P.O. Box 1046, Shelbyville, TN 37162	(931) 684-7496	American breed descended from Standardbred, Mustang, and Tennessee Walking Horses. All around pleasure riding horse. Usually 14.3-16 hands. Gaited, colorful horses.
Standardbred	US Trotting Association	750 Michigan Avenue, Columbus, OH 43215-1191	(614) 224-2291	Among the world's finest harness racehorses. May be raced as trotters or as pacers. A medium-sized horse standing between 15.2 and 16 hands.
Tarpan	American Tarpan Studbook Association	1658 Coleman Avenue, Macon, GA 31201-6602	(912) 741-2062	This extremely rare breed is a genetic re-creation of the original wild Tarpan. Between 13 and 13.2 hands; mouse dun or grullo. There are only approximately 100 in the world.
Tennessee Walking Horse	Tennessee Walking Horse Breeders' & Exhibitors' Association	P. O. Box 286, Lewisburg, TN 37091	(615) 359-1574	Claimed to be the most comfortable ride in the world. A characteristic feature of this breed is its peculiar four-beated gait that is half walk and half run. Stands approximately 15 to 15.2 hands.

BREED CHART—*cont'd.*

Breed	Association	Phone/Fax	Address	Description
Thoroughbred	Jockey Club	(606) 224-2700	821 Corporate Drive, Lexington, KY 40503-2794	Bred extensively for flat racing, but its athleticism allows it to be successful in all equestrian sports. Any color is permissible, and the height can vary from as little as 14.2 to well over 17 hands.
Trakehner	American Trakehner Association	(740) 344-1111; (Fax) (740) 344-3225	1520 West Church Street, Newark, OH 43055	Excellent performance horse standing between 16 and 17 hands. Popular for show jumping and dressage.
Welsh Pony and Cob	Welsh Pony and Cob Society of America	(703) 667-6195	P.O. Box 2977, Winchester, VA 22604	A courageous and intelligent riding pony. The height limit is 13.2 hands, and any color is permissible except piebald or skewbald.

Equivalents

NEEDLE AND CATHETER REFERENCE CHART

Gauge	Regular ID	Thin ID	Inches OD	French Size	Inches OD
36	0.002	0.003	0.004		0.109
35	0.002	0.003	0.005		0.118
34	0.003	0.004	0.007		0.12
33	0.004	0.005	0.008		0.131
32	0.004	0.005	0.009		0.134
31	0.005	0.006	0.01		0.144
30	0.006	0.007	0.012		0.148
29	0.007	0.008	0.013	1	0.158
28	0.007	0.008	0.014		0.165
27	0.008	0.01	0.016		0.17
26	0.01	0.012	0.018		0.18
25	0.01	0.012	0.02		0.184
24	0.012	0.014	0.022		0.197
23	0.013	0.015	0.025		0.203
22	0.016	0.018	0.026	2	0.21
21	0.02	0.022	0.028		0.223
20	0.023	0.025	0.032		0.236
19	0.027	0.031	0.035		0.249
18	0.033	0.042	0.039	3	0.263
17	0.041	0.046	0.042		0.276
16	0.047	0.052	0.05		0.288
15	0.054	0.059	0.053	4	0.302
14	0.063	0.071	0.059		0.315
13	0.071	0.077	0.065		0.328
12	0.085	0.091	0.066	5	0.341
11	0.094	0.1	0.072		0.354
10	0.106	0.114	0.079	6	0.367
9	0.118	0.126	0.083		0.38
8	0.135	0.143	0.092	7	0.393
7	0.15	0.158	0.095		0.407
6	0.173	0.181	0.105	8	0.42
					0.433
					0.446

ID, Inner diameter; *OD*, outer diameter.

PHYSICAL EQUIVALENTS
Weight Equivalents

1 lb	453.6 g = 0.4536 kg = 16 oz
1 oz	28.35 g
1 kg	1000 g = 2.2046 lb
1 g	1000 mg = 0.0353 oz
1 mg	1000 µg = 0.001 g
1 µg	0.001 mg = 0.000001 g

1 µg/g or 1 mg/kg is the same as 1 ppm.

Volume Equivalents

1 drop (gt)	0.06 milliliter (ml)
15 drops (gtt)	1 ml (1 cc)
1 teaspoon (tsp)	5 ml
1 tablespoon (tbs)	15 ml
2 tablespoons	30 ml
1 teacup	180 ml (6.0 oz)
1 glass	240 ml (8.0 oz)
1 measuring cup	240 ml (½ pint)
2 measuring cups	480 ml (1 pint)
1 fluid ounce (fl oz)	29.57 ml
1 pint (pt)	0.473 L
1 pint	16 fluid ounces
1 gallon	3.785 L
1 gallon (US)	0.833 gallon (Imperial)
1 ml	0.03382 fluid ounce
1 L	2.1134 pints
1 L	0.26417

Pressure Equivalents

1 centimeter water (cm H_2O) = 0.736 mm Hg = 0.098 kPa
1 millimeter mercury (mm Hg) (Torr) = 1.36 cm H_2O = 0.133 kPa
1 kilopascal (kPa) = 7.5 mm Hg = 10.2 cm H_2O
1 atmosphere (atm) = 760 mm Hg = 1033.6 mm H_2O

TEMPERATURE CONVERSION

Degrees Celsius to degrees Fahrenheit: (C)(9/5) + 32°
Degrees Fahrenheit to degrees Celsius: (F − 32)(5/9)

WEIGHT-UNIT CONVERSION FACTORS

Unit Given	Unit Wanted	For Conversion Multiply By
lb	g	453.6
lb	kg	0.4536
oz	g	28.35
kg	lb	2.2046
kg	mg	1,000,000
kg	g	1000
g	mg	1000
g	μg	1,000,000
mg	μg	1000
mg/g	mg/lb	453.6
mg/kg	mg/lb	0.4536
μg/kg	μg/lb	0.4536
Mcal	kcal	1000
kcal/kg	kcal/lb	0.4536
kcal/lb	kcal/kg	2.2046
ppm	μg/g	1
ppm	mg/kg	1
ppm	mg/lb	0.4536
mg/kg	%	0.0001
ppm	%	0.0001
mg/g	%	0.1
g/kg	%	0.1

CONVERSION FACTORS

1 milligram	1/65 grain (1/60)
1 gram	15/43 grains (15)
1 kilogram	2.20 pounds (avoirdupois)
	2.65 pounds (troy)
1 milliliter	16.23 minims (15)
1 liter	1.06 quarts (1+)
	33.80 fluid ounces (34)
1 grain	0.065 g (60 mg)
1 dram	3.9 g (4)
1 ounce	31.1 g (30+)
1 minim	0.062 ml (0.06)
1 fluid dram	3.7 ml (4)
1 fluid ounce	29.57 ml (30)
1 pint	473.2 ml (500–)
1 quart	946.4 ml (1000–)

Resources for the Veterinarian for Information on Terrorist Attacks and Emergency Preparedness

FOR GOVERNMENT INFORMATION

FirstGov, Deborah Diaz, Deputy Associate Administrator, 750 17th Street NW, Suite 200, Washington, DC 20006-4634; (202) 634-0053; www.firstgov.gov

FOR BIOTERRORISM AND CHEMICAL WARFARE INFORMATION

Centers for Disease Control and Prevention, Bioterrorism and Preparedness Response, 1600 Clifton Road, Atlanta, GA 30333; (404) 639-3311; www.bt. cdc.gov/. To report an event call (770) 488-7100.

Chemical and Biological Information Analysis Center, an information analysis center sponsored by the Department of Defense, Ronald L. Evans, Director, Aberdeen Proving Ground, Edgewood Area, P.O. Box 195, Gunpowder, MD 21010-0196; (410) 676-9030; www.chiac.apgea.army.mil/

VETERINARY, PUBLIC HEALTH, EMERGENCY RESPONSE RESOURCES

Department of Agriculture, Office of Communications, 1400 Independence Avenue, SW, Washington, DC 20250-1300; (202) 720-4623; www.usda.gov

Department of Health and Human Services, 200 Independence Avenue, SW, Washington, DC 20201; (877) 696-6775; www.hhs.gov

Federal Emergency Management Agency (FEMA) 500 C Street, SW, Washington, DC 20472; (202) 646-4600; www.fema.gov

American Veterinary Medical Association, Emergency/Disaster Response, Dr. Cindy Lovern, Assistant Director, Emergency Preparedness and Response, 1931 N. Meacham Road, Suite 100, Schaumburg, IL 60173; (800) 248-2862, ext. 261; clovern@avma.org/vmat/default.asp. The AVMA also publishes *Zoonosis Updates*.

FOR CONTINUING EDUCATION

FEMA Emergency Management Institute, 16825 S. Seton Avenue, Emmitsburg, MD 21727; (301) 447-1200; www.fema.gov/emi/crslist.htm. Independent study courses on animals in disaster and emergency preparedness that can be downloaded.

The U.S. Army Medical Research Institute of Infectious Disease, 1425 Porter St., ATTN: MCMR-UIM-0, Fort Detrick, MD 21702-5011; (301) 619-4563; scott.stanek@det.amedd.army.mil; www.usarmriid.army.mil/education. Training courses on biological warfare and terrorism and the medical and public health response.

Decision System Alternatives & Technologies, 528 N. 7th Ave., Royersford, PA 19468-3335; (877) TRY-DSAT; www.dsat.com. Course on terrorism training.

Chemical Casualty Care Division, 3100 Rickets Point Road, Aberdeen Proving Ground, MD 21010-5400; (410) 436-2230; ccc@apg.amedd.army.mil; http://cehmdef.apgea.army.mil. The Department of Defense/U.S. Army offers a course on field management of chemical and biological casualties.

The USDA Animal and Plant Health Inspection Service veterinary service, (301) 734-5750; www.aphis.usda.gov/vs/training.htm. Telephone and Internet conferencing and satellite seminars on a variety of animal-related topics.

Compiled by the Publications Division, AVMA.

Susceptibility Patterns of Organisms Isolated from Equine Submissions

PERCENTAGE SUSCEPTIBLE OF TOTAL NUMBER OF ISOLATES

Organism	AMK	AMP	NXL	CF	C	E	ENRO	GM	P	RIF	SDM	TE	TIC	TIM	SXT	VA
GRAM-NEGATIVE																
Actinobacillus equuli, other Actinobacillus organisms	100	88	100	94	100	NA	100	100	NA	NA	81	100	94	100	94	NA
Pantoea agglomerans	95	90	95	85	95	NA	100	90	NA	NA	80	100	70	95	100	NA
Enterobacter organisms (all others)	88	63	72	53	75	NA	81	69	NA	NA	56	81	53	75	72	NA
Escherichia coli	97	62	84	56	83	NA	87	78	NA	NA	29	63	65	86	49	NA
Klebsiella pneumoniae	71	14	57	43	43	NA	100	57	NA	NA	14	43	NA	43	29	NA
Other Klebsiella organisms	92	17	75	50	58	NA	100	58	NA	NA	17	50	8	67	50	NA
Pseudomonas aeruginosa	92	0	0	0	0	NA	46	46	NA	NA	0	80	54	54	8	NA
GRAM-POSITIVE																
β-Streptococci, group C	0	100	94	88	NM	82	82	59	100	88	35	59	94	94	88	100
Streptococcus equi	0	100	100	100	MN	100	25	100	100	100	25	100	100	100	100	100
Streptococcus zooepidemicus	14	100	100	100	NM	86	71	71	100	100	14	29	100	100	100	100
Enterococcus species	NM	94	26	20	69	20	49	NM	89	11	0	43	63	60	NM	100
Rhodococcus equi	100	13	63	50	100	100	100	100	59	100	67	92	92	100	50	100
Staphylococcus, coagulase-positive*	100	44	78	78	94	83	100	72	44	89	78	78	44	6	89	100

AMK, amikacin; AMP, ampicillin; NXL, ceftiofur; CF, cephalothin; C, chloramphenicol; E, erythromicin; ENRO, enrofloxacin; GM, gentamicin; P, penicillin; RIF, rifampin; SDM, sulfadimethoxine; TE, tetracycline; TIC, ticarcillin; TIM, timentin; SXT, trimethoprim/sulfamethoxazoles; VA, vancomycin; NA, not applicable; NM, not approved for use by National Committee for Clinical Laboratory Standards.

Bacterial isolates tested were from submissions to the diagnostic microbiology laboratory, Department of Pathobiology, University of Pennsylvania.

Data were obtained with the Sensititre microdilution broth technique for in vitro susceptibility testing. Response to antimicrobial therapy depends on the integrity of the host defenses, the site and the nature of the infection, and the pharmacokinetics of the antimicrobial agent. The statistics in this report may be misleading because drug appropriateness and contraindications are not specified.

"Extra label" use of an antimicrobial agent is defined as use of a compound in an animal for which there is no approved indication or for management of a disease in an animal other than that disease for which the compound is approved. Extra label use of antimicrobial agents in food animals can result in violative residues. Antimicrobial susceptibility test results are meant only to be a guide in selecting the most appropriate compound for the indicated animal. It is the responsibility of the submitting clinician to select the most appropriate compound for the indicated animal.

*Four of the 18 Staphylococcus isolates are methicillin resistant.

Miscellaneous Notes from the National Committee for Clinical Laboratory Standards Document M31T: *Performance Standards for Antimicrobial Disk and Dilution Susceptibility Tests for Bacteria Isolated from Animals*

Some organisms have predictable susceptibility to antimicrobial agents. Susceptibility testing is seldom necessary when the infection is due to a microorganism that is susceptible to a highly effective drug. The universal susceptibility of group C Beta hemolytic Streptococci and *Actinomyces pyogenes* to Penicillin G are such examples.

Coagulase-positive staphylococci that test resistant to Oxacillin/Methicillin should be considered resistant to Penicillin, Ampicillin, Timentin, Ticarcillin, and all the cephalosporins, including Ceftiofur.

The drug of choice for serious enterococcal infections is a combination therapy of Ampicillin or Penicillin G plus an aminoglycoside. This combination provides synergistic killing activity. Results of susceptibility testing against other agents such as cephalosporins should not be recorded due to lack of clinical correlation.

Treatment of foal pneumonia due to *Rhodococcus equi* usually requires a combination of Erythromycin or Azithromycin, and Rifampin. However, there is no established protocol for testing the susceptibility of *Rhodococcus* against this combination.

Enrofloxacin, the fluoroquinolone approved only for cats and dogs, may cause erosion of cartilage of weight bearing joints and therefore should not be administered to actively growing animals.

Review of Nomenclature Changes

Previous Designation	Current Designation
Actinomyces pyogenes	*Arcanobacterium pyogenes*
Enterobacter agglomerans	*Pantoea agglomerans*
Pasteurella haemolytica	*Mannheimia haemolytica*
Pseudomonas cepacia	*Burkholderia cepacia*
Pseudomonas maltophilia	*Stenotrophomonas maltophilia*
Pseudomonas paucimobilis	*Sphingomonas paucimobilis*
Streptococcus equi	*Streptococcus equi* subsp. *equi*
Streptococcus zooepidemicus	*Streptococcus equi* subsp. *zooepidemicus*

Long Bone Physeal Fusion Times and Growth Plate Closures

Physeal fusion times are important for radiographic interpretation and are not always indicative of true growth-plate closure. The fusion times listed are for the long bones of the thoracic and pelvic limbs. Breed variations occur (i.e., the growth plates of lighter breeds close earlier than those of heavier breeds). The bones also differ in terms of fusion age, and the proximal and distal growth plates close at different periods.

➤ *Key Points*

- The most rapid growth period in foals is from birth to 10 weeks.
- The distal radius has continuous growth up to 60 weeks.
- Angular limb deformities should be recognized and managed early in life (<70 days for fetlock deformities).
- The radiographic appearance of the growth plate does not directly reflect the ability of chondrocytes to proliferate.
- Growth plates determine bone length and, to some extent, bone shape.
- Endochondral ossification abnormalities affect bone length, axial alignment of bone ends, and joint contour.

GROWTH PLATE CLOSURES

Bone	Closure Time (Months of Age)
THORACIC LIMB	
Humerus	
Proximal	24-36
Distal	12-24
Radius	
Proximal	12-24
Distal	24
Ulna	24-36
Metacarpal III	
Proximal	Fused at birth
Distal	6-9
Proximal Phalanx (PI)	
Proximal	6-12
Distal	Fused at birth
Middle Phalanx (PII)	
Proximal	8-12
Distal	Fused at birth
PELVIC LIMB	
Femur	
Proximal	24-36
Distal	24-30
Tibia	
Proximal	24-30
Distal	17-24

GROWTH PLATE CLOSURES—*cont'd.*

Bone	Closure Time (Months of Age)
Metatarsal III	
Proximal	Fused at birth
Distal	9-12
Proximal Phalanx (PI)	
Proximal	6-12
Distal	Fused at birth
Middle Phalanx (PII)	
Proximal	8-12
Distal	Fused at birth

Trade*/Generic Names Used in Equine Practice

DRUGS USED IN EQUINE PRACTICE

Trade Name	Generic Name
Adequan (EENT)	Polysulfated glycosaminoglycans
Adequan (unclassified)	Polysulfated glycosaminoglycans
Adrenalin Chloride	Epinephrine
Albon	Sulfadimethoxine
Amicar	Aminocaproic acid
Amiglyde	Amikacin
Amoxi-Mast	Amoxicillin (intramammary)
Amp-Equine	Ampicillin sodium
Ancef; Kefzol	Cefazolin
Antirobe	Clindamycin
Apresoline	Hydralazine
Aquasol E	Vitamin E
Arquel	Meclofenamic acid
Aspirin	Acetylsalicylic acid
Atarax	Hydroxyzine
Atrovent	Ipratropium
Azium	Dexamethasone
Bactocill, Banamine	Flunixin meglumine
Baytril	Enrofloxacin
Beclovent; Vanceril	Beclomethasone
Benadryl	Diphenhydramine
Brethine	Terbutaline
Carafate	Sucralfate
Carbocaine-V2%	Mepivacaine hydrochloride
Cefa-Lak	Cephapirin (intramammary)
Ceftin	Cefuroxime
Cetacaine	Benzocaine
Chorulon	Gonadotropin-releasing hormone (Human Chorionic Gonadotropin [hCG])
Chronulac	Lactulose
Ciloxan	Ciprofloxacin
Corophyllin; Palaron	Aminophylline
Corrective mixture	Bismuth subsalicylate
Cuprimine	Penicillamine
Cytotec	Misoprostol
Dantrium	Dantrolene
Daraprim	Pyrimethamine
Delta-Cortef	Prednisolone
Deltasone	Prednisone

*There may be other trade names used for the same drug. These listings are intended as a guide only and do not suggest completeness and/or preference in the naming of drugs.

862

DRUGS USED IN EQUINE PRACTICE—*cont'd.*

Trade Name	Generic Name
Dibenzyline	Phenoxybenzamine
Diflucan	Fluconazole
Dilantin	Phenytoin
Dobutrex	Dobutamine
Domoso solution	Dimethyl sulfoxide
Domoso GBC	Dimethyl sulfoxide
Dopram	Doxapram HCl
Dormosedan	Detomidine HCl
DSS, DOSS	Dioctyl sodium succinate
ECP	Estradiol
Efudex	5-Fluorouracil
Enacard	Enalapril
Epsom salts	Magnesium sulfate
EQ-Stim	Propionibacterium acnes
Equipoise	Boldenone undecylenate
Erythro-100; Erythro-200	Erythromycin lactobionate
Erythrocin	Erythromycin stearate
Estrumate	Cloprostenol
Excenel **in the United States**	Ceftiofur hydrochloride (Excenel is sodium ceftiofur in Canada and Europe)
Flagyl; Metizol	Metronidazole
Follutein	hCG
Fortaz	Ceftazidime
Fulvicin	Griseofulvin
Fungizone	Amphotericin B
Gastro-Cote	Bismuth subsalicylate
Gastrogard; Prilosec	Omeprazole
Gentocin	Gentamicin
Geopen; Pyopen	Carbenicillin
Hespan	Hetastarch
Histavet-P	Pyrilamine maleate
Imodium	Loperamide
Imuran	Azathioprine
Inderal	Propranolol
Intal	Sodium-cromoglycate
Intropin	Dopamine
Inulin	Insulin
KCL	Potassium chloride
Keflex	Cephalexin
Keflin	Cephalothin
Kefzol, Ancef	Cefazolin
Ketofen	Ketoprofen
Lanoxin	Digoxin
Lasix	Furosemide
Liquamycin-200	Oxytetracycline (injectable)
Lutalyse	Dinoprost
Meta-Dote	Calcium-EDTA
Metamizole; Novin	Dipyrone
Metamucil	Psyllium hydrophilic mucilloid
Metizol; Flagyl	Metronidazole
Molypen	Ammonium molybdate
Mydriacyl	Tropicamide
Narcan	Naloxone

Continued

DRUGS USED IN EQUINE PRACTICE—*cont'd.*

Trade Name	Generic Name
Naropin	Rupivacaine
Natacyn	Natamycin
Naquasone	Trichlormethiazide-dexamethasone
Naxcel	Ceftiofur sodium
Neomycin; Neovet	Neomycin
Neo-Synephrine	Phenylephrine
Nitro-Bid	Nitroglycerine
Novin; Metamizole	Dipyrone
Novo	Colchicine
Ocufen	Flurbiprofen
Optimmune	Cyclosporine
Ovuplant	Deslorelin
Palaron; Corophyllin	Aminophylline
Palosein	Orgotein
Parlodel	Bromocriptine
Penicillin or Potassium USP	Penicillin (Benzathine & Procaine)
Pen-P 110, Pen-P 100	Penicillin G Procaine
Pepcid AC	Famotidine
Pepto-Bismol	Bismuth subsalicylate
Periactin	Cyproheptadine
Permax	Pergolide
Platinol	Cisplatin
Poly-Flex	Ampicillin trihydrate
Prilosec, Gastrogard	Omeprazole
Primaxin	Imipenem-cilastatin
Priscoline	Tolazoline
Pronestyl	Procainamide
Prostigmin	Neostigmine
Proventil	Albuterol
Pyopen; Geopen	Carbenicillin
Pyridium	Phenazopyridine
Quinidex	Quinidine sulfate, quinidine gluconate
Re-Covr	Tripelennamine
Reglan	Metoclopramide
Regu-Mate	Altrenogest
Rifadin	Rifampin
Rimadyl	Carprofen
Robaxin-V	Methocarbamol
Robinul-V	Glycopyrrolate
Rocephin	Ceftriaxone
Rompun; Sedazine	Xylazine HCl
Serevent	Salmeterol
Serosporin	Polymixin B sulfate
Solganal	Aurothioglucose
Solu-Delta-Cortef; Delta-Cortef	Prednisolone
Sporanox	Itraconazole/DMSO
Tagamet	Cimetidine
Terramycin	Oxytetracycline ophthalmic
Thermazene	Silver sulfadiazine
Thyro-L	Levothyroxine
Timentin	Ticarcillin-clavulanic acid
Tobrex	Tobramycin
Tofranil	Imipramine HCl

DRUGS USED IN EQUINE PRACTICE—*cont'd.*

Trade Name	Generic Name
Torbugesic	Butorphanol tartrate
Trental	Pentoxifylline
Tribrissen	Trimethoprim-sulfamethoxazole
Urecholine	Bethanechol
Valium	Diazepam
Vanceril; Beclovent	Beclomethasone
Vancocin	Vancomycin
Ventipulmin	Clenbuterol
Vetalog	Triamcinolone
Winstrol-V	Stanozolol
Yocon	Yohimbine
Zantac	Ranitidine

TRADE NAMES

Index

Note: Page numbers followed by f indicate figures; those followed by t indicate tables.

HOTLINE NUMBERS EVERY VETERINARIAN SHOULD KNOW

Veterinary Practitioners' Reporting Program:
Veterinary product failure and adverse reaction reporting—(800) 487-7776
US Pharmacopeia: To report or request reporting forms for product quality problems, medication mishaps, and adverse reactions regarding drugs, biologics, chemicals, pesticides, medical devices, and other products used for companion, food, zoo, and exotic animals. (Reports may be submitted anonymously.)

FDA/CVM:
Drug Interactions Only—(888) FDA-VETS; ([888] 332-8387)
Line for health professionals to report adverse events, particularly with drugs (collect; after hours, record a message).

USDA: Veterinary Biologics and Diagnostics Hotline—(800) 752-6255
(Weekdays 7:30 AM to 4 PM CST; message service available other hours.)
A 24-hour hotline to report adverse reactions involving veterinary diagnostic and biologic products.

USDA-APHIS Health Requirements Worldwide Web: www.aphis.usda.gov/vs/sregs

National Animal Poison Control Center Hotlines:
(888) 232-8870—Animal Poison Hotline. Fee is $35 per incident, payable by credit card. No charge for follow-up calls.
(900) 680-0000—ASPCA National Animal Poison Control Center. Fee is $45 per case. Follow-up calls at no additional charge can be made to (888) 426-4435.

DEA toll-free number for Office of Diversion Control, Registration Section—(800) 882-9539
A registration assistant is available from 8:30 AM to 5 PM EST. Leave a voicemail message after hours to request registration and order forms.

HEMOPET—(949) 252-8455
A national, full-service, nonprofit blood bank and educational network for animals in Irvine, Calif. Accessible 24 hours.

Animal Blood Bank Hotline—(800) 243-5759
A 24-hour hotline that focuses on transfusion medicine (particularly blood component therapy) and recommending dosages and infusion rates, at no cost to caller.

Eastern Veterinary Blood Bank—800-949-EVBB; ([800] 949-3822)
A 24-hour commercial blood bank that focuses on transfusion medicine; gives recommendations and referrals to distribution centers when it cannot ship the requested product; for complicated cases, offers a paid consultation service; available to callers nationwide except for California and Oregon.

National Pesticide Telecommunications Network—(800) 858-7377 or 7378
Service sponsored by the EPA and Oregon State University provides information about pesticide products and poisonings, toxicology, environmental chemistry, and other pesticide-related issues.

USDA Voice Response Service—(800) 545-8732
Up-to-date interstate shipping regulations, emergency notices, and animal care regulations for shipping pets on airlines.

Impaired Veterinarians Information Line—(800) 321-1473
Information on, and referrals for, assistance with chemical impairment; sponsored by the AVMA.